DIMENSIONS
OF
PROFESSIONAL
NURSING

Lucie Young Kelly, R.N., Ph.D., F.A.A.N.

DIMENSIONS OF PROFESSIONAL NURSING

FIFTH EDITION

Macmillan Publishing Company
New York
Collier Macmillan Canada, Inc.
Toronto
Collier Macmillan Publishers
London

Macmillan Publishing Company
866 Third Avenue, New York, New York 10022

Collier Macmillan Canada, Inc.

Collier Macmillan Publishers • London

Library of Congress Cataloging in Publication Data

Kelly, Lucie Young.
   Dimensions of professional nursing.

   Includes bibliographies and index.
   1. Nursing. 2. Nursing—United States. I. Title.
[DNLM: 1. Nursing. WY 16 K33d]
RT82.K4 1985   610.73   84–29478
ISBN 0-02-362580-5

Printing: 1 2 3 4 5 6 7 8   Year: 5 6 7 8 9 0 1 2

Preface

DIMENSIONS OF PROFESSIONAL NURSING is what the late Cordelia Kelly, author of the first two editions, called, "an overview of the nonclinical aspects of nursing in sufficient detail to be adaptable for use at all stages in all types of preservice programs in professional nursing," and also, as I maintain, in the continuing education of all professional nurses. This book is directed particularly toward educational programs whose philosophy includes the belief that if nurses are to be professional practitioners, they must not only be knowledgeable and skilled in the clinical aspects of nursing, but also understand what the profession is and work toward making it what it could be. In addition, many teachers have found that various sections can serve as a basic text for more than one course such as in history, law, health care delivery, trends and issues in nursing, and career development, adding only the supplementary readings found in the references and bibliography.

Because *Dimensions of Professional Nursing* is intended for use by a diverse readership and for reference even after the end of a course, the references and bibliography are extensive. Thus students, RNs and others can further research what is of interest and importance to them. References giving more than one point of view on a controversial issue are included wherever possible. Besides the standard nursing journals, references from other professional journals and books give a different flavor to familiar issues.

In using the book, readers will find that cross references are frequent. For instance, different aspects of collective bargaining are discussed in Chapter 19 (components of the various labor laws); in Chapter 22 (the right of the nurse to organize and engage in collective bargaining and the process used), and in Chapter 25 (the role of the ANA in collective bargaining). Another major issue, continuing education, is referred to in Chapter 2 (Nightingale's concept), Chapter 6 (the consumer movement and educational trends), Chapter 10 (accountability for competent practice), Chapter 12 (issues), Chapter 13 (types), Chapter 20 (mandatory continuing education), and Chapter 31 (where and how to get it). Such cross references are noted in both the text and footnotes. In this 5th edition the references and bibliography are completely updated. For some chapters, the bibliography contains almost totally new citations due to the plethora of new information available. (Examples are the sections on law and health care delivery). Some classical citations are referred to in each chapter's reference list and the fourth edition can continue to be used for other references. The bibliography is now at the end of the book; the references follow each chapter.

Other than the chapters on history, no chapter is without some revision, primarily updating to include current information. Although in the fourth edition I had anticipated trends in nursing and health care that have indeed come to fruition, it seemed more appropriate to integrate rather than "tack on" these events. To make the text more visually attractive and readable, a number of useful drawings and other exhibits have been added. Reports of pertinent surveys and research also add a special dimension.

A summary of other major changes might

be helpful. In Chapter 5, the most important recent studies on nursing done by private and governmental groups are presented in some detail. In Chapter 6, increased emphasis is given to how these external factors affect nursing, including the new population profile, the health of the people, technological changes, and the environment. In Chapters 7 and 8, the issues relating to health care delivery and predictions for the future are discussed. This includes changes in the education and practice of others in the health care team. In Chapter 9, nursing theories are given more attention and the ANA Social Policy Statement is discussed. Both the areas of ethics and accountability are expanded in Chapter 10 with practical examples of ethical dilemmas. In the next section, the changes in nursing education and research and their implications for the future of nursing are considered.

Besides describing the many career opportunities available to nurses, Chapter 15 reports on the effects of health economics on nursing practice. With these economic pressures, the need for autonomous practice of nursing acquires even greater importance. Therefore Chapter 16 is expanded considerably with increased emphasis on leadership, and professionalism as an attitude. Also expanded are the chapters on law, especially 20, 21, and 22, with many practical applications and examples. Chapter 19 on federal legislation is still one of a kind in nursing literature.

In the last section, *Dimensions of Professional Nursing* again presents the most comprehensive description of the major organizations and agencies available anywhere, as well as a consideration of how this growth of organizational entities affects nursing. Equally comprehensive is the listing of nursing journals; and because of the growing interest in publication, an augmented section on writing. Also in response to reader demand, Chapter 30 (on employment guidelines) has been totally rewritten and expanded, adding useful examples of a resumé and application letter. Finally, the "Challenge of Professionalism" is intended to assist the new graduate and even the more experienced nurse in professional development and dealing with the stresses, but also with the opportunities created by a competitive health care system.

If there has ever been a turning point for nursing, it is this period in our history—a time that offers unparalleled opportunity for those who would seize it. To do so, nurses must understand their profession and the elements that affect it. While recognizing the problems and rising to the challenges, they must nurture the pride and joy their profession can bring them. Again, it is my hope that this book will help nurses to understand and care about the continually new dimensions of professional nursing.

LUCIE YOUNG KELLY

Acknowledgments

Writing *Dimensions of Professional Nursing* has been one of the most stimulating, challenging, and rewarding professional activities of my nursing career. But a book that has as many facets as *Dimensions of Professional Nursing* requires the author to call on colleagues many times for some special insight about nursing or for information that is not readily available. I wish to give special recognition to Dr. Melanie Dreher, now Associate Professor at the University of Miami School of Nursing, who wrote most of the section on Nursing Theories, Concepts, and Models in Chapter 9; Sister Rosemary Donley, Dean, Catholic University School of Nursing for her suggestions in Chapters 12 and 13 and for "A Final Word" in Chapter 31; Sandy Wisener, a doctoral student at the University of Alabama School of Nursing, now a member of the graduate faculty of the University of Arkansas College of Nursing, who wrote the section on accountability in Chapter 10; Carol Shanik, doctoral student at Columbia University, School of Public Health who wrote the descriptions of some of the newer clinical nursing organizations.

For reviewing and updating information about their organizations, services, or agencies, I thank their respective staffs and presidents, and especially Brigadier General Connie L. Slewitzke and staff, Army Nurse Corps; Commodore Mary J. Nielubowiez and staff, Navy Nurse Corps; Brigadier General Diann Hale and staff, U.S. Air Force Nurse Corps; Ms. Vernice Ferguson, Deputy Assistant Chief Medical Director, and staff, Veterans Administration; Ms. Jo Eleanor Elliott, Director, Dr. Mary F. Hill, Mr. Thomas Phillips; Dr. Virginia Saba, Dr. O. Marie Henry, Dr. Doris Bloch, and Ms. Evelyn Moses, Division of Nursing, DHHS; Dr. Faye Abdellah, Deputy Surgeon General, U.S. Public Health Service DHHS, and her associate, Helen V. Foerst, Deputy Chief Nurse Officer; Ben Santaiti, Financial Management Officer, Bureau of Health Professions, DHHS (who developed the charts on the budget process in Chapter 18); Leah Brock, Deputy Director for National League for Nursing; Dr. Eileen Jacobi, Third Vice President, International Council of Nursing and Dean, University of Texas-El Paso College of Nursing; Robin Kriegel, Director of Organizational Affairs, National Student Nurses' Association; Katherine Goldring, Director, Marketing, American Nurses' Association; Gretchen Gerds, Vice President, Editorial, American Journal of Nursing Company, and the editors of the AJN Company magazines. I am also grateful to Ms. Cosy Brown, of the American Journal of Nursing Company's Sophia Palmer Library who gave me a tremendous amount of help in locating essential references; and to Georgia Serrapica, who typed almost all of the manuscript—not an easy task! And to Carol Wolfe, Senior Editor at Macmillan, who nagged gently and organized efficiently, a medal for patience and fortitude.

Finally, I would like to thank those for whom this book was written—the teachers, students and other colleagues whom I have met as I travelled around the country and who have shared with me their concerns and interests in nursing "trends and issues." Equally appreciated are the efforts of those who answered a questionnaire seeking input into the new edition and others who made so many helpful suggestions. This is as much their book as mine.

LUCIE YOUNG KELLY

Contents

Part

III

PROFESSIONAL COMPONENTS AND CAREER DEVELOPMENT

DEVELOPMENT OF MODERN NURSING

EARLY
HISTORICAL
INFLUENCES

1

Care of the Sick:
A Historical Overview

The clinical practice of nursing is quite rightly the major focus of most of its practitioneers and the prime concern of students. Therefore, there is a tendency to greet nursing history with a "What good is it to me?" attitude. Undoubtedly, nurses can give good nursing care even if they have never heard of Florence Nightingale, Isabel Hampton Robb, Lavinia Dock, or Lillian Wald. But one of the major differences between an occupation and a profession is its practitioners' long-term commitment to the profession, which includes working toward its development. To do so without some understanding of its past is possibly to repeat errors.

Nursing today was formed by its historical antecedents. Its development since ancient times, within the social contexts of those times, explains many things: its power or lack of power, its educational confusion, and the makeup of its practitioners. The changing relationships between nursing and other health care professions, nursing and other disciplines, and nursing and the public can be traced and better understood with the knowledge of past history. The impact of social and scientific changes on nursing and nursing's impact on society are ongoing processes that need to be studied; nursing does not exist in a vacuum. Sometimes there is a repetition of history, with the answer to the problems apparently not much clearer now than a hundred years ago. For instance, a 1901 editorial in the *Journal of the American Medical Association* said, "The usefulness of the nurse is and always will be gauged by her faithfulness as a subordinate intelligently carrying out the directions of the physician. . . ."[1] In 1977, a major medical organization noted, "An independent, autonomous nurse practitioner is inconsistent with [the organization's position that nurses and other health care personnel work under the physician's direction] and must lead to second-class medical care."[2] A hundred years ago, there was objection from within and without nursing to nurses having more education; the scenario is repeated today. Seventy-five years ago, the question of nursing licensure was hotly debated; today, it is again a major concern. These issues affect the practice of every nurse; in some cases, they are a factor in determining whether the nurse even chooses to stay in the profession. An understanding of the past can bring additional clarity to the decisions that shape the future.

This chapter and those that follow in Part I are not intended in any way as a substitute for the many fine texts that are available on nursing history. Instead, they provide an overview to set the stage for the more detailed study of nursing history an individual may undertake for professional reasons or personal satisfaction. In this book's fourth edition, Appendix A presents vignettes of distinguished nurses of the past.

PRIMITIVE SOCIETIES

Although historians sometimes advance theories and cite an occasional archaeological discovery to prove that prehistoric civilization practiced crude medicine and nursing, the supporting evidence about nursing is somewhat inconclusive. It must be assumed, however, that in most tribes there were some individuals who were more adept than others at caring for the sick and injured and helping the medicine men or witch doctors. It seems reasonable to assume further that some of these men and women taught their sons and daughters and certain members of the tribes to give this care, for these people were able to communicate; they wanted to survive; they were human beings with some ability to think, to recall, and to teach by example, if not by coherent explanation.

Indirect evidence of some of the beliefs and practices of ancient man concerning illness has evolved from recent studies of primitive cultures. Apparently, many concepts of health and illness were related to belief in the supernatural. Everything in nature was seen as being alive, with invisible forces and supernatural power. There were good spirits and evil spirits that must be placated. Primitive man believed that a person became sick (1) when an evil spirit entered the body; (2) when a good spirit within the body that was ordinarily able to fend off diseases left, either because some-

one or something had taken it away or of its own accord; and (3) because witchcraft had been performed upon the affected part of the body, either directly or through some object that had been given to the person.

Thus, although it was probably recognized how heat, cold, certain foods, wounds, and strains were related to health and empirical treatments developed for them, serious illness called for the services of a medicine man (witch doctor, shaman, root doctor). This mysterious figure, sometimes a woman but usually a man, functioned through a ritualistic mystique, frequently a shock or fright technique that was intended to induce evil spirits to leave the body. Included were the use of frightening masks and noises, incantations, vile odors, charms, spells, sacrifices, and fetishes. In a primitive version of modern trephining, the medicine man cut a hole in the skull to let the evil spirit out. Purgatives, emetics, deodorants, applied hot and cold substances, cauterization, massage, cupping, and blistering were frequently used.

A woman in abnormal labor was treated by similarly drastic measures, such as placing a lighted fire between her outstretched legs to hasten delivery. Needless to say, patients did not always survive this treatment, and if they did, there is no evidence that any daily ongoing care was given by the shaman. Probably a relative gave this "nursing" care. Women generally assisted other women in childbearing. But whether treatment of illness and injury by use of herbs and other "natural" means was carried out by all men and/or women, or by specially designated individuals, is not known.

EARLY CIVILIZATIONS

In the written records of the early civilizations (5000 B.C. to A.D. 476), there is very little reference to nursing as such. However, if there is evidence of a high standard of living, a good sanitation system, architectural achievement, interest in education and culture and scientific medicine, or even two or three of these, it is reasonably certain that the health of the inhabitants was of paramount importance and that nurses were not only present but were trained in some fashion to prepare them for the work they did.

The Babylonians

Babylonia was the center of ancient Mesopotamian culture, which was in ruins by the time the Christian era began. Located between the eastern Mediterranean Sea and the Persian Gulf and nourished by the Tigris and Euphrates rivers, this land was very fertile, offering a good life to its settlers. Coveted by many peoples, it was for thousands of years first under the rule of one master and then another who took possession by force. Each influenced the others' development intellectually, socially, and scientifically. Their many wars brought misery and suffering, and, even in that abundant country, there must have been many illnesses and injuries in the normal course of life.

There is evidence that a legalized medical service was instituted and that some type of lay nurse cared for patients. They may have been men, but if they were women, their status was probably quite low, and they must have been subservient to physicians because the women of Babylonia were dominated by men who controlled their every action.

Herodotus, a Greek historian called the "Father of History," recorded that it was customary in Babylon for the sick to go to the marketplace where passersby could see them and stop and inquire into the "nature of their distemper." Those who had knowledge of how to treat a condition (knowledge acquired principally through experience) advised the ill on therapy that had helped them. This was hardly a scientific method of treatment, but it no doubt was effective in many instances.

Excavations made in 1849 of 700 medical tablets show that the Babylonian physician-priest allowed his patient to choose whether he wanted to be treated with medicine or charms. If he selected medicine, the physician had many vegetable and mineral preparations to employ. If he selected charms, the doctor told him which ones to wear for his particular illness and probably uttered a few incantations to accompany them, for they still believed that disease was caused by sin and displeasure of the gods.

However, some of the treatments indicate a realistic attitude toward illness, for they included diet, rest, enemas, bandaging, and massaging plus emphasis on the importance of good personal hygiene. This care might be given by family or a "nurse."

The first Babylonian Empire was founded by King Hammurabi, who developed a code of laws for the whole empire. The code is engraved on a huge stone, unearthed in 1902, and shows Hammurabi worshipping a sun god from whom he is receiving instructions about the laws. Included are laws concerned with the fees that a physician was allowed to charge for his services and also punishment for the physician who committed "malpractice." Payments were to be made in *shekels* of silver—usually two, five, or ten, depending upon whether the patient was a master or a slave. Punishment for causing a patient to lose his life or an eye was to "cut off the physician's hands if the patient was a nobleman." (This kind of punishment was reserved for surgeons, not physician-priests.) Wet nurses were also regulated as to remuneration and responsibility.

The Ancient Hebrews

Much of the story of the ancient Hebrews is told in the Talmud and the Old Testament. The Hebrews, alone of their contemporaries, believed in one God, Yahweh, not many.

Their misfortunes and illnesses they attributed to God's wrath, and they depended upon Him more than on man to restore them to health when they were sick. One facet of their religion was that it was their duty to be hospitable to strangers as well as to their own people, and they were obliged to give a tithe to augment their personal service in visiting the sick and needy.

The Hebrews brought many hygienic practices from Babylonia, where they had been in captivity, but under the leadership of Moses they also developed principles and practices of hygiene and sanitation. Moses decreed that all meat must be inspected, the selection and preparation of all foods must be carefully supervised, and cleanliness in all areas of living was absolutely essential. This has been called the first sanitary legislation. It represented one of the first public health movements on record.

Their people were taught to help prevent the spread of communicable diseases by burning an infected person's garments and sometimes even his house, and by scrubbing the room in which he was ill and the utensils he used. They were often able to diagnose and control the spread of leprosy and gonorrhea. They performed trephining operations skillfully and humanely, giving the patient a sleeping potion before surgery to dull the pain. They also did cesarean sections, splenectomies, amputations, and circumcisions and set fractures. They dressed wounds with oil, wine, and balsam and used sutures and bandages.

From these operations and careful examination of animals made primarily for sanitary purposes, they developed a body of knowledge about anatomy and physiology, although we know now that some of their information was understandably superficial and inaccurate.

The nurse is mentioned occasionally in the Old Testament and the Talmud, but in what capacity she served, except as wet nurse, is not entirely clear. It does appear that the "nurse" visited and possibly cared for the sick in their homes. She probably also had a role in health teaching.

The Persian Contribution

Between c. 550 and 500 B.C., Cyrus the Great, king of Persia, and his son, Cambyses, acquired a vast empire in the Near East. They adopted many of the medical practices and much of the culture from the great lands they conquered—Asia Minor, Babylonia, Syria, Mesopotamia, Egypt, and several others.

In Egypt, the Emperor Darius, successor of Cambyses, restored a school for training priest-physicians and, in effect, established a government-controlled medical center, the first of its kind recorded in history. It is also known that there were practitioners who healed with holy words, with herbs, and with the knife—in decreasing order of practice.

The Art of Medicine in Egypt

There are references to nurses in accounts of Egyptian medicine as it was practiced in the pre-Christian era. The medical papyri discovered during excavations contain descriptions of such nursing procedures as feeding a tetanus patient and dressing wounds. The extent of the nurse's duties is not clear, however.

Egyptian medicine, on the other hand, is revealed by graven inscriptions, the papyri, and other literature as having been rather far advanced. In spite of the Egyptians' ideas about the origins of life, the journey that man took after death, the causes of disease, and the catastrophic effects of incurring the wrath of the gods, they also practiced some very good medicine, although it may not have been based on scientific principles. Priests and physicians were identical in early Egyptian civilization, and in healing temples, rest, rituals, and prayer were part of the treatment. Later there emerged physicians who were concerned only with matters of health and hygiene.

Medical specialization became so common that a physician usually spent his entire career in caring for diseases of one particular part of the body. Members of the profession were organized to protect their medical secrets.

It was in ancient Egypt that the great physician Imhotep lived in about 2980 B.C. Skilled in architecture, magic, and priestcraft as well as medicine, he became so famous that he was never forgotten. More than two and a half centuries after his death, he became the god of medicine, identified by the Greeks with their famous god of healing, Asclepios (Latin, Aesculapius).

In Egypt, as in most countries, one of the important areas of concern was the health of the people.

The Egyptians formulated regulations about diet, baths, purgatives, and other matters of personal hygiene. They initiated laws of health suited to Egypt's climate and terrain. They developed diagnostic procedures (which differed in some respects from those of other ancient civilizations) for the common illnesses of their people. Examinations of mummies indicate that the Egyptians suffered many bone diseases and injuries. Osteoarthritis was apparently very common, and there must also have been ailments all humans are subject to such as abdominal, gynecological, and genitourinary conditions.

There were medical schools and at least one school of midwifery for women, the graduates of which taught physicians about "women's conditions." They became quite well informed about some aspects of anatomy and physiology. For example, the papyri reveal that Egyptian physicians may have had reasonably accurate knowledge of the circulatory system, which was not described accurately and completely by modern man until the sixteenth century A.D., when William Harvey studied it. Taking the pulse was a common practice, and the quality of both the heartbeat and the pulse was considered important in understanding a patient's condition. Treatments included the use of a kind of adhesive plaster for closing small wounds, swabs, bandages, and tampons made from linen ravelings, sutures, and molded splints. The papyri also contains records of the preparation of pills, ointments, snuffs, gargles, and emollients that have continued, at least in name, until modern times. Drugs included opium, castor oil, hemlock, salts of copper, and many others.

Dentistry was practiced skillfully, if the gold-filled teeth of mummies of wealthy citizens are to be accepted as evidence. Egyptians developed the art of embalming the body to provide a home for the soul as it went on its journey after death.

The Ancient Hindus

The history of pre-Christian India reports the establishment of hospitals, probably the first in the world, and also the first special nursing group of which we have accurate information. These male attendants (perhaps more accurately called physician's assistants instead of nurses) staffed the hospitals to which surgeons with remarkable skills sent their patients for care. The Indian philosophy which assigned women to an inferior role in society would not allow them to work outside the home environment. The "nurses" qualifications were stated as follows in the *Charhaka Samhita*, a medical manuscript:

> . . . there should be secured a body of attendants of good behavior, distinguished for purity or cleanliness of habits, attached to the person for whose services they are engaged, possessed of cleverness and skill, endowed with kindness, skilled in every kind of service that a patient may require . . . clever in bathing or washing a patient . . . well skilled in making or cleaning beds . . . and skillful in waiting upon one that is ailing, and never unwilling to do any act that they be commanded to do.

One does not know who did the "commanding" of these workers—patients or doctors, or both. The nurse's status is also unclear (it appears that he might have become a physician after training), but we at least know that he performed some nursing functions.

The knowledge about Indian medicine derives principally from several of their books and writings (in contrast to the reliance on archeological discoveries for data about the Mesopotamian and Egyptian civilizations and others). Of these, the sacred writings called the Vedas, a compendium of surgical works (*Susruta Samhita*), and another of medical works (*Charaka Samhita*) are most informative.

From the Vedas, which were the oldest scriptures of Hinduism, it is learned that the Indian people of ancient times were highly religious and believed in divine control of health and disease. They worshipped many gods, especially the sun god Brahma, until Buddhism originated in the sixth century B.C. They used charms and invocations and other primitive methods to quell the wrath of the gods, but from abut 800 B.C. to A.D. 1000, all of India flourished and progressed, and medicine also advanced. It was during this period that the hospitals mentioned earlier were built.

The two outstanding physicians of ancient times were Susruta and Charaka, who in their writings revealed that physicians were members of the upper castes and were required to be pure of mind and body and ethical in every respect. Their knowledge of anatomy and physiology was often inaccurate, but they evolved some theories that persisted for centuries. Among these was the belief that disease might be caused by impurities in the body fluids or humors. They used bloodletting procedures to rid the body of the impure fluids. This theory of humoral pathology was accepted subsequently by Greek physicians and became a basic concept of European medicine. The Indian physician had a great many drugs and other pharmaceutical preparations to help him in his work.

The surgery practiced in India was particularly outstanding for the time. With instruments they designed themselves, under the cleanest conditions possible, without the aid of effective antiseptics or the benefits of anesthesia, the surgeons performed tonsillectomies, herniorrhaphies, tumor excisions, cataract operations, and other forms of surgery.

To help prevent disease, the Hindus formulated religious laws covering particularly matters of hygiene and diet suitable to the tropical climate.

Scientific medicine in India eventually lost its momentum, and during the Mohammedan era beginning about A.D. 622 it began to decline and became almost completely extinguished, a genuine loss to world medicine.

Ceylon, an island just off India's southeast coast, also enjoyed an advanced standard of living during the period of India's greatest achievement. History has recorded the establishment of many hospitals in which well-prepared physicians and nurses attended the sick. Hospitals for animals also were founded in India as well as Ceylon.

The Chinese

As in other ancient cultures, magic, demons, and evil spirits were part of Chinese medical beliefs. The beginning of a more modern medicine is credited to the emperor Shen Nung (c. 2700 B.C.), who apparently originated drug therapy and acupuncture. These were incorporated into the theory of yang and yin, which still exists. Yang, the male principle, is light, positive, full of life; yin, the female principle, is dark, cold, lifeless. When the two are in harmony, the patient is in good health. Originally, acupuncture consisted of inserting needles into areas called meridians, which controlled the flow of yang and yin. (With new interest in acupuncture, American medicine is trying to determine its anatomic and physiological basis.)

Other Chinese contributions include the use of many still pertinent drugs and further refinement of ancient measures of hydrotherapy, massage, cupping (bloodletting), moxa (a form of counterirritation) cautery, and the promotion of systematic exercise to maintain physical and mental well-being.

Sources of information include a book on medicine written by Shen Nung, and later works, notably the classic *Canon of Medicine*, which is a complete discussion of anatomy and physiology with many details about blood circulation and pulse. Another outstanding book was the *Essay on Typhoid*, written in the first century A.D. by Chang Chung Ching, often regarded as China's greatest physician.

There is little mention of any type of hospital, perhaps because of strong family traditions that would naturally include giving care to the sick within the family circle. Thus, nursing care was probably given in the home.

The Great Achievements of Greece

Whenever ancient Greece is mentioned, one immediately thinks of education, progress, philosophy, and democracy. But Plato, Aristotle, Socrates, Herodotus, Homer, Sophocles, Pericles, Euripides, and other great names of Greece were not typical of its earliest times, for this country too began under primitive conditions in about 2000 B.C.

The first of the great philosophers, Socrates, was born in 469 B.C.; his pupil Plato was born in 427 B.C.; and Aristotle, Plato's famous pupil, in 384 B.C. Herodotus, the great historian, was born in 484 B.C.; Homer, the epic poet, in c. 1000 B.C.

The ancient Greeks represented many peoples, principally the Achean, Dorian, Aegean, Ionian, Arcadian, and Aeolian, who came from the mountains, from fertile valleys where they had engaged in agriculture, and from the seacoast where seafaring was their occupation. Collectively they called themselves the Hellenes (after their ancestor Hellen, a legendary king of Phthia).

They were barbaric peoples at first, with the superstitions and practices of primitive peoples, but gradually there emerged the well-known Grecian character with a thirst for truth and knowledge. Because of their geographical location and the ease of maritime travel, they were able to visit such comparatively advanced countries as Crete and Mesopotamia and to borrow or usurp their culture.

They were also eager to expand their geographical borders, and were so successful that within a few centuries their culture extended from Greece to India. Gradually they developed their own Hellenic civilization, and by 500 B.C., if not before, they displayed the keen intellect, independence of thought, and democratic action for which they are famous. They also enjoyed religious freedom. Their great center of civilization was Athens, which was at its peak in the fourth century B.C. Athenian culture spread to other beautiful cities, principally along the Mediterranean coast, some of which eventually surpassed Athens in brilliance.

In such a vital society, the art of medicine naturally kept pace with advances in other fields. But, like other ancient cultures, Greece went through centuries of belief in demons and spirits as causes of human ills, but with an element of greater complexity (not known to some simple primitive peoples) because of its acquisition of other cultures and a divergence of beliefs and practices among them. Here, too, the Greeks gradually evolved their own ideas about the relationships of the gods to health and illness. The famous Greek myths told in story and poem show a mixture of common sense and mysticism in their medical attitudes.

Aesculapius, the classical god of medicine, is part of one such myth. Whether he actually lived or not seems uncertain, for his origin is obscure, but it is generally conceded that he did exist in person and that the mystery that surrounds him stems largely from his deification. A parallel is seen in the deification of Imhotep by the Egyptians. Hygieia, the goddess of health, is reputed to have been the daughter of Aesculapius.

His contributions, real or imagined, were further recognized by the founding of temples in his honor in localities suitable for rest and restoration to health. Sometimes referred to as hospitals, they were much more like the spas and health resorts of modern times, with mineral springs, baths, gymnasiums, athletic fields, and treatment and consultation rooms.

They differed from modern resorts, however, in that they were controlled by priests and were essentially religious institutions. Prayers, sacrifices, rituals, and thank offerings were part of every patient's regimen in one of these sanitoria. (However, pregnant women and individuals with incurable diseases were not admitted.) The therapeutic effects of the earthly facilities were considerable, however, and knowledge of them was significant in later medical practice. Priestesses served as attendants and waited upon the sick, but they could not be considered nurses. The best-known of these temples was Epidauros, about 30 miles from Athens, the ruins of which can still be seen.

To Aesculapius can also be traced the origin of the symbol of the medical profession—a serpent entwined on a staff—known as the caduceus. The staff was the staff of Aesculapius; the serpent since primitive times had represented wisdom and knowledge.

The greatest name in Greek medicine—and possibly in all medicine—is Hippocrates. Born in Cos in 460 B.C, he is frequently seen as the epitome of the ideal physician both personally and professionally. Humane, brilliant, progressive, a great physician, teacher, and leader, he is often known as the "Father of Medicine."

Hippocrates' medical achievements can be grouped into four major areas:

1. *Rejection of all beliefs in the supernatural origin of disease.* He divorced medicine from religion, philosophy, and the remaining traces of magic and taught that illness was caused by a breach of natural laws. He did not accept the theories of others who preceded him, but made his diagnosis on the basis of symptoms he observed in his patients. His emphasis was on the whole patient, and he advocated constant and continuous bedside care.
2. *Development of thorough patient assessment and recording.* He thoroughly examined his patients and then made a systematic recording of his findings: general appearance, temperature, pulse, respiration, sputum, excreta, ability to move about, and so on. Never before had physicians prepared good clinical records.
3. *Establishment of the highest ethical standards in medicine.* Hippocrates considered medicine one of the noblest of arts and believed that the conduct of the physician should be above reproach. He must be loyal to his profession and never bring dishonor upon it. He must be equally loyal to his patients and never injure them in any way. The Hippocratic Oath (probably written after his death) is reproduced in part on pages 204–205 and presumably encompasses some of his convictions.
4. *Author of medical books.* Although it is thought that much of the writing was actu-

ally done by contemporaries or possibly his students, the information is supposed to be based on Hippocrates' teachings. The works include his case histories, descriptions of techniques such as bathing and bandaging, treatises on fractures and dislocations, diet in acute diseases, ulcers, epidemic diseases, and others. He reported on treatments that did not work as well as those that did to avoid repetition of errors.

Also attributed to him by some authorities (questioned by others) is a *Book of Decorum*, from which this oft-quoted excerpt is taken:

> Let one of your pupils be left in charge, to carry out instructions without unpleasantness, and to administer the treatment. Choose out one who has already been admitted into the mysteries of the art, so as to add anything that is necessary and to give treatment with safety. He is there also to prevent those things escaping notice that happen in the intervals between visits. Never put a layman in charge of anything, otherwise if a mischance occurs the blame will fall on you, but achievement will bring you pride.
> [From a translation by W. H. S. Jones.]

It is assumed that the author was not referring to nurses but probably to medical students or attendants, who might also have taught and supervised care of the sick in the patient's home. This kind of care was probably done by the women of the family.

Little is known of nursing as an occupation in pre-Christian Greece. However, because the Greeks never established hospitals, in spite of nominal advances in surgery, Greek physicians did not need the assistance of nurses to the degree that the surgeons of India did, for example, and that may have been an important factor. Through the ages, the development of nursing seems to have been greatly influenced by the physician's need for assistance, the quality of help that he wanted, and the amount of responsibility he was willing to delegate to others. If there were nurses who worked outside the home in Greece, they must have all been men because women held a very inferior position and were denied education as well as participation in community activities, both civil and humanitarian, except for the few instances in which women became midwives or physicians.

Advances in Alexandria

After Alexander the Great conquered Greece in about 338 B.C., he spread Greek civilization throughout the known world. It reached a particularly high point in Alexandria, an Egyptian city on the Mediterranean Sea. Here the arts and sciences, including medicine, flourished for about 300 years.

In c. 300 B.C., the first great medical school of this period was established in Alexandria with clinics, laboratories, and a huge library of 500,000 volumes. The physicians were supported by the state and did not have to depend on their practice to make a living. Dissections were permitted, and this resulted in tremendous advances in the knowledge of anatomy and physiology. The studies made by the Alexandrian physicians are considered the first medical research worthy of the name. After Cleopatra was defeated by the Romans in 30 B.C., Alexandria's place in the sun dimmed considerably, and the art of and interest in research declined.

Roman Hospitals and Sanitation

When the Etruscans conquered Rome in about 750 B.C., they brought new arts to this farming community, particularly the use of bronze, skill in building stone edifices, and a written language. In about 500 B.C., the Romans overthrew the Etruscans and became powerful masters of the Western world. Rome soon became a thriving commercial center and, through later conquests, a vast empire. Much emphasis was placed on government administration and related activities, on pleasures for the well-to-do, sometimes at the expense of the less fortunate, and on beautifully constructed public buildings, aqueducts, and roads.

Gradually Rome assimilated what it wanted

of the Greek culture, and in some fields that was considerable. Although a temple of Aesculapius was built, Romans were somewhat wary of the Greek methods of treating disease, believing that their own deities, folklore, and magic were functioning well enough. Moreover, they were reluctant to accept advice and direction from the Greek physicians who, they thought, might poison or assassinate them in the name of medicine. They considered them social inferiors and thought them mercenary because they charged fees for their services.

Nevertheless, Greek medicine gradually replaced or supplemented Roman practices, and medicine was soon considered part of the necessary education of upper-class Roman men. Celsus (c. first century A.D.), in his lay work *De Medicina*, reported on, among other things, dietetics, pharmacy, medical conditions (particularly dermatological), surgical conditions (including cataract surgery and the use of ligatures), and mental illness. It might be added that physicians of ancient times had little interest in the care of childbearing women. Soranus, another Greek of this period, did write some treatises on obstetrics and gynecology, which is the first indication of a male physician's interest in these matters. Galen later referred to some of the techniques used by the midwives in delivery and care of the newborn, and it can be assumed that midwives were the key figures in the care of women. Galen (A.D. 130–201), considered one of the greatest of Greek physicians, practiced in Rome after receiving an education in many cities, including Alexandria. He wrote some 100 treatises on medicine, so comprehensive that for 200 years they remained unchallenged. He is seen as the greatest scientific experimentalist before the seventeenth century and perhaps the originator of scientific medicine.

Major Roman contributions to health were in public health sanitation and law. Their aqueducts, sewage systems, and baths were unequaled for centuries, and their city planning included the appointment of both a water commissioner and a public health official. In addition, they may be credited with the development of hospitals. *Valetudinaria* were detached buildings or just a large room designated for the care of valuable slaves on Roman estates. Apparently attendants watched over the sick, possibly with the attention of a physician. There is some indication that, at a later time, individuals other than slaves might have been cared for in *valetudinaria*. Given even more attention was the care of sick and injured soldiers. Originally, they were billeted with local Roman families, who tried to outdo each other in the quality of care. But as the Roman wars expanded to new frontiers, permanent convalescent camps succeeded temporary mobile hospitals. Modern excavations along the Rhine and Danube show the remains of hospitals that could accommodate 200 patients, with wards, recreation areas, baths, pharmacies, and rooms for attendants. Roman historians report that military discipline prevailed and, although the patients received good care, they were also required to conduct themselves "quietly."

Thus, it appears that the Romans took Greek medicine an additional step to the care of the sick by both male and female attendants.

THE FIRST FIVE CENTURIES OF CHRISTIANITY

After centuries of vilification, Christianity became the official religion of Rome in A.D. 335. The early Christian era brought another dimension to the care of the sick. Christian charity, based to a great extent on the Hebrew model as well as on the teachings of Christ, was reinforced by the persecution suffered by the early followers. Their beliefs included a strong emphasis on the sanctity of human life, and infanticide and abortion were considered murder. In the institutionalization of these ideals, bishops were given responsibility for the sick, the poor, widows, and children, but deacons and deaconesses were designated to

carry out the services. (Deaconesses, found almost entirely in the Eastern church until the eighth century and always fewer in number, had almost disappeared in the East by the eleventh century.)

The duties were not the same in all churches, but a deaconess usually assisted with such church services as the baptism of women, visiting sick women of the church in their homes, acting as ushers for women attending church, carrying messages for the clergy, and visiting prisoners when they could be helped through counseling. Not all were ordained by the church fathers, who resisted giving women too much recognition or freedom. Nor were they permitted to form orders with rules until somewhat later in history. The role of women was seen as marriage and the begetting of children. Young widows were encouraged to remarry. Widows over sixty (which in those days of early death must have restricted the number considerably) were designated to, among other things, watch over the sick. Some virgins also chose to take vows of service. It is not certain to what extent the early deaconesses were involved in such care, but it is clear that a group of specially designated women, whether deaconesses, widows, virgins, or matrons, cared for the sick.

Noted Women

Among the fabled women who made noted contributions to the care of the sick were the following:

Phoebe (spelled *Phebe* in the Bible) of Cenchrea in southern Italy, who lived about A.D. 60, was the first deaconess who performed nursing functions that were referred to in records of such early times. St. Paul, in Romans 16:1–2 (King James Version), commends her to authorities in Rome—to which she traveled—as a "succorer of many and of myself, also."

The **Empress Helena**, mother of Constantine the Great of Rome, lived c. 248–328. In c. 312, she converted to Christianity and made a pilgrimage to Jerusalem reportedly to expiate the sins of her son. In the Holy Land, she built two churches and a Christian hospital. An influential personage, she won support for the Christian church and especially for its humanitarian aspects.

Olympias, an aristocratic and beautiful young woman of Constantinople, was born in 368. Widowed at nineteen, she became a deaconess and devoted the rest of her life to work among the sick and poor. She was an excellent organizer, and the 40 deaconesses who worked under her accomplished a great deal in alleviating suffering, caring for orphans and the aged, and converting others to Christianity.

Perhaps unfortunately, Olympias is remembered in history chiefly for her extreme asceticism. She denied herself the luxury of a bath, dressed as the lowliest of beggars, and refused to observe any of the rules of hygienic living. Fabiola, Paula, and others (both men and women) of the early Christian era had ascetic tendencies, but none to the degree that Olympias demonstrated. Largely because of her personal neglect, she contracted many illnesses and thus lessened the effectiveness of her work.

Fabiola, a beautiful and wealthy matron of Rome, founded the first free hospital in that city in c. 390. Twice married and twice divorced, she embraced Christianity and spent her fortune and the rest of her life in service to the poor and sick. She personally nursed the sickest and filthiest people who came to her hospital, and was so gentle and kind that she was beloved by all Romans. Following her death, St. Jerome wrote a letter about her, sometimes called "the first literary document in the history of nursing."

Paula, a friend of Fabiola, widowed at twenty-three, learned and wealthy, also became a Christian. In about 385, she sailed from Rome to Palestine, where she built hospitals and inns for pilgrims and travelers along the route to Jerusalem, a monastery in Bethlehem, and a convent for women in Jerusalem. She, like Fabiola, performed nursing duties.

Hospitals

Following the closing of the temples of Aesculapius, in those same early centuries, another form of hospital emerged, the *diakonia*, providing a combination of outpatient and welfare service, managed by the deacons and supervised by the bishop. This was replaced in time by "a house for the sick" as there was a house for the poor and for the old. Generally, only the poor, the destitute, or the traveler, those who could not be cared for in their own homes, chose this alternative, an attitude that persisted to a great extent into the eighteenth and nineteenth centuries. One of these hospitals may have been the Basilias outside Caesarea, built in the third century by St. Basil, one of the Four Fathers of the Greek Church, and his sister Macrina. Huge and apparently magnificent, it had special rooms or areas for patients with different conditions, a separate building for lepers, and a special area where the physically handicapped could learn a new trade. There were homes for physicians and nurses, for convalescent patients, for the elderly, and schools and workshops for foundlings. Presumably, some kind of attendant had to be present. Some of these were the women cited earlier, who probably came from their homes to give care. A brotherhood known as *parabolani*, organized in the third century during a great plague in Alexandria, gave care to the sick and buried the dead.

The most regrettable fact in the history of this period is the attitude of the Christians toward science and education—an attitude that stultified progress in all intellectual pursuits, including medicine, and permeated the so-called Dark Ages, which continued for another 500 years.

THE MIDDLE AGES

The term *Middle Ages* usually is applied to the years from approximately A.D. 500 to 1500, of which roughly the first half has been called the *Dark Ages*, to distinguish it from the periods of classical civilization preceding and following it. Some historians acknowledge that the Dark Ages may have been more enlightened than was formerly believed. Certainly there were many areas allied to nursing in which the era might have been termed "light gray" rather than "dark," for progress was made that influenced the later development of nursing as a profession for both women and men.

Politically, the world changed greatly during the Middle Ages. The early centuries brought invasions against the Roman Empire by "barbarians" (to the Romans anyone outside the pale of the Empire), which resulted in the formation of many smaller kingdoms within the empire. By the twelfth century, many kingdoms existed, chiefly England, Scotland, France, Denmark, Poland, Hungary, Sicily, and several in Spain. In the meantime, the Vikings had settled in the Scandinavian areas and in parts of Russia, and expanded rapidly. Trade routes were established between principal cities, and new occupations developed to meet the needs of a rapidly increasing population and changing economies and goals.

The barbarians were all pagans, and not until the thirteenth and fourteenth centuries were they converted to Christianity. Most of the work of conversion was carried out under the direction of the pope, and Roman Catholicism quite naturally was the principal religion of the world at that time.

Also significant in the general picture of the known world during medieval times was the rise and fall of feudalism in Central Europe, with its devastating effects on the welfare of the common man. It was a time of famine and pestilence, with accompanying miseries and serious illnesses. Medical and nursing care was needed, but unfortunately was not available in either sufficient quality or quantity. Beginning in the thirteenth century, feudalism gradually disappeared.

During the Middle Ages, the deaconesses, suppressed by the Western churches in particular, gradually declined and became almost extinct. However, a small spark remained that has been fanned into a flame every now and then during history, resulting in the formation of a new order of deaconesses, the most important of which are mentioned later.

As the deaconesses declined, the religious orders grew stronger. Known as *monastic orders* and comprised of monks and nuns (though not in the same orders), they controlled the hospitals, running them as institutions concerned more with the patients' religious problems than their physical ailments. However, monks and some nuns were better educated than most people in those times, and their liberal education may well have included some of the medical writings of Celsus and Galen.

Later, with the coming of the Renaissance in the fourteenth century, separation of hospital and church began, effecting spectacular improvement in the scientific and skillful treatment of the sick and injured. It was within the monasteries, however, that education in general progressed significantly during this earlier period.

Lay citizens banded together to form secular orders. Their work was similar to that of the monastic orders in that it was concerned with the sick and needy, but they lived in their own homes, were allowed to marry, and took no vows of the church. They usually adopted a uniform, or habit. Nursing was often their main work.

The military nursing orders, known as the Knights Hospitallers, were the outcome of the Crusades, the military expeditions undertaken by Christians in the eleventh, twelfth, and thirteenth centuries to recover the Holy Land from the Moslems.

The most prominent of these three types of orders—religious, military, and secular—during the Middle Ages are described in the following paragraphs.

The **Order of St. Benedict**, the foremost religious order, was founded by St. Benedict of Nursia (c. 480–543) on the beautiful mountain Monte Cassino, about halfway between Rome and Naples. It became a great and powerful center which sent workers throughout Europe, raising standards of education and culture and providing better care for the sick and poor. St. Benedict's rule placed the care of the sick (in which bathing was stressed, a departure from the ascetic practices of some other orders) above and before every other duty of the monks. He established infirmaries within the monasteries primarily for the care of sick members of the order, but also to help centralize and organize the care of pilgrims, wayfarers, and "refugees." With war, famine, and pestilence common occurrences, such service was sorely needed.

The **Knights Hospitallers**, an outgrowth of the Crusades, was the first military order of nurses. The first Crusade (there were nine in all) originated in 1095 when disorganized hordes of men and women of every age, type, and description answered Pope Urban II's call to march to Jerusalem and recover the Holy Land from the Moslems, who had taken it by force from the Byzantine Empire in the seventh century A.D. Ill prepared physically and psychologically for such a journey, disorganized and inadequately equipped, the crusaders (whose symbol was an eight-pointed cross) died by the thousands along the way.

The later Crusades were essentially expeditions to assist the earlier crusaders in the Holy Land. It was during the first Crusade that the military order, the Knights Hospitallers, was established for the original purpose of bringing the wounded from the battlefield to the hospitals and caring for them there, which explains the name of the order. Later, two other branches of the Knights were formed, one to defend the wounded from the enemy while they were being brought to the hospital, and the other to defend the pilgrims when they were attacked.

There were three principal orders of the Knights of Hospitallers: St. John of Jerusalem; the Teutonic Knights; and the Knights of St. Lazarus, whose principal mission was to care for victims of leprosy, one of the major health problems from the eleventh to the mid-thirteenth century. Women had their own branches of the Knights Hospitallers. They performed their services principally in hospitals to which only women patients were admitted.

The story of the Knights Hospitallers is both colorful and interesting. Wealthy and influential, these orders had their successes and failures for approximately seven centuries.

The **Hospital Brothers of St. Anthony** was a secular order founded about 1095 by a grateful man who had been miraculously cured of St. Anthony's fire, which was probably erysipelas. The men and women who joined the order cared only for patients with this disease in special hospitals to which no other patients were admitted. Thus they succeeded in curtailing the spread of erysipelas and no doubt became specialists of a sort in the treatment of this disease.

The Antonines later became a religious order and, when these orders were suppressed, the character of their contribution to nursing changed. They took care of patients with other illnesses, the special hospitals for St. Anthony's fire closed, and erysipelas became a major problem for several centuries, especially among surgical and obstetric patients in general hospitals.

The **Beguines of Flanders**, believed to have been founded in about 1184 by a priest, was one of the most important secular orders. The widows and unmarried women who comprised its membership (at one time numbering 200,000) devoted their lives to helping others. Their nursing duties included the care of the sick in their homes and in hospitals, serving soldiers and civilians during the Battle of Waterloo, caring for victims of cholera during the dreadful epidemics of the nineteenth century, and responding to calls for assistance in times of disastrous fires, floods, and famines.

These sisterhoods spread to Germany, Switzerland, and France and became so numerous, strong, and popular that they were able to resist attempts to abolish them by monastic orders and religious leaders.

The **Third Order of St. Francis** is one of three orders founded by St. Francis of Assisi (1182–1226), probably the best known of the saints connected with nursing. A compassionate young man who loved people, birds, and animals, he was also a fanatic and ascetic with marked qualities of leadership, attracting the influential and learned as well as the humble and lowly to his orders.

The Third Order of St. Francis, also called the *Franciscan Tertiaries*, worked principally among the lepers. They were assisted by the women of the Order of Poor Clares, the second order formed by St. Francis, whose members were largely young women who had left their noble families for a life of service.

After the death of St. Francis at the age of forty-four, the ideals of the Franciscan friars changed considerably, improving in some respects, degenerating in others. But the friars extended their work to the sick and poor, particularly in the slum areas of Europe's large cities, and rendered remarkable service.

The Order of Poor Clares became an enclosed order, which greatly changed the lives of the sisters. They continued their work in some ways, however. It was the Franciscan sisters who helped Dr. W. W. Mayo, a Civil War surgeon, to found the famous St. Mary's Hospital in Rochester, Minnesota, in 1889.

Order of the Holy Ghost (Santo Spirito), a secular order, was founded in Montpellier, France, in the late twelfth century. Initiated by a knight known as Guy de Montpellier, its members included both men and women. They nursed the poor in the community and assumed responsibility for all of the nursing at the Santo Spirito Hospital in Rome in 1204. They later extended their service to other large hospitals in Italy, France, and Germany. They cared for lepers in shelters outside the hospitals and for persons with other infectious diseases. The order later became monastic and eventually almost disappeared.

Guy de Montpellier established this order in connection with a medical school which had existed in Montpellier since the eighth century, and which became famous as a center of medical education, reaching its period of greatest achievement in the thirteenth and fourteenth centuries. Patients flocked to Montpellier seeking cures under the care of renowned physicians, one of the most outstanding being the surgeon Guy de Chauliac (1298–1368).

The **Grey Sisters**, an order of uncloistered nuns which originated in about 1222, ministered to the poor and the sick in homes and hospitals for many years. In the fourteenth and fifteenth centuries when the plague invaded Europe, they worked closely with the Alexian Orders in meeting the nursing needs.

The **Alexian Brotherhood** came into being in about 1348 in the Netherlands when the "Black Death" was sweeping Europe. The brothers took no vows, adopted no rule at the time, bending all their efforts to caring for the stricken and burying the victims of plague.

Nearly a century later, in 1431, they organized as a religious order, taking vows of obedience, poverty, and chastity and choosing as their patron saint Alexus, a man of noble birth who in the fifth century had worked in a hospital in Syria. They were among the pioneers of organized nursing in Europe.

There were several outstanding personalities of the Middle Ages who were not members of orders, but who nonetheless made significant contributions to the health and welfare of the masses. Some of these were canonized, notably Elizabeth of Hungary, Catherine of Siena, and Hildegard of Bingen. The most prominent women were abbesses or members of royalty who nursed the sick, established educational programs for nurses, and sometimes wrote books and treatises. Hildegarde of Bingen (1098–1178) was educated in a Benedictine monastery and years later became its abbess. Several of her writings were related to medicine and the care of the sick, including general diseases of the body, their causes, symptoms and treatment, aspects of anatomy and physiology, and human behavior. Many of these things were unknown to physicians of the time.

Medicine

The Dark Ages on the Continent halted the promising progress of medicine, and except for Galen, who died about A.D. 200, no great physician practiced medicine in Europe during this period. The Christian church, obsessed with its belief that man's main purpose on earth was to prepare for a future life, saw little need for the science and philosophy of the Greeks or the hygienic teachings and sanitation systems of the Romans. Plagues swept Europe periodically for centuries. Medical knowledge survived and developed in only three areas.

In the eastern Roman Empire, Byzantine physicians nourished the teachings of Hippocrates and Galen, refusing to let them become obsolete; in Salerno in southern Italy, an educational ideal was fostered for medicine as well as for other areas of learning, a medical school was established, and laymen in Salerno translated many Greek manuscripts of importance in medical history; and vigorous medical activity was carried on in the Moslem empires. Although there was warfare there, as in Europe, the conquerors preserved rather than destroyed the culture they found and encouraged further development. Within 100 years they had achieved a standard of culture that took the Germanic tribes who invaded the Roman Empire ten times as long to develop.

The Arabs translated the works of Hippocrates, Galen, Aristotle, and others. Physicians adopted the Hippocratic method of careful observation of patients. One of the outstanding physicians was Rhazes (850–932) of Baghdad, who was especially interested in communicable diseases and gave an accurate account of smallpox. Another and far more prominent physician was Avicenna (980–1037), a Persian whose *Canon of Medicine* was studied in the medical schools of Europe from the twelfth to the seventeenth century. Moses ben Maimon (Maimonides), born in Moslem-controlled Spain of a Jewish family

descended from King David, was an excellent clinician who became the court physician to Sultan Saladin.

Medical centers that included hospitals were founded in Cairo, Alexandria, Damascus, and Baghdad. There the Arabs made advances in physiology, hygiene, chemistry, and particularly pharmacy. Because their religion prohibited human dissection, their knowledge of anatomy changed little during this time. Men probably gave care in these hospitals, because women were kept in seclusion.

Hospitals and Hospital Care

Hospitals in which the sick received care were established as the need increased and the wherewithal became available. At the close of the Middle Ages, there were hospitals all over Europe, particularly in larger cities such as Paris and Rome, and in England, where several hundred had been established. Most of these have long since been eliminated or abandoned, but a few have remained. The oldest of these is the Hotel Dieu of Lyons (House of God's Charity), built in 542, in which both men and women nursed the patients.

The Hotel Dieu of Paris, founded in c. 650, has a less favorable record as far as nursing is concerned. Staffed by Augustinian nuns who did the cooking and laundry as well as the nursing, and who had neither intellectual nor professional stimulation, the hospital was not distinguished for its care of patients. In 1908 the nuns were expelled from the Hotel Dieu. The records of nursing kept by this hospital were well done, however, and have been a source of enlightenment for historians. Still in existence in Rome is the Santo Spirito Hospital, established in 717 by order of the pope, to care only for the sick.

Hospitals in England during the Middle Ages differed from those on the Continent in that they were never completely church controlled, although they were founded on Christian principles and accepted responsibility for the sick and injured. The oldest and best-known English hospitals from a historical point of view are St. Bartholomew's founded in 1123; St. Thomas's, founded in 1213; and in 1247, Bethlehem Hospital, originally a general hospital that later became famous as a mental institution, referred to frequently as Bedlam.

An interesting sidelight here is the treatment of the mentally ill. In Bedlam, as in similar institutions, the inmates were treated with inhumane cruelty. Beatings and starvation were not uncommon. However, in Gheel, Belgium, reports of miraculous cures at the tomb of St. Dymphna, an Irish princess murdered by her mad father, brought the mentally ill hope of healing. The people of Gheel took in the pilgrims as foster families and gave them care and affection. The therapy persists to this day in Gheel.

The nursing care in most early hospitals was essentially basic: bathing, feeding, giving medicines, making beds, and so on. It was rarely of high quality, however, largely because of the retarded progress of nearly all civilization and the shortsighted attitude toward women that was typical of the Dark Ages.

THE RENAISSANCE

The word *renaissance* as used in history refers to both a movement and a period of time. In years, it is generally conceded to have lasted from 1400 to 1550, the years during which there was a transitional movement toward revival of the arts and sciences in Europe, culminating in the modern age in which we still live. Also during this period great explorations were made, including the discovery of America.

New impetus was given to literature and art, to bookbinding, to the founding of libraries, universities, and medical schools—but not nursing schools. These came more than three centuries later. Merchants made huge fortunes in trade. Bankers likewise became wealthy by making loans, especially to kings and princes.

The Age of Discovery, 1450–1550, a part of this period, brought great increase in geographical knowledge. Man became excited about the world around him and about the prospect of finding gold in other lands, particularly America. New passageways were sought to old countries, and the acquisition of new colonies and territories became extremely important to the established kingdoms and empires.

The Renaissance saw the birth and death of Leonardo da Vinci, Michelangelo, and other great artists. And to medicine it gave Paracelsus, Vesalius, and Paré.

Theophrastus Paracelsus (1493–1541), a Swiss physician and exceptional chemist, made contributions chiefly in the area of pharmaceutical chemistry.

Andreas Vesalius (1514–1564), a Belgian, made detailed anatomical studies in universities and hospitals, disproving by his practical methods some of the classical theories of Galen and others. One of his many published works was a voluminous illustrated book, *De Corporis Humani Fabrica Libri Septem (Seven Books on the Structure of the Human Body)*, in which he displayed his great fund of knowledge and also criticized and corrected Galen. For this he was berated by advocates of Galen. He gradually lost his tremendous energy and initiative and settled down to a routine physician's life.

Ambroise Paré (1510–1590), a Frenchman, served as an apprentice to a barber-surgeon and later became the first surgeon of the Renaissance. A student of Vesalius, he became a great military surgeon who reintroduced the use of the ligature instead of the cautery to occlude blood vessels during surgery, adopted a simple technique of wound dressing to replace the oil-boiling method in wide use, improved obstetrical techniques, designed artificial limbs, and wrote books on surgery.

Barber-surgeons were men in France who not only did barbering but also performed such procedures as bleeding, cupping, leeching, giving enemas, and extracting teeth—procedures that the physicians of medieval times prescribed for their patients but considered undignified to perform. The barber-surgeon was required to wear a short robe, whereas the regular surgeons, of whom there were very few, were entitled to wear a long one.

There was understandable friction among the three groups—physicians, barber-surgeons, and surgeons—and the problems were not completely resolved until the practice of surgery improved greatly and the Royal College of Surgeons was established in 1800.

The striped barber pole, symbol of the present-day barber, dates from the time when the patient being bled clung to a staff; the bloody bandage that covered his wound is represented by the red stripe on the barber's pole.

Nursing apparently continued in a way similar to that established in the earlier Middle Ages. The charter of St. Bartholomew's Hospital called for a matron and twelve other women to make beds, wash, and attend the poor patients. They were to receive about two pounds a year and room and board, with the matron receiving more. All slept in one room at the hospital. They cared for about 100 patients. However, whether this arrangement was typical is not known.

FROM REFORMATION TO NIGHTINGALE

The Reformation was a religious movement beginning early in the sixteenth century that resulted in the formation of various Prostestant churches under leaders who had revolted against the supremacy of the pope. Monasteries were closed; religious orders were dispersed, even in Catholic countries. Because many of these orders were involved in the care of the sick, nursing and hospital care suffered a severe setback. A startling effect was the almost total disappearance of male nurses. Almost all Catholic nursing orders after 1500 were made up of women. In Protestant countries, too, women and nursing became almost synonymous, for Protestant leaders recognized the vacuum in care of the sick and urged the hiring of nurse deaconesses and other elderly women to nurse the sick.

William Hunter (1718–1783) and his brother **John** (1728–1793), of Scotland, obstetrician and surgeon, respectively, conducted meticulous anatomical research and thus founded the science of pathology.

William Tuke (1732–1822), an English merchant and philanthropist, instituted long overdue reforms in the care of the mentally ill. Chief founder of the York Retreat (1796), he had important influence on subsequent treatment of the mentally ill.

Edward Jenner (1749–1823), an English physician, friend and pupil of John Hunter, in 1796 originated vaccination against smallpox.

Rene Laennec (1781–1826), of France, invented the stethoscope in 1891. Before this, the physician had listened to the patient's heartbeat by placing his ear against the patient's chest wall.

Even with these advances, medical education was still sketchy. Some practicing physicians had no medical education. An MD degree required apprenticeship with a physician, surgeon, or apothecary, some university classes, some dissecting at an anatomical school or hospital—or any variation of these. There were a few noted schools in Italy, Germany, and Scotland; the English colonies had none until 1765. A practical apothecary school started earlier, but most often pharmacists were also physicians.

By the end of the eighteenth century, nurses of some kind functioned in hospitals. Conditions were not attractive, and much has been written about the drunken, thieving women who tended patients. However, some hospitals made real efforts to set standards. One set of criteria included such attributes as good health, good sight and hearing (to make pertinent observations), nimbleness, quietness, good temper, diligence, temperance and "to have no children, or other to come much after her."[4] Already a hierarchy of nursing personnel had begun, with helpers and watchers assigned to help the *sisters*, as the early English nurses were called.

In other parts of Europe, nursing was becoming recognized as an important service.

Diderot, whose *Encyclopedia* attempted to sum up all human knowledge, said that nursing "is as important for humanity as its functions are low and repugnant." Urging care in selection, since "all persons are not adapted to it," he described the nurse as "patient, mild, and compassionate. She should console the sick, foresee their needs, and relieve their tedium."[5]

Another progressive step was the first nursing textbook, which had been published in Vienna early in the eighteenth century.

Midwifery, too, was gaining new attention. In England in 1739, a small lying-in infirmary was started for the education of medical students and midwives, and soon other lying-in hospitals began to appear. In London, poor women also benefited in home deliveries when a famous physician began to teach medical students midwifery and also taught women to become nurse-midwives at the bedside. (His students had to contribute funds to the care and support of these women.)

Nevertheless, it should be remembered that even with the tremendous increase in hospital building at that time, most care was still given in the home by wives and mothers.

The advent of the Industrial Revolution in England saw the development of power-driven machinery to do the spinning, weaving, and metal work that had previously been done manually in the home. Improvement in the steam engine as a source of power improved mining procedures and resulted in the development of factories, which the English called *mills*. The cotton, woolen, and iron industries grew rapidly, and there was a corresponding improvement in agriculture.

Also out of this era came noted Catholic orders devoted to care of the sick.

The Sisters of Charity were founded by St. Vincent de Paul (1576–1660) of France, a Catholic priest. He was ably assisted by Mlle. Louise La Gras, a woman of noble birth greatly interested in nursing and social work.

Once a prisoner himself, having been captured by pirates, St. Vincent de Paul became vitally interested in lessening the suffering of all slaves and prisoners. This interest expanded to include the sick and poor in his small country parish, and to help him in his work, he organized a society of women. This small group was so successful that similar groups were formed in other localities in France. The most famous of all, the Sisters of Charity, was organized in Paris under the direction of Mlle. La Gras. A younger group, the Daughters of Charity, was formed later. A noncloistered order, the Sisters were free to go wherever they were needed.

The Sisters of Charity were always carefully selected, and from the beginning their ideals and standards were very high. Members of this order took over the nursing service in many European hospitals, and came to Canada and the United States to give similar service during the early history of these countries.

In Spain, the **Brothers Hospitallers of St. John of God** was founded by a man who gave care to the sick, with special attention to the mentally ill. The order spread throughout the world, and its members opened and staffed hospitals wherever they went, including the Americas. The care given in their hospitals in Goa, as described by a sixteenth-century traveler, seemed to be a model of its time, perhaps even ahead of its time.

In Italy, Camillus, also to be canonized, trained and supplied nurses (men) for hospital care and founded an order dedicated to care of the sick and dying.

In the New World, Cortez founded the first hospital (in Mexico City); within 20 years, most major Spanish towns had one. It was 100 years later that a Hotel Dieu was founded in Sillery (Canada) and another at Montreal. In the latter, care was given by a young lay woman and three nursing sisters who came from France, but perhaps the first "nurse" in Canada was Marie Herbert Hobau in Nova Scotia, the widow of the surgeon and apothecary who accompanied Champlain.[3]

Records in Jamestown, Virginia, also tell of the selection of certain men and women to care for the sick. There were numerous health problems in the early American colonies, in part the result of the difficult living conditions. Hospitals of some type existed; one was described as accommodating fifty patients—if they slept two in a bed (not uncommon in Europe either).

The seventeenth and eighteenth centuries were periods of continuing change in Europe, and scientific advances had an enduring influence on medicine and health. Of the creative scientists of those times, the following are key figures:

William Harvey (1578–1657), an English physician generally regarded as the father of modern medicine, was the first to describe completely (except for the capillary system) and accurately the circulatory system, replacing the earlier explanations which, though remarkable at the time, actually were at least partially incorrect.

Thomas Sydenham (1624–1689), an Englishmen educated at Oxford and Montpellier, revived the Hippocratic methods of observation and reasoning and in other ways "restored" clinical medicine to a sound basis.

Antonj van Leeuwenhoek (1632–1723), of Holland, improved on Galileo's microscope and produced one that permitted the examination of body cells and bacteria.

The industrialization of Europe did not begin until the mid-nineteenth century, when England had already assumed international leadership, its empire was growing, and British trade was the center of world marketing.

People of means lived a most luxurious life. Graciousness and elegance prevailed, and woman's mission in life was to carry on these traditions. For this she was educated and carefully prepared by her parents.

The common women worked largely as servants in private homes or not at all. With the coming of factories, men, women, and children worked under cruel conditions. Caring for the sick in hospitals and homes were the "uncommon" women—prisoners, prostitutes—unkempt, unsavory, disinterested. Health conditions were still dreadful, with epidemics such as cholera sweeping whole countries. Children orphaned in these epidemics were finally put in almshouses, which provided no improvement in their lot. The situation was no different in America but was probably worst in England, and a number of social reformers began to work for change.

Culturally, great progress was made, particularly on the Continent. The demand for intellectual liberty brought marked advancement in educational facilities for men, but not for women. This was also true in the United States where, for example, Harvard University, established at Cambridge, Massachusetts, in 1636, admitted only men, a policy it steadfastly maintained into the twentieth century. Columbia University in New York City, founded in 1754, followed a similar policy but lowered its ban on women with the founding of Barnard College in 1889. Teachers College was founded as a coeducational institution in 1888.

Out of this confused century came scientists and physicians who made dramatic breakthroughs in medical science:

Oliver Wendell Holmes (1809–1894), a Boston physician, furthered safe obstetric practice, pointing out the dangers of infection. He is author of the famous treatise "The Contagiousness of Puerperal Fever," published in 1843.

Crawford W. Long (1815–1878), an American physician, excised a tumor of the neck under ether anesthesia in 1832 but did not make his discovery public until after Dr. William T. Morton announced his in 1846. This led to one of medicine's most enduring controversies: Who should receive the credit for discovering the anesthetic properties of ether?

Ignaz P. Semmelweis (1818–1865), of Vienna, is famous for his advances in the safe practice of obstetrics.

Louis Pasteur (1822–1895), of France, chemist and bacteriologist, became famous for his germ theory of disease, the development of the process known as *pasteurization*, and the discovery of a treatment for rabies. His work overlapped that of Robert Koch.

Lord Joseph Lister (1827–1912), English

surgeon, developed and proved, in 1865, his theory of the bacterial infection of wounds on which modern aseptic surgery is based.

Robert Koch (1843–1910), of Germany, founded modern bacteriology. He originated the drying and staining method of examining bacteria. His most important discovery was the identification of the tubercle bacillus, which led eventually to tremendous reductions in loss of life from tuberculosis.

Wilhelm Röntgen (1845–1923), a German physicist, discovered x-rays in 1895 and laid the foundation for the science of roentgenology and radiology.

Sir William Osler (1849–1919), a renowned Canadian teacher and medical historian, was associated with McGill University, the University of Pennsylvania, Johns Hopkins University, and Oxford University, England. He was knighted in 1911.

Pierre Curie (1859–1906), a French chemist, and his Polish wife, **Marie** (1867–1934), discovered radium in 1898.

NURSING IN THE NINETEENTH CENTURY

The dreary picture of secular nursing is not totally unexpected, given the times. Because proper young women did not work outside the home, nursing had no acceptance, much less prestige. Even those nurses not in the Dickens' Sairy Gamp mold or those desiring to nurse found themselves in competition with workhouse inmates, who were cheaper workers for hospital administrations.

It was acceptable to nurse as a member of a religious order, when the motivation was, of course, religious and the cost to the hospital was little or none.

During the nineteenth century, several nursing orders were revived or originated that had substantial influence on modern nursing. In most instances, these orders cared for patients in hospitals that were already established, in contrast to the orders of earlier times, which had founded the hospitals in which they worked. The most influential are the following:

The **Church Order of Deaconesses**, an ancient order, was revived by Theodor Fliedner (1800–1864), pastor of a small parish in Kaiserswerth, Germany, to care for the patients in a hospital he opened in 1836. At first he had only one deaconess, whom he trained in nursing. Although the training was quite superficial, the work expanded, more deaconesses joined the staff, and the deaconess institute at Kaiserswerth became famous. (Florence Nightingale obtained her only "formal" training in nursing there.) Four of the deaconesses and Pastor Fliedner journeyed to Pittsburgh, Pennsylvania, in 1849, to help establish a hospital under the leadership of Pastor William Passavant; and similar assistance was given to the founders of institutions on the Kaiserswerth plan in London, Constantinople, Beirut, Alexandria, Athens, and other localities.

Pastor Fliedner's work began with discharged prisoners (rather than the sick poor), in whom he became greatly interested through the reforms effected in England under Elizabeth Fry. Aided by both his first and second wives, he also established an orphanage and a normal school. The Kaiserswerth institute still exists and still conducts a school of nursing.

The **Protestant Sisters of Charity** was founded by Elizabeth Fry (1780–1845) of England, whose work among prisoners and the physically and mentally ill was based on reforms that had been instituted by John Howard (1726–1790) a quarter of a century before. Mrs. Fry became interested in the deaconesses at Kaiserswerth and visited the hospital to observe how they functioned. She then organized a small group of "Nurses" in London to do similar work among the sick poor. She first called the group the Protestant Sisters of Charity, later changing it to Institute of Nursing Sisters. (Unofficially they often were called the Fry Sisters or Fry Nurses.) The sisters were not affiliated with any church. Their training for nursing was extremely elementary. This group was in no way connected with the Sisters of Charity established earlier by Saint Vincent de Paul.

The **Sisters of Mercy** was a Roman Catholic society formed by Catherine McAuley (1787–1841) in Dublin, which later became an order and adopted a rule. The sisters visited in Dublin hospitals and nursed victims of a cholera epidemic in 1832; their work grew rapidly and spread throughout the world, including the establishment of several Mercy hospitals in the United States.

The **Irish Sisters of Charity**, also a Roman Catholic group, was started by Mary Aikenhead (1787–1858). The sisters visited the sick in their homes and did volunteer nursing in the community during emergencies. They had limited nurses' training and, in 1892, founded a training school for lay persons in St. Vincent's Hospital, in Dublin, in which they previously had assumed all nursing duties. They opened additional St. Vicnent's hospitals in other areas of the world, including the United States, to which they had come in 1855 to nurse victims of a cholera epidemic in San Francisco.

Also during this period, several nursing sisterhoods were established under the auspices of the Church of England. One of these, the **Sisters of Mercy in the Church of England**, was organized about 1850. The sisters had little if any formal preparation, but through practical experience acquired in district "nursing" and work in a cholera epidemic, they became quite proficient.

Another Anglican sisterhood, **St. Margaret's of East Grinstead**, was founded by a doctor in 1854. The sisters worked entirely among the sick in the community; they were not associated with hospitals in any way.

The Anglican order that did the most to improve hospital nursing during this period was **St. John's House**, founded in 1848 by the Church of England. Named for the parish in which it was located—St. John the Evangelist in St. Pancras, London—its purpose was to instruct and train members of the Church of England "to act as nurses and visitors to the sick and poor."[6] The original plan also stipu-

lated that the order should be connected with "some hospital or hospitals, in which the women under training, or those who had already been educated, might find the opportunity of exercising their calling or of acquiring experience."[7]

The first training program was successful, as were the twenty-five subsequent ones developed by St. John's House to meet changing needs, and the graduates were always in great demand.

Progress in medicine and science during these centuries was accompanied by accelerated interest in better nursing service and nurses' training. Neither was achieved to a significant degree, however, despite the fine work of dedicated men and women who belonged to the several nursing orders of the time. Limited in numbers and inadequately prepared for their nursing functions, the members of these orders could not begin to meet the need for their services. Such care as patients received in the majority of institutions was grossly inadequate.

In the mid-nineteenth century, therefore, the time was right—perhaps overdue—for the revolution in nursing education that originated under the leadership of Florence Nightingale and that influenced so greatly and so quickly (from an historical point of view) the nursing care of patients and, indeed, the health of the world.

REFERENCES

1. Thelma Ingles, "The Physicians' View of the Evolving Nursing Profession—1873–1913," *Nursing Forum*, **15**,2:141–2 (1976).
2. Committee on Medical Education, "Nursing Education: Status or Service Oriented?" *Bull. N.Y. Acad. Med.*, **53**:502 (June 1977).
3. Josephine A. Dolan, *Nursing in Society*, 14th ed. (Philadelphia: W. B. Saunders, 1978), p. 98.
4. Bonnie Bullough and Vern Bullough, *The Care of the Sick: The Emergence of Modern Nursing* (New York: Prodist, 1978), p. 57.

5. Ibid., p. 69.
6. Lucy Ridgely Seymer, *A General History of Nursing*, 4th ed. (London: Faber & Faber, 1956), p. 74.
7. Ibid., p. 75.

2

The Influence of Florence Nightingale

It has been said that Florence Nightingale, an extraordinary woman in any century, is the most written-about woman in history. Through her own numerous publications, her letters, the writings of her contemporaries, including newspaper reports, and the numerous biographies and studies of her life, there emerges the picture of a sometimes contradictory, frequently controversial, but undeniably powerful woman who probably had a greater influence on the care of the sick than any other single individual.

Called the founder of modern nursing, Nightingale was a strong-willed woman of quick intelligence who used her considerable knowledge of statistics, sanitation, logistics, administration, nutrition, and public health not only to develop a new system of nursing education and health care but also to improve the social welfare systems of the time. The gentle, caring lady of the lamp, full of compassion for the soldiers of the Crimea, is an accurate image, but no more so than that of the hard-headed administrator and planner who forced changes in the intolerable social conditions of the time, including the care of the sick poor. Nightingale knew full well that

a tender touch alone would not bring health to the sick or prevent illness, so she set her intelligence, her administrative skills, her political acumen, and her incredible drive to achieve her self-defined missions. In the Victorian age when women were almost totally dominated by men—fathers, husbands, brothers—and it was undesirable for them to show intelligence or profess interest in anything but household arts, this indomitable woman accomplished the following:

1. Improved and reformed laws affecting health, morals, and the poor.
2. Reformed hospitals and improved workhouses and infirmaries.
3. Improved medicine by instituting an army medical school and reorganizing the army medical department.
4. Improved the health of natives and British citizens in India and other colonies.
5. Established nursing as a profession with two missions—sick nursing and health nursing.[1]

The new nurse and the new image of the nurse that she created, in part through the nursing schools she founded, in part through her writings, and in part through her international influence, became the model that persisted for almost 100 years. Today, some of her tenets about the "good" nurse seem terribly restrictive, but it should be remembered that in those times not only the image but also the reality of much of secular nursing was based on the untutored, uncouth workhouse inmates for whom drunkenness and thievery were a way of life. It was small wonder that each Nightingale student had to exemplify a new image.

> The Nightingale nurse had to establish her character in a profession proverbial for immorality. Neat, ladylike, vestal, above suspicion, she had to be the incarnate denial that a hospital nurse had to be drunken, ignorant, and promiscuous.[2]

These historical idiosyncrasies should not, and do not, detract from the many Nightingale precepts that are not only pertinent today but remarkably far-sighted.

EARLY LIFE

Florence Nightingale was born on May 12, 1820, in Florence, Italy, during her English parents' travels there. She was named for the city in which she was born, as was her older sister, Parthenope, who was born in 1819 in Naples (known in ancient times by the Greek name Parthenope).

The family was wealthy and well educated, with a high social standing and influential friends, all of which would be useful to Nightingale later. Primarily under her father's tutelage, she learned Greek, Latin, French, German, and Italian, and studied history, philosophy, science, music, art, and classical literature. She traveled widely with her family and friends. The breadth of her education, almost unheard of for women of the times, was also considerably more extensive than that of most men, including physicians. Her intelligence and education were recognized by scholars, as indicated in her correspondence with them.

Nightingale was not only bright, but, according to early portraits and descriptions, slender, attractive, and fun-loving, enjoying the social life of her class. She differed from other young women in her determination to do something "toward lifting the load of suffering from the helpless and miserable."[3] Later she said that she had been called by God into His service on four separate occasions, beginning when she was seventeen. This strong religious commitment remained with her, although she had increasingly little patience with organized religion or with traditional biblical exhortations. At one point she stated, "God's scheme for us was not that He should give us what we asked for, but that mankind should obtain it for mankind."[4] Apparently, the encouragement of Dr. Samuel Gridley Howe and his wife, Julia Ward Howe (who wrote "The Battle Hymn of the Republic"), during a visit to the Nightingale family home in 1844 helped to crystallize Florence's interest in hospitals and nursing. Nevertheless, her intent to train in a hospital was strongly opposed by her family, and she limited herself to nursing family members. There is some indication that this was the genesis of her firm belief that nursing required more than kindness and cold compresses.

Later, in *Notes on Nursing*, she wrote, "It has been said and written scores of times that every woman makes a good nurse. I believe, on the contrary, that the very elements of nursing are all but unknown."[5] At the same time, she added a few tart remarks about the need for education.

> It seems a commonly received idea among men and even some women themselves that it requires nothing but a disappointment in love, the want of an object, a general disgust, or incapacity for other things to turn a woman into a good nurse. This reminds one of the parish where a stupid old man was set to be schoolmaster because he was 'past keeping the pigs.' . . . The everyday management of a large ward, let alone of a hospital—the knowing what are the laws of life and death for men,

and what the laws of health for wards (and wards are healthy or unhealthy, mainly according to the knowledge or ignorance of the nurse)—are not these matters of sufficient importance and difficulty to require learning by experience and careful inquiry, just as much as any other art? They do not come by inspiration to the lady disappointed in love, nor to the poor workhouse drudge hard up for a livelihood.[6]

Although remaining the obedient daughter, Nightingale found her own way to expand her knowledge of sick care. She studied hospital and sanitary reports and books on public health. Having received information on Kaiserswerth in Germany, she determined to receive training there—more acceptable because of its religious auspices. On one of her trips to the Continent, she made a brief visit and was impressed enough to spend three months in training and observation there in 1851 while her mother and sister went to Carlsbad to "take the cure." (The Nightingales were considered appropriately delicate Victorian ladies, although all lived past eighty.) At the time she wrote positively about Pastor Fliedner's program, but she later described the nursing as "nil" and the hygiene as "horrible."[7] Her later effort to study with the Sisters of Charity in Paris was frustrated, although she got permission to inspect the hospitals there, as she had in other cities during her tours. She examined the general layout of the hospital, as well as ward construction, sanitation, general administration, and the work of the surgeons and physicians. Apparently, these observational techniques and her analytical abilities then and later were the basis of her unrivaled knowledge of hospitals in the next decade. Few of her contemporaries ever had such knowledge.

In 1853 Nightingale assumed the position of superintendent of a charity hospital (probably more of a nursing home) for ill governesses run by titled ladies. Although she had difficulties with her intolerant governing board, she did make changes considered revolutionary

for the day and, even with the lack of trained nurses, improved the patients' care. And she continued to visit hospitals. Just as Nightingale was negotiating for a superintendency in the newly reorganized and rebuilt King's College Hospital in London, England and France, in support of Turkey, declared war on Russia in March 1854.

CRIMEA—THE TURNING POINT

The Crimean War was a low point for England. Ill-prepared and disorganized in general, the army and the bureaucracy were even less prepared to care for the thousands of soldiers both wounded in battle and prostrated by the cholera epidemics brought on by less than primitive conditions. Not even the most basic equipment or drugs were available, and, as casualties mounted, Turkey turned over the enormous but bare and filthy barracks at Scutari across from Constantinople to be used as a hospital. The conditions remained abominable. The soldiers lay on the floor in filth, untended, frequently without food or water because there was no equipment to prepare or distribute either. Rats and other vermin came from the sewers underneath the building. There were no beds, furniture, basins, soap, towels, or eating utensils, and few provisions. There were only orderlies, and none of these at night. The death rate was said to be 60 percent.

In previous wars, the situation had not been much different, and there was little interest on the battle sites, for ordinary soldiers were accorded no decencies. But now, for the first time, civilian war correspondents were present and sent back the news of these horrors to an England with a newly aroused social conscience. The reformers were in an uproar; newspapers demanded to know why England did not have nurses like the French Sisters of Charity to care for its soldiers, and Parliament trembled. In October 1854, Sidney Herbert, Secretary of War and an old friend of Florence Nightingale, wrote begging her to lead a group of nurses to the Crimea under government authority and expense. "There is but one person in England that I know of who would be capable of organizing such a scheme . . . your own personal qualities, your knowledge, and your power of administration, and, among greater things, your rank and position in society give you advantages in such work which no other person possesses."[8] Nightingale had already decided to offer her services, and the two letters crossed. In less than a week, she had assembled thirty-eight nurses, the most she could find that met her standards—Roman Catholic and Anglican sisters and lay nurses from various hospitals—and embarked for Scutari.

Even under the miserable circumstances found there, Nightingale and her contingent were not welcomed by the army doctors and surgeons. Dr. John Hall, chief of the medical staff, and his staff, although privately acknowledging the horrors of the situation, resented outside interference and refused the nurses' services. Hall and Nightingale soon developed a mutual hatred for each other. When Dr. Hall was honored with the KCB—Knight Commander of the Order of the Bath—she referred to him as "Knight of the Crimean Burial Grounds."[9]

Nightingale chose to wait to be asked to help. To the anger of her nurses, she allowed none of them to give care until one week later, when scurvy, starvation, dysentery, exposure, and more fighting almost brought about the collapse of the British army. Then the doctors, desperate for any kind of assistance, turned to the eager nurses.

Modern criticisms of Florence Nightingale frequently refer to her insistence on the physician's overall authority and her own authoritarian approach to nursing. The first criticism may have originated with her situation in the Crimean War. In mid-century England her appointment created a furor; she was the first woman ever to be given such authority. Yet, despite the high-sounding title that Herbert insisted she have—General Superintendent of the Female Nursing Establishment of the Mili-

tary Hospitals of the Army—her orders required that she have the approval of the Principal Medical Officer "in her exercise of the responsibilities thus vested in her. The Principal Medical Officer will communicate with Miss Nightingale upon all subjects connected with the Female Nursing Establishment, and will give his directions through that lady."[10] Although no "lady, sister, or nurse" could be transferred from one hospital to another without her approval, she had no authority over anyone else, even orderlies and cooks. What she accomplished had to be done through sheer force of will or persuasion. Her overt deference to physicians was probably the beginning of the doctor-nurse game.

Whatever the limitations of her power, Florence Nightingale literally accomplished miracles at Scutari. Even in the "waiting" week, she moved into the kitchen area and began to cook extras from her own supplies to create a diet kitchen, which for five months was the only source of food for the sick. Later, a famous chef came to the Crimea at his own expense and totally reorganized and improved military cooking. Nightingale managed to equip the kitchen and the wards by various means. One report is that when a physician refused to unlock a supply storehouse, she replied, "Well, I would like to have the door opened, or I shall send men to break it down."[11] It was opened, and he was recalled to London.

Miss Nightingale had powerful friends and control over a large amount of contributed funds—a situation that gained her some cooperation from most physicians after a while. Through persuasion and the use of good managerial techniques, she cleaned up the hospital; the orderlies scrubbed and emptied slops regularly; solders' wives and camp followers washed clothes; and the vermin were brought under some control. (Wrote Nightingale to Sidney Herbert, "the vermin might, if they had but unity of purpose, carry off the four miles of beds on their backs and march them into the War Office.")[12] Before the end of the war, the mortality rate at Scutari declined to 1 percent. When the hospital care improved, Nightingale began a program of social welfare among the soldiers—among other things, seeing to it that they got sick pay. The patients adored her. She cared about them, and the doctors and officers reproached her for "spoiling the brutes." The soldiers wrote home, "What a comfort it was to see her pass even; she would speak to one and nod and smile to as many more, but she could not do it all, you know. We lay there by hundreds, but we could kiss her shadow as it fell, and lay our heads on the pillow again content." And, "Before she came, there was cussin' and swearin', but after that it was holy as a church." And, "She was all full of life and fun when she talked to us, especially if a man was a bit downhearted."[13] News correspondents wrote reports about the "ministering angel" and "lady with the lamp" making late rounds after the medical officers had retired—which inspired Longfellow later to write his famous poem "Santa Filomena." England and America were enthralled, and she was awarded decorations by Queen Victoria and the Sultan of Turkey.

But all did not go well. The military doctors continued in their resentment and tried to undermine her. There were problems in her own ranks, dissension among the religious and secular nurses, and problems of incompetence and immorality. Later, she wrote:

> Rebellion among some ladies and some nuns, and drunkenness among some nurses unhappily disgraced our body; minor faults justified *pro tanto* the common opinion that the vanity, the gossip, and the insubordination (which none more despise than those who trade upon them) of women make them unfit for, and mischievous in the Service, however materially useful they may be in it.[14]

Her problems increased with the unsolicited arrival of another group of nurses under another woman's leadership, although the problem was eventually resolved. No doubt Night-

ingale was high-handed at times, and despite praise of her leadership, she was also called "quick, violent-tempered, positive, obstinate, and stubborn."[15]

Certainly she drove herself in all she did. When the situation at Scutari was improved, she crossed the Black Sea to the battle sites and worked on the reorganization of the few hospitals there—with no better support from physicians and superior officers. There she contracted Crimean fever (probably typhoid or typhus) and nearly died. However, she refused a leave of absence to recuperate and stayed in Scutari to work until the end of the war. She had supervised 125 nurses and forced the military to recognize the place of nurses.

From her experiences, and to support her recommendations for reform, Nightingale wrote a massive report entitled *Notes on Matters Affecting the Health, Efficiency, and Hospital Administration of the British Army*, crammed with facts, figures, and statistical comparison. On the basis of this and her later well-researched and well-documented papers, she is often credited with being the first nurse researcher. Reforms were slow in coming but extended even to the United States when the Union consulted her about organizing hospitals. In 1859 she wrote a small book, *Notes on Nursing: What It Is and What It Is Not*, intended for the average housewife and printed cheaply so that it would be affordable. These and other Nightingale papers are still amazingly readable today—brisk, down-to-earth, and laced with many a pithy comment. For instance, in *Notes on Hospitals*, written in the same year, she compared the administration of the various types of hospitals and characterized the management of secular hospitals under the sole command of the male hospital authorities as "all but crazy." And her words were prophetic: "If we were perfect, no doubt an absolute hierarchy would be the best kind of government for all institutions. But, in our imperfect state of conscience and enlightenment, publicity, and the collision resulting from publicity are the best guardians of the interests of the sick."[16]

Her knowledge was certainly respected, and she was consulted by many, including the Royal Sanitary Commission on the Health of the Army in India. When asked by the members of the commission what hospitals she had visited, she listed those in England, Turkey, France, Germany, Belgium, Italy, and Egypt, including all hospitals in some cities, and even Russian military hospitals. Her reforms in India extended beyond the medical and nursing facilities to raising the sanitary level of India. Again, her insights were uncanny. In describing the proper method of analyzing the problem of sanitation and disease, she also suggested checking on "unwholesome trades fouling the water."

What is particularly astonishing is that all of this was done from her own quarters. On her return from the Crimea, she took to her bed or at least to her rooms and emerged only on rare occasions. There is much speculation on this illness—whether it was a result of the Crimea fever, neurasthenia, or a bit of both, or whether she simply found it useful to avoid wasting time with people she did not want to see. For she was famous now and had been

---

Duties of Probationer under the "Nightingale Fund." St. Thomas's Hospital, 1860.

You are required to be

Sober.	Punctual.
Honest.	Quiet and Orderly.
Truthful.	Cleanly and Neat.
Trustworthy.	Patient, Cheerful, and Kindly.

You are expected to become skillfull

1. In the dressing of blisters, burns, sores, wounds and in applying fomentations, poultices, and minor dressings.
2. In the application of leeches, externally and internally.
3. In the administration of enemas for men and women.
4. In the management of trusses, and appliances in uterine complaints.
5. In the best method of friction to the body and extremities.
6. In the management of helpless patients, i.e., moving, changing, personal cleanliness of, feeding, keeping warm, (or cool), preventing and dressing bed sores, managing position of.
7. In bandaging, making bandages, and rollers, lining of splints, etc.
8. In making the beds of the patients, and removal of sheets whilst patient is in bed.
9. You are required to attend at operations.
10. To be competent to cook gruel, arrowroot, egg flip, puddings, drinks, for the sick.
11. To understand ventilation, or keeping the ward fresh by night as well as by day; you are to be careful that great cleanliness is observed in all the utensils; those used for secretions as well as those required for cooking.
12. To make strict observation of the sick in the following particulars: The state of secretions, expectoration, pulse, skin, appetite; intelligence, as delirium or stupor; breathing, sleep, state of wounds, eruptions, formation of matter, effect of diet, or of stimulants, and of medicines.
13. And to learn the management of convalescents.

given discretion over the so-called Nightingale Fund, to which almost everyone in England had subscribed, including many of the troops.

THE NIGHTINGALE NURSE

In 1860, Nightingale utilized some of the 45,000 pounds of the Nightingale Fund to establish a training school for nurses. She selected St. Thomas's Hospital because of her respect for its matron, Mrs. S. E. Wardroper. The two converted the resident medical officers to their plan, although apparently most other physicians objected to the school. The students were chosen, and the first class in the desired age range of twenty-five to thirty-five years and with impeccable character references numbered only fifteen. It was to be a one-year training program, and the students were presented with what could be called terminal behavioral objectives that they had to reach satisfactorily. Students could be dismissed by the matron for misconduct, inefficiency, or negligence. However, if they passed the courses of instruction and training satisfactorily, they were entered in the "Register" as certified nurses. The Committee of the Nightingale Fund then recommended them for employment; in the early years, they were obligated to work as hospital nurses for at least five years (for which they were paid).

The students' time was carefully structured, beginning at six in the morning and ending with a nine o'clock bedtime, which included a semimandatory two-hour exercise period (walking abroad must be done in twos and threes, not alone). Within that time there was actually about a nine-hour work and training day (a vast difference from future American schools). This included bedside teaching by a teaching sister or the Resident Medical Officer and elementary instruction in "Chemistry, with reference to air, water, food, etc.; Physiology, with reference to a knowledge of the leading functions of the body, and general instruction on medical and surgical topics,"[17] by professors of the medical school attached to

St. Thomas's, given voluntarily and without remuneration. The keys to the Nightingale school were that it was not under the control of the hospital and had education as its purpose. The Nightingale Fund paid the medical officers, head nurses, and matron for teaching students, beyond whatever they earned from the hospital in their other duties. Both the head nurses and matron kept records on each student, evaluating how she met the stated objectives of the program. The students were expected to keep notes from the lectures and records of patient observation and care, all of which were checked by the nurse-teachers. At King's College Hospital, run by the Society of St. John's House, an Anglican religious community, midwifery was taught in similar style and with similar regulations, again under the auspices of the Nightingale Fund Committee. And, at the Royal Liverpool Infirmary, nurses were trained for home nursing of the sick poor under a Nightingale protocol but were personally funded by a Liverpool merchant-philanthropist. As Nightingale said in 1863, "We have had to introduce an entirely new system to which the older systems of nursing bear but slight resemblance. . . . It exists neither in Scotland nor in Ireland at the present time."[18]

The demand for the Nightingale nurses was overwhelming. In the next few years, requests also came for them to improve the workhouse (poorhouse) infirmaries and to reform both civilian and military nursing in India. In response to these demands, Nightingale wrote many reports, detailing to the last item the system for educating these nurses and for improving patient care, including such points as general hygiene and sanitation, nutrition, equipment, supplies, and the nurses' housing conditions, holidays, salaries, and retirement benefits. (For India, she suggested that they had better pay good salaries and provide satisfactory working and living conditions, or the nurses might opt for marriage, because the opportunities there were even greater than in England.) She constantly reiterated that she could not supply enough nurses but, when possible, she would send a matron and some other nurses, who would train new Nightingale nurses. She warned that one or two could not change the old patterns. "Good nursing does not grow of itself; it is the result of study, teaching, training, practice, ending in sound tradition which can be transferred elsewhere."[19]

Although Nightingale never headed a school herself, she selected the students and observed their progress carefully; with some she carried on correspondence for years. One of her favorites, Agnes Jones, was recommended to reform nursing at the Liverpool Workhouse Infirmary, which, with twelve other nurses, she did admirably, proving to the economy-minded governor that this kind of nursing also saved money. Nightingale often said that conditions there were as bad as those at Scutari; and indeed her young protégé died of typhus there. Nevertheless, reform of this pesthole showed England an example of what nursing care could be.

Despite her reputation and her personal acquaintance with Queen Victoria, her cabinet, and every prime minister during this time, Nightingale and her ideas ran into opposition. Although some doctors who understood what this new nurse could do were supporters, the idea of the nurse as a professional was not commonly accepted. Said one physician, "A nurse is a confidential servant, but still only a servant. . . . She should be middle-aged when she begins nursing, and if somewhat tamed by marriage and the troubles of a family, so much the better."[20] Maintaining standards was a constant struggle; even St. Thomas's Hospital slipped, and Nightingale, who had been immersed in the Indian reforms, had to take time to reorganize the program. What evolved over the years, from the first program, was one of preparation for two kinds of nursing practitioners: the educated middle- and upper-class ladies who paid their own tuition, and the still carefully selected poor women who were subsidized by the Nightingale Fund. The first were given an extra year or two of education to prepare them to become teachers or superintendents; a third choice was district nursing. "This nurse must be of a yet higher class and of a yet fuller training than a hospital nurse, because she has not the doctor always at hand and because she has no hospital appliances at hand."[21] The special probationers were expected to enter the profession permanently. The second group were prepared to be the hospital ward nurses.

In Nightingale's later years, she came into conflict with the very nurses who had been trained for leadership. In 1886, some of these nurses, now superintendents of other training schools, wanted to establish an organization that would provide a central examination and registration center, the forerunner of licensure. Nightingale opposed this movement for several reasons: nursing was still too young and disorganized; national criteria would not be as high as those of individual schools; and the all-important aspect of "character" could not be tested. She fought the concept with every weapon at her disposal, including her powerful contacts, and succeeded in limiting the fledgling Royal British Nurses' Association to maintaining a "list" instead of a "register." (Nurse licensure came to South Africa before it came to England.) Nevertheless, it was a beginning and, although she was probably right about the standards, recognition of nurses was facilitated with the setting of national standards, however minimal.

Nightingale's prolific writings on nursing have survived, and some of them are still surprisingly apt. Often they reflected her concern about the character of nurses and her own determination that their main focus be on nursing. For instance, in her early writings on hospitals (before the Nightingale schools), she reluctantly conceded that the nurse would have to be permitted visitors on her time off, distracting though that might be, and that spying on the nurse when she went out in her limited free time, although it had some advantages, was "no blessing in the long run and degrading to all concerned." Yet, nurses were to be held strictly to rules that limited their outside excursions to their exercise period, and it was preferred that they live adjacent to the patient wards. Nightingale's views moderated over the years, but her emphasis on morality and other personal qualities never wavered.

It was a time when salaries were low and petty thievery was common, and an accepted, desirable fringe benefit of a job (also recommended by Nightingale for nurses) was a daily allowance of beer, or even wine and brandy. But a Nightingale nurse who was found to be dishonest and drunken was dismissed instantly and permanently.

One principle from which Nightingale did not swerve was that nurses were to nurse, not to do heavy cleaning ("if you want a charwoman, hire one"); not to do laundry ("it makes their hands coarse and hard and less able to attend to the delicate manipulation which they may be called on to execute"); and not to fetch ("to save the time of nurses; all diets and ward requisites should be brought into the wards"). Then, as in many places

now, status and promotion came through assumption of administrative roles, but Nightingale recognized that "many are valuable as nurses, who are yet unfit for promotion to head nurses." Her alternative, however, would not be greeted favorably today—a raise after ten years of good service!

Nightingale also commented on other issues considered pertinent today. Continuing education was a must, for she saw nursing as a progressive art, in which to stand still was to go back. "A woman who thinks of herself, 'Now I am a full nurse, a skilled nurse. I have learnt all there is to be learned,' take my word for it, she does not know what a nurse is, and she will never know: she has gone back already."[22] Although there is no evidence that she took any action to help end discrimination against women, Nightingale believed that women should be accepted into all the professions, but she warned them, "qualify yourselves for it as a man does for his work." She

---

What a Nurse Is to Be

A really good nurse must needs be of the highest class of character. It need hardly be said that she must be—(1) Chaste, in the sense of the Sermon on the Mount; a good nurse should be the Sermon on the Mount in herself. It should naturally seem impossible to the most unchaste to utter even an immodest jest in her presence. Remember this great and dangerous peculiarity of nursing, and especially of hospital nursing, namely, that it is the only case, queens not excepted, where a woman is really in charge of men. And a really good trained ward "sister" can keep order in a men's ward better than a military ward-master or sergeant. (2) Sober, in spirit as well as in drink, and temperate in all things. (3) Honest, not accepting the most trifling fee or bribe from patients or friends. (4) Truthful—and to be able to tell the truth includes attention and observation, to observe truly—memory, to remember truly—power of expression, to tell truly what one has observed truly—as well as intention to speak the truth, the whole truth, and nothing but the truth. (5) Trustworthy, to carry out directions intelligently and perfectly, unseen as well as seen, "to the Lord" as well as unto men—no mere eye-service. (6) Punctual to a second and orderly to a hair—having everything ready and in order before she begins her dressings or her work about the patient; nothing forgotten. (7) Quiet, yet quick, quick without hurry; gentle without slowness; discreet without self-importance; no gossip. (8) Cheerful, hopeful; not allowing herself to be discouraged by unfavourable symptoms; not given to depress the patient by anticipations of an unfavourable result. (9) Cleanly to the point of exquisiteness, both for the patient's sake and her own; neat and ready. (10) Thinking of her patient and not of herself, "tender over his occasions" or wants, cheerful and kindly, patient, ingenious and feat.

Source: From a Nightingale article on "Nurses, Training of, and Nursing the Sick," in *A Dictionary of Medicine,* edited by Sir Robert Quain, Bart., M.D., 1882.

believed that women should be paid as highly as men, but that equal pay meant equal responsibility. In a profession with as much responsibility as nursing, it was particularly important to have adequate compensation, or intelligent, independent women would not be attracted to it. Until the end, she was firm on the need for nurses to obey physicians in medical matters; however, she stressed the importance of nurse observation and reporting because the physician was not constantly at the patient's bedside, as the nurse was. She was adamant that a nurse (and woman) be in charge of nursing, with no other administrative figure having authority over nurses, including physicians. She knew the importance of a work setting that gave job satisfaction. In words that are a far-off echo of nurses' plaints today, she wrote:

> Besides, a thing very little understood, a good nurse has her professional pride in results of her Nursing quite as much as a Medical Officer in the results of his treatment. There are defective buildings, defective administrations, defective appliances, which make all good Nursing impossible. A good Nurse does not like to waste herself, and the better the Nurse, the stronger this feeling in her. Humanity may overrule this feeling in a great emergency like a cholera outbreak; but I don't believe that it is in human nature for a good Nurse to bear up, with an ever-recurring, ever-useless expenditure of activity, against the circumstances which make her nursing activity useless, or all but useless. Her work becomes slovenly like the rest, and it is a far greater pity to have a nurse wasting herself in this way than it would be to have a steam engine running up and down the line all day without a train, wasting coals.
>
> Perhaps I need scarcely add that Nurses must be paid the market price for their labor, like any other worker; and that this is yearly rising.[23]

Obviously, Nightingale is eminently quotable, in matters of health care and nursing today, in part because she was so far ahead of her time, and in part, unfortunately, because the errors of omission and commission in the field have a tendency to reappear or remain uncorrected.

Planner, administrator, educator, researcher, reformer, Florence Nightingale never lost her interest in nursing. As nearly as can be determined, her actual clinical nursing was limited to her early care of sick families, the short period at Kaiserswerth, a briefer interim of caring for victims of a cholera epidemic before the war, and then, of course, her experience in the Crimea. Yet, her perception of patients' needs was uncanny for the time and frequently is still applicable today. In her *Notes on Nursing*, not only is there careful consideration of "Observation of the Sick" and crisp comments on "Minding Baby," but also pertinent directions on hygiene, nutrition, environment, and the mental state of the patient. At age seventy-four, in her last major work on nursing, she differentiated between sick nursing and health nursing, and emphasized the primary need for prevention of illness, for which a lay "Health Missioner" (today's health educator?) would be trained.

When Nightingale died on August 13, 1910, she was to be honored by burial in Westminster Abbey. However, she had chosen instead to be buried in the family plot in Hampshire, with a simple inscription: "F.N. Born 1820, Died 1910."

REFERENCES

1. Evelyn R. Barritt, "Florence Nightingale's Values and Modern Nursing Education," *Nursing Forum,* **12**,4:10(1973).
2. Ibid., p. 34.
3. Vern Bullough and Bonnie Bullough, *The Care of the Sick: The Emergence of Modern Nursing* (New York: Prodist, 1978), p. 86.
4. Barritt, op. cit.
5. Lucy Ridgely Seymer, *Selected Writings of Florence Nightingale* (New York: Macmillan Publishing Co., Inc., 1954) p. 124.
6. Ibid., pp. 214–15.
7. Bullough, op. cit., p. 86.
8. Josephine A. Dolan, *Nursing in Society:*

A Historical Perspective, 14th ed. (Philadelphia: W. B. Saunders Company, 1978) p. 159.

9. Philip Kalisch and Beatrice Kalisch, *The Advance of American Nursing* (Boston: Little, Brown and Company, 1978), p. 37.
10. Seymer, op. cit., p. 28.
11. Dolan, op. cit., p. 161.
12. Kalisch and Kalisch, op. cit., p. 37.
13. Kalisch and Kalisch, op. cit., p. 39.
14. Seymer, op. cit., p. 28.
15. Barritt, op. cit., p. 8.
16. Seymer, op. cit., pp. 222–223.
17. Seymer, op. cit., p. 244.
18. Ibid., p. 234.
19. Ibid., p. 229.
20. Dolan, op. cit., p. 169.
21. Seymer, op. cit., p. 316.
22. Agnes E. Pavey, *The Story of the Growth of Nursing* (London: Farber & Farber, Ltd., 1938), p. 296.
23. Seymer, op. cit., p. 276.

NURSING IN THE UNITED STATES

3

The Evolution of the Trained Nurse, 1873–1903

Nursing in the United States between the American Revolution and the Civil War was probably no better or worse than that in Europe. As noted in Chapter 1, nurses from both Catholic and Protestant nursing orders came to America, and their nursing care, although semitrained, was the best offered. But there were not enough of them. Even given the occasional compassionate lady who might have ventured into hospitals to help with care in an epidemic or other emergency, the quality of lay nurses was probably about the same as that in England.

Early hospitals, privately managed and funded by endowments or public subscription, were modeled after those in Europe, with no improvement in quality; the mentally ill were confined in insane asylums or poorhouses and prisons.

Yet, by the time of the Civil War, social reforms had also reached America. One of the key figures was Dorothea Lynde Dix (1802–1887), a gentle New England schoolteacher, who became interested in the conditions under which the mentally ill existed when she went to teach a Sunday school lesson in a jail. She began to survey the needs of those forgotten people, and her descriptive reports and careful documentation eventually resulted in the construction of state psychiatric institutions (the first in Trenton, New Jersey) and the lessening of inhumane care, even if no improvement in the understanding of the illnesses.

THE CIVIL WAR

When the Civil War began in April 1861, there was no organized system to care for the sick and wounded. There never had been. In the American Revolution, for instance, such basic care as existed was given by camp followers, a few wives, women in the neighborhood, and "surgeons' mates." It is possible that some of these women were employed by the army, for there are female names on the payroll lists as "nursing the sick."[1]

American women, considered by American men to be just as delicate and proper and unsuited for unpleasant service as their European counterparts, nevertheless rushed to volunteer. Within a few weeks, 100 women were given a short training course by physicians and surgeons in New York City, and Dorothea Dix, well known by then, was appointed by the Secretary of War to superintend these new "nurses." Meanwhile, members of religious orders also volunteered, and nursing in some of the larger government hospitals was eventually assigned to them because of the inexperience of the lay volunteers.[2]

Except for that group, almost none of the several thousand women who served as nurses during the war had any kind of training or hospital experience. They can be categorized as follows:

1. The nurses appointed by Miss Dix or other officials as legal employees of the army for forty cents and one ration a day.
2. The sisters or nuns of the various orders.
3. Those employed for short periods of time for menial chores.
4. Black women employed under general orders of the War Department for $10 a month.
5. Uncompensated volunteers.
6. Women camp followers.
7. Women employed by the various relief organizations.[3]

It is estimated that some 6,000 women performed nursing duties for the Northern armies. The South used only about 1,000 because of the attitude that prevailed for some time that caring for men was unfit for Southern ladies. (Nevertheless, a number of these ladies, such as Kate Cummings, who recorded her experiences, gave distinguished service under severe conditions in Southern hospitals.)[4]

U.S. Army medical officers were no more pleased with the presence of females in their domain than were the British in the Crimea. It was not that Miss Dix didn't try for the serious-minded; her recruiting specified only plain-looking women over thirty-five who wore gray, brown, or black dresses with no bows, curls, jewelry, or hoop skirts, and who were moral and had common sense. Presumably, those who did not qualify were among the many unofficial and unpaid volunteers. Some of the information on what the Civil War nurses did comes from the writings of Louisa May Alcott and Walt Whitman, both volunteers. In her journal, Alcott described her working day, which began at six. After opening the windows, because of the bad air

in the makeshift base hospital, she was "giving out rations, cutting up food for helpless boys, washing faces, teaching my attendants how beds are made or floors are swept, dressing wounds, dusting tables, sewing bandages, keeping my tray tidy, rushing up and down after pillows, bed linens, sponges, and directions. . . ."[5] Volunteers also read to the patients, wrote letters, and comforted them. Apparently, even the hired nurses did little more except, perhaps, give medicines. But so did the volunteers, sometimes giving the medicine and food of their choice to the patient, instead of what the doctor ordered.

By 1862, enormous military hospitals, some with as many as 3,000 beds, were being built, although there were still some makeshift hospitals, former hotels, churches, factories, and almost anything else available. There was even a hospital ship, the *Red Rover*, a former Mississippi steamer captured from the Confederates and staffed by nuns. Other floating hospitals were inaugurated and served as transport units, with nurses attending the wounded.[6] Discipline in the hospitals was rigid for nurses and patients alike, with the latter given strict orders to be respectful to the nurses. According to one Army hospital edict, the nurses, under the supervision of the "Stewards and Chief Wardmaster," were responsible for the administration of the wards, but many of their duties appeared to be related more to keeping the nonmedical records of patients and reporting their misbehavior than to nursing care. If the patient needed medical or surgical attendance, the doctor was to be called.[7]

Georgeanna Woolsey wrote that the surgeons treated the nurses without even common courtesy because they did not want them and tried to make their lives so unbearable that they would leave. The surgeons were often incompetent. As a temporary expedient, contract surgeons were employed with no position, little pay, and only minimal rank. Jane, another Woolsey sister who was also a volunteer nurse, wrote that although some were highly skilled, "faithful, sagacious, tenderhearted,'' others were drunken, refused to attend the wounded, or injured them more because of their incompetence.[8]

It was surgeons and officers of the latter type that the formidable nurse Mary Ann (Mother) Bickerdyke attacked. She managed to have a number of them dismissed (in part because of her friendship with General Grant and General Sherman). About this tough "Soldier's Friend," one physician stated, "Woe to the surgeon, the commissary, or quartermaster whose neglect of his men and selfish disregard for their interests and needs come under her cognizance."[9]

Another fighter was Clara Barton, who early in the war cared for the wounded of the Sixth Massachusetts Regiment. One story told about her is that while supervising the delivery of a wagonload of supplies for soldiers, she neatly extricated an ox from a herd intended for the Army, so that the wounded would have food.[10]

Only in recent years has attention been given to the black nurses of the Civil War. Harriet Tubman, the "Moses of her people," not only led many black slaves to freedom in her underground railroad activities before the war but also nursed the wounded when she joined the Union Army. Similarly, Sojourner Truth, abolitionist speaker and activist in the women's movement, also cared for the sick and wounded. Susie King Taylor, born to slavery and secretly taught to read and write, met and married a Union soldier and served as a battlefront nurse for more than four years, although she received no salary or pension from the Union Army.[11]

There were other heroines, untrained women from the North and South, caring for the sick and wounded with a modicum of skills but much kindness, and, as in the Crimea, the soldiers were sentimentally appreciative, if not discriminating.

Even when paid, Civil War nurses had little status and no rank. One exception was Sally Tomkins, a civic-minded Southern woman, who efficiently took charge of a makeshift hospital and was made a captain of the cav-

alry by Confederate President Jefferson Davis so that she could continue her work. An investigative report by the United States Sanitary Commission noted that nurses had not been well treated or wisely used.

> They have not been placed, as they expected and were fitted to be, in the position of head nurses. On the contrary, with a very inefficient force of male nurses, they have been called on to do every form of service, have been overtaxed and worn down with menial and purely mechanical duties, additional to the more responsible offices and duties of nursing.[12]

Nevertheless, the Civil War opened hospitals to massive numbers of women, well-bred "ladies," who would otherwise probably not even have thought of nursing. Some of these, such as Abby, Jane, and Georgeanna Woolsey, later helped lead the movement to establish training schools for nurses.

THE EARLY TRAINING SCHOOLS

The nursing role of women in the Civil War, however unsophisticated, and probably the fame of Florence Nightingale brought to the attention of the American public the need for nurses and the desirability of some organized programs of training. There had been previous elementary efforts in this direction; an organized school of nursing, founded in 1839 by the Nurse Society of Philadelphia under Dr. Joseph Warrington, awarded a certificate after a stated period of lectures, demonstrations, and experience at a hospital; a school of nursing for a "better type" of woman connected with the Women's Hospital in Philadelphia in 1861 gave a diploma after six months of lectures.

More physicians became interested in the training of nurses and, at a meeting of the American Medical Association in 1869, a committee to study the matter stated that it was "just as necessary to have well-trained, well-instructed nurses as to have intelligent and skillful physicians." The committee recommended that nursing schools be placed under the guardianship of county medical societies, although under the immediate supervision of lady superintendents; that every lay hospital should have a school; and that nurses be trained not only for the hospital but for private duty in the home.[13]

In 1871, the editor of *Godey's Lady's Book*, the most popular woman's magazine of the time, wrote an editorial on "Lady Nurses" that was remarkably farsighted.

> Much has been lately said of the benefits that would follow if the calling of sick nurse were elevated to a profession which an educated lady might adopt without a sense of degradation, either on her own part or in the estimation of others. . . .
>
> There can be no doubt that the duties of sick nurse, to be properly performed, require an education and training little, if at all, inferior to those possessed by members of the medical profession. . . . The manner in which a reform may be effected is easily pointed out. Every medical college should have a course of study and training especially adapted for ladies who desire to qualify themselves for the profession of nurse; and those who had gone through the course, and passed the requisite examination, should receive a degree and a diploma, which would at once establish their position in society. The graduate nurse would in general estimation be as much above the ordinary nurse of the present day as the professional surgeon of our times is above the barber-surgeon of the last century.[14]

Unfortunately, this idea of an educated nurse with professional status was a long time in coming.

Nevertheless, in 1892, the New England Hospital for Women and Children, staffed by women physicians who were interested in the development of a school, acted upon a statement in its bylaws of 1863 "to train nurses for the care of the sick." It was a one-year program in which the students provided round-the-clock service for patients; there was no classwork (although a few lectures were given

during the winter months), and the duty extended from 5:30 A.M. to 9 P.M., with a free afternoon every second week from 2 to 5 P.M. At the end of the year, one student graduated—Melinda Ann (Linda) Richards, thereafter called America's first trained nurse, probably because of all of the nurses who graduated from this primitive early program, she moved on to be a key figure in the development of nursing education. Richards, like some of the other students in the schools that evolved, had been a nurse in a hospital, although some schools would not accept them because they wanted to set a new image. This indicates that despite the frequent descriptions of criminal and thieving women who nursed, some nurses, although untrained in the later sense, must have been at least respectable, intelligent women.

Another outstanding graduate of the New England Hospital for Women and Children (1879) ws Mary Mahoney, the first trained black nurse. A tiny, dynamic, charming woman, she worked primarily in private duty in the Boston area but was apparently always present at national nurses' meetings. In her honor, the Mary Mahoney Medal was initiated by the National Association of Colored Graduate Nurses, and the award was later continued by the American Nurses' Association.

In 1873, three schools supposedly based on the Nightingale model were established.[15] The Bellevue Training School in New York City was founded through the influence of several society ladies who had been involved in Civil War nursing, including Abby Woolsey. Appalled by the conditions—900 patients, 3 to 5 occupying strapped-together beds, tended by ex-convict nurses and night watchmen who stole their food and left them in filth—these women sent a young physician to England to confer with Nightingale. Then they raised funds to set up a nurses' training class for which they were given six wards. The hospital agreed to place these students under the direction of a female superintendent, provided that they also did the scouring and cleaning that had been done by the other ''nurses''; they would not hire anyone to clean. Although the school attempted to follow Nightingale principles and reported that it was attracting educated women, its overall purpose was to improve conditions in a great charity hospital, and much of the learning was on a trial-and-error basis. Nevertheless, Bellevue had a lot of interesting firsts: interdisciplinary rounds where nurses reported on the nursing plan of care; patient record keeping and writing of orders, initiated by Linda Richards, who became night superintendent; and the first uniform, by stylish and aristocratic Euphemia Van Rensselaer, which started a trend. And of course, two of nursing's greatest leaders were Bellevue graduates—Lavinia Dock and Isabel Hampton Robb.

The Connecticut Training School was started through the influence of another Woolsey, Georgeanna, and her husband, Dr. Francis Bacon. Through negotiation with the hospital, the superintendent of nurses was designated as separate from, and not responsible to, the steward (administrator) of the hospital, and teaching outside the wards was permitted. However, the threatened steward managed to make life so miserable for a series of superintendents that each resigned; but control remained with nursing. Meanwhile, all good intentions notwithstanding, the students soon were sent to give care in the homes of sick families, with the money going to the School Fund—and the school could boast that for thirty-three years it was not financed or directed by the hospital.

The Boston Training School was the last of that first famous triumvirate. Again, a group of women associated with other educational and philanthropic endeavors spearheaded its organization, but this time to offer a desirable occupation for self-supporting women and to provide good private nurses for the community. After prolonged negotiations that allowed the director of the school, instead of the hospital, to maintain control, the Massachusetts General Hospital assigned ''The Brick''

building to the school because it (The Brick) ''stands by itself; represents both medical and surgical departments; and offers the hard labor desirable for the training of nurses.''[16] Apparently, there was rather poor leadership, and nurses continued to do dishwashing and other menial tasks, with little attention to training. When Linda Richards became the third director, she reorganized the work, started classes, and set out to prove that trained nurses were better than untrained ones. As an example, she cared for some of the sickest patients herself. By the end of 1876, she had charge of all of the nursing in the hospital.

Other major training schools that were to endure into the next century were founded in the next fews years, somewhat patterned after Nightingale's precepts. Their success and the popularity of their graduates resulted in a massive proliferation of training schools. In 1880, there were 15; by 1900, 432; by 1909, 1,105 hospital-based diploma schools. Hospitals with as few as twenty beds opened schools, and the students provided almost totally free labor. Usually the only graduate nurses were the superintendent and perhaps the operating room supervisor and night supervisor. Students earned money for the hospital, for after a short period they were frequently sent to do private nursing in the home, with the money reverting to the hospital, not the school. Except for the few outstanding schools, all Nightingale principles were forgotten: the students were under the control of the hospital and worked from twelve to fifteen hours a day—twenty-four if they were on a private case in a home—and lessons, if any, were scheduled for an hour late in the evening when someone was available to teach (it wasn't necessary for all students to be available). Moreover, if the ''pupils'' lost time because of sickness, which was almost always contracted from patients or caused by sheer overwork, the time had to be totally made up before they could graduate. Why then did training schools draw so many applicants? Because the occupational opportunities for untrained women were limited to domestic service, factory work, retail clerking, or prostitution. Even with the strict discipline, hard work, long hours, and almost no time off, after a year or two of training (the second year unabashedly free labor to the hospitals), the trained nurse could do private duty at a salary ranging from $10 a week to the vague possibility of $20 (if she could collect it), a far cry from the $4 to $6 average of other women workers. Of course, on these cases, she was a twenty-four-hour servant to the family and patient, lucky to have time off for a walk, and because there were necessarily months with no employment, even an excellent nurse was lucky to gross $600 a year.[17] Higher education for women was limited to typewriting or teaching, but these were seldom taught in universities. Those colleges and universities that did admit women rarely prepared them for professions. So the more famous hospital schools, particularly, had hundreds and even thousands of applicants a year. On the other hand, there were a multitude of hospitals and sanitoriums of all kinds that were looking for students to meet their staffing needs, and for these, high-quality applicants were frequently lacking. Consequently, application standards were lowered rapidly. Apparently, most schools admitted a class of thirty to thirty-five[18] (in some cases determined by their staffing and financial needs). Attrition, caused in part by the tremendously high rate of student illness and the unpleasant working and living conditions, was often 75 percent.

Student admission requirements varied, but all nurse applicants were female. Some hospitals accepted men in programs but gave them only a short course and frequently called them *attendants*. In 1888, at Bellevue Hospital, the Mills School was established with a two-year course, but for a long time its graduates were also called *attendants*. Other early schools admitting men were at Grace Hospital, Detroit; Battle Creek Sanitorium, Battle Creek, Michi-

gan; Boston City Hospital, Carney, and St. Margaret's, Boston; Pennsylvania Hospital in Philadelphia; and the Alexian Brothers hospitals in Chicago and St. Louis.[19] At first, the minimum age for all students was about twenty-five, later lowered to twenty-one, to prevent losing young women to other fields. Eight or fewer years of schooling were common, but usually good health and good character were absolute prerequisites. Obedience in training was essential, and a student could be dismissed as a troublemaker if the overworked girl grumbled, talked too much, was too familiar with men, criticized head nurses or doctors, or could not get along "sweetly" wherever placed. Married women and those over thirty were frequently excluded because they could not "fall in with the life successfully." And, of course, if they were divorced, they were naturally eliminated—"too self-centered with interests elsewhere." Blacks were also generally silently excluded. Over the years, training schools for black nurses were founded, the first organized in 1891 at the Provident Hospital in Chicago.

In the 1890s, only 2 percent of nurse training was theory, containing some anatomy and physiology, materia medica, perhaps some chemistry, bacteriology, hygiene, and lectures on certain diseases. The leading schools developed their own institutional manuals, such as the simply written *Hand-Book of Nursing for Family and General Use*, written by a committee of nurses and physicians at the Connecticut Training School and published in 1878. The other great pioneering texts were *A Textbook of Nursing for the Use of Training Schools, Families, and Private Students*, by Clara Weeks Shaw (1885); *Nursing: Its Principles and Practice for Hospital and Private Use,* by Isabel Hampton (1893); *The Textbook on Materia Medica for Nurses*, by Lavinia Dock (1890); and the first scientific book written by a nurse, a textbook on anatomy, by Diana Kimber (1893). Almost from the beginning, there were physicians who objected to so much education for nurses and devoted con-

siderable medical journal space to their fulmi-
nations about the "overtrained nurse."

> Training, as we understand it, is drilling,
> and a person who is to carry out the instruc-
> tions of another cannot be too thoroughly
> drilled. Pedagogy is another matter. We have
> never been able to understand what great
> good was expected from imparting to nurses a
> smattering of medicine and surgery. . . . To
> feed their vanity with the notion that they are
> competent to take any considerable part in or-
> dering the management of the sick is certainly
> a most erroneous step.

> The work of a nurse is an honorable "call-
> ing" or vocation, and nothing further. It im-
> plies the exercise of acquired proficiency in
> certain more or less mechanical duties, and is
> not primarily designed to contribute to the
> sum of human knowledge or the advancement
> of science. . . .[20]

One physician even suggested a correspondence course for training nurses to care for the
"poor folks,"[21] and a New York newspaper
editorial proclaimed, "What we want in
nurses is less theory and more practice." But
then, this was at a time when a leading Harvard physician held that serious mental exercise would damage a woman's brain or cause
other severe trauma, such as the narrowing of
the pelvic area, which would make her unable
to deliver children.[22]

However, there were also farsighted physicians who supported not "teaching a trade,
but preparing for a profession," as Dr. Richard Cabot noted in 1901. He listed reforms
that included the following: (1) nurses should
pay for their training and be taught by paid instructors; (2) nursing should be taught by
nurses, medicine by physicians; (3) the nurse's
training should not be entirely technical. He
added, "Subjects like French literature and
history, which tend to give us a deeper and
truer sympathy with human nature, are surely
as much needed in the education of the nurse,
who is to deal exclusively with human beings,
as in the curriculum of the chemist or engineer, who deals primarily with things and not

persons."[23] But, meanwhile, students continued to live a slavelike existence, without outward complaint, poorly housed, overworked,
underfed ("rations of a kind and quality only
a remove better than what we might place before a beggar," said a popular journal), and
unprotected from life-threatening illness (80
percent of the students in the average hospital
graduated with positive tuberculin tests).[24] If
they survived all this, no wonder they were expected to graduate as "respectful, obedient,
cheerful, submissive, hard-working, loyal, pacific, and religious."[25] It was not professional
education; it was not even a respectably run
apprenticeship, because learning was not derived from skilled masters, but rather from
their own peers, who were but a step ahead of
them. These principles of sacrifice, service,
obedience to the physician, and ethical orientation are embodied in the Nightingale
Pledge, written in 1893 by Lystra E. Gretter,
superintendent of the school at Harper Hospital in Detroit, a pledge still frequently recited
by students today.

> I solemnly pledge myself before God and in
> the presence of this assembly;
> To pass my life in purity and to practice my
> profession faithfully;
> I will abstain from whatever is deleterious
> and mischievous and will not take or know-
> ingly administer any harmful drug; I will do
> all in my power to maintain and elevate the
> standard of my profession, and will hold in
> confidence all personal matters committed to
> my keeping and all family affairs coming to
> my knowledge in the practice of my calling;
> With loyalty will I endeavor to aid the phy-
> sician in his work, and devote myself to the
> welfare of those committed to my care.[26]

THE NURSE IN PRACTICE

In the late eighteenth and early nineteenth
centuries, the graduate trained nurse had two
major career options: she could do private
duty in homes or, if she was exceptional (or

particularly favored), gain one of the rare positions as head nurse, operating room supervisor, night supervisor, or even superintendent. The latter positions were, of course, much more available before the flood of nurses reached the market. Even so, in private duty, trained nurses often competed with untrained nurses who were not restrained from practicing in many states until the middle of the twentieth century. And, given the long hours and taxing physical work in home nursing, most private nurses found themselves unwanted at forty, with younger, stronger nurses being hired instead. Some of the more ambitious and perhaps braver nurses chose to go west to pioneer in new and sometimes primitive hospitals.

The practice of nursing was scarcely limited to clinical care of the patient. Job descriptions of the time appear to have given major priority to scrubbing floors, dusting, keeping the stove stoked and the kerosene lamps trimmed and filled, controlling insects, washing clothes, making and rolling bandages, and other unskilled housekeeping tasks, as well as edicts for personal behavior.[27] Nursing care responsibilities included "making beds, giving baths, preventing and dressing bedsores, applying friction to the body and extremities, giving enemas, inserting catheters, bandaging, dressing blisters, burns, sores, and wounds, and observing secretions, expectorations, pulse, skin, appetite, body temperature, consciousness, respiration, sleep, condition of wounds, skin eruptions, elimination, and the effect of diet, stimulants, and medications," and carrying out any orders of the physician.[28] One of the more interesting treatments to modern nurses might be the vivid description of leeching, which included placing leeches, removing them from human orifices where they may have disappeared, and emptying them of excess blood.[29]

At the end of the nineteenth century, the growth of large cities was marked in the United States. Although the cities had their beautiful public buildings, parks, and mansions, they also had their seamy sides—the festering slums where the tremendous flow of immigrants huddled. Between 1820 and 1910, nearly 30 million immigrants entered the United States, with a shift in numbers from Northern European to Southern European by the early 1900s. Health and social problems multiplied in the slum areas. In New York, for instance, it was not unusual to house thirty-six families in a six-story walk-up on a narrow 25 × 90 foot lot. Vermin, lack of sanitation, and the fact that many immigrants converted their crowded rooms into sweatshops made it easy for epidemics to rage through the neighborhoods, and death from tuberculosis was common.[30]

Somehow, Americans did not seem to feel a great need to serve the sick poor in their homes; after all, there were public dispensaries and charity hospitals. Nevertheless, in 1877, the Women's Board of the New York City Mission sent nurses, who received their training at Bellevue, into the homes of the poor to give care. In 1886, the Visiting Nurse Society of Philadelphia sent nurses not only to the poor but also to those of moderate means who could pay. In the same year, the nurses of the Boston Instructive District Nursing Association formally included patient teaching in their visits—principles of hygiene, sanitation, and aspects of illness. Other such agencies followed, but by 1900 it was estimated that only 200 nurses were engaged in public health nursing.

One of the key figures in community health nursing was Lillian Wald. After graduating from New York Hospital School of Nursing and working a short time, she decided to enter the Women's Medical College. When she and another nurse, Mary Brewster were sent to the Lower East Side to lecture to immigrant mothers on the care of the sick, they were shocked at what they saw; neither had known such abject poverty could exist. Wald left medical school, moved with Mary Brewster to a top-floor tenement on Jefferson Street, and began to offer nursing care to the poor. After a short while, the calls came by the hundreds from families, hospitals, and physicians. People were cared for, whether or not they could afford to pay. The concern of these nurses was not just giving nursing care but seeing what other services could be made available to meet the many social needs of the poor. Challenging the entire community to assume responsibility for these conditions of "poverty and misery" was an attitude strongly advocated by Lavinia Dock, who wrote in 1937:

> As I recollect it, this point of view turned rather toward exploration and discovery than simply toward good works alone, when Lillian D. Wald and Mary Brewster went in 1893, free from every form of control, "without benefit of" managers, committees, medical encouragement, or police approval, into Jefferson Street (at first, then later into Henry Street), there to do what they could do; to see what they could see; and to publicize all that was wrong and remediable by making their findings known as widely as possible. . . .
>
> If I am not mistaken, it was Lillian Wald who first used the term *public health nursing*—adding the one word *public* to Florence Nightingale's phrase *health nursing*—in order to picture her inner vision of the possibilities of nursing services as widely and as effectively organized as were state and federal health services, and acting in harmonious cooperation with them, if not a part of them.[31]

After two years of such success, larger facilities, more nurses, and social workers were needed. In 1895, Wald, Brewster, Lavinia Dock, and other nurses moved to what was eventually called the Henry Street Settlement, a house bought by philanthropist Jacob H. Schiff. By 1909, the Henry Street staff had thirty-seven nurses, all but five providing direct nursing service. Each nurse was carefully oriented to the customs of the immigrants she served and was able to demonstrate the value of understanding the family and the environment in giving good nursing care. Each nurse kept two sets of records, one for the physician and another recording the major points of the nurse's work.[32]

The establishment of school nursing was also started by Lillian Wald, who suggested that placing nurses in schools might help solve the problem of the schools having to send home so many ill children. (Health conditions in New York Schools were so bad that in 1902 10,567 children were sent home from school; local physicians did little in these settings.) Wald sent a Henry Street nurse, Lina L. Rogers, to a school on a one-month demonstration project, which proved so successful that by 1903 the school board began to appoint nurses to the schools. It was not an easy job, and on occasion the schools were the sites of riots because mothers misunderstood the preventive measures that needed to be taken by the nurses. One amusing tale is found in the Children's Bureau records. On being notified that her child needed a bath, a mother wrote, "teacher, Johnny ain't no rose. Learn him, don't smell him."[33]

Industrial nursing also began to provide job opportunities for trained nurses. Its beginnings are generally credited to the president of the Vermont Marble Company in Proctor, Vermont, who in 1895 employed a trained nurse, Ada M. Stewart, to give "district nursing" service to the employees of the company. No public health nursing service was available at that time.

Miss Stewart often traveled about the town on a bicycle, wearing her nurse's uniform and a plain coat and hat, teaching company employees and sometimes other members of the community "habits for healthy living," caring for minor injuries, calling the doctor when indicated, and, at the schoolteacher's request, talking to schoolchildren about hygiene and first aid. Miss Stewart's service was so helpful that in 1895 the marble company employed her sister, Harriet, to give similar service in other Vermont communities in which the company had mills and quarries.[34]

The century ended with another war, in which nurses again proved their worth. The Spanish-American War lasted less than a year, but there was considerable loss of life. The army was completely unprepared for it, and the hospital corpsmen were even less ready to cope with the sick and wounded. The National Society of the Daughters of the American Revolution offered to serve as an examining board for military nurses. The task of separating the fit from the unfit and the trained from the untrained among the 5,000 applicants was overwhelming. Significant questions asked the volunteers were, "Are you strong and healthy?" and "Have you ever had yellow fever?" Although only a small percentage of the soldiers ever left the camps in the South to fight in Cuba, at one point fully 30 percent became ill from malaria, dysentery, and typhoid. Once more, some Army surgeons, particularly the Surgeon General, objected to the presence of trained women nurses, but their efforts to recruit male nurses were unsuccessful because glory, rank, and decent salary were lacking. Consequently, nursing was done by the dregs of the infantry squads. Finally, with serious outbreaks of typhoid killing the enlistees, women nurses from many training schools took over. Wearing their own distinctive school uniforms and caps, they included superintendents of nursing on leave from their noted schools, as well as new, young graduates. Their letters and journals relate the horrible conditions under which they worked. Some literally worked themselves to death in the Army hospitals in the South.

Meanwhile, a hospital ship, the *U.S.S. Relief,* sailed to Cuba with supplies, medicines, and equipment—and Esther Hasson of New London, Connecticut, who would later become the first superintendent of the Navy Nurse Corps. They were just in time to receive the wounded of a naval battle, but again, the greatest problem was diseases. Among these was yellow fever, about which little was known. In testing the theory that the disease was caused by a certain type of mosquito, nursing gained its first martyr. Twenty-five-year-old Clara Maas of East Orange, New Jersey, volunteered to be bitten by a carrier mosquito. After being bitten several times, she died of yellow fever and is still considered a heroine in helping to prove the source of the disease.

The conditions under which soldiers and sailors were cared for continued to be horrendous. An investigation after the war indicated that the only redeeming aspect was the quality of the services of the women nurses, even though they were insufficient in number and were forced to work inefficiently. A recommendation was made for "a corps of selected trained women nurses ready to serve when necessity shall arise, but, under ordinary circumstances, owing no duty to the War Department, except to report residence at determined intervals."[35] Still, the attitude of military authorities was hostile. One hospital commander surgeon objected to retaining women nurses, citing their "coddling" of patients, not letting the Army private (orderly) nurse, and the difficulty in preserving "good military discipline with this mixed personnel." So, although the number of women Army nurses had reached 1,158 in September 1898, by the next July there were only 202. Despite this setback, a group of influential women, including some prominent nurses, eventually lobbied through a bill, and the Army Nurse Corps was established on February 2, 1901. Dita H. Kinney, Head Nurse of the U.S. Army Hospital at Fort Bayard, New Mexico, became the first nurse superintendent. It took longer for the Congress to act on a Navy Nurse Corps, although it had the support of the Navy's Surgeon General, but finally it too became a reality in 1908.[36]

THE IMPACT OF NURSING'S EARLY LEADERS

Perhaps it was said best by Isabel Hampton Robb as she spoke to other early nursing leaders. "We are the history makers of trained nurses. Let us see to it that we work so as to leave a fair record as the inheritance of those who come after us, one which may be to them an inspiration to even better efforts."[37]

It was an amazing period of coordinated female leadership in what was barely becoming an accepted, respectable occupation in the last quarter of the nineteenth century. Yet, before the new century was far along, this intrepid coterie of nurses was responsible for setting nursing standards, improving curricula, writing textbooks, starting two enduring professional organizations and a nursing journal, inaugurating a teacher training program in a university, and initiating nursing licensure. They were a mixed group, but with certain commonalities: usually unmarried but, except for Lavinia Dock, not feminist; graduates of the better training schools; later functioning in some teaching and/or administrative capacity, most often as superintendent of a school; and involved in the early nursing organizations. Fortunately, many were also great letter writers and letter savers as well as authors, so that there are many fascinating insights into their lives.*

Nursing's first trained nurse Linda Richards, had a continuing impact on the training schools because she spent much of her career moving from hospital to hospital in what seems to have been an improvement campaign. In those earliest days, almost any graduate was considered a prime candidate for starting another program, and some undoubtedly lacked the intellectual and leadership qualities needed, so that the new schools, if not actual disasters, were frequently of poor quality. Linda Richards apparently had the skill and authority to upgrade both the school and the nursing service which were, after all, almost inseparable. However, she seemed willing to accept school management that tied the economics of the hospital to student education, usually to the detriment of the latter.

One of the most noted nursing figures is Isabelle Hampton, who left teaching to enter the Bellevue Training School in 1881. Not only was she attractive and charming, but she was "in every sense of the word a leader, by nature, by capacity, by personal attributes and qualities, by choice, and probably to some extent by inheritance and training; a fol-

*See particularly the Christy series in *Nursing Outlook*, listed in the bibliography.

lower she never was."[38] In her two major superintendencies, she made a number of then radical changes—cutting down the students' workday to ten hours and eliminating their free private duty services. At Johns Hopkins, which she founded, she recruited fractious Lavinia Dock, who was still at Bellevue, to be her assistant. They must have made an interesting pair, for Lavinia, also a "lady," was outspoken and frequently tactless, particularly with physicians. Later, she was to say:

A quite determined movement on the part of our masculine brothers to seize and guide the helm of the new teaching is . . . most undeniably in progress. Several . . . have lately openly asserted themselves in printed articles as the founders and leaders of the nursing education, which so far as it has gone, we all know to have been worked out by the brains, bodies and souls of women . . . who have often had to win their points in clinched opposition to the will of these same brothers and solely by dint of their own personal prestige as women. . . .[39]

M. Adelaide Nutting graduated in that first Hopkins class, and the three became friends. Nutting followed Hampton as principal of the school when in 1894 Isabel was married to one of her admirers, Dr. Hunter Robb, and, as was the custom, retired from active nursing. (Letters of the time reveal the anger, dismay, and even sadness of her colleagues at her marriage. They were sure Dr. Robb was not nearly good enough for her, and, besides, she was betraying nursing by robbing the profession of her talents.) Nevertheless, Isabel Hampton Robb maintained her interest in nursing and continued to be active in the development of the profession. In 1893, she had been appointed chairman of a committee to arrange a congress of nurses under the auspices of the International Congress of Charities, Correction, and Philanthropy at the Chicago World's Fair. There, before an international audience of nurses, she voiced her concern about poor nursing education and stated that the term *trained nurse* meant "anything, everything, or next to nothing" in the absence of educational standards. At the same time, Dock pointed out that the teaching, training, and discipline of nurses should not be provided at the discretion of medicine. Similar themes were reiterated in other papers, as well as the notion that there ought to be an organization of nurses. Shortly after the Congress, eighteen superintendents organized the American Society of Superintendents of Training Schools for Nursing (later to become the National League of Nursing Education) to promote the fellowship of members, establish and maintain a universal standard of training, and further the best interests of the nursing profession. The first convention of the society elected Linda Richards president.

Another attendee at those early meetings was Sophia Palmer, descendant of John and Priscilla Alden and a graduate of the Boston Training School, who, after a variety of experiences, organized a training school in Washington, D.C., over the concerted opposition of local physicians who wanted to control nursing education. She approved the steps that were taken but was impatient with what seemed to be blind acceptance of hospital control of schools. "She had a very intense nature and, like all those who are born crusaders, had little patience with the slower methods of persuasion. . . . She was like a spirited racehorse held by the reins of tradition."[40] Within a short time, she and some of the others in the Society, including Dock and the new Mrs. Robb, recognized the need for another organization for all nurses. Although some of the training schools had alumnae associations, they were restrictive; in some cases, their own graduates could not be members, and any "outsider" could not participate. Therefore, if a nurse left the immediate vicinity of her own school, there was no way in which she had any organized contact with other nurses. In a paper given in 1895, Palmer stressed that the power of the nursing profession was dependent upon its ability to organize individuals who could influence public opinion. Dock also made recommendations for a na-

tional organization. In 1896, delegates representing the oldest training school alumnae associations and members of an organizing committee of the Society selected a name for the proposed organization—Nurses' Associated Alumnae of the United States and Canada (to become the American Nurses' Association in 1911), set a time and place for the first meeting (February 1897 in Baltimore), and drafted a constitution. At the end of that February meeting, held in conjunction with the fourth annual Society convention, the constitution and by-laws were adopted and Isabel Hampton Robb was elected president. Among the problems discussed at those early meetings were nursing licensure and the creation of an official nursing publication.

There were a number of nursing journals: the *British Journal of Nursing*, established by one of England's nursing leaders, Ethel Gordon Fenwick; and in the United States, the short-lived *The Nightingale*, started by a Bellevue graduate; *The Nursing Record* and *The Nursing World*, also short-lived; and *The Trained Nurse and Hospital Review*, which Palmer edited for a time, and which continued for seventy years. But the leaders of the new organizations wanted a magazine that would promote nursing, owned and controlled by nursing.

For several years there was discussion but no action, until another committee on the ways and means of producing a magazine was formed. In January 1900, they organized a stock company and sold $100 shares only to nurses and nurses' alumnae associations. By May, they had a promise of $2,400 in shares, and almost 500 nurses had promised to subscribe. Admittedly, they had overstepped their mandate, they reported to the third annual convention of the Nurses' Associated Alumnae, but they were given approval to establish the magazine along the lines formulated. The J. B. Lippincott Company was selected as publisher, and Sophia Palmer became editor, which she did on an unpaid basis for the first nine months. (She had become director of the Rochester City Hospital in New York.) As the first issues went for mailing in October, it was discovered that the post office rules prevented its being mailed because the journal's stockholders were not incorporated. M. E. P. Davis and Sophia Palmer assumed personal responsibilities for all liabilities of the new *American Journal of Nursing*, and it went out. The *Journal* was considered the official organ of the nursing profession, but the stock was still held by alumnae associations and individual nurses. It was Lavinia Dock who donated the first share of stock to the association, and by 1912 the renamed American Nurses' Association had gained ownership of all the stock of the American Journal of Nursing Company, which it still retains.[41]

One other major organization, the American Red Cross, was established by a nurse, Clara Barton, the school teacher who had volunteered as a nurse and directed relief operations during the Civil War and served with the German Red Cross during the Franco-Prussian War in 1870. (The establishment of the International Red Cross as a permanent international relief agency that could take immediate action in time of war had occurred in Geneva in 1864 with the signing of the Geneva Convention guidelines.) After her return to the United States, Barton organized the American Red Cross and persuaded Congress in 1882 to ratify the Treaty of Geneva so that the Red Cross could carry on its humanitarian efforts in peacetime. Clara Barton, however, was not an active part of the nursing leadership that was molding the profession.

That group had another immediate goal. The society recognized that the nurses were at a disadvantage because they had no postgraduate training in administration or teaching, so a committee consisting of Robb, Nutting, Richards, Mary Agnes Snively, and Lucy Drown was formed to investigate the possibilities. At the sixth Society convention, they reported their success. James Russell, the farsighted dean of Teachers College, Columbia University, in New York, had agreed to start a course for nurses if they could guarantee the enrollment of twelve nurses, or $1,000 a year. The Society agreed. Members of the Society screened the candidates, contributed $1,000 a year, and taught the course—hospital economics. Later, the students were also allowed to enroll in psychology, science, household economics, and biology. Anna Alline, one of the two graduates of the first class, then took over the total administration of the course.

There was one more major goal to be reached—licensure of nurses. Not only did the 432 hospital-based schools vary greatly in quality, but the market was also flooded with "nurses" who had been dismissed from schools without graduating, "nurses" from six-week private and correspondence courses, and a vast number of those who simply called themselves nurses. It was inevitable that people became confused, for when they hired nurses for private duty in their homes, the "nurse" could present one of the elaborate diplomas from a $13 correspondence course that guaranteed that anyone could become a nurse, a real or forged reference, or a genuine diploma from a top-quality school. How could they judge? Consequently, because of the abysmal care given by individuals representing themselves as nurses, the public was once more disenchanted with the "nurse." Therefore, nursing's leaders were determined that there must be legal regulation, both to protect the public from unscrupulous and incompetent nurses and to protect the young profession by establishing a minimum level of competence, limiting all or some of the professional functions to those who qualified. The idea was not new; medicine already had licensing in some states, and many aspiring professions were also moving in that direction.

In September 1901, at the first meeting of the newly formed International Council of Nurses, which was held in Buffalo, a resolution was passed, stating that "it is the duty of the nursing profession of every country to work for suitable legislative enactment regulating the education of nurses and protecting the interests of the public, by securing State examinations and public registration, with the proper penalties for enforcing the same.''[42]

In the United States, such licensing was a state function, so to gain the necessary legislative lobbying power, it was recommended that state or local nurses' associations be formed. In many ways the disagreements that arose in their formation were the forerunners of those that would center on the licensure process. Who should be eligible? In New York, for instance, Sylveen Nye, who became the state association's first president, thought that *all* nurses should be included and that standards could be raised later. Sophia Palmer, another key figure in its formation, believed that only ''qualified'' nurses should be permitted to belong—those who graduated from certain types of schools. Later, the question was "Who should be eligible for licensure?''

As it was, New York had become the early leader in the licensure drive, for it had in place a Board of Regents that regulated education and licensure. In 1897, Palmer, in a smart political move, had already presented nursing's case to another emerging group of women who were gaining power and prestige—the New York Federation of Women's Clubs. They passed a resolution supporting her licensure concept, which included two major points—the need for a diploma from a school meeting certain standards, and insistence that the examining board consist only of nurses, as in other professions. Immediately Palmer organized a meeting with the secretary of the Board of Regents, who then and later was helpful and supportive, suggesting guidelines for action. (For instance, the licensed nurse needed to be called something. Among the titles suggested by nurses were *graduate nurse*, trained nurse, *certified nurse, registered nurse*, and *registered graduate nurse*.) The Regents also suggested the formation of a state nurses' association. Once formed, the New York State Nurses' Association developed a licensure bill and embarked on a campaign to gain support for the proposed legislation. Opposition was foreordained. In a circular addressed to the women's clubs, Palmer accurately pinpointed the sources:

> The New York State Nurses' Association is preparing to apply for legislative enactments which will place training schools for nurses under the supervision of the Regents of the University of the State, with a view to securing by the authority of the law a minimum basis of education for the nurse, beyond which the safety of the sick and the protection of the public cannot be assured.
>
> While such a law cannot prevent the public from employing untaught women as nurses, if it so desires, it will prevent such women from imposing themselves upon the public as fully trained nurses.
>
> In this movement the Nurses' Association will meet with opposition: First, from the trained nurses of the State who are afraid to make an independent stand for their own and the public protection. Second, from all of the managers and proprietors of institutions which are not equipped for giving this minimum education, and which now conduct so-called training schools, for commercial advantages, and third, from all the vast army of so-called nurses who, without adequate nursing experience and education, undertake the grave responsibility of a nurse's work.[43]

And there was just that kind of opposition and more, for there were 15,000 untrained nurses in New York at the time, opposed to 2,500 who were trained. In addition, some physicians objected to their lack of representation on the proposed nursing board, as did some nurses, including Nye. Moreover, some physicians did not see the necessity for any fancy standards and worried about overeducation of nurses. Said one, ''Nursing is not, strictly speaking, a profession. Any intelligent, not necessarily educated, woman can in a short time acquire the skill to carry out with explicit obedience the physician's directions.''

Nevertheless, the bill became law on April 24, 1903. It was pitifully weak by today's standards, but daring for the times. Educational standards were set. A training school for nurses had to give at least a two-year program and be registered by the regents. The board of five nurses was to be chosen by the regents from a list submitted by the New York State Nurses' Association. The regents, on the advice of the board, were to make rules for the examination of nurses and to revoke licensure for cause. The New York State Nurses' Association was given the right to institute proceedings and prosecute those violating the law, a responsibility that was not changed for some years. It should be remembered, though, that this, like all nurse licensure laws in those times, was permissive, not mandatory. That is, only the RN title was protected. Untrained nurses could continue to work as nurses as long as they did not call themselves RNs.

New York was not the first state to register nurses. On March 3, 1903, North Carolina, and on April 1, 1903, New Jersey had passed laws. It was said that both were inspired by New York's initiative. (Virginia followed New York on May 14.) However, New York's law was the strongest. For instance, New Jersey's law omitted a board of any kind; North Carolina had a mixed board of nurses and doctors and allowed a nurse to be licensed without attending a training school, if vouched for by a doctor. Partially because New York had the greatest number of trained nurses and because of the experience in regulation of the board of regents, the state's nurses were looked to as leaders in the further developments. The prestige, power, and authority of the board of regents was such that later many training schools in other states and other countries sought and received approval under New York's law—an action that also upgraded schools in those states. In fact, by 1906, more schools were registered outside the state than within it.

The enactment of the first nursing licensure laws was soon followed by like actions in other states; in a sense, it was the end of one era and the beginning of another. Nursing's leaders had shown themselves to be, as a whole, dedicated, strong, and remarkably bold. They set standards for nursing at a time when standards in long-established medicine were still quite weak. Despite internal dissension and the opposition of some powerful hospital administrators and physicians, they had had a licensing law passed—at a time when women had no vote. They literally created a young profession out of a woman's occupation. But the struggle to achieve full professionalism was far from over.

REFERENCES

1. Ida C. Selavan, "Nurses in American History: The Revolution," *Am. J. Nurs.*, **74**:592–594 (Apr. 1975).
2. Josephine A. Dolan, *Nursing in Society*, 14th ed. (Philadelphia: W. B. Saunders Company, 1978), p. 175.
3. Philip Kalisch and Beatrice Kalisch, "Untrained But Undaunted: The Women Nurses of the Blue and Gray," *Nurs. Forum*, **15**,1:25–26 (1976).
4. Ibid., pp. 22–25.
5. Ibid., p. 17.
6. Anne Austin, "Nurses in American History—Wartime Volunteers—1861–1865," *Am. J. Nurs.*, **75**:817 (May 1975).
7. Kalisch and Kalisch, op. cit., pp. 15–16.
8. Vern Bullough and Bonnie Bullough, *The Care of the Sick: The Emergence of Modern Nursing* (New York: Prodist, 1978), p. 113.
9. Dolan, op. cit., pp. 176–177.
10. Ibid., pp. 175–176.
11. Joyce Ann Elmore, "Nurses in American History: Black Nurses: Their Service and Their Struggle," *Am. J. Nurs.*, **76**:435 (Mar. 1976).
12. Kalisch and Kalisch, op. cit., p. 27.
13. Dolan, op. cit., p. 194.
14. Ibid.
15. Josephine Dolan, "Nurses in American History: Three Schools—1873," *Am. J. Nurs.*, **75**:991 (June 1975).
16. Dolan, op. cit., p. 206.
17. Phililp Kalisch and Beatrice Kalisch, *The Advance of American Nursing* (Boston: Little, Brown, and Company, 1978), pp. 188–189.
18. Ibid., pp. 135–136.

19. Dolan, *Nursing in Society*, op. cit., pp. 308–309.

20. Thelma Ingles, "The Physician's View of the Evolving Nursing Profession—1873–1913," *Nurs. Forum,* **15**,2:147 (1976).

21. Ibid , p. 148.

22. Bonnie Bullough and Vern Bullough, "Sex Discrimination in Health Care," *Nurs. Outlook,* **23**:44 (Jan. 1975).

23. Ingles, op. cit., pp. 139–140.

24. Beatrice Kalisch and Philip Kalisch, "Slaves, Servants, or Saints (An Analysis of the System of Nurse Training in the United States, 1873–1948)," *Nurs. Forum,* **14**,3:230–231 (1975).

25. Ibid., p. 228.

26. Kalisch and Kalisch, *The Advance of American Nursing*, op. cit., pp. 141–142.

27. Ibid., pp. 173–174.

28. Ibid., p. 174.

29. Ibid., pp. 176–177.

30. Ibid., pp. 225–228.

31. "Our First Public Health Nurse—Lillian D. Wald," *Nurs. Outlook,* **19**:660 (Oct. 1871).

32. Kalisch and Kalisch, *The Advance of American Nursing*, op. cit., pp. 230–236.

33. Ibid., pp. 236–240.

34. Ada Stewart Markolf, "Industrial Nursing Begins in Vermont," *Publ. Health Nurs.,* **37**:125 (Mar. 1945).

35. Kalisch and Kalisch, *The Advance of American Nursing*, op. cit., p. 216.

36. Ibid., pp. 217–220.

37. Lyndia Flanagan, *One Strong Voice: The Story of the American Nurses' Association* (Kansas City, Mo.: American Nurses' Association, 1976), p. 292.

38. M. A. Nutting, "Isabel Hampton Robb—Her Work in Organization and Education," *Am. J. Nurs.,* **10**:19, 1910.

39. Ashley, Jo Ann, "Nurses in American History: Nursing and Early Feminism." *Am. J. Nurs.,* **75**:1466 (Sept. 1975).

40. Teresa Christy, "Portrait of a Leader: Sophia F. Palmer," *Nurs. Outlook,* **23**:746–747, (Dec. 1975).

41. Flanagan, op. cit., pp. 35–38.

42. Kalisch and Kalisch *The Advance of American Nursing*, p. 260.

43. Mary Lucile Shannon, "The Origin and Development of Professional Licensure Examinations in Nursing: From a State-Constituted Examination to the State Board Test Pool Examination" (unpublished Ed.D. dissertation, Teachers College, Columbia University, 1972), pp. 57–58.

4

The Emergence of the Modern Nurse, 1904–1965

The period between 1904 and 1965 was a time of multiple changes for nursing, many again precipitated by external forces, including the Depression, two world wars, and various social movements. But the changes were created within nursing by nurses. They included major shifts in education—type, location, curriculum, student body, and alterations in practice—responsibility, economic status, and degree of autonomy. In 1903, the passage of the first nursing licensure laws set standards for nursing education and practice; in 1965, development of new nursing roles and the American Nurses' Association (ANA) position paper on nursing education opened the door for major revisions of those licensure laws and the emergence of the modern nurse.

NURSING BEFORE WORLD WAR I

After the licensure breakthrough, the leaders of nursing continued to look toward improvement of nurse training programs and, consequently, the improved practice of graduates of those programs. Most training schools remained under the control of hospitals, and the needs of the hospital superseded those of the school. For instance, it was not until 1912 that an occasional nurse received release time from hospital responsibilities in order to organize and teach basic nursing, and superintendents were warned not to "neglect" patient care in favor of the school or they would face punishment. There was little support for improvement from physicians. Before the Flexner Report of 1910, the education of the physician, although different, was sometimes less organized than that of the nurse. In the 1870s few of the medical schools required high school diplomas and courses were completed in two years, whereas the nurses' program was being lengthened to three years. For the next 100 years, physicians complained of "overtrained nurses." Moreover, nursing was dominated by and primarily made up of women; it was not considered a profession, in part because it was not situated in an academic, collegiate setting. But to get into that setting as women, much less nurses, was a battle in itself. In essence, then, there were no major changes in the quality of education in the years that followed licensure, once those very limited standards were met. The hours were still long, and the students continued to give free service, with "book learning" as an afterthought.

The public, beginning to be aroused by

poor conditions in factory sweatshops, showed surprisingly little interest in the exploitation of nursing students. Only in California, where an Eight-Hour Law for Women was passed in 1911, was there any movement to include student nurses (not even graduate nurses). Yet, when the bill was introduced in 1913, it was fought bitterly not only by hospitals, as might be expected, but also by physicians and nurses. No doubt, some were influenced by a sentiment voiced by physicians who were saying that nursing would be debased by being included in a law enforced by the State Bureau of Labor. Stated one physician to nurses, "The element of sacrifice is always present in true service. The service that costs no pains, no sacrifice, is without virtue, and usually without value." Retorted Lavinia Dock, "I think nurses should stand together solidly and resist the dictation of the medical profession in this as in all other things. Many MD's have a purely commercial spirit toward nurses . . . and would readily overwork them. . . . If necessary, do not hesitate to make alliances with the labor vote, for organized labor has quite as much of an 'ideal' as the MD's have, if not more."[1] Although the bill finally passed, thanks to the persistence of Senator Anthony Caminetti, delegations of hospital representatives and physicians went to the governor to ask him to withhold his signature. When he asked where the people were who favored the law, a woman reporter told him that *they* were in the hospitals caring for the sick and unable to plead their own cause; he signed.[2] But, for years, superintendents of nursing complained about the expense of hiring nurses who were now necessary to do the work students had done.

While the Flexner Report was bringing about reform in medical schools, eliminating the correspondence courses and the weaker and poorer schools, Adelaide Nutting and other leaders were agitating for reform in nursing education. In 1911, the American Society of Superintendents of Training Schools for Nurses presented a proposal for a similar survey of nursing schools to the Carnegie

Foundation. Then President Pritchitt, stating that the foundation's energies were centered elsewhere and ignoring nursing, directed a considerable amount of the foundation funds in such studies for dental, legal, and teacher education.

Although women were having a little more success in being accepted in colleges and universities, there was only limited movement to make basic nursing programs an option in academic settings. Apparently, before 1900 there was a short-lived program at Howard University, but it was almost immediately taken over by Freedman's Hospital Nursing School. There is also some evidence that the School of Medicine at the University of Texas in 1896 "adopted" a hospital school of nursing to prevent its closing for lack of funds. However, the University of Minnesota program, founded in 1903 by Dr. Richard Olding Beard, a physician who was dedicated to the concept of higher education for nurses, became the first enduring baccalaureate program in nursing. Even this was more similar to good diploma programs than other university programs. Although eventually the students had to meet university admission standards and took some specialized courses, they also worked a fifty-six-hour week in the hospital and were awarded a diploma instead of a degree after three years. Similar programs were started by other universities which took over hospitals or started new ones, in part to obtain student services for their hospitals. Just prior to World War I, several hospitals and universities, such as Presbyterian Hospital of New York and Teachers College, offered degree options. These developed into five-year programs with two years of college work and three years in a diploma school. This became a common pattern that lasted through the 1940s, but in 1916, when Annie Goodrich reported that sixteen colleges and universities maintained schools, departments, or courses in nursing education, they were an assortment of educational hybrids.

Nursing practice had also not developed to any extent, with most graduate nurses still doing private duty in homes. A nurse, unless she became the favorite of one or more doctors who liked her work, found her cases through registries, established by alumnae associations, hospitals, medical societies, or commercial agencies. The first two frequently limited the better jobs to their graduates; commercial agencies not only charged the nurse a fee, but did not distinguish between trained and untrained nurses. Finally, a county nurses' association gained control of a registry in Minnesota in 1904, and others followed. Nevertheless, private duty was an individual enterprise, with long hours, no benefits, and limited pay. (In 1926, some nurses were still working a twenty-four-hour day at what averaged out to forty-nine cents an hour, less than cleaning women made.)

However, in 1915, it is estimated, no more than 10 percent of the sick received care in the hospitals, and the majority of people could not afford private duty nurses. From this need, a public health movement emerged that increased the demand for nurses. At first most of these nurses concentrated on bedside care, but others, like those coming from the settlement houses, took broader responsibilities. Nevertheless, there were no recognized standards or requirements for visiting nurses. Therefore, in June 1912, a small group of visiting nurses, representing unofficially some 900 agencies and almost four times that many colleagues, founded the National Organization for Public Health Nursing (NOPHN), with Lillian Wald as the first president.* It was an organization of nurses and lay people engaged in public health nursing and in the organization, management, and support of such work. The leaders of the group selected the term *public health nursing* as more inclusive than *visiting nursing;* it was also reminiscent of Nightingale's health nursing, which had focused on prevention. One of its first goals was

to extend the services to working and middle-class people as well as to the poor.

The Visiting Nurse Quarterly, the first American publication dealing exclusively with public health nursing, was offered to the NOPHN by its founder, the Cleveland Visiting Nurse Association. It became *Public Health Nursing,* the official journal of NOPHN until 1952–1953, when it was absorbed by *Nursing Outlook.* Also in 1912, the Red Cross established the Rural Nursing Service. Wald, at a major meeting on infant mortality, had cited the horrible health conditions of rural America, the high infant and maternal mortality rates, the prevalence of tuberculosis, and other serious health problems, and suggested that the Red Cross operate a national service, similar to that of Great Britain. Later, the name was changed to Town and Country Nursing Service in order to include small towns that had no visiting nurse service, and it was headquartered in Washington. Although the Service provided nurses to care for the sick, do health teaching, and otherwise improve health conditions, it was not wholly successful. Many communities did not choose to call in a national organization for assistance or could not afford the salaries of the nurses. (For a while, a wealthy woman contributed financial support to salaries, but withdrew funds because the rural nurses were not "ladies.") Nevertheless, the rural nurses carried on and proved to be a remarkably resourceful group, coping with an almost total lack of ordinary supplies and equipment. The service survived primarily because the Metropolitan Life Insurance Company decided to use rural nurses for services to their policy-holders, for many local Red Cross chapters had no interest in or understanding of the service. (Red Cross involvement gradually decreased until, with increased government involvement in public health, it discontinued the program altogether in 1947.)

By 1916, public health nurses were being called on to be welfare workers, sanitarians, housing inspectors, and health teachers as well. A number of universities began offering

---

*Changes had also occurred in the first two nursing organizations. In 1911, the Associated Alumnae changed its name to the American Nurses' Association (ANA) and in 1912, the Society of Superintendents adopted the name National League of Nursing Education (NLNE).

courses to help prepare nurses to fulfill this multifaceted role, and Mary Gardner, one of the founders of NOPHN and an interim director of the Rural Nursing Service, authored the first book in the field, *Public Health Nursing*. One of the observations she made was that although broad-minded physicians recognized that public health nurses helped them produce results that would not have been possible alone, the more conservative feared interference by nurses and were resentful of them. She noted that a service had a better chance of success if it was started with the cooperation of the medical profession, and pointed out ways nurses could avoid friction with physicians and still be protected from the incompetents.

Another outstanding public health nurse of that period was Margaret Higgins Sanger. She became interested in the plight of the poorly paid industrial workers, particularly the women. Herself married with three children when she decided to return to work in public health, she was assigned to maternity cases on the Lower East Side of New York, where she found that pregnancy, often unwanted, was a chronic condition among the women. One of her patients died from a repeated self-abortion, after begging doctors and nurses for information on how to avoid pregnancy. That was apparently a turning point for Sanger. After learning everything she could about contraception, she and her sister, also a nurse, opened the first birth control clinic in America in Brooklyn. She was arrested and spent thirty days in the workhouse, but continued her crusade.[3] She fought the battle for free dissemination of birth control information for decades, against all types of opposition, until today, birth control education is generally accepted as the right of women and one nursing role.

A new specialty for nurses that endured was give anesthesia at Mayo Clinic. After she married Charles Mayo, another nurse was trained to take over, for the Mayos had found a nurse more useful than an intern who was also trying to learn surgery. In 1909, a course for nurse anesthetists was established in Oregon, as were others, and these nurses were promptly as exploited by the hospitals as their sisters. it was not until 1917 that the question was officially raised of whether nurse anesthetists were practicing medicine, and it was ruled then that they were not, if paid and supervised by a physician. However, the legal answer was murky for more than sixty years, and the education of nurse anesthetists remained under the control of hospitals and doctors.[4]

NURSES AT WAR

The First World War was different from other wars fought by the United States, both because of its international proportions and the kinds of weapons that were used. Immediately, the demand for nurses was increased. The Army Nurse Corps expanded greatly, as did the Navy Nurse Corps (although to a lesser extent). As the war continued, recruitment standards dropped, and applicants were accepted from nursing schools attached to hospitals with fewer than 100 beds. All nurses needed was certification of moral character and professional qualifications by their superintendent of nurses—and, of course, they had to be unmarried. Once more, untrained society girls were clamoring to be Red Cross volunteer nurses, without knowing what training was required or being willing to accept it. Afraid that Army nursing would fall into untrained hands, as it had in Europe, Nutting, Goodrich, Wald, and others formed a Committee on Nursing to devise "the wisest methods of meeting the present problems connected with the care of the sick and injured in hospitals and homes; the educational problems of nursing; and the extraordinary emergencies as they arise."[5] Some weeks later, the committee was given governmental status and limited financial backing; most funds were contributions from nursing. The committee was able to estimate the number of available nurses and those in training, but, obviously, these were insufficient for both military and civilian needs.

The American Red Cross served as the unofficial reserve corps of the Army Nurse Corps. When these nurses, as well as those who were part of total multidisciplinary base units originating in hospitals, went to Europe, the home situation became desperate. Recruiting efforts were stepped up, first to attract educated women into nursing and then to encourage schools of nursing to somehow increase their capacity, even if it meant the unheard of—having local students live at home for part of their training. Interestingly enough, even though there were male nurses, and they did volunteer, they were usually put in regular fighting units and their skills went unused. Neither, apparently, did the Army choose to use black nurses. Only in mid-1917 would the Red Cross accept them, and then only if the Army Surgeon General agreed. Their eventual acceptance is credited to the efforts of Adah Thom, a black nurse.

Even with the patriotic fervor generated by the war, it was not easy to entice young women into nursing. High school students, queried about their interest in nursing, objected to the life of drudgery, strenuous physical work, poor education, severe discipline, lack of freedom and recreation as a student, and what they saw as limited satisfactory options of employment. However, schools did increase their capacity some 25 percent, and the pressures of the war brought about some educational changes. One of the more daring experiments of the times was the Vassar Training Camp. The idea came from a Vassar alumna and member of the board of trustees to establish at Vassar in the summer of 1918 a preparatory course in nursing, from which the students would move to selected schools of nursing to complete the program in little more than two additional years. As attested to by graduates of the program, it was the spirit of patriotism that attracted more than 400 young women aged fourteen to forty, schooled in many professional fields, and representing more than 100 colleges. They were to be known as Vassar's Rainbow Division because the students wore the various colored student uniforms of the schools they had selected. A large percentage of the women completed the program and entered the nursing schools they had selected, and many of nursing's leaders arose from this group. Soon, five other universities opened similar prenursing courses and also admitted high school students. Because these programs were generally of considerably higher quality than those of the training schools, the movement of nursing education toward an academic setting received another nudge.

Meanwhile, nursing conditions in American military camps were reported as atrocious, and the Committee on Nursing convinced the Surgeon General to appoint Annie Goodrich to evaluate the quality of nursing service. Miss Goodrich, then an assistant professor at Teachers College, had had experience inspecting training schools for New York State. She minced no words in her report—conditions were much worse than in civilian hospitals, because there were not enough nurses to care for the patients, and they found it impossible to deal with a constantly changing group of disinterested corpsmen. Goodrich recommended that nurse training schools be set up in each military hospital, where the students, under careful supervision, would give better care than aides or corpsmen. The suggested Army School of Nursing was to be centralized in the Surgeon General's Office under the supervision of a dean. After some dispute, but with the support of the nursing organizations and influential Frances Payne Bolton of Cleveland, the Army School was approved in May 1918, with Annie Goodrich appointed Dean. The three-year course was based on the new *Standard Curriculum for Schools of Nursing,* published by the National League of Nursing Education. Unlike civilian hospitals, duty hours did not exceed six to eight hours. The military hospitals provided all medical and surgical experience, and gynecology, obstetrics, diseases of children, and public health were provided through affiliations in the second and third year. The response to the school was overwhelming, and it attracted many more students than it could accommodate.

The service of the nurse in the nightmarish battle conditions of World War I, coping with the mass casualties, dealing with injuries caused by the previously unknown shrapnel and gas, and then battling influenza at home and abroad, is a fascinating and proud piece of nursing history.[6]

BETWEEN THE WARS

In the twenty-three years between World Wars I and II, nursing was affected by the Great Depression and adoption of the Nineteenth Constitutional Amendment in August 1920, granting women the right to vote. Of the two, the latter had less immediate impact. Nurses showed relatively little interest in fighting for women's rights, and only one, Lavinia Dock, can be called an active feminist. "Dockie" was a maverick of the times. A tiny woman who loved music and was an accomplished pianist and organist, she also seemed to take on the whole world in her battle for the underdog. Early on, she decided that nurses could have no power unless they had the vote. Her speeches and writings were brilliant, but she did not move her colleagues. Nevertheless, she devoted a good part of her life to working for women's rights. In England, she joined the Pankhursts and landed in jail. Back in the United States, she picketed the White House, seizing the nearest, if not most appropriate, banner, "Youth to the Colors" (she was almost sixty then). Wrote her colleague, Isabel Stewart, "They all went into the cooler for the night. I think it just pleased her no end."[7]

For all her devotion to women's rights, Dock remained committed to nursing. She was editor of the *Journal's* Foreign Department from 1900 to 1923, during which she quarreled regularly with Editor Sophia Palmer and managed to ignore World War I because she was a pacifist. She was also involved with the International Council of

Nursing and was the author of a number of books, including *Health and Morality* in 1910, in which she discussed venereal disease. She was equally outspoken on the forbidden subject in open meetings. A number of nurses had become infected because physicians frequently refused to tell nurses when patients had the disease. Dock also regularly castigated her profession for withholding its interest, sympathy, and moral support from "the great, urgent throbbing, pressing social claims of our day and generation."[8]

But nursing had problems of its own. Immediately after the war, there was a shortage of nurses, because many who had switched careers "for the duration" returned to their own field, and others appeared not to be attracted. In part, it was an image problem, one that was to continue to haunt nursing,* but another quite real aspect was that nursing education was in trouble. As Isabel Stewart said, "The plain facts are that nursing schools are being starved and always have been starved for lack of funds to build up any kind of substantial educational structure."[9] Later, this problem was clearly pinpointed by a prestigious committee. In 1918, Nutting had approached the Rockefeller Foundation to seek endowment for the Johns Hopkins School of Nursing, stressing the need for improvement in the education of public health nurses. The meeting resulted in a committee to investigate the "proper training" of public health nurses, an investigation that quickly concluded that the problem was nursing education in general. The findings of the Goldmark Report (presented in more detail in Chapter 5) concluded that schools of nursing needed to be recognized and supported as separate educational components with not just training in nursing, but also a liberal education. Although the report had little immediate impact, it did result in Rockefeller Foundation support for the founding of the Yale School of Nursing (1924), the first in the world to be established

_____

*See Chapter 11.

as a separate university department with its own dean, Annie Goodrich. Although a few other such programs followed, progress lagged, for many powerful physicians reached the public media with their notions that nurses needed only technical skills, manual dexterity, and quick obedience to the physician. Charles Mayo, for instance, deciding that city-trained nurses were too difficult to handle, too expensive, and spent too much time getting educated, wanted to recruit 100,000 country girls.[10] But even popular journals recognized that student nurses were being exploited by hospitals and that the kind of student being encouraged into nursing by school principals was one seen as not too bright, not attractive enough to marry, and too poor to be supported at home.[11]

A study following close on the heels of the Goldmark Report soon reaffirmed the inadequacy of nursing schools and practicing nurses. *Nurses, Patients, and Pocketbooks* (see Chapter 5) pointed out that the hasty postwar nurse-recruiting efforts had not improved the lot of the patient or nurse; in 1928, problems included an oversupply of nurses, geographic maldistribution, low educational standards, poor working conditions, and some critically unsatisfactory levels of care.

How could education be so poor with licensure in effect? Ten years after the passage of the first acts, thirty-eight states had also passed such laws, but all were permissive, and although the title RN was protected, others could designate themselves nurses and work.* At one point, Annie Goodrich cited a correspondence school that had turned out 12,000 "graduates" in ten years. In addition, hospital schools of all sizes felt no need to meet standards that might deprive them of free student labor. Even those schools that chose to follow state board standards found them not too difficult, and follow-up was almost totally absent; most were approved on the basis of paper credentials. The states that did employ nurse "inspectors" ran into problems in with-

holding approval; members of the boards of nurse examiners were frequently as poorly qualified as the heads of schools, and the political pressures to avoid embarrassing hospitals were overwhelming.

Even in New York State, where the state board was considered a model, the pressures and responsibilities of board members who also held jobs were unbelievable. They not only wrote all the licensing examination questions, but corrected all the papers and traveled throughout the state to give the practical exams. Writing about grading the lengthy open-ended questions, one board member complained, "The monotony is horrible; it stultifies the brain and one finds it impossible to work long at a sitting. So tiresome is it that one welcomes the diversion of a stupid answer."[12] By 1940, New York board members were each forced to grade 1,994 tests as well as the practicals. Not until 1943 were exams scored by machine. Aside from grading fatigue, neither the test-writing skills of the authors nor the state of the art of testing gave any assurance that state boards guaranteed minimum levels of safe and effective practice for the newly licensed practitioner. Many nursing leaders were calling for grading of training schools as a starting point, but the Depression aborted any such action, although there were continued efforts to strengthen the licensing laws.

Unemployment after the stock market crash of 1929 also affected nursing. People who had no jobs could not afford private-duty nurses. It was estimated that 8,000 to 10,000 graduate nurses were out of work, and notices warning nurses not to come to find work in specific areas became frequent in the *Journal*. A 1932 campaign by the ANA to promote an eight-hour day for nurses, hiring of nurses by hospitals, and discontinuance of some nursing schools met a cold reception. Even though they complained of the cost of training students, hospital administrators clung to the schools, perhaps because, despite financial figures to the contrary, students were obviously an economic asset. If one compared

---

*The first mandatory law was passed in New York in 1938 and implemented in 1944.

what the American Hospital Association said the students gave to hospitals in service—$1,000—with an average of 7,000 hours that the students gave—the hospital seemed to be crediting their contribution at about fourteen cents an hour. This was of questionable accuracy at best.[13] However, even directors of nursing showed a reluctance to hire graduate nurses, and 73 percent of hospitals employed no graduates at all on floor duty. By 1933, the desperate straits of unemployed nurses finally forced many to work in hospitals for room and board. Even then, although some administrators believed this was taking advantage of unfortunate nurses, others thought that they were not worth food and lodging.

Some help finally came with the Roosevelt Administration, when relief funds were allocated for bedside care of the indigent and nurses were employed as visiting nurses under the Federal Emergency Relief Administration (FERA). Ten thousand unemployed nurses were put to work in numerous settings under the Civil Work Administration (CWA) in public hospitals, clinics, public health agencies, and other health services. The follow-up Works Progress Administration (WPA) then continued to provide funds for nurses in community health activities. A few nurses also entered a new field that opened—airline stewardess.

By 1936, the number of diploma nursing schools had decreased from more than 2,200 in 1929 to a little less than 1,500 state-accredited programs. There were about seventy "collegiate" programs, most merely of the liberal arts plus hospital school pattern. Many were still floundering. At this point the NLNE presented its third revision of the *Curriculum Guide for Schools of Nursing,* with input from thousands of nurses around the country. A guide that was to endure (probably beyond its optimum usefulness), its major assumptions were that the primary function of the school was to educate the nurse and that the community to be served extended beyond the hospital. Numbers of academic and clinical hours as well as content were suggested.

An obvious problem was the lack of qualified teachers; even in so-called university programs, nurses did not meet the usual requirements for teaching. One outcome was that baccalaureate programs for diploma nurses began to offer specialized degrees in education, administration, or public health nursing. The other was a very slow movement to graduate education. For years, most of the graduate degrees held by nurses were in education, in part because Teachers College and other universities began to accept baccalaureate graduates for graduate preparation in education. In fact, some of the greatest leaders in nursing education either graduated from Teachers College or held teaching positions. One such was Isabel Stewart, who arrived in 1908 for one semester and stayed for thirty-nine years.[14] She succeeded M. Adelaide Nutting, who was the first nurse ever to receive a professorship in a university (1910) and who remained until 1925.[15] As early as 1932, Catholic University offered graduate courses in nursing, but that was uncommon. Apparently, the first, or nearly first, nurse to earn a doctoral degree was Edith S. Bryan; it was in psychology and counseling from Johns Hopkins.

Another slow starter in American nursing was nurse-midwifery. In the 1920s, legislation such as the Sheppard-Tanner Act paid for nurses to give maternity and infant care, but nurse-midwives were not included. Still, a considerable amount of maternity care, particularly deliveries, was done by lay midwives, some competent, some dangerously incompetent. When, in 1925, Mary Breckenridge founded the Frontier Nursing Service (FNS) in rural Kentucky, its staff was a mix of British nurse-midwives and American nurses trained in midwifery in Britain. (The rule was that if the husband could reach the nurse, the nurse could make it back to the patient by some means.) The outstanding services of the nurses on horseback (later in jeeps), who gradually increased their services to include other aspects of primary care, is an ongoing success story.[16] The FNS also founded one of the early nurse-midwifery schools (1936); the first was at the maternity center of New York City in 1932. Also formed was a professional association (see Chapter 27).

Of all the entrants into nursing, two groups got particularly short shrift—men and blacks. The prejudice against men was specifically related to nursing and has persisted to some extent (see Chapter 11). As the distorted image of the female nurse evolved, men did not seem to fit the concepts held by powerful figures in and out of nursing. Therefore, although men graduated from acceptable nursing schools, usually totally male, and attempted to become active members of the ANA, even forming a men's section, their numbers and influence remained small until the post-World War II era.

Black nurses, on the other hand, were caught in the overall common prejudice against their race. Individual black nurses, as noted earlier, broke down barriers in various nursing fields. As early as 1908, they organized the National Association of Colored Graduate Nurses (NACGN), both to fight against discriminatory practices and to foster leadership among black nurses. Although the ANA had a nondiscriminatory policy, some state organizations did not and a rule that the nurse must have graduated from a state-approved school to be an ANA member eliminated even more black nurses.* In 1924, it was reported that only fifty-eight state-accredited schools admitted blacks, and most of these were located in black hospitals or in departments caring for black patients in municipal hospitals. Of these schools, 77 percent were located in the South; twenty-eight states offered no opportunities in nursing education for black women. Most of the southern "schools" that trained black nurses were totally unacceptable, and many of those approved barely met standards. Moreover, there were some 23,000 untrained black midwives in the South, but no one made the effort to combine training in nursing and midwifery, which

would have been a distinct service. In 1930, there were fewer than 6,000 graduate black nurses, most of whom worked in black hospitals or public health agencies that served black patients. Opportunities in other fields either were not open to them or could not admit them because they did not, understandably, have the advanced preparation necessary. Middle-class black women were usually not attracted to nursing, because teaching and other available fields offered more prestige and better opportunities. It was not until a 1941 Executive Order and the corresponding follow-through that any part of the federal government made any effort to investigate grievances and redress complaints of blacks. The subsidized Cadet Nurse Corps of World War II also proved to be a boon for black nurses. Of the schools participating, 20 were all-black and enrolled 600 black students; the remaining 400 were distributed among 22 integrated schools. However, it was clear that approved black schools were being held to lower standards for a variety of reasons, some political. There were also overt and covert methods in the North and South to prevent the more able black nurses from assuming leadership positions—some as simple as advancing the least aggressive. And for all the desperate need for nurses, the armed forces balked at accepting and integrating black nurses. Not until the end of the war and after some aggressive action by the NACGN and the National Nursing Council for War Service did this change.[17]

THE EFFECTS OF WORLD WAR II

Not just black nurses but nurses in general found that the exigencies of war created new opportunities, freedom, and also problems for nurses that proved to be long-lasting. As usual in wartime, nurses were in demand in the armed services. There were not enough nurses for both the home front and the battlefield, even with stepped-up efforts to encourage women to enter nursing programs. Finally, legislation was passed in 1943 estab-

*Finally, in 1951, the NACGN was absorbed into the ANA, which required nondiscrimination for all state associations as a prerequisite for ANA affiliation.

lishing the Cadet Nurse Corps. The Bolton Act, the first federal program to subsidize nursing education for school and student, was a forerunner of future federal aid to nursing. For payment of their tuition and a stipend, students committed themselves to engage in essential military or civilian nursing for the duration of the war. The students had to be between seventeen and thirty-five years old, in good health, and with a good academic record in an accredited high school. This new law brought about several changes in nursing. For instance, it forbade discrimination on the basis of race and marital status and set minimum educational standards. The first, theoretically accepted, was not always implemented in good faith. The second, combined with the requirement that nursing programs be reduced from the traditional thirty-six months to thirty, forced nursing schools to reassess and revise their curricula.

Two other major efforts to relieve the nursing shortage had long-range effects in the practice setting. One was the recruitment of inactive nurses back into the field. For the first time, married women and others who could work only on a part-time basis became acceptable to employers and later became part of the labor pool. The other change was the training of volunteer nurse's aides. Although such training was initiated by the Red Cross in 1919, it was discouraged later by nurses, particularly during the Depression. During World War II, both the Red Cross and the Office of Civilian Defense trained more than 20,000 aides. At first, they were used only for non-nursing tasks, but the increasing nurse shortage forced them to take on basic nursing functions. After the war, with a continued shortage, trained aides were hired as a necessary part of the nursing service department. Their perceived cost effectiveness stimulated the growth of both aide and practical nurse training programs and eventually increased federal funding for both.

Finally, major changes occurred within the armed forces. Nurses had held only relative rank, meaning that they carried officers' titles but had less power and pay than their male counterparts. In 1947, full commissioned status was granted, giving them the right to manage nursing care. At the same time, as noted previously, discrimination against black nurses ended but, oddly enough, in the male-controlled armed services, it was not until 1954 that male nurses were admitted to full rank as officers.

As in all previous wars, nurses proved themselves able and brave in military situations. Many were in battle zones and some became Japanese prisoners of war. Their stories have been told in films, books, plays, and historical nursing research, and are well worth reading. (See bibliography.)

TOWARD A NEW ERA

The usual postwar nurse shortage occurred after World War II, but this time for different reasons. Only one of six Army nurses planned to return to her civilian job, finding more satisfaction in the service. Poor pay and unpleasant working conditions discouraged civilian nurses as well. In 1946, the salary for a staff nurse was about $36 for a forty-eight-hour work week, less than that for typists or seamstresses (much less men). Salaries were supposed to be kept secret, and hospitals, particularly, held them at a minimum, with such peculiarities as a staff nurse earning more than a head nurse. Split shifts were common, with nurses scheduled to work from seven to eleven and from three to seven, with time off between the two shifts. The work was especially difficult because staffing was short and nurses worked under rigid discipline. It was small wonder than in one survey only about 12 percent of the nurses queried planned to make nursing a career; more than 75 percent saw it as a pin-money job after marriage, or planned to retire altogether as soon as possible. Unions were beginning to organize nurses, so in 1949 the ANA approved state associations as collective bargaining agents for nurses. However, because the Taft-Hartley Act excluded nonprofit institutions from collective bargaining, hospitals and agencies did not need to deal with nurses. In addition, the ANA no-strike pledge took away another powerful weapon.

As noted previously, one answer that administrators saw was the hiring of nurses's aides. The use of volunteers and auxiliary help—that is, anyone other than licensed or trained nurses, practical nurses, aides, or orderlies—increased tremendously.

One group of workers that proliferated in the postwar era was practical nurses, defined by ANA, NLNE, and NOPHN as those trained to care for subacute, convalescent, and chronic patients under the direction of a physician or nurse. Thousands who designated themselves as practical nurses had no such skills, and their training was simply in caring for their own families, or, at most, aide work. Whereas the first school for training practical nurses appeared in 1897, by 1930 there were only eleven, and in 1947, still only thirty-six. With the new demand for nurse substitutes, 260 more practical nurse schools opened by 1954, mostly in hospitals or long-term care institutions, and a few in vocational schools. Aiding the movement was funding from federal vocational education acts. There were, unfortunately, also a number of correspondence courses and other commercialized programs that did little more than expose the student to some books and manuals and present her with a diploma. By 1950, there were 144,000 practical nurses, 95 percent of them women, and, although their educational programs varied, their on-the-job activities expanded greatly—to doing whatever nurses had no time to do. By 1952, some 56 percent of the nursing personnel were nonprofessionals, and some nurses began to fear that they were being replaced by less expensive, minimally trained workers.

Nevertheless, with working and financial conditions not improving, the nursing shortage persisted. Soon, a team plan was developed with a nurse as a team leader, primarily responsible for planning patient care, and less prepared workers carrying it out. Although the plan persisted for years, it did little to improve patient care; rather, it kept the nurse mired in paper work, away from the patient or required to make constant medication rounds. Often practical nurses carried the primary responsibilities for patient units on the evening and night shift, with the few nurses available stretched thin, "supervising" these workers.

There were more nurses than ever at midcentury, but there were also tremendously expanded health services, a greater population to be served, growth of various insurance plans that paid for hospital care, a postwar baby boom with in-hospital deliveries, new medical discoveries that kept patients alive longer, and a proliferation of nurses into other areas of health care. Hospitals still weren't the most desirable places to work, and economic benefits were slow in coming. Moreover there were now more married nurses who chose to stay home to raise families. Studies done in 1944, 1947, and 1948,* all of which pointed out some of the economic and status problems of nurses, particularly in hospitals, went largely ignored.

When the Korean War broke out in 1950, the Army again drew nurses from civilian hospitals, this time from their reserve corps. War nursing on the battlefront was centered to an extent on the Mobile Army Surgical Hospitals (MASH), located as close to the front lines as possible. Flight nurses, who helped to evacuate the wounded from the battlefront to military hospitals, also achieved recognition. When that war was over and nurse reservists returned to their civilian jobs, it is possible that their experiences increased their discontent with working situations at home.

This was also a period of great medical and scientific discoveries, and physicians became increasingly dependent on hospitals for supportive services. As physicians cured or prolonged the lives of patients, the corollary care required of nurses became more complex. It was not just a matter of patient comfort, but crucial life-and-death judgment. In the 1950s,

---

*See Chapter 5.

Frances Reiter began to write about the nurse clinician, a nurse who gave skilled nursing care on an advanced level. This concept developed into the clinical specialist,* a nurse with a graduate degree and specialized knowledge of nursing care, who worked as a colleague of physicians. At the same time, the development of coronary and other intensive care units called for nurses with equally specialized technical knowledge, formerly the sole province of medical practice.* In Colorado in 1965, a physician, in collaboration with a school of nursing, was pioneering another new role for nurses in ambulatory care. As the nurses easily assumed responsibility for well-child care and minor illnesses, they called upon their nursing knowledge and skills as well as a medical component. What emerged was the "nurse practitioner."*

Nursing education was also going through a transition period in those decades. In the years immediately after World War II, the quality of nursing education was under severe criticism. There was no question that in the diploma schools, where most nurses were educated, there were frequently poor levels of teaching, inadequately prepared teachers, and a major dependence on students for services; often two-thirds of the hours of care were given by students.

The Brown Report† in 1948 and a follow-up study in 1950† that attempted to implement that report made it clear that nursing education was anything but professional. It was on the basis of findings of the latter report that national accreditation for nursing by nursing was strengthened.

With the reorganization of the nursing organizations, the National League for Nursing (NLN) assumed the responsibility for all accrediting functions in nursing. Dr. Helen Nahm, director of the accrediting service for the first seven years, saw it as the culmination of all previous efforts to raise nursing education standards—and as a last chance. Those

schools that chose to go through the voluntary process and met the standards were placed on a published list, which for the first time gave the public, guidance counselors, and potential students some notion of the quality of one school compared with another. Eventually, accreditation proved a significant force in improving good schools and closing poor ones (although it has also been accused of rigidity throughout the years).

An impetus for collegiate nursing education was an advisory service funded by the Russell Sage Foundation for institutions of higher learning that were interested in enriching and improving their programs. The 1953 report by Dr. Margaret Bridgman, "Collegiate Education for Nursing," helped to stimulate baccalaureate nursing programs to improve academically. In many cases, they were still quite similar to diploma programs, whose quality had improved considerably in the 1950s. The slow rate of growth of collegiate programs resulted in part from the uncertainty of nursing about what these programs should be and how they should differ from diploma education and in part from the anticollegiate faction in nursing that saw no point in higher education—a faction that was cheered and nurtured by a large number of physicians and administrators. At times, it seemed to be a moot question whether any nurses were necessary. A postwar survey of the American College of Surgeons indicated that the vast majority believed, with few exceptions, that the needs of the sick could be met by nurse's aides, or, at most, by practical nurses, and administrators were not averse to the "cheap is best" concept.

Introduction of a different kind of nurse was a startling breakthrough. The development of the nurse technician in community colleges was the most dramatic change in nursing education since its beginning. Based on a study by Dr. Mildred Montag at Teachers College, and funded by the W. K. Kellogg Foundation, pilot programs were established in a number of sites around the country in 1952. It was an idea whose time had come, for

---

*See Chapter 15.
†See Chapter 5.

not only were community colleges the most rapidly expanding educational entities of the time, but the late bloomer, the mature man and woman, and the less affluent student found this opportunity for a career in nursing and a college degree highly desirable. Follow-up studies showed that these nurses performed well in what they were prepared to do—provide care at the intermediate level in the continuum of nursing functions as defined by Montag. It was probably partially the influence of the associate degree (AD) programs, which were nondiscriminatory and generally nonpaternalistic in their relations with students, that helped loosen the tight restrictions on nursing students' personal lives in both diploma and some baccalaureate programs. Still, even into the late 1960s, some diploma schools excluded married students and men. The growth of AD programs ultimately outran all others in nursing except practical nurse programs.

Graduate education for nurses progressed slowly. Most degrees continued to be in education, in part because of the great shortage of teachers of nursing with graduate degrees and in part because graduate schools of education had part-time programs. In 1953, only 36 percent of nursing faculties had earned master's degrees, and some had no degree at all. In 1954, it was estimated that 20 percent of the positions held by nurses should require master's degrees and at least 30 percent baccalaureate degrees. Yet, only 1 percent of all nurses held master's and about 7 percent baccalaureate degrees, many not in nursing.

Part of the problem, of course, was financial and, although private foundations, such as the Commonwealth Fund, provided some support for graduate education, federal funding made the crucial difference. It also controlled the direction of nursing education. Its funding for the study of public health nursing from 1936 on created more baccalaureate-prepared nurses in public health than in any other field; its support of psychiatric nursing in-creased the volume of nurses educated in that field.[18] In 1956, the passage of the Federal Nurse Traineeship Act, which authorized funds for financial aid to registered nurses for full-time study to prepare for teaching, supervision, and administration in all fields, opened the door for advanced education for nurses at both the baccalaureate and graduate levels. Short-term traineeships also provided for continuing education programs. Another boost was the 1963 Surgeon General's Report* that specifically pointed out differences in the quality and quantity of nurses and their education and recommended both recruitment and advanced education. Following this, there was a new surge of federal aid to nursing. Nurse Traineeship programs continued to be enacted until the present although the struggle for funds, depending on the administration, was sometimes most difficult (see Chapters 12 and 19).

Master's programs for nurses still tended to focus on administration or education even in schools of nursing, and not until the 1960s did clinical programs develop. Clinical doctoral programs in nursing were nonexistent until the 1960s.

Nursing research also tended to take a slow path. Although there were studies of nursing service, nursing education, and nursing personality, most were done with or by social scientists. When nurses assisted physicians and others in medical research, it was just that—assisting. Nursing leaders realized that nursing could not develop as a profession unless clinical research focusing on nursing evolved. One of the first major steps in that direction was the 1952 publication of *Nursing Research,* a scholarly journal that reported and encouraged nursing research. The other was the ANA's establishment of the American Nurses' Foundation* in 1955 for charitable, educational, and scientific purposes. The Foundation conducts studies, surveys, and research, funds nurse researchers and others, and publishes scientific reports.

*See Chapter 5.

*See Chapter 25.

In 1956, the federal government also began to fund nursing research. Federal support in the 1960s provided research training through doctoral programs, including the nurse scientist program, and funding for individual and collaborative research efforts.

In all of these changes, it can be seen that the professional organizations of nursing had varied influence. At the same time, as organizations, they too were examining their roles and relationships. A study to consider restructuring, reorganizing, and unifying the various organizations was initiated shortly after World War II. In 1952, the six major nursing organizations—ANA, NLNE, NOPHN, NACGN, the Association of Collegiate Schools of Nursing (ACSN), and the American Association of Industrial Nurses (AAIN)—finally came to a decision about organizational structure. Two major organizations emerged, the ANA, with only nurse members, and the renamed National League for Nursing, with nurse, non-nurse, and agency membership. The AAIN decided to continue, and the National Student Nurses' Association was formed. (Practical nurses had their own organization.) (See Chapters 24, 25, 26, and 27 for details of the organizations.) Although there was an apparent realignment of responsibilities, the relationships between the ANA and NLN ebbed and flowed; sometimes they were in agreement and sometimes they were not; sometimes they worked together, and at other times each appeared to make isolated unilateral pronouncements. Some nurses longed for one organization, but there seemed to be mutual organizational reluctance to go in that direction. Yet, it must be said that in those changing times each had some remarkable achievements—NLN in educational accreditation; ANA in its lobbying activities, its development of a model licensure law in the mid-1950s, and its increased action in nurses' economic security.

Then, in 1965, ANA precipitated (or inflamed) an ongoing controversy. After years of increasingly firm statements on the place of nursing education in the mainstream of Amer-

ican education, ANA issued its first Position Paper on Education for Nursing. It stated, basically, that education for those who work in nursing should be in institutions of higher learning, that minimum education for professional nursing should be at least at the baccalaureate level; for technical nursing, at the associate degree level; and for assistants, in vocational education settings.

Although there had been increased complaints by third-party payers about diploma education, and diploma schools had declined as associate and baccalaureate degree programs increased, there was an outpouring of anger by diploma and practical nurses and those involved in their education. It was a battle that persisted and became another divisive force in nursing. But, then, so was the beginning of the nurse practitioner movement. There were nurses who feared it or saw it as pseudomedicine, detracting from pure nursing professionalism. The issues remain unresolved.

Therefore, whether or not 1965 can be considered the gateway to a new era of nursing, it was the beginning of dramatic and inevitable changes in the education and practice of nursing and in the struggle for nursing autonomy.

REFERENCES

1. Philip Kalisch and Beatrice Kalisch, *The Advance of American Nursing* (Boston: Little, Brown and Company, 1978), pp. 285–286.
2. Ibid., pp. 281–284.
3. Ibid., pp. 398–406.
4. Vern Bullough and Bonnie Bullough, *The Care of the Sick: The Emergence of Modern Nursing* (New York: Prodist, 1978), pp. 201–202.
5. Kalisch and Kalisch, op. cit., p. 297.
6. Ibid., pp. 295–325.
7. Teresa E. Christy, "Portrait of a Leader: Lavinia Lloyd Dock," *Nurs. Outlook,* **17**:74 (June 1969).
8. Ibid.
9. Kalisch and Kalisch, op. cit., p. 332.
10. Bullough and Bullough, op. cit., p. 156.
11. Dorothy D. Bromley, "The Crisis in

Nursing," *Harper's Magazine,* **161**:159–160 (July 1930).

12. Mary Lucille Shannon, "The Origin and Development of Professional Licensure Examinations in Nursing: From a State-Constituted Examination to the State Board Test Pool Examination," Unpublished Ed.D. dissertation, Teachers College, Columbia University, 1972, p. 127.

13. Beatrice Kalisch and Philip Kalisch, "Slaves, Servants, or Saints? An Analysis of the System of Nurse Training in the United States, 1873–1948," *Nurs. Forum,* **14,** 3:248 (1975).

14. Teresa Christy, "Portrait of a Leader: Isabel Maitland Stewart," *Nurs. Outlook* **17**:44–48 (Oct. 1969).

15. Teresa Christy, "Portrait of a Leader: M. Adelaide Nutting," *Nurs. Outlook,* **17**:20–24 (Jan. 1969).

16. Helen Tirpak, "The Frontier Nursing Service: Fifty Years in the Mountains," *Nurs. Outlook,* **23**:308–310 (May 1975).

17. Kalisch and Kalisch, *The Advance of American Nursing,* op. cit., pp. 553–569.

18. Ibid. p. 591.

Major Studies of the Nursing Profession

Although a great many of the studies in nursing that have been done in this country have helped to advance the profession as well as to solve local or immediate problems, comparatively few have marked a definite trend or greatly influenced the progress of nursing. Described here are the reports of research and studies that have guided nursing in the past and will always be considered milestones in the development of nursing.

The Educational Status of Nursing (1912). Conducted under the leadership of M. Adelaide Nutting, chairman of the education committee of the American Society of Superintendents of Training Schools for Nurses, and published by the U.S. Bureau of Education, this report resulted from a questionnaire study of what schools of nursing throughout the country were actually teaching their students at that time and the techniques employed. It also covered the students' working and living conditions. Although this study revealed many appalling practices, it did not create the stir in nursing or in the public that it should have. However, it did begin to establish nursing as a profession and to set a precedent for later studies. It also highlighted the need for continued investigation of educational prac-

tices in nursing, and—even as early as 1912—the need for schools of nursing to be independent from hospitals.

Nursing and Nursing Education in the United States. The Goldmark Report (1923). Also stimulated by Nutting, the Rockefeller Foundation funded a Committee for the Study of Nursing Education to investigate "the proper training of the public health nurse." It was chaired by Dr. C. E. A. Winslow, professor of public health, Yale University, and included ten physicians (two of whom were hospital superintendents), six nurses (Nutting, Goodrich, Wald, Clayton, Beard, and Ward), and two lay representatives. Secretary and chief investigator was Josephine Goldmark, who had already done a recognized field study. It soon became apparent that the scope of the study needed to be expanded to encompass nursing education in general. Goldmark gathered and synthesized the opinions of leading nurse educators and also surveyed and studied twenty-three schools of nursing and forty-nine public health agencies, seeking answers to questions about the preparation of teachers, administrators, and public health nurses, clinical and laboratory experience for students, financing of schools of nursing, licensure for nurses, and the development of university schools.

As the study pointed out, education of nurses was still on an apprenticeship basis, a method abandoned by other professionals. Moreover, the quality of the teachers was poor; formal instruction was erratic, uncoordinated, and frequently sacrificed to the needs of the hospital; and students were often poorly selected. In essence, there was little training and almost no education. The conclusions of this landmark study did not result solely from the survey but also from the firm opinions of its prestigious committee members and the opinions of nursing leaders interviewed. Because some have still not been implemented, they have a remarkably contemporary ring:[1]

Conclusion 1. That, since constructive health work and health teaching in families is best done by persons:

(a) capable of giving general health instruction, as distinguished from instruction in any one specialty; and

(b) capable of rendering bedside care at need; the agent responsible for such constructive health work and health teaching in families should have completed the nurses' training. There will, of course, be need for the employment, in addition to the public health nurse of other types of experts such as nutrition workers, social workers, occupational therapists, and the like.

That as soon as may be practicable all agencies, public or private, employing public health nurses, should require as a prerequisite for employment the basic hospital training, followed by a post-graduate course, including both class work and field work, in public health nursing.

Conclusion 2. That the career open to young women of high capacity, in public health nursing or in hospital supervision and nursing education, is one of the most attractive fields now open in its promise of professional success and of rewarding public service; and that every effort should be made to attract such women into this field.

Conclusion 3. That for the care of persons suffering from serious and acute disease, the safety of the patient and the responsibility of the medical and nursing professions demand the maintenance of the standards of educational attainment now generally accepted by the best sentiment of both professions and embodied in the legislation of the more progressive states; and that any attempt to lower these standards would be fraught with real danger to the public.

Conclusion 4. That steps should be taken through state legislation for the definition and licensure of a subsidiary grade of nursing service, the subsidiary type of worker to serve under practising physicians in the care of mild and chronic illness, and convalescence, and possibly to assist under the direction of the trained nurse in certain phases of hospital and visiting nursing.

Conclusion 5. That, while training schools for nurses have made remarkable progress, and while the best schools of today in many respects reach a high level of educational attainment, the average hospital training school is not organized on such a basis as to conform to the standards accepted in other educational fields; that the instruction in such schools is frequently casual and uncorrelated; that the educational needs and the health and strength of students are frequently sacrificed to practical hospital exigencies; that such shortcomings are primarily due to the lack of independent endowments for nursing education; that existing educational facilities are on the whole, in the majority of schools, inadequate for the preparation of the high grade of nurses required for the care of serious illness and for service in the fields of public health nursing and nursing education; and that one of the chief reasons for the lack of sufficient recruits of a high type to meet such needs lies precisely in the fact that the average hospital training school does not offer a sufficiently attractive avenue of entrance to this field.

Conclusion 6. That, with the necessary financial support and under a separate board or training school committee, organized primarily for educational purposes, it is possible, with completion of a high school course or its equivalents as prerequisite, to reduce the fundamental period of hospital training to 28 months, and at the same time, by eliminating unessential, noneducational routine, and adopting the principles laid down in Miss Goldmark's report, to organize the course along intensive and coordinated lines with such modifications as may be necessary for practical application; and that courses of this standard would be reasonably certain to attract students of high quality in increasing numbers.

Conclusion 7. Superintendents, supervisors, instructors, and public health nurses should in all cases receive special additional training beyond the basic nursing course.

Conclusion 8. That the development and strengthening of university schools of nursing of a high grade for the training of leaders is of fundamental importance in the furtherance of nursing education.

Conclusion 9. That when the licensure of a subsidiary grade of nursing service is provided for, the establishment of training courses in preparation for such service is highly desirable; that such courses should be conducted in special hospitals, in small unaffiliated general hospitals, or in separate sections of hospitals where nurses are also trained; and that the course should be of 8 or 9 months' duration; provided the standard of such schools be approved by the same educational board which governs nursing training schools.

Conclusion 10. That the development of nursing service adequate for the care of the sick and for the conduct of the modern public health campaign demands as an absolute prerequisite the securing of funds for the endowment of nursing education of all types; and that it is of primary importance, in this connection, to provide reasonably generous endowment for university schools of nursing.

Although the recommendations related to education are usually given the most attention, the Goldmark Report did not neglect its original focus on public health nursing.

Among other things, it was concluded that both bedside nursing care and health teaching for preventive care could be combined in one generalized service, as opposed to the separated services and agencies that were more common at the time.

Although the 500-page report was published, it did not have the wide dissemination, interest, or impact of the Flexner Report. Only a few of the recommendations were given serious consideration on a wide scale at the time. One important result of the study, however, was the establishment of the Yale Unversity School of Nursing in 1923, financed by the Rockefeller Foundation. This represented a significant forward step in education for nursing.

Nurses, Patients, and Pocketbooks (1928). This study was conducted by the Committee on the Grading of Nursing Schools, composed of twenty-one members representing the American Nurses' Association, National League of Nursing Education, National Organization for Public Health Nursing, the American Medical Association (which later withdrew), American College of Surgeons, American Hospital Association, American Public Health Association, and representatives of general education. Nurses contributed about one-half of the $300,000 needed to finance the study; the remainder came from foundations and friends of nursing, such as Frances Payne Bolton, who also served on the committee. May Ayres Burgess, a statistician, directed the study.

The committee focused on three separate studies: supply of and demand for graduate nurses; job analysis of nurses; and grading of nursing schools. The first report, *Nurses, Patients, and Pocketbooks,* showed that there was an oversupply of nurses, with serious unemployment problems; that there was a geographic maldistribution, with most nurses remaining in large cities; that salaries and working conditions were poor; and that although in general both patients and physicians were satisfied with nurses' services (which were, of course, primarily in the private duty sector), there was evidence of some serious incompetence.

An Activity Analysis of Nursing (1934). This is a report of the second study sponsored by the Committee on the Grading of Nursing Schools. The principal purpose of this study, conducted by Ethel Johns and Blanche Pfefferkorn at the committee's request, was to gather facts about nurses' activities that could be used as a basis for improving the curricula in schools of nursing. It represents the first large-scale attempt to find out what nurses were actually doing on the job—in hospitals, in public health agencies, and on private duty—and this focused attention on nursing service as well as on nursing education and encouraged a closer correlation of theory and practice.

Nursing Schools Today and Tomorrow (1934). This was the final report of the eight year study conducted under the auspices of the Committee on the Grading of Nursing Schools. It gave statistics on the number of "trained and untrained" nurses and answered such questions as: What should a professional nurse know and be able to do? How can hospitals provide nursing service? It described the nursing schools of the period and recommended essentials for a basic professional school of nursing.

A number of startling facts were brought to light. For instance, 42 percent of teachers in schools of nursing had not even graduated from high school; only 16 percent had a year or more of college. Again, it was pointed out that nursing was the only profession in which the student essentially provided all the service for her "learning" institution. Moreover, a large number of the existing schools were so small that student education was totally inadequate. The need for consistent evaluation of programs was urgent.

A Study on the Use of the Graduate Nurse for Bedside Nursing in the Hospital (1933).

This was the first study done by the NLNE Department of Studies, which was established in 1932, with Blanche Pfefferkorn as its director. Prompted by previous findings of the Grading Committee, Miss Pfefferkorn and her co-workers made a comparative study of the bedside activities of the graduate and student nurse in the hospital to lend support to the gradually emerging belief (somewhat reluctantly accepted by hospital administrators) that nursing care should be given principally by graduate staff nurses, not by nursing students. The study helped clarify the issues and laid a foundation for further reduction in the number of noneducational assignments given to students of nursing.

A Curriculum Guide for Schools of Nursing (1937). Although in style and format this publication does not appear to be a report of a study, the content was so much influenced by a study that it is sometimes referred to as such. The purpose of the study, directed by Isabel Stewart, chairman of the NLNE Committee on Curriculum, was to

> . . . gather evaluate, and present in usable form the most progressive ideas and practices in relation to the basic nursing curriculums that have been successfully tried out or are considered by competent judges to be suitable for use and practicable in nursing schools.

The need for this study was recognized following the issuance of two NLNE publications containing recommendations on curriculum content and method: *Standard Curriculum for Schools of Nursing,* (1917) and *A Curriculum for Schools of Nursing,* (1929). Although it was extremely helpful to directors and others responsible for schools of nursing, the curricula advocated in these first two publications proved to be too rigid to meet the changing emphasis on broader education for nurses. The word *guide* in the 1937 publication was, therefore, highly significant. The new guide, intended, according to Stewart, for students of professional caliber preparing themselves for a profession, placed much greater emphasis on application of the sciences. The role of the clinical instructor was stressed, and all faculty members were encouraged to use newer and more creative methods of teaching. The guide was never revised again but was used in many schools for another quarter-century.

Study of Incomes, Salaries and Employment Conditions Affecting Nurses (Exclusive of Those Engaged in Public Health Nursing) (1938). The ANA initiated this questionnaire survey, which was launched in 1936 and conducted through state studies sponsored by the twenty-three state nurses' associations that agreed to participate. The data obtained from more than 11,000 private duty, institutional, and office nurses were presented in the published report as state summaries, national findings, and recommendations. This study undoubtedly had considerable bearing on the development of the ANA's economic security program.

Administrative Cost Analysis for Nursing Service and Nursing Education (1940). Blanche Pfefferkorn directed this study, which was sponsored jointly by NLNE and AHA in cooperation with ANA. The major objectives of the study, as stated in the report (p. 4), were

1. To find out the cost to an individual hospital of
   a. Operating the nursing service without a school;
   b. Operating the nursing service with a school.
2. To develop methods and criteria which will make possible a valid comparison of costs in one institution with the costs in another.

This study, which focused on the purely business side of nursing service and education, produced some interesting and potentially usable data on the cost to the hospital of conducting a school of nursing and the economic value of the service rendered by nursing students, estimated in terms of graduate service.

Hospital administrators and nurse educators were greatly enlightened by this study, although it appears doubtful that many institutions actually adopted cost accounting for nursing education and service at that time.

The General Staff Nurse (1941). As it became more and more common for hospitals to employ graduate professional nurses to provide bedside nursing care, formerly given almost entirely by students, the organizations most concerned—ANA, NLNE, AHA, and CHA—felt the need to determine the status of general staff nurses as seen by directors of nursing, the nurses themselves, and others. A joint committee of these organizations was formed to make such a study. The report indicates that general staff nurses had little status at the time. This was reflected in their hours of duty, their salaries, and personnel policies. This study gave impetus to a movement to try to upgrade the status of the general staff nurse.

Hospital Care in the United States (1947). Although this study, conducted by the Commission on Hospital Care, a national group appointed by the AHA representing a wide variety of occupations and professions, was primarily concerned with hospitals in this country, it necessarily touched upon nurses and nursing because they are such an integral part of hospitals and the services they render.

An introductory statement noted:

We have boasted of our fine institutions, of the number of hospital beds per unit of population, and of the high standards of hospital care that exist in the United States. Yet, both physical facilities and the arrangements under which they operate leave much to be desired. Many of our hospitals are old and outmoded. Some are housed in makeshift adaptations of buildings designed for other purposes. In many urban communities, there is wasteful duplication of facilities created and continued by special interests, individual ambitions, and prejudices. There are many regions in the United States in which hospital care is quite inadequate. It is wholly lacking in some rural areas.

The survey was far-reaching in scope and recommendations, many of which applied to nursing service and education. The findings were of great interest to legislators, and it is generally agreed that the Hill-Burton Hospital Construction Act was influenced by this study. The report, published by the Harvard University Press for the Commonwealth Fund, is still considered a valuable source book.

Nursing for the Future (1948). Esther Lucile Brown, a social anthropologist with the Russell Sage Foundation, conducted this study for the National Nursing Council, a large group of representatives of many health organizations and services, which had functioned under other titles before and during World War II to recruit nursing students and coordinate military and civilian nursing needs.

The study, funded by the Carnegie Foundation for the Advancement of Teaching and the Sage Foundation (which published it), was to analyze the changing needs of the profession. Brown, who had already studied nursing as an emerging profession, gathered data by visiting nursing schools, attending workshops, and consulting with individual physicians and hospital administrators, as well as using both a nursing and a lay advisory committee.

The report of her findings was, ironically, not much different from those of earlier studies, indicating the slow progress of nursing education. At one point, Brown pondered "why young women in any large numbers would want to enter nursing as operated today."[2] Once more, the same inadequacies were pointed out and, once more, the closing of the several thousand small, weak schools was urged. In particular, Brown emphasized the necessity for official examination of all schools, publication and distribution of lists of accredited schools, and public pressure to eliminate the nonaccredited schools.[3]

In addition, she strongly recommended

"that effort be directed to building basic schools of nursing in universities and colleges, comparable in number to existing medical schools, that are sound in organizational and financial structure, adequate in facilities and faculty, and well-distributed to serve the needs of the entire country."[4] Noting that many diploma schools still operated for the staffing benefit of the hospital, she found nursing education not professional.

Although Brown was undoubtedly also influenced by her nursing advisors, many of whom had already made similar statements, the report was the first to make the point that nursing education as a whole, not just an elite part, should be part of the mainstream of education, and that nurses could be divided into professional and practical groups.

The report received mixed reviews. Many nurses felt threatened, and some physicians and hospital administrators considered it a subversive document, fearing that it had economic security implications for nurses. (Nor did they appreciate the fact that the authoritarianism of hospitals was pinpointed, as was the dilemma of the nurse caught between the demands of physicians and administrators.)

Therefore, although the Brown report prompted a reexamination of beliefs and attitudes about professional education and practice, relationships with practical nurses, and discrimination in the selection of students based on race, religion, sex, marital status, and economic background, in 1970, Lysaught found that many of the recommendations were still unfulfilled—and still valid.

A Program for the Nursing Profession (1948). Actually an account of the extended deliberations and thinking of a Committee on the Functions of Nursing rather than a report of study or research, this report was accorded the attention and had the immediate influence of a scientific presentation. Under the direction of Eli Ginzberg, a professor of economics at Columbia University, the committee, which originated in the Division of Nursing Education of Teachers College, Columbia University, with representatives from nursing, medicine, and the social sciences, undertook to identify the problems confronting nursing and to suggest their solutions. The group found the shortage of personnel to be the outstanding problem in nursing at that time and attributed that shortage to minimal economic incentives in nursing, the public's increasing need for health care and more nurses, the "apparent financial weakness" of voluntary hospitals, and inefficient use of available nursing personnel. The committee recommended a number of broad and specific solutions related to both nursing education and service, encompassing both practical and professional nurses.

Nursing Schools at the Mid-Century (1950). Current national accreditation procedures for schools of professional nursing were influenced by the findings of this study of practices (in 1949) in more than 1,000 schools of nursing. The study represented one attempt to implement the Brown Report, previously described. Conducted under the auspices of the National Committee for the Improvement of Nursing Services (a committee of the joint board of the six national nursing associations in existence at that time), the study covered such areas as organization of the schools, the cost of nursing education, curriculum content, clinical resources, student health, and others. The report contained statistics, tables, and graphs that schools used to evaluate their own performance as compared with that of others.

Patterns of Patient Care (1955). This study was conducted under the direction of Frances L. George and Dean Ruth Perkins Kuehn of the University of Pittsburgh. Its main purposes were to determine how much nursing service was needed by a group of nonsegregated medical and surgical patients in a large general hospital and how much of this service could safely be delegated to nursing aides and other nonprofessional personnel. The report, published by the Macmillan Publishing Company, New York, contained much practical information about staffing patterns and the allocation of duties which was helpful to other nursing service administrators and of interest to all nurses. Variations of these suggested staffing patterns were used in a number of hospitals for years.

Twenty Thousand Nurses Tell Their Story (1958). This is a report of a five-year program of studies of nursing functions, initiated by ANA and the American Nurses' Foundation (ANF), made possible by the financial support of individual nurses throughout the country, and made meaningful by the 20,000 nurses who were "guinea pigs" in one way or another for the study. The report of results, prepared under the direction of Everett C. Hughes, professor of sociology at the University of Chicago, who also helped with some of the thirty-four studies, was published by the J. B. Lippincott Company, Philadelphia.

These studies, intended to produce better care for patients, revealed what nurses actually were doing on the job, their attitude toward their role as they saw it, and their satisfaction in their work.

The results formed the basis for the development of stated functions, standards, and qualifications of nurses prepared by each ANA section for its members. The studies also indicated that further research was needed in many rapidly developing areas of nursing practice, both clinical and nonclinical.

Community College Education for Nursing (1959). Mildred Montag wrote Part I of this report of a five-year Cooperative Research Project in Junior and Community College Education for Nursing. Part II was written by Lasser G. Gotkin. The project was sponsored by the Institute of Research and Service in Nursing Education at Teachers College, Columbia University, New York, and the report was published by McGraw-Hill Book Company, New York.

This was an "action research" project in that a program was developed with methods of evaluating its effectiveness built into the planning. Seven junior/community colleges cooperated in the study by establishing two-year programs leading to an associate degree in nursing. Dr. Montag participated in the planning of all programs.

Part II of the report gives data obtained from 811 graduates of the junior/community colleges, presenting persuasive arguments for the establishment of more associate degree programs to prepare nurses for first-level positions in nursing.*

Toward Quality in Nursing: Needs and Goals (1963). The Consultant Group on Nursing, a twenty-five-member panel of representatives from nursing, medicine, hospital administration, other areas of the health field, and the public, was appointed in 1961 by the Surgeon General of the U.S. Public Health Service to advise him on nursing needs and to identify what role the federal government should take in assuring adequate nursing services for the nation. The report of this group discussed major problem areas and recommended a number of measures for their solution.

Quantitative and qualitative shortages of various levels of nursing personnel were emphasized; deficiencies in the educational preparation for nursing were summarized; recruitment needs to assure adequate personnel by 1970 were projected; problems in attracting, retaining, utilizing, and upgrading personnel through improved nursing administration were identified; and the need for augmentation and support of nursing research was stressed.

One recommendation urged the nursing profession, with the aid of federal and private funds, to begin a study of the present system of nursing education; the remaining recommendations were directed specifically toward areas requiring federal financial assistance.

An Abstract for Action (1970). This study

_____
*See Chapter 13 for more detail on the original Montag dissertation and its effect on nursing education.

was a direct result of a recommendation by the Surgeon General's Consultant Group on Nursing in its 1963 report, *Toward Quality in Nursing.* These experts recommended a national investigation of nursing education with special emphasis on the responsibilities and skills required for high-quality patient care. Although provision of funds for such a study was also recommended, no government funds were forthcoming.

Shorty thereafter, the ANA and National League for Nursing (NLN) established a joint committee to determine ways to conduct and finance such a study. The scope of the proposed study was enlarged to examine not only the changing practices and educational patterns of current nursing, but also probable future requirements. Confident that the problems of nursing ranged beyond the manpower problem, which the President's National Advisory Committee on Health Manpower was about to investigate, the ANF in the fall of 1966 voted to grant up to $50,000 to help launch a study. Impressed by this willingness of nursing to back its conviction that the study was needed, both the Avalon Foundation and the Kellogg Foundation granted $100,000 each to support the investigation. At the same time, an anonymous benefactor contributed $300,000.

In a meeting with the proposed head of the study, W. Allen Wallis, president of the University of Rochester and of the joint committee, it was decided that the study group to be set up would be an independent agency, functioning as a self-directing group with the power to plan and conduct its investigations as it saw fit. No participants would be selected to represent an interest group or a particular position, but would be chosen for their broad knowledge of nursing, their skills in related disciplines, such as medicine and health administration, or their competency in relevant fields, such as economics, education, management, and social research. By January 1968, the new National Commission for the Study of Nursing and Nursing Education (NCSNNE) was fully established with twelve commissioners (three of whom were nurses); a project director, Jerome P. Lysaught; an associate director, Charles H. Russell; and a small staff. A timetable for the three-year study was set, including the provision for a contingency operation (until January 1971) to initiate implementation of the recommendations.

Basically, the study focused on the supply of and demand for nurses, nursing roles and functions, nursing education, and nursing careers. After reviewing the emerging trends affecting the health care system, the commission set as its major objective to "improve the delivery of health care to the American people, particularly through the analysis and improvement of nursing, and nursing education." To meet this objective, two general approaches were used—the analysis of current practices and patterns and the assessment of future needs.

The methods of study included observational and descriptive tasks, combined with collection and analysis of findings from other studies. The findings and recommendations, plus projections for the future, were then subjected to the scrutiny of groups and individuals involved in the delivery of health care. The project staff likened this approach to the work of Flexner in his study of American medicine, refined by the experience of professional studies conducted in the last quarter century. A nursing advisory panel of ten was appointed to advise on plans for the study, suggest locations for site visits, and generally review and criticize each stage of the study. In addition, a health professions advisory panel, consisting of individuals with broad experience and understanding, was selected to ensure a rounded analysis of each content area. The two panels also provided a means for reaching a consensus and a reasonable compromise in terms of the needs of the health field when rival solutions to problems were presented.

Overall, there was an extensive search of the literature, questionnaires and surveys, 100 site visits, and a number of invitational confer-

ences and meetings involving leaders in nursing service, nursing education, medicine, health administration, consumer groups, and third-party payers, to react to preliminary recommendations.[5] The final report, entitled *An Abstract for Action,* was published in mid-1970, followed by a second volume of *Appendices* in 1971. A total of some fifty-eight specific recommendations and subsumed recommendations emerged from the report, with four priorities cited:

> Increased research into the practice of nursing and education of nurses; improved educational systems and curricula based on the results of that research; clarification of roles and practice conjointly with other health professions to insure the delivery of optimum care; and increased financial support for nurses and for nursing to ensure adequate career opportunities that will attract and retain the number of individuals required for quality health care in the coming years.[6]

The report concluded with four central recommendations:

1. The federal Division of Nursing, the National Center for Health Services Research and Development, other government agencies, and private foundations appropriate grant funds or research contracts to investigate the impact of nursing practice on the quality, effectiveness, and economy of health care.

2. Each state have or create, a master planning committee that will take nursing education under its purview, such committees to include representatives of nursing education, other health professions, and the public, to recommend specific guidelines, means for implementation, and deadlines to ensure that nursing education is positioned in the mainstream of American educational patterns.

3. A National Joint Practice Commission, with state counterpart committees, be established between medicine and nursing to discuss and make recommendations con-

cerning the congruent roles of the physician and the nurse in providing quality health care, with particular attention to the use of the nurse clinician; the introduction of the physician's assistant; the increased activity of other professions and skills in areas long assumed to be the concern solely of the physician and/or the nurse.

4. Federal, regional, state and local governments adopt measures for the increased support of nursing research and education. Priority should be given to construction grants, institutional grants, advanced traineeships and research grants and contracts. Further, we recommend that private funds and foundations support nursing research and educational innovations where such activities are not publicly aided. We believe that a useful guide for the beginnings of such a financial aid program would be in the amounts and distribution of funds authorized by Congress for fiscal 1970, with proportional increases from other public and private agencies.[7]

The report was received with mixed reactions, and continued to be controversial. Some stated that the research was poorly done; others that many of the recommendations were not valid; still others that there was little that was new.

Eventually, however, all the major nursing organizations, the AMA, AHA, and other health groups either published a statement of support for the report or endorsed it "in principle." An NLN Task Force studied the National Commission report in depth, and in early 1973 its report was published. Each recommendation had been evaluated and either endorsed or revised and restated, with a rationale for the suggested revision. The greatest concerns were with the concept of "episodic" and "distributive" care and specific recommendations for nursing education.[8]

The determination of the commission and the project staff to begin implementation of the recommendations resulted in a commitment of funds for one year of implementation by ANA and NLN. Thereupon the Kellogg

Foundation agreed to underwrite the project for two years and share with nursing the support for a third year, a total of $361,000 of Kellogg support and $25,000 each from ANA and NLN. In 1973 the status of the implementation effort was reported in *From Abstract into Action*.

At the beginning of this new phase, there was a reconstitution of the commission, which had fulfilled its task, with some members moving to a National Advisory Board. Leroy C. Burney, MD, president of the Milbank Memorial Fund, became president of the commission. In addition, five advisory committees of varied makeup, including other disciplines, were also established. Nine target states were designated to begin involvement and demonstration of the practical tasks of implementation, and regional associates were appointed to aid in these efforts. The priority items of implementation were set as nursing roles and functions, nursing education, and nursing careers.

The timetable of the staff included emphasis on educational and informational activities for various "publics" the first year, development of a National Joint Practice Commission between nursing and medicine and state counterparts the second year, and concentration on generation of statewide master planning committees and changes in patterns of education and practice the third year.

During the first year, numerous articles, reviews, and commentaries were written about the report, the recommendations, and implementation by staff and interested individuals. Sixteen pamphlets were developed and printed by NCSNNE on particular concerns that grew out of the implementation phase. There were also frequent general speaking engagements and meetings with target state groups. By the summer of 1971, a newly organized National Joint Practice Commission (NJPC) had been established with ten nurses and ten physicians, each a practitioner engaged in direct patient care approximately 50 per cent of the time. The group developed a number of specific objectives, focused on the basic charge of the commission's recommendation. Subsequently, NCSNNE attention was given to models of "episodic" and "distributive" care in education and practice, study of new utilization patterns, and progress in nursing research. In terms of educational changes, much interest was focused on open curriculum, preparation of nurses in the expanded role, and some aspects of graduate education. In terms of careers, the commission looked at economic and social satisfactions, new approaches to extend the horizons of nursing, the impact of organizations, and the licensure dilemma.[9]

In summarizing the effect of the National Commission report on nursing and health care, it is necessary to recognize that it is difficult to differentiate between changes that may have occurred through a normal process of evolving trends and those that could have been a direct result of NCSNNE recommendations. For instance, there has been an upsurge of action in continuing education, open curriculum programs, and increase in AD and baccalaureate programs. It is entirely possible that the report at least accelerated, if it did not initiate, action.

One specific action that occurred was the formation of the NJPC and its counterparts on the state, local, and institutional levels. Most states began, or continued, formalized nurse–physician dialogue, although some eventually dissolved, frequently because of lack of physician interest or inadequate organization. The national organization, funded in part by the Kellogg Foundation, early on made important statements.[10] It remained active until 1981.

Other NCSNNE interests did not have as long-lasting an impact. Many statewide master planning committees were formed, but actual results of their planning are not as evident. A few diploma programs made progress toward becoming independent educational programs; a limited number of educational programs revised their curriculums to incorporate the concepts of episodic and distributive care. Particularly disappointing was that,

after the major increase in federal support to nursing in 1972, there was a totally negative attitude on the part of the administration and a consequent cutback of funds.

Lysaught concluded that there was still much to be accomplished but indicated "faith and hope" that continued progress would ensue.

In 1977, he conducted a national survey of nursing service directors to determine how much progress had been made on four selected projections of the final report: joint practice committees, a reward system for increased nursing competence, enhancement of career perspectives through recognition of advanced clinical competence, and increase of ties and joint responsibilities between nursing education and nursing service. The results showed minimum progress toward these goals on the grass-roots level. Perhaps remembering that the Commission had repeated some of the recommendations of Brown's report, Lysaught suggested that the next years "should be characterized not by further search but by accomplished fulfillment."[11]

Extending the Scope of Nursing Practice: A Report of the Secretary's Committee to Study Extended Roles for Nurses (1971) At the request of the Secretary of Health, Education, and Welfare (HEW), a multidisciplinary committee was formed to study potential and actual new roles for nursing. The committee, which was chaired by Dr. Roger O. Egeberg, then Special Assistant for Health Policy at DHEW, consisted of thirteen physicians and thirteen nurses, as well as administrators and trustees of hospitals, administrators of schools of allied health, and knowledgeable DHEW staff. The purpose was to "examine the field of nursing practice, to offer some suggestions on how its scope might be extended, and to clarify the many ambiguous relationships between physicians and nurses."[12] The committee elected to view the subject from the perspective of the consumers of health services. The preface of the report ended with the statement:

We believe that the future of nursing must encompass a substantially larger place within the community of the health professions. Moreover, we believe that extending the scope of nursing practice is essential if this nation is to achieve the goal of equal access to health services for all its citizens. . . . [13]

The report reviewed many current responsibilities of nurses, from simple tasks to expert, professional techniques necessary in acute life-threatening situations, and noted the nurse's role on the health team, as leader of the nursing team, and in counseling, teaching, planning, and assessing. The committee delineated major elements of nursing practice in primary, acute, and long-term care, indicating those elements for which nurses already had primary responsibility, those for which responsibility was exercised by either physicians or nurses or a member of the allied health professions, and those responsibilities for which some nurses were already prepared and others could be prepared. Although recognizing that most nurses were not currently educationally prepared to assume extended roles and that some were reluctant to accept these roles, the committee arrived at certain conclusions and recommendations it believed significant in achieving extended roles for nursing. Legal considerations of the role were also reviewed (see Chapter 20).

Because of the impact of the report and the specific recommendations on both nursing practice and education, and subsequent DHEW financial support to programs and individuals willing to carry out these recommendations, they are cited here:

Health education centers should undertake curricular innovations that demonstrate the physician-nurse team concept in the delivery of care in a variety of settings under conditions that provide optimum opportunity for both professions to seek the highest levels of competence. Financial support should be made available for programs of continuing nurse education that could prepare the present pool of over one million active and inactive nurses to function in extended roles. The continuing education of nurses should be structured to encourage professional advancement among and through all nursing education programs and to encourage the use of equivalency examinations to evaluate competence, knowledge, and experience.

Increased attention should be paid to the commonality of nursing licensure and certification and to the development and acceptance of a model law of nursing practice suitable for national application through the States. The nursing profession should undertake a thorough study of recertification as a possible means of documenting new or changed skills among practicing nurses.

Collaborative efforts involving schools of medicine and nursing should be encouraged to undertake programs to demonstrate effective functional interaction of physicians and nurses in the provision of health services and the extension of those services to the widest possible range of the population. The transfer of functions and responsibilities between physicians and nurses should be sought through an orderly process recognizing the capacity and desire of both professions to participate in additional training activities intended to augment the potential scope of nursing practice. A determined and continuing effort should be made to attain a high degree of flexibility in the interprofessional relationships of physicians and nurses. Jurisdictional concerns per se should not be permitted to interfere with efforts to meet patient needs.

Cost–benefit analyses and similar economic studies should be undertaken in a variety of geographic and institutional settings to assess the impact on the health care delivery system of extended nursing practice.* Toward the same objective, attitudinal surveys of health care providers and consumers should be conducted to assess the significance of factors that might affect the acceptance of nurses in

---

*An appendix to this paper listed more than thirty locations in which nurses were being prepared for or were practicing in extended roles at that time.

extended care roles which they do not now normally occupy.

The Study of Credentialing in Nursing: A New Approach (1979). There were two major considerations that precipitated a study of credentialing in nursing: an ongoing disagreement and/or confusion between ANA and NLN on their respective roles in credentialing nurses, which was becoming somewhat acidulous by the mid-1970s, and increased activity by state and federal governments, presumably indicating public disaffection on the whole matter of health manpower credentialing (see Chapter 20). It was the action of the 1974 ANA House of Delegates "to examine the feasibility of accreditation of basic and graduate education" that stimulated two conferences on credentialing, under the sponsorship of the ANA Commission on Education. The outcome of these conferences, in which NLN and the American Association of Colleges of Nursing (AACN) were also involved, was a recommendation that a feasibility study should encompass more than accreditation, that it should be broadened to include assessment of credentialing mechanisms for organized nursing services, certification, and licensure, and "to formulate a proposal for studying the adequacy of these mechanisms, and to recommend future directions."[14]

In August 1975, ANA contracted with the Center for Health Research, College of Nursing, Wayne State University, to complete a proposal that had been developed in draft form at the second credentialing conference. The proposal that was developed had as its stated purposes (1) to assess the adequacy of current credentialing mechanisms in nursing, including accreditation, certification, and licensure, for providing quality assurance to the public served, and (2) to recommend future directions for credentialing in nursing. The study was to include nursing service and nursing education, but was not to attempt to demonstrate the relationship between credentials and the quality of care. The proposal was accepted by the ANA Board of Directors in De-

cember 1975. When the NLN declined to co-sponsor the study, the ANA proceeded to do so alone in August 1976. At that time, the Committee for the Study of Credentialing in Nursing (CSCN) was appointed—ten nurses and five others, with the later addition of Dr. Margretta Styles, former dean of the Wayne State College of Nursing, as chairperson. A project director, Inez G. Hinsvark, professor in the School of Nursing, University of Wisconsin, Milwaukee, was selected as project director. The twenty-four-month contract negotiated by ANA specified that the study committee have responsibility for the program, and the university, the administrative responsibility.

The purposes of the study remained essentially the same, with the addition of "to suggest ways for increasing the effectiveness of credentialing." It was a complex task of some magnitude. The study began with a comprehensive review of the literature and information, position papers, documents, and laws that were offered by various state agencies, nursing associations, and credentialing agencies. Groups of nursing and related health organizations and agencies concerned about nursing credentialing were invited to participate as cooperating groups and became a useful source of information. A model was constructed, composed of three areas identified for analysis: governance, policy, and control of credentialing within nursing; credentialing in the job market; and credentialing in nursing education. In addition, a set of principles appropriate to guide all credentialing endeavors was created, and current issues in credentialing and barriers to change were identified with position statements formulated. The methodologies used in the study included interviews, meetings, a modified Delphi technique, content analysis of written materials, and surveys.

The committee's final recommendations encompassed the following: principles to be applied to credentialing in nursing; position statements concerning definitions of nursing, entry into practice, control and cost of credentialing, accountability, and competence; credentialing definitions and their application to nursing (licensure, registration, certification, educational degrees, accreditation, charter, recognition, approval); the establishment of a national nursing credentialing center; and a statement that "the professional society in nursing, currently called the American Nurses' Association, make provision for categories of memberships for credentialed nursing personnel and students of nursing."[15] Plans for follow-up were also suggested.

In 1979, an independent task force for implementation of the report was established by the ANA Board of Directors. Despite stated concerns by some members of the 1980 House of Delegates that the independence of the task force threatened the possibility of ANA "control" of nursing credentialing, a resolution was passed supporting implementation "based on continuing review, development, and necessary modification" as well as cooperation of appropriate nursing groups. The task force of fifteen distinguished individuals (including eleven nurses) began its work with funding from ANA, one SNA and some specialty nursing organizations.

The Task Force on Credentialing in Nursing worked for two and a half years, cooperating with 146 groups that were willing to be "resource groups." These included national, state, and regional nursing associations, nursing certification boards, other health professional associations, educational associations, boards of nursing, the Armed Services Nurse Corps, Veterans Administration Nursing Service, and subgroups of ANA. A small percentage of these groups and some individuals made financial contributions, but ANA bore the major burden of support for the activities of the Task Force. ANF assumed administrative responsibility.

An early accomplishment of the Task Force was an informational packet and audiotape entitled "Credentialing Issues and Answers," both of which were sold at cost. A speaker's bureau, available to groups on request, was also maintained. However, after considerable study of the original report, the major focus

of the Task Force was the development of alternative structures and models of a credentialing center. The final recommendations described sixteen design parameters for a center, but the crucial points were that the center should be separately incorporated, established within the private, voluntary sector, with support and involvement of (but not separate control by) current credentialers of nursing, as well as the public and the "community of interests" (such as the American Hospital Association), and that the center must be involved in all aspects of nursing credentialing, including licensure. Specific recommendations were also made on how the center could be implemented immediately through a coalition of nursing organizations.

This report was presented to representatives of national nursing organizations considered potential coalition members and some of the nursing press on April 24, 1982. Although seventy-three resource groups had endorsed the *principle* of a national nursing credentialing center, it was immediately clear that if implementation meant giving up control of their own credentialing activities, the national organizations including ANA were not interested. Although all groups expressed interest in continued dialogue and some still endorsed the concept or principle of a center, only the Public Health Nursing Section of the American Public Health Association reiterated its support, and the National Council of State Boards of Nursing (NCSBN) expressed no position on a free-standing center as proposed. It was finally agreed that ANA, NLN, NCSBN, the National Association for Practical Nurse Education and Service (NAPNES), and the National Federation for Specialty Nursing Organizations (NFSNO) would co-convene a meeting of the credentialing organizations within four months. However, this did not occur.

Currently, the nurse credentialing mechanisms continue as they did before the original study. As noted in the ANA statement given at that final meeting and later affirmed by the House of Delegates, the ANA moved to the establishment of a separately incorporated credentialing center under the aegis of ANA, but no other organization is participating. The Task Force dissolved itself after the meeting; its final report was distributed through ANF.[16] Nurse credentialing remains in the same state of confusion.

In the last decade, the number of studies about and important to the nursing profession have increased. Some are national studies that are federally funded and include such topics as the career patterns of nurses, trends in RN supply, job availability for new graduates, and the distribution, salaries, and job responsibilities of nurse practitioners. For instance, one major study of this kind, *Analysis and Planning for Improved Distribution of Nursing Personnel and Services,* which was contracted to the Western Interstate Commission for Higher Education by the then Department of Health, Education, and Welfare in 1975, was geared to strengthen nurses' abilities to analyze and plan for improved distribution of nursing personnel and services, explore ways to reduce uneven distribution, and involve nurses in health planning. One of the most complex activities was the development of a state model for planners to project nursing manpower resources and requirements—a major breakthrough in the field.[17]

For a number of reasons, the early 1980s produced especially significant nursing studies. Ironically, all began and may have been somewhat influenced by the nursing shortage then at its peak, and almost all the reports were released as the shortage *appeared,* at least, to be subsiding. Whether or not this situation will eventually dilute their impact is yet to be seen.

A report released in late 1980, although not directly related to nursing, created a stir in the nursing community because of its implications for the profession. The Graduate Medical Education National Advisory Committee (GMENAC) had been charged by the Secretary of the Department of Health and Human Services (DHHS) to advise on "the number of physicians required in each specialty to bring supply and requirements into balance, methods to improve the geographic distribution of physicians, and mechanisms to finance graduate medical education."[18] The committee consisted primarily of physicians. The overall conclusion was that there would be an oversupply of physicians by the year 2000, and many recommendations were related to this point. As noted by a nurse member in a dissenting opinion, the focus on "non physician health care practice" centered primarily on the question of physician service substitutability and delegation of medical services as these affect physician manpower requirements, and the attitude was described as skeptical and negative. The recommendations repeatedly stated that the number of physician assistants (PAs), nurse practitioners (NPs), and nurse-midwives being graduated from educational programs each year should not be increased until the need for them could be determined. The desired numbers were those needed to attain the delegation levels which had been deemed desirable by the GMENAC. The "medical" services of NPs and PAs were to be under the supervision of a physician, and third-party reimbursement was to be made only to the employing institution or physician in relation to the physician manpower. While not all the recommendations were so negative, the report was seen by many nurses as one more act of interference by medicine with nursing's professional development.

One study referred to frequently during this time was related to nurse employment in Texas. [19,20] Released in 1980, it was replicated in many other states and helped to stimulate national studies exploring the factors that affected nurses' employment satisfaction, particularly in hospitals. Spurred by the severe nursing shortage, the purpose of *Conditions Associated with Registered Nurse Employment in Texas* was to determine the reasons for nurses' working or not working in nursing and to decide how they might be attracted back into the work force. By means of a questionnaire and interviews, more than 10,000 Texas nurses were asked to describe their feelings about nursing. In addition, administrators, educators, and nurses participated in a nominal group conference to generate innovative and practical ideas for attracting and keeping nurses.

The findings of the study indicated that the chief component of job dissatisfaction was that structural elements in the job (hospital policies and administration attitudes) kept nurses from providing patients with professional care.

It was determined that the following professional prerogatives were not accommodated:

- Autonomy of practice and respect for the judgment of the professional.
- Determination of standards of quality of care and determination of staffing needs and work schedules to achieve the standards.
- Educational programs and support (financial and time) for updating knowledge and skills.
- Participating with full vote in establishing policy related to patient care, personnel benefits, and working conditions.
- Work responsibilities that are nurse related, with elimination of requirements for nurses to perform tasks that are responsibilities of other services.
- Opportunities for professionals to share expertise with other professionals in other agencies, on hospital time.
- Recognition and personnel benefits comparable to those accorded other health care professionals.[21]

Major dissatisfactions cited were inadequate salaries and benefits, the amount of paper work, and lack of both hospital and nursing administrative support; specific conditions distressing to nurses were listed. Satisfied nurses were also able to pinpoint those factors that created a good working environment. Much had to do with the way their nurse administrators (properly qualified) functioned and their own ability to function as autonomous professionals.

Innovative ideas generated by the nominal group included the following: encourage self-scheduling by RN's with appropriate accountability; delineate nursing functions and eliminate nonnursing functions; develop a career ladder; plan recognition and merit awards for high-quality nursing care; establish group peer review; establish a joint practice committee with physicians; provide nursing residencies; give recognition to high-stress areas; provide for flexible schedules (a structured work week with ten- to twelve-hour days); develop pools of part-time nurses; provide child-care facilities; give bonuses to staff nurses who recruit inactive nurses.

One immediate outcome of the study was that a number of hospitals across the country initiated some of these innovative suggestions, with some evidence of success.

Almost simultaneously with the Texas study, several other extensive studies were undertaken. Two, federally funded, examined the effect of federal funding on nursing. The third, a multidisciplinary study, looked at nursing from the viewpoint of its relationship to health care delivery, particularly hospitals. The fourth was initiated by the American Academy of Nursing (AAN) to identify factors that attract and hold nurses in hospitals. Together, these studies present a view of nursing that has some interesting areas of agreement and disagreement and has a real potential for influencing the direction of the profession.

Effects of Federal Support for Nursing Education on Admissions, Graduations, and Retention Rates at Schools of Nursing. In some ways, the report *Effects of Federal Support for Nursing Education on Admissions, Graduations, and Retention Rates at Schools of Nursing* was overshadowed by the congressionally mandated Institute of Medicine (IOM) report. Prepared by Abt, a professional consultant company, for the Health Resources Administration, the study examined federal assistance to nursing education from only one perspective: its impact on the number of students entering, continuing in, and graduating from basic nurse training programs. The authors blamed limitations of available data for their inability to report also on the effect of federal funds on advanced training, educational quality, access for minorities, and other areas of intended impact that were included in the objectives that the legislation of 1964 and subsequent years was intended to achieve.

The study used year-by-year data on the admission, attrition, and graduation of individual nursing schools from 1969 (1968 for associate degree programs) to 1979. Although there were frequent references to lack of data and problems in the statistical analysis of the data, it was clearly stated that federal funds had certain important effects: 47,000 additional admissions and 32,800 to 42,200 additional graduates in basic programs in the ten years studied, and a higher than average retention rate among those entering nursing school as a result of federal funding. It was also noted that although it was unrealistic to expect federal support to produce massive changes in the size of the nursing workforce in a short time, the impact over the decade had been appreciable.

Nursing and Nursing Education: Public Policies and Private Actions. The findings of a significant study mandated by Public Law 96-76, the Nurse Training Act Amendments of 1979 (NTA), and contracted to the IOM by DHHS were presented in 1983 as *Nursing and Nursing Education: Public Policies and Private Actions.* A six-month interim report in July 1981 had raised strong protests in the nursing community.

The original purpose of this study was in some ways similar to that of the Abt study in that it was prompted by the question of whether further substantial outlays for nursing education were needed to assure an adequate supply of nurses. However, it went further. As expressed in the legislative history, the intent of the mandate was to secure an objective assessment of the need for continued federal support, to make recommendations

for improving the distribution of nurses in medically underserved areas, and to suggest actions to encourage nurses to remain active in their profession.

The study committee was composed of Institute members and recognized experts in public policy in disciplines related to nursing. Out of the twenty-six members, nine were nurses. Neither the chairman nor the staff were nurses, but some were included on the ad hoc advisory panels established. Because new data collection was apparently discouraged by a key congressional committee, the study's findings were based primarily on the synthesis and interpretation of data secured from existing sources. This became a controversial point when the interim report was released, since much of the same data, including that garnered from open hearings, was the basis of the Commission on Nursing study, and that interim report, presented only months later, contained very different recommendations. Included in the IOM data were seventy-five recent state-level studies of nursing, as well as national survey and inventory data about RNs and licensed practical nurses (LPNs). The interim report contained summaries of useful information about nursing in 1981 but raised provocative questions. Frequently, the reports of data analysis were the same as those in other studies. For example, the information on nurses' job dissatisfaction was almost identical to that contained in the Texas study and the Commission report. Some of the findings, while not necessarily palatable to organized nursing, were certainly issues already discussed within the profession. Criticism by nursing focused primarily on the fact that, as compared to the GMENAC committee, controlled by physicians, here nurses were in the minority, which could suggest "a view of nursing as an occupation that is not clinically valued and that must have others assume leadership and major input in making recommendations regarding what is best for it."[22]

Moreover, while no actual recommendations were made, certain statements were interpreted to mean that the IOM Committee tended to see nursing in relation to resource allocation and cost rather than quality. There was the implication that the minimum baccalaureate degree advocated by nursing might result in increased salaries, fewer nurses, and a lower quality of care. A major concern, of course, was that the IOM report, being mandated by Congress, would also greatly influence legislation affecting nursing, and nursing education and research are both highly dependent on federal funds.

Whether or not these statements were only intended to raise questions for further exploration, or whether nursing's negative attitude toward the report, or the follow-up of additional data from varied sources affected the attitude of some members of the committee, may never be known. Nevertheless, the final report presented some farsighted recommendations. Significantly, the addition of considerable new information received in the interim between the reports was noted.

The recommendations are presented in full because of their potential impact on nursing. For instance, within six months, legislation was introduced to place a National Institute of Nursing within the National Institutes of Health. Most persons traced this unprecedented action directly to the IOM statement that lack of adequate funding for nursing research had inhibited the development of nursing investigations and that the federal government should establish an organizational entity in the mainstream of scientific investigation.

The IOM report recommendations are as follows:

1. No specific federal support is needed to increase the overall supply of registered nurses, because estimates indicate that the aggregate supply and demand for generalist nurses will be in reasonable balance during this decade. However, federal, state, and private actions are recommended throughout this report to alleviate particular kinds of shortages and maldistributions of nurse supply.

2. The states have primary responsibility for analysis and planning of resource allocation for generalist nursing education. Their capabilities in this effort vary greatly. Assistance should be made available from the federal government, both in funds and in technical aid.

3. The federal government should maintain its general programs of financial aid to postsecondary students so that qualified prospective nursing students will continue to have the opportunity to enter generalist nursing education programs in numbers sufficient to maintain the necessary aggregate supply.

4. Institutional and student financial support should be maintained by state and local governments, higher education institutions, hospitals, and third-party payers to assure that generalist nursing education programs have capacity and enrollments sufficient to graduate the numbers and kinds of nurses commensurate with state and local goals for the nurse supply.

5. To assure a sufficient continuing supply of new applicants, nurse educators and national nursing organizations should adopt recruitment strategies that attract not only recent high school graduates but also nontraditional prospective students, such as those seeking late entry into a profession or seeking to change careers, and minorities.

6. Licensed nurses at all levels who wish to upgrade their education so as to enhance career opportunities should not encounter unwarranted barriers to admission. State education agencies, nursing education programs, and employers of nurses should assume a shared responsibility for developing policies and programs to minimize loss of time and money by students moving from one nursing education program level to another.

7. Closer collaboration between nurse educators and nurses who provide patient services is essential to give students an appropriate balance of academic and clinical practice perspectives and skills during their educational preparation. The federal

government should offer grants to nursing education programs that, in association with the nursing services of hospitals and other health care providers, undertake to develop and implement collaborative educational, clinical, and/or research programs.

8. The federal government should expand its support of fellowships, loans, and programs at the graduate level to assist in increasing the rate of growth in the number of nurses with master's and doctoral degrees in nursing and relevant disciplines.* More such nurses are needed to fill positions in administration and management of clinical services and of health care institutions, in academic nursing (teaching, research, and practice), and in clinical specialty practice.

9. To alleviate nursing shortages in medically underserved areas, their residents need better access to all types of nursing education, including outreach and off-campus programs. The federal government should continue to cosponsor model demonstrations of programs with states, foundations, and educational institutions, and should support the dissemination of results.

10. To meet the nursing needs of specific population groups in medically underserved areas and to encourage better minority representation at all levels of nursing education, the federal government should initiate a competitive program for state and private institutions that offers institutional and student support under the following principles:

    • Programs must be developed in close collaboration with, and include commitments from, providers of health services in shortage areas.

    • Scholarships and loans contingent on commitments to work in shortage areas

---

*Two members of the committee wished to delete the words "and relevant disciplines." Their statement of exception is in Chapter V of the report.

should be targeted, though not limited, to members of minority and ethnic groups to the extent that they are likely to meet the needs of underserved populations, including non-English-speaking groups.

11. Differential allowances in payment should take into account the special burdens of inner-city hospitals that demonstrate legitimate difficulties in financing services because of disproportionate numbers of uninsured or Medicaid and Medicare patients. Federal, state, and local governments and third-party payers should pay their fair shares of amounts necessary to prevent insolvency and to support acceptable levels of service, including nursing care.

12. The rapidly growing elderly population requires many kinds of nursing services for preventive, acute, and long-term care. To augment the supply of new nurses interested in caring for the elderly, nursing education programs should provide more formal instruction and clinical experiences in geriatric nursing. Federal support of such efforts is needed, as well as funding from states and private sources.

13. Nursing service staffs in nursing homes certified as "skilled nursing facilities" and in other institutions and programs providing care to the elderly often lack necessary knowledge and skills to meet the clinical challenges presented by these patients. Such facilities, in collaboration with nursing education programs and other private and public organizations, should develop and support programs to upgrade the knowledge and skills of the aides, LPNs, and RNs who work with elderly patients. States should assist vocational and higher education programs to respond to these needs. Federal support of such programs should be maintained.

14. The federal government (and the states, where applicable) should restructure Medicare and Medicaid payments so as to encourage and support the delivery of

long-term care nursing services provided to patients at home and in institutions. For skilled nursing facilities, such payment policies should encourage the continuing education of present staffs and the recruitment of more licensed nurses (RNs and LPNs), and should permit movement toward a goal of 24-hour RN coverage.

15. There is a need for the services of nurse practitioners, especially in medically underserved areas and in programs caring for the elderly. Federal support should be continued for their educational preparation. State laws that inhibit nurse practitioners and nurse midwives in the use of their special competencies should be modified. Medicare, Medicaid, and other public and private payment systems should pay for the services of these practitioners in organized settings of care, such as long-term care facilities, free-standing health centers and clinics, and health maintenance organizations, and in joint physician–nurse practices. (Where state payment practices are broader, this recommendation is not intended to be restrictive.)

16. The proportion of nurses who choose to work in their profession is high, but examination of conventional management, organization, and salary structures indicates that employers could improve both supply and job tenure by the following:
   • providing opportunities for career advancement in clinical nursing as well as in administration
   • ensuring that merit and experience in direct patient care are rewarded by salary increases
   • assessing the need to raise nurse salaries if vacancies remain unfilled
   • encouraging greater involvement of nurses in decisions about patient care, management, and governance of the institution
   • identifying the major deterrents to nurse labor force participation in their

own localities and responding by adapting conditions of work, child care, and compensation packages to encourage part-time nurses to increase their labor force participation and to attract inactive nurses back to work.

17. Lack of precise information about current costs and utilization of nursing service personnel makes it difficult for nursing service administrators and hospital managers to make the most appropriate and cost effective decisions about assignment of nurses. Hospitals, working with federal and state governments and other third-party payers, should conduct studies and experiments to determine the feasibility and means of creating separate revenue and cost centers for case-mix costing and revenue setting, and for other fiscal management alternatives.

18. The federal government should establish an organizational entity to place nursing research in the mainstream of scientific investigation. An adequately funded focal point is needed at the national level to foster research that informs nursing and other health care practice and increases the potential for discovery and application of various means to improve patient outcomes.

19. Federal and private funds should support research that will provide scientifically valid measurements of the knowledge and performance competencies of nurses with various levels and types of educational preparation and experience.

20. As national and regional forums identify promising approaches to problems in the organization and delivery of nursing services, there will be a need for wider experimentation, demonstration, and evaluation. The federal government, in conjunction with private sector organizations, should participate in the critical assessment of new ideas and the broad dissemination of research results.

21. To ensure that federal and state policymakers have the information they need for

future nurse manpower decisions, the federal government should continue to support the collection and analysis of compatible, unduplicated, and timely data on national nursing supply, education, and practice, with special attention to filling identified deficits in currently available information.[23]

The budgetary impact of the committee's recommendations was presented as a modest increase in NTA funding to alleviate certain nurse shortages, holding the line against possible erosion of federal and state funding for higher education, and modifying payment systems of public and third-party payers to permit (nurse) providers of service to the poor and elderly to become financially secure.

The National Commission on Nursing Study. The National Commission on Nursing was formed as an independent commission sponsored by the American Hospital Association, the Hospital Research and Educational Trust, and the American Hospital Supply Corporation. Composed of thirty leaders in the fields of nursing, hospital management, medicine, government, academia, and business, it was charged, during its three-year charter, with developing and implementing action plans to provide practical solutions for institutions and organizations confronting nursing problems. One-half of the group were nurses. In part because of its sponsorship and because a hospital administrator (distinguished though he was) was chairman, organized nursing at first regarded the National Commission with some suspicion. Once more, there was concern about a nonnursing-sponsored group potentially making decisions about nursing. Yet the commission did, indeed, prove to be an independent entity. With a respected nurse as staff director, the commission began, like the IOM group, to study data about nursing, relying primarily on the literature, policy statements, surveys and studies, and hearings (in this case held in six major cities). A variety of interested people testified. The testimony, published in mid-1981, stressed that nursing, although closely meshed with other health care disciplines, has the professional right and responsibility to define the nature and scope of nursing practice. To be recognized as independent professionals, nurses themselves must understand, value, and promote their professional identity and role in providing high-quality care. Also highlighted was the need for a highly visible, effective nursing leadership promoting a strong, unified image of the profession. There was disagreement on collective bargaining as a mechanism to improve working conditions and control over practice.

The *Initial Report and Preliminary Recommendations,* published in September 1981, was received with considerable enthusiasm and perhaps some astonishment by nursing. The report was seen as much more positive than the IOM report of the same period. Although the National Commission on Nursing recognized that nursing was practiced in a variety of settings, emphasis was on the hospital, where the largest percentage of nurses practice. When viewed from a national perspective, the issues were seen as more similar than different, regardless of settings and geographic areas. Forty different factors were mentioned frequently and consistently as related to the shortage of nursing. Foremost were salaries, flexible scheduling, nurse–physician relationships, the image and status of nurses and their roles in decision making, career mobility, nursing education, and the relationship of nursing education and nursing practice.

All of these factors were summarized and discussed in five major categories from which recommendations evolved:

- Status and image of nursing, including changes in the nursing role in response to new variations in health care delivery and professional growth as well as the corresponding changes in interprofessional relationships and public image

- Interface of nursing education and practice, including current and potential models for basic and graduate education and continuing nursing education to prepare nurses for practice and professional interaction in health care delivery

- Effective management of the nursing resource, including the mix of organizational factors required for nursing job satisfaction (such as the issues of staffing, scheduling, salary and benefits, support services, modes of care delivery, and career development) as well as manpower planning and recruitment and retention strategies
- Relationships among nursing, medical staff, and hospital administration, including nurses' ability to participate through organizational structures in decision-making as it relates to nursing care, the value and development of collegial relationships among health care professionals, and the development and operation of interdisciplinary patient care teams
- Maturing of nursing as a self-determining profession, including nursing's right and responsibility to define and determine the nature and scope of its practice, the need for and role of nursing leadership, the potential of collective action to increase decision-making in nursing practice, and the need for unity in the nursing profession[24]

In summary, the key recommendations focused on nurses and physicians participating in a collaborative relationship in which nurses are included in clinical decision making and have authority and responsibility for their own practice; administrators establishing a suitable practice environment, including involvement of the nurse administrator as part of the top management team; establishment of salaries, benefits, and educational opportunities for nurses, commensurate with their responsibilities as professionals; the need for diverse nursing constituencies to join together to formulate and support common policies in education, credentialing, and standards of practice; promotion of accessibility and educational mobility in higher education through educational articulation for undergraduate

nurses and RNs; continuation of funding for nursing education; appropriate utilization of nurses related to the competency obtained in the specific educational program; collaboration between educational institutions and practice agencies to provide good clinical experience for students, practice opportunities for faculty, and continuing education for RNs; and implementation and maintenance of nationally accepted standards for licensure. On the controversial issue of baccalaureate education for professional nursing practice, it was seen as a "desirable goal," with consideration given to regional differences in availability of programs, funds, faculty, and students. Specific goals for each set of recommendations were presented, with concomitant demonstration and research projects recommended.

In the interim between reports, the National Commission published the results of a survey of innovative nursing programs and projects, and sponsored an invitational conference to learn about evolving trends and innovative approaches to nursing in hospitals, to which chief executive officers, trustees, medical directors, and chief nurses from hospitals with successful models came as a team and discussed strategies and solutions to nursing problems. There were also surveys to discover trends in relationships between nursing education and practice, meetings with various groups, and site visits, as well as review and study of new literature and responses to the *Initial Report.*

Of the major groups interested in the *Initial Report,* it appeared that nursing responded positively (with hesitation by some educators in relation to the educational recommendations). The AMA, with a very positive attitude, bought multiple copies of the document for its most influential member to study. The AHA also distributed copies, but received a less than positive response from some of its constituent organizations and administrators.

When the final report was released, some disappointment by nurses was inevitable since certain recommendations were seen as less strong. For instance, in relation to nursing education, there were new recommendations stating:

> Current trends in nursing toward pursuit of the baccalaureate degree as an achievable goal for nursing practice and toward advanced degrees for clinical specialization, administration, teaching, and research should be facilitated.
>
> All types of nursing education programs, which continue to be needed, increasingly operating within the mainstream of higher education and in accordance with local circumstances and statewide planning, should hasten progress toward availability of baccalaureate and higher degrees for those desirous and capable of achieving them. Educational mobility and reentry opportunities should be promoted within the educational system. Accreditation processes should respond to these needs and trends.
>
> In recognition of these trends toward higher education for general and specialty practice, and in anticipation of further changes in the practice field, the nursing profession must periodically assess and project the need for assisting personnel in nursing and specify the competency, accountability, education, and credentialing requirements of such personnel.[25]

Omitted was the statement urging appropriate utilization of nurses according to educational background. On the other hand, a new recommendation strongly urged that a high priority be given to nursing research and to preparation of nurse researchers in order that "nurses can test, refine and advance the knowledge base on which education and practice must rest."[26]

Under "Nursing and the Public," the suggestion for nationally accepted standards of licensure was eliminated, but participation of nurses in community activities and public forums was encouraged.

Why the changes? New data, new analysis, new discussion might be one answer. But another is pragmatic: Nurses alone cannot bring about the recommended changes, however desirable they may be; they need the cooperation of physicians and hospital administrators—especially to support changes in the practice setting. The fine art of compromise is necessary to get most plans moving, and the National Commission was certainly concerned that its work not be filed away as simply another report never acted upon, particularly since one of the primary motives for the study was the nursing shortage, which by 1983 was no longer considered serious. Strategies for action concluded the report, and there were tentative plans for assessment of results later, although the commission recognized that many recommended actions had already gained impetus from forward-looking individuals.

The chairman summarized their conclusions:

> . . . if we are going to make any progress at all, the first priority would seem to be better educated, more highly qualified nurses; reformed relationships among health professionals; and new types of organizational structures. Action must be long-range. Short-term solutions alone are difficult and costly; they hamper nursing's ability to keep up with the present, let alone prepare for the future.[27]

In late 1984 the W. K. Kellogg funded a three year project to carry out selected recommendations of the commission related to nursing education, nursing administration, and nursing research. Named as collaborating sponsors were: the American Nurses' Association, the American Society for Nursing Service Administrators, and the National League for Nursing. Representatives of these nursing organizations, the American Hospital Association, the American Medical Association, the National Congress for Hospital Governing Boards, and the National Consumers' League, formed a 12 member governing body to direct the project.

MAGNET HOSPITALS: ATTRACTION AND RETENTION OF PROFESSIONAL NURSES

In 1981, the Governing Council of the American Academy of Nursing (AAN) appointed a Task Force on Nursing Practice in Hospitals, charging it "to examine characteristics of systems impeding and/or facilitating professional nursing practice in hospitals." The interim report of both the IOM and the National Commission on Nursing had been studied, and the prestigious nurse administrators who comprised the task force were also aware of the identified causes of the hospital nurse shortage. They chose, instead, to focus on those hospitals across the country that seemed to have created nursing practice organizations that served as "magnets" for professional nurses: that is, they were able to attract and retain a staff of well-qualified nurses and consistently provided high-quality care.

The purpose of the study they developed was basically to identify magnet hospitals in eight regions of the country, to identify, describe, and analyze the organizational variables that promote job satisfaction, to explicate replicable variables for use by others, and to publish the report. Bureau of Labor Statistics (BLS) regions, combining Regions I and II and Regions VII and VIII, were used, and selected fellows of the Academy were asked to nominate and describe potential magnet hospitals in their region. Specific criteria were as follows: nurses considered the hospital a good place to work and practice; the hospital had the ability to recruit and retain professional nurses; and it was in a geographic area in which it had competition for staff. The Center for Health Care Research and Evaluation (CHCRE) at the School of Nursing, the University of Texas at Austin, was selected as the site for data collection, tabulation, and analysis.

A total of 165 institutions was nominated. All the directors of nursing received a letter explaining the project, including a data collection instrument that asked for descriptive personnel and hospital statistics, as well as delineating what was expected of hospitals and their representatives if selected. The four task force members independently reviewed and evaluated the recruitment and retention records of the 155 hospitals that responded and ranked their ten top choices. At CHCRE, a numerical score was calculated for each, and on the basis of the rankings, forty-six institutions were selected as magnet hospitals. The final sample was forty-one.

The magnet hospitals were primarily private, nonprofit institutions, with the majority in the 201- to 700-bed range. Only four were under and three over that size. The occupancy rate was 72 to 98 percent. At least 85 percent of their budgeted RN positions were filled throughout the year. There was an average of 1.1 RNs per occupied bed, an RN:LPN ratio of 10:1, RN:aide ratio of 12:1, and RN:unit clerk ratio of 9:1. The educational preparation of the directors of nursing was primarily at the master's level, with about 12 percent holding doctorates and about 7 percent baccalaureates. Associates or clinical directors were also primarily prepared at the master's or doctorate level, although 19 percent held no degree. About one-half of the head nurses and about 43 percent of the area supervisors held no degree.

Interviews were conducted by the task force members in each of the eight areas. The director of nursing and a director-selected staff nurse from each magnet hospital were grouped according to position and interviewed separately. Each group was interviewed in such a way as to assure participation of each individual. The answers were both recorded on tape and typed. Questions asked each group were:

1. What makes your hospital a good place for nurses to work?
2. Can you describe particular programs in your situation that you see leading to professional/personal satisfaction?
3. How is nursing viewed in your hospital and why? (Image of nursing.)

4. Can you describe nurse involvement in various ongoing programs/projects whose goals are quality of patient care?

5. Can you identify activities and programs calculated to enhance, both directly and indirectly, recruitment/retention of professional nurses in your hospital?

6. Could you tell us about nurse–physician relationships in your hospital?

7. Please describe staff nurse–supervisor (various levels) relationships in your hospital.

8. Are some areas in your hospital more successful than others in recruitment/retention? Why?

9. What single piece of advice would you give to a director of nursing who wishes to do something about high registered nurse vacancy and turnover rates in her hospital?[28]

On a Post-Interview Comments form, the participants were asked to indicate those activities, programs, and policies that they believed were effective in enhancing professional and personal satisfaction and their individual assessments of factors that contribute to staff retention.

The perceptions of the staff nurses can be summarized as follows:

High standards, clearly enunciated, with adequate administrative support to ensure that standards can be met:

• Visibility, accessibility, support of the director of nursing
• Strength and knowledge of the director
• Practice of participatory management, including effective two-way communication
• Clear philosophy that is based on caring not only for patients and family, but also the staff
• Responsibility is decentralized
• Committee membership of nurses involve them in hospital and nursing service affairs
• Low patient to RN ratio with qualified staff, and consultation from clinical specialists available

Personnel policies that reflect the hospitals' concern with employees' needs and interests:

• Flexible work schedules
• Competitive salaries and benefits
• Social and recognition programs

Opportunities for professional practice:

• Professional practice models, particularly primary nursing, that allow for independent judgment and freedom to function (autonomy)
• Participation in quality assurance programs
• Involvement in community outreach
• Opportunities to teach patients and families
• Positive nurse image in the hospital and the community
• Mutual respect for each other's knowledge by nurses and physicians
• Good orientation, inservice education, and opportunities for continuing education (formal or informal)
• Development and operation of a career ladder[29]

The nurse administrators, while taking more of a conceptual view and being somewhat more abstract in answering the same questions, seemed to agree almost entirely with the staff nurses about what created the positive environment that made their nursing services a magnet for RNs. Although recognizing the importance of their own leadership, they freely acknowledged the importance of supervisors and head nurses in decentralization, especially in the areas of support and communication. They also cited collaboration with schools of nursing, including the beginning of joint appointments, as adding to the professional milieu. Nor did the directors underrate the importance of staffing patterns, policies, salaries, and benefits. They, too, mentioned the strong RN ratios, schedule flexibilities, competitive salaries, and such popular benefits as tuition reimbursement and paid time-off programs. Here, too, there was strong emphasis on the positive image nurses had, their good relationship with physicians (including joint practice committees), career ladder and educational opportunities, and particularly the autonomy to practice nursing professionally. They also identified the opportunity to participate in nursing research as a good educational opportunity for the nurses.

The report concluded that change was possible, since some of these hospitals had enjoyed magnet status for some time, while others had changed rather dramatically in a relatively short time prior to the study. This positive change seemed to have followed a change in key leadership people such as the hospital administrator and the director of nursing.

Although the magnet hospitals had certain differences, there were certain critical similarities. First, the shared values of administration and staff were clearly evident. Second, both staff and directors recognized their own changing roles, and the continued need to interpret these roles and the needs of patients and to stand up for one's principles. Finally, rather than a voiced concern about power per se, what came through on all sites was a sense of what might be called a lack of powerlessness. Nurses recognized the locus of control in the director and the power held by the physicians in admitting patients to the hospital, but recognized that this could be balanced by the nurses' power as coordinators of care—the care needed by patients. There was also a "fit" of vision and competence between the nurse administrator and the hospital's chief executive office (and presumably the board of trustees). Without such a balanced power structure, change cannot occur.[30]

REFERENCES

1. Josephine Goldmark, *Nursing and Nursing Education in the United States* (New York: Macmillan Publishing Co., Inc., 1923).
2. Esther Lucile Brown, *Nursing for the Future* (New York: Russell Sage Foundation, 1948), p. 45.
3. Ibid., pp. 132–170.
4. Ibid., pp. 48, 178.
5. Jerome Lysaught, *An Abstract for Action* (New York: McGraw-Hill Book Company, 1970), pp. 1–23.
6. Ibid., p. 155.
7. Ibid., pp. 156–161.
8. "Report of the Task Force," *Nurs. Outlook,* 21:111–118 (Feb. 1973).
9. Jerome Lysaught, *From Abstract into Action* (New York: McGraw-Hill Book Company, 1973), pp. 1–21.
10. "Nurse and Medical Practice Act Must Permit Flexibility, NJPC Says," *Am. J. Nurs.,* 74:602 (Apr. 1974).
11. Jerome Lysaught et al., "Progress in Professional Service: Nurse Leaders Queried," *Hospitals,* 52:120 (Aug. 16, 1978).
12. U.S. Department of Health, Education, and Welfare, *Extending the Scope of Nursing Practice* (Washington, D.C.: The Department, 1971), p. 2.
13. Ibid., p. 4.
14. "The Study of Credentialing in Nursing: A New Approach," A report of the Committee Milwaukee, Jan. 1979, p. 3. (mimeographed.)
15. Ibid., pp. 82–92.
16. Rheba de Tornyay, *Report of the Meeting Convened by the Task Force on Credentialing in Nursing* (Kansas City, Mo.: American Nurses Foundation, 1983).
17. Jean Lum, "WICHE Panel of Expert Consultants Report: Implications for Nursing Leaders," *J. Nurs. Admin.* 9: 11–19 (July 1979).
18. *Report of the Graduate Medical Education National Advisory Committee to the Secretary, Department of Health and Human Services,* Vol. VII (Washington, D.C.: USDHHS, 1981), pp. 19–20.
19. Mabel Wandelt, et al., *Conditions Associated with Registered Nurse Employment in Texas* (Austin, Tex: Center for Research, School of Nursing, the University of Texas at Austin, 1980).
20. Mabel Wandelt et al., "Why Nurses Leave Nursing and What Can Be Done About It," *Am. J. Nurs* 81:72–77 (Jan. 1981).
21. *Conditions Associated with Registered Nurse Employment in Texas,* op. cit., p. 7.
22. Ada Jacox, "Significant Questions About IOM's Study of Nursing," *Nurs. Outlook* 31:28–33 (Jan.–Feb. 1983).
23. *Nursing and Nursing Education: Public Policies and Private Actions.* (Washington, D.C.: National Academy Press, 1983), pp. 1–226.

24. *Initial Report and Preliminary Recommendations* (Chicago, Ill.: National Commission on Nursing, Sept. 1981), p. 5.

25. *Summary Report and Recommendations* (Chicago, Ill.: National Commission on Nursing, Apr. 1983), p. 5.

26. Ibid., p. 11.

27. Ibid., p. xi.

28. Task Force on Nursing Practice in Hospitals, *Magnet Hospitals: Attraction and Retention of Professional Nurses* (Kansas City, Mo.: American Academy of Nursing, 1983), 8–9.

29. Ibid., pp. 14–98.

30. Ibid., pp. 103–104.

CONTEMPORARY PROFESSIONAL NURSING

THE
HEALTH CARE
SETTING

6

The Impact of Social and Scientific Changes

As a part of society, and as one of the health professions, nursing is affected by the changes, problems, and issues of society in general, as well as those that specifically influence the health care scene. Some of the changes, such as the civil rights of minority groups and women, have been developing for amost 100 years but seem to have reached the point of real action. Others, such as the new life-styles and technological and scientific advances, have appeared to emerge on the scene with a suddenness that has created what Toffler calls "future shock," the shattering stress and disorientation induced in individuals when they are subjected to too much change in too short a time.[1]

Surrounded by constant change, nurses (and others, for that matter) are tempted to ignore the potential effects on the profession, or at best to cope with the problems only when they become inescapable. Professions that ignore the pervasiveness of social trends find themselves scrambling to catch up, rather than planning to advance; reacting, rather than acting. When the public justifiably accuses the professions of unresponsiveness to their needs, it is, in part, because those professions have not been acute enough to observe patterns of future development or have been too insular to see the necessity to become a part of them. It is a luxury that no profession, least of all nursing with its intimate person-to-person contact, can afford. The purpose of this chapter, therefore, is to review some of the major changes in the last decade or two to determine their impact on nursing.

WORLD POPULATION: PROBLEMS AND PROGRESS

In 1980, the *Global 2000 Report* from the State Department and the Council on Environmental Quality stated, "If present trends continue, the world will be more crowded, less stable ecologically and more vulnerable to disruption. . . . Despite greater material output, the world's people will be poorer in many ways than they are today."[2] Among the predictions were:

• Production and consumption of food will rise, but in the less developed countries (LDCs) and particularly in Southern, East, and Southeast Asia, poor areas of North Africa and the Middle East, and especially central Africa, "the quantity of food available to the poorest people will be insufficient to permit children to reach normal body weight and intelligence and to permit normal activity and good health in adults.'' As the population rises, the number of malnourished people in the world will rise from 400–600 million in the 1970s to 1.3 billion in the year 2000.

• Crowding and urban growth will bring about a decrease in living standards.

Clearly, the problem of population growth, a major societal concern for a number of years, is no less urgent now. By 1972, world population had reached 3.7 billion; a little over a decade later, it was estimated at almost 4.7 billion. At a predicted growth rate of about 1.7 percent per year, with 28 births and 11 deaths for every 1,000 persons in the world, population at the turn of the century will be over 6 billion people, mostly in the LDCs.[3] In 1980, the populations in these areas outnumbered those in the developed world by three to one. Experts predict that world population will not stabilize until it reaches 8 to 10 billion sometime in the next two centuries.

The most recent comparison of seventy countries in relation to income, gross national product (GNP) per capita, population growth, and daily calorie supply per capita shows that with rare exceptions, the poorer countries have the greater population growth (2 to 5.6 percent) and less than the required number of calories per person. The industrialized nations, with the highest GNP per capita, have a growth rate that averages considerably under 1 percent, and the number of calories per person is well over the minimum requirement.[4]

Because the ''hunger belt'' of the world tends to be in the Southern Hemisphere, it is natural that population control has been given increased attention in many underdeveloped and/or overpopulated countries, with more or less success. A world fertility study, based on interviews with 343,000 women in forty-two developing and twenty developed countries showed that contraceptive use is increasing in most of the Third World, except for Africa. Fertility has dropped by at least one child per

woman in Asia, Latin America, and the eastern Mediterranean, but not at all in sub-Saharan Africa. Fertility ranges from 4.6 children in Latin America to 6.7 in sub-Saharan Africa. An average of 2.2 to 2.5 children per woman is needed to end population growth in these countries. Nearly half of the women surveyed in most of the developing countries said they wanted no more children (although as many as nine was considered the preferred number). There was a clear relationship between contraceptive use and the availability of family planning services.[5] Other surveys show that it is generally the least educated and the poor who are unaware of or resist using family planning techniques.

Whereas most such activities were once funded by private groups, the designation by the United Nations of 1974 as World Population Year signified a change in population control activities to international organizations (the United Nations, the Organization for Economic Cooperation and Development, and the World Bank). One expert made the following observation:

> This organization expansion has been facilitated by the weakening of traditional sources of resistance to population control policies. Marxist, Nationalist, and Catholic opposition has been countered by arguments about the importance of population control for economic development and the increase of freedom of choice. Furthermore, the proliferation of family planning activity in rural Chinese communes and American ghettos suggests that family planning is becoming ''internationalized'' and ''depoliticized.''[6]

The development of pills, injections, and intrauterine devices (IUDs), and societal acceptance of (and sometimes governmental pressure for) family planning, including sterilization and abortion, have also had an impact. In China, for instance, with a current population of over 800 million, there is strong governmental pressure for one-child families, a plan more successful with the urban families than with the peasants. A report from the

Guttmacher Institute has stated that contraceptive practice the world over could be revolutionized in the next decade, but that current levels of funding for such research, which have been decreasing, prevent such a revolution. Potential contraceptive measures under research which could be significant in increasing the use of contraception include a nonsurgical method of female sterilization, several reversible methods for male contraception, an antipregnancy vaccine, a self-administered menses inducer, and a postpartum sterilization device.[7] Also needed is social service research devoted to understanding the sources of resistance to family planning and methods of overcoming it, particularly in the seriously overpopulated and poverty-stricken countries.

More than a decade ago, problems such as the energy crisis, pollution, housing, crime, illiteracy, hunger, crowding, deforestation, overgrazing, unemployment, endangered species, restrictions on individual freedom, and health threats were identified as being created by, or related to, overpopulation. In relation to health alone, the World Health Organization has reported that four-fifths of the world's population do not have any form of health care, and that almost 1 billion—almost one-quarter of the persons alive—suffer from combined long-term malnutrition and parasitic diseases, and thus are handicapped in their ability to work. Even though smallpox appears to have been conquered, the other infectious diseases are making a comeback, and deaths due to dysentery, diarrhea, and pneumonia, all closely related to malnutrition and poor housing conditions, are rising. In fact, the developing world's progress in combatting high death rates may be slowing down, and in some cases reversing. Life expectancy in the Third World is still up to twenty years below the sixty- to sixty-five-year-life expectancy level at which Western nations' progress slowed and which is considered the natural "ceiling" level. No improvement is anticipated. Among threats cited in the *Global 2000 Report* were the hampering of agriculture because of soil erosion, loss of nutrients in the soil, and rising air and water pollution, the last a problem in itself. Also noted was the fact that things could be different if national policies around the world were to change. While some nations are making such efforts, they are seen as far from adequate.

A president of the American Public Health Association put it well:

> Biologically, we know that population will ultimately be controlled by some stress such as war, famine, pestilence, pollution or congestion, if not by rational behavior. People must curb population growth, not for whimsical aesthetic reasons, but for the very self-serving reason that we must protect our environment because it literally gives us life. The Earth and its resources are finite.[8]

UNITED STATES POPULATION

In the United States, the census clock at the Commerce Building in Washington, D.C., recorded more than 220 million Americans in the year before the official 1980 census. The clock adds a person every nineteen seconds, taking into account the birth rates, death rates, and patterns of movement of people in and out of the country. The census, completed with some disagreement about its accuracy, showed a new diversity in population makeup. The white majority has been diminished somewhat by a tide of immigrants of other races. Of the approximately 226.5 million people in the United States, about 83.2 percent were white; 11.7 percent black; 0.6 percent American Indian, Eskimo, or Aleuts; 1.5 percent Chinese, Filipinos, Japanese, Asian Indians, Koreans, Vietnamese, Hawaiians, Somoans, and Guamanians; and 3 percent included other Asians, Mexicans, Puerto Ricans, Cubans, Africans, and many other groups not listed in the census forms. A little over 6 percent identified themselves as Hispanic. Illegal aliens who did not respond to the census make up an additional layer of population, but not many are believed to be white Europeans. In the decade before the census, European and

Canadian immigration decreased, but Asian, African, South American, and Mexican immigration increased. Moreover, the acknowledged undercount of legal residents is presumed to be among black and brown people.

This change has been increasing in every region of the country, with every indication that it will grow. There is a question of whether these immigrants will be as easily assimilated as the Europeans, and controversies rage over the proposed reimposition of restrictive quotas. However, cultural diversity brings new dimensions to American life.[9]

By 1983, the United States population had increased to 232.6 million, a 2.7 percent increase over that reported in the 1980 census. Besides increasing cultural diversity, there were other changes in population patterns. The number of one-parent families doubled from 1971 to 1981, comprising 20 percent of the nation's 31.6 million families with children present. About 90 percent of the one-parent households were headed by mothers; nearly three-fourths of all persons maintaining such families were separated or divorced. Although 68 percent of such families were headed by whites, the proportion was considerably higher among blacks—51 percent compared with 17 percent.

The average household size of 2.72 persons in 1982 was down from 3.14 in 1970. Contributing factors were relatively low birth and marriage rates, high levels of separation and divorce, and a 78 percent increase in those living alone. Another significant change was the population's age structure. Between 1970 and 1981, there were strong shifts toward more young adults and elders and fewer minors. The largest drop was in the five- to thirteen-years age group. Persons sixty-five or over increased by 31.4 percent, from 20.0 to 26.3 million.

A potentially critical political factor is that the voting-age population is both expanding and getting younger—29 million more in 1982 than in 1972. This reflects the movement of the baby boom generation into adulthood; two out of five voting-age persons are twenty-five to forty-eight years old, and one in five is under twenty-five. Nationally, women represent 52.4 percent of the voting-age population, outnumbering men by 8 million. Women are the majority in all states except Alaska, Hawaii, Nevada, and Wyoming. They represent about 60 percent of those sixty-five years and over. Blacks comprise about 10.5 percent of the electorate, with the highest black proportions in the South but the largest numbers in New York, California, Texas and Illinois. Nearly 70 percent of the Hispanic electorate is located in California, Texas (about half), New York, and Florida.

As might be expected, people completing four years of college had greater lifetime earnings (about 40 percent higher) than high school graduates. However, male college graduates had more than twice as high lifetime earnings as women, although it was suggested that continuity of work life is a factor.

Both advanced education and occupation seemed to influence birth rates among women. First births for women between eighteen and forty-four who had completed four or five years of college was 47 as opposed to the national average of 38 percent. The fertility rate for women in professional and managerial positions in 1981 was 37.2 per 1,000, compared to 70.9 for all women; 19 percent said they expected no children. The average lifetime birth expectancy of women eighteen to thirty-four declined from 3.1 in the 1960s to 2.2 in 1981. Single women had a 1.8 rate.[10]

It can be seen that, after the spectacular two-decade population explosion after World War II, the birth rate in the United States has also gradually declined and the rate of growth has slowed. But the fact that those who are already poor, undernourished, undereducated, and underemployed tend to have the most children brings international emphasis down to national and local practical concerns, particularly those related to health. For instance, the most economically depressed members of the population have converged in the urban areas. As the middle class made a hasty exodus from the deteriorating inner cities, blacks,

Spanish-speaking persons, and the poor from Appalachia moved in. For some, it was merely an exchange of rural poverty with fresh air to urban poverty with polluted air.

By 1984, another dimension of poverty and displacement was evident in the number of homeless persons in urban areas. The makeup included not only the classic alcoholic drifter but also the young, unemployed, homeless male, often black; the mentally incompetent, discharged from institutional care without appropriate follow-through and unable to cope with the outside world; and, during the time of the deepest depression, whole families who lived in tents or makeshift shelters on public lands. Public and private facilities were opened for "temporary housing." Soup kitchens, not seen since the Great Depression of the 1930s were crowded daily. It appeared that not only the Third World had a hunger problem, but also the wealthy United States. Nevertheless, a commission appointed by the Reagan Administration, which had been consistently cutting funding for the needs of the poor and near-poor, reported that these cutbacks for food had not harmed the poor. The members averred that hunger among Americans could not be documented, although it probably "does persist."

Regardless of the accuracy of this report, there is little doubt that the poor not only lack adequate housing, nutrition, and jobs but also have a multitude of health problems for which they may not seek help until there is a serious need. A whole series of specific needs related to health has emerged because of their particular social-ethnic-economic problems. The need is for readily available health services, such as neighborhood family health centers, health workers who understand the problems of the people and are able to communicate with them, understandable health teaching, and coordination of the multiple services required. Some of the more urgent health needs that have been cited are preventive, diagnos-

tic, referral, and counseling services for pregnant women, infants, and preschool children, and community mental health services to alleviate problems or redirect deviant behavior of individuals, families, or groups.

Population control and family planning are also issues in the United States.* Although the concept of population control is acceptable to most in the abstract, the specific methods are controversial for various reasons. Use of contraceptive measures may be against the moral, religious, or cultural mores of a group, and there is particular opposition by some to any form of sterilization. Abortion, made legal for the first trimester of pregnancy by a Supreme Court decision, has been bitterly opposed by the Catholic Church and various right-to-life groups. Both pro-choice and anti-abortion groups have been active politically. A study of the activists in both groups showed that their populations tended to be overwhelmingly white, but otherwise were quite different from each other. About 70 percent of the pro-life group was Catholic, and the women seemed more likely to have had problems connected to fertility (inability to conceive, miscarriages, unplanned pregnancies); most members opposed making birth control information available to teenagers and saw extramarital sex for anyone as always wrong. They also had more children than the pro-choice group.[11]

The influence of the two groups seems to wax and wane. In each congressional session and in many state legislatures since the 1973 decision, there have been pressures and subsequent actions to restrict severely the cases in which abortions are paid for by tax dollars. In 1977, the Supreme Court ruled that states were under no obligation to pay for elective abortions with Medicaid funds and that municipal hospitals were not required to provide elective abortions. The Hyde amendment, which had triggered that action, was then implemented and effectively cut off 99 percent of federal Medicaid funding for abortions. On the other hand, attempts to have the right to life guaranteed from the moment of fertiliza-

---

*See Chapter 22 for further discussion of the legal aspects of these issues.

tion have been unsuccessful, and requirements that parents be notified if minors seek birth control information or abortion are consistently challenged in court.

Because of the Medicaid cuts, there was concern about the ethics of discriminating against poor women. However, five years later, a survey revealed that most poor women who sought abortions were able to obtain them. Sixty-five percent of those who needed but could not afford an abortion used state Medicaid funds. Where these funds were not available, they relied on combinations of personal funds, reduced provider fees, county hospital services, and philanthropic contributions.

In general, while these legal struggles continue, the number of abortions is increasing. Most are obtained by women under twenty-four, most of whom are unmarried. (The U.S. abortion rate is about the middle range of those countries where the procedure is legal and statistics are available.)

Adolescent sexuality and pregnancy are still major health and social problems. The U.S. rate of teenage pregnancies is among the highest in all developed countries. One out of ten female teenagers has a baby before age eighteen, with blacks having three times as high a rate as whites. Although only 18 percent of all sexually active women who can get pregnant are adolescents, they have 46 percent of out-of-wedlock babies and 31 percent of all abortions. Sex education by schools and/or families still seems to be lacking. Only a portion of the downward trend of teenage births, which began in the late 1970s, is due to contraceptive use. Most of it is caused by an increase in abortion. The lack of contraceptive use has been identified as being due to ignorance about reproduction and lack of maturity. For instance, some teenagers are not concerned about the social, economic, or health consequences of illegitimate births. Yet, studies have shown that young parenthood has adverse effects on the young parents' educational attainment and economic self-sufficiency, and that infants born to young

mothers may show deficits in physical health, cognitive development, social/emotional development, and school achievement.[12]

THE NATION'S HEALTH

The health status of the U.S. population as a whole is, according to health statistics, better than ever. A report by the American Council on Science and Health[13] asserts that although there is popular concern about man-made epidemics due to life-style, dietary habits, food additives, pesticides, and pollutants, technological and life-style changes that have occurred in the past eight decades have improved rather than harmed Americans' health.

Health status is determined in several ways: using mortality statistics (life expectancy and death rates), which are easily obtained, and morbidity statistics (the incidence and prevalence of illness). The latter are much more difficult to obtain and are less accurate because most diseases are not reportable, and reports, surveys, and research can be interpreted in a number of ways.

The Council's 1983 report presents some interesting information. The life expectancy of the newborn is now 75.5 years, with females still living longer. The leading causes of death are heart disease (although this has declined in the last few years); cancer; cerebrovascular disease (strokes); accidents, particularly motor vehicle; chronic obstructive pulmonary diseases and allied conditions; pneumonia and influenza; diabetes mellitus, chronic liver disease, and cirrhosis; atherosclerosis; and suicide. Whereas infectious diseases once claimed the lives of thousands of Americans, only sexually transmitted infections have increased in recent years. Of special concern is genital herpes because, unlike the other venereal diseases, adequate treatment has not yet been found. The most recent and most serious infectious disease, because of the high incidence of fatality, is acquired immune deficiency syndrome (AIDS). It appears to affect primarily homosexuals and drug addicts. Experts also warn that the unwarranted reluctance of some parents to have their children immunized could pose a serious threat to public health, since these childhood diseases have not been eliminated, but only controlled, by immunization.

One logical way to review American health is by age group. The mortality rate is higher than reported in some other industrialized countries, but this may be due to differences in the way statistics are gathered. There is some evidence that the higher incidence of low-birth-weight infants in the United States caused (in part) by poor maternal nutrition and poor physical condition, smoking, and lack of prenatal care may be responsible for a greater death rate. The infant mortality rate for blacks is nearly twice that of whites. Cancer is the leading cause of disease-related deaths in children, but since the late 1960s, more school-age children have died from accidents and violence than from disease.

The death rate of adolescents and young adults fell until 1960 but is now higher than it was twenty years ago. The chief causes are accidental death, homicide, and suicide; unwanted pregnancies and sexually transmitted disease are cited as major threats to the well-being of young people. Alcohol and drug abuse, besides their inherent dangers, also contribute to accidental death. Cancer, the leading cause of natural death, accounted for only 5 percent of all deaths in this age group.

Accidents, primarily motor vehicle accidents, are also the leading cause of death in adults twenty-five to forty-four years old, with the overall death rate of men being twice that of women. Most women in this age group die of cancer (chiefly breast and genital); besides accidents, men die of heart disease, other accidents, cancer, homicide, and suicide. For the next age group, heart disease, although lessening, is still the major killer. Cancer deaths have increased primarily due to the rise in lung cancer.

The age-adjusted death rate of Americans sixty-five and over has dropped since 1950,

primarily due to the decrease in heart disease mortality. Cancer deaths have increased, with lung, colon, genital organ, and breast cancer (among women) accounting for more than half of all cancer deaths. About 75 percent of the mortality in this age group is due to heart disease, cancer, and stroke. However, despite other diseases and their own feeling that their health is declining, most older Americans are reported to maintain their vigor and independence.

No doubt, scientific discoveries and technology have had an impact on the mortality and morbidity rates. More sophisticated diagnostic tools allowing for early diagnosis, new drugs, sophisticated surgery, and the nursing care that is essential to recovery are all elements to be considered. Nevertheless, prevention is seen as the one factor that will make the difference from now on. One-third of the deaths caused by heart disease, cancer, strokes, accidents, and pulmonary disease could have been prevented by modifying just three risk factors: smoking, hypertension, and alcohol abuse. There are data showing that a balanced diet and exercise also reduce cardiac-pulmonary disease. Another life-style choice, the use of addictive drugs, with its potentially serious social as well as health problems, is of particular concern because of its early beginnings. Nearly two-thirds of high school seniors report using an illicit drug during their lifetime, and dropouts may well have a much higher rate. Although general drug use by young adults may be falling, their use of stimulants and hard drugs, especially cocaine, has increased. Smoking, called a drug addiction by the U.S. Public Health Service, and less socially acceptable than it once was, still seems to have increased in women and teenagers. A newly discovered hazard is that of exposure of nonsmokers to cigarette smoke, particularly in the workplace, where the smoke may interact with other agents.

Perhaps one of the most controversial health issues in the last decade has been the effect of "toxic agents" on the public's health. The morbidity and mortality caused by such agents are often difficult to document, since the effect on health may not be seen for decades, and there may not be a clear indication of which of the many interacting factors is clearly responsible for an illness or death. Some occupational illnesses have been identified, and to varying degrees, safety standards have been set and enforced by the Occupational Safety and Health Administration (OSHA) and the Environmental Protection Agency (EPA). Consumer groups and unions have claimed that such protection is generally insufficient and limited because of political considerations, while industry complains that it is so overregulated that expenses for compliance are unreasonable. Some conditions, such as byssinosis (brown lung disease), caused by cotton dust in the textile industries, and silicosis (black lung disease) caused by silica, particularly in mining, are clearly recognized as job-related diseases. It is generally accepted that other occupation-related disabilities are caused by benzine, asbestos, ethylene oxide (a sterilizing agent in hospitals and medical products industries), diisocyanate (a chemical used to produce plastic products), vinyl chloride, lead, and radiation, to name a few. Considered a major public health issue is the trend to exclude women, especially those of childbearing age, from positions involving possible exposure to chemical and physical agents with known or suspected teratogenic (birth defect-causing) properties. Men have not been excluded, although there are data suggesting that paternal exposure to these toxic agents may also be teratogenic. It is estimated that 100,000 jobs are closed to women because of these policies. The argument is that instead of such action, the environment could and should be made safe for all workers.

Other environmental hazards are also cited by public health experts and environmentalists. The depletion of the stratospheric ozone layer caused by chlorofluorocarbons (CFC) used in sprays, refrigeration, and air-conditioning systems, industrial blowing agents, insulating foams, metal cleaning and drying, garment cleaning, sterilization of medical supplies, and liquid fast freezing causes skin cancer and potential changes in the world's climate. Limitations have been set by the Clean Air Act for sulfur oxides, suspected particulate matter, nitrogen oxides, carbon monoxides, hydrocarbons, lead, and other pollutants emitted by various industries and automobiles, but there is a constant battle to determine what that limit should be.

Acid rain, resulting from emissions from coal-burning plants and factories—chiefly sulfur dioxide and nitrogen oxides that are chemically changed in the atmosphere—is suspected of destroying freshwater life, damaging forests and crops, and possibly threatening human health. Cited by the EPA as probably the most serious environmental problem in the United States is that of hazardous wastes. These are by-products of the manufacturing process of many products, but the large-scale generators are chemical manufacturers, petroleum refiners, and metal-production companies. Careless dumping of these wastes, for instance, in areas where they leak into a water supply or cause an explosion, has resulted in serious danger to whole communities. A report by the National Academy of Science contends that it is possible to contain wastes safely if certain caveats are observed, and some manufacturers are making an effort to clean up sites. Meanwhile, dangerous old waste dumps are continually being discovered.

The deadly chemical dioxin, an unwanted by-product of herbicides, pesticides, and other industrial products, has been given considerable attention, particularly since the question was raised as to its effect on soldiers and civilians in Vietnam, where it was a chemical contaminant of the defoliant Agent Orange. There is some belief that others, such as the inhabitants of the Love Canal area and those exposed to dioxin in train wrecks or factory explosions, have suffered from a variety of conditions, including kidney and liver ailments, birth defects, and cancer. In other environmental situations, contamination by polybrominated biphenyls (PPBs) and polychlorinated biphenyls (PCBs), now banned, has resulted in the expensive destruction of food products because of danger to human beings. One of the most recently publicized chemicals being regulated is ethylene dibromide (EDB), found in cereals, cake mixes, and other ready-to-eat foods.

Almost daily, there is some report in the media about product or environmental dangers, whether noise, food additives, safety failure of equipment, toys, autos, or even clothing, hazardous wastes, acid rain, radioactive leaks, unsafe drinking water, or even human destruction from nuclear weapons or plants. Some feel that this is a hysterical reaction to unproven claims. Others ignore the entire issue. Still others feel that with or without more definitive data, a stronger effort must be made to improve the environment. Certainly, the clearly visible smog in so many urban areas is evidence that there is room for improvement.

Several years ago, one scientist commented, "The new danger to our well-being, if we continue to listen to all the talk, is in becoming a nation of healthy hypochondriacs, living gingerly, worrying ourselves half to death."[14] Between that fate and the danger of living sick or dying prematurely because of danger created by people's indifference, carelessness, and ignorance lies the answer to the nation's health problems.

TECHNOLOGICAL, SCIENTIFIC, AND MEDICAL ADVANCES

There is little question that the technological advances of the last quarter century have been extraordinary and, combined with scientific–medical advances, the beginnings of a new health care system have been emerging. Some of the most significant technological changes affecting patient care facilities can be categorized as follows:

1. Developments in diagnosis and patient care, such as automated clinical laboratory equipment, artificial human organs, improved surgical techniques and equipment, and the use of the electronic computer in diagnosis.

2. Hospital information handling—mainly coming from application of the electronic computer for patient billing, accounting, medical research, and diagnostic applications. These are being developed to control the flow of information so that health practitioners can have ready access to necessary data and can have information transmitted quickly and accurately to all affected departments. (In the area of community health, a complete physical with all necessary laboratory and other diagnostic tests is possible in less time and usually for less cost than by traditional methods—all with the help of computers.)

3. Developments affecting hospital supply and services, such as widespread adoption of plastic and other inexpensive materials, and adoption of improved materials and such equipment as specialized carts, conveyers, and pneumatic tubes.

4. Improvement in the management and structural design of health facilities all aimed at more efficient utilization of personnel, equipment, and space. This involves improved concepts of management and construction of health facilities, putting into effect concepts of progressive patient care and other advances in organizing health services.

5. Mass communication, making possible speedy transmission of health information and new knowledge, and exerting a powerful influence in molding public opinion. It can bring about positive results, such as providing information on communicable diseases and ways in which to get help; it can provide knowledge about other social and health problems, and even provide formal educational programs. Unfortunately, entertainment for the masses appears to take overwhelming precedence over any kind of positive teaching-learning process.

Although there is undeniable progress in health care directly attributable to technology, there is also great fear that the more machines do, the less human interaction there will be. In addition, the fear of loss of privacy becomes particularly acute with revelations of how the government and others could gain access to information about an individual's private life. Some sociologists predicted a few years ago that man would soon carry one card, containing a record of his name, age, address, date and place of birth, blood type, IQ, religion, marital status, salary, credit rating, political affiliation, and personality traits, all carefully coded and stored by a computer (accurately, one hopes). Actually this exists today in Sweden, with almost all of these data correlated with the citizen's personal number, which is given at birth.

In the United States, the computer is playing a growing role in people's lives. Not only are computers used in almost every phase of business, the professions, and education but they have also become popular in the home for those who can afford them. There they are used for everything from game playing to job- or school-related projects. Children are being taught to work with computers in some schools, and a major report on education recommended that a half-year of computer science be required for high school graduation.[15] Predicted within a decade are the Japanese-designed knowledge information-processing systems (KIPS), a new generation of computers so immensely powerful as to constitute a revolutionary form of wealth. They will be so much more powerful that, whereas today's machines can handle 10,000 to 100,000 logical inferences per second (LIPS), the next generation of computers will be capable of handling 100 million to 1 billion LIPS. They will be able to interact with people using normal language, speech, and pictures, transform talk into print, and translate one language into another.

While such computers are on the drawing board, several immediate problems of current computer usage have alarmed the public. First is the question of security of information. In the early 1980s, young computer experts made headlines with their ability to invade the computers of banks, hospitals, industry, and even the government, in some cases changing or erasing data. While others had already used the computer to commit crimes (and were not always caught and punished), this new danger reinforced earlier concerns about the confidentiality of computer-stored information. Would an employer, or simply a curious individual, be able to review another individual's credit record or hospital record? For that matter, would the record be accurate? Anyone who has had to deal with the unresponsive computer of businesses and the government knows the difficulty of catching and correcting errors; computer input still has a human component.

For those in the health field, computer use is a reality in many health care agencies. For nurses, this means learning to use the new technology for the benefit of the patient, but continually maintaining the emphasis on individuality and human contact, which no machine can provide, as well as protecting the patient's privacy.

There are other issues. Computerization may take much of the routine paperwork off nurses' hands, theoretically giving them more time for patient care—patient care that is also assisted by computer monitoring. But, given the financial pressures of most hospitals, for instance, will they replace labor costs with capital investments in such technology as a hedge against inflation? Will a choice be made between a computer that monitors continuously with 84 percent accuracy and coronary care nurses who monitor perhaps 30 to 50 percent of the time with close to 100 percent accuracy? There are some predictions that high-technology computers, micro-electronics, satellite communications, and robotics, seen by business and government as the nation's economic solution, will actually have a negative impact on the female workforce. Women already perform most of the low-skilled, high-technology labor at low wages and are even being displaced in their traditional stronghold, the office. It has been noted that job loss for women is high for stenographers, bank tellers, keypunch operators, insurance clerks, and telephone operators when computerization is introduced. On the other hand, there are predictions of increased jobs in specialized areas.

Computers have had a definite impact on organizational structures such as hospitals. Farlee[16] notes that although the goals of any organization include efficiency and productivity, these have not been characteristics of hospital organization. Hospital information systems (HIS) are expected to promote efficiency, but their introduction may prove to be both disturbing and disruptive to those already employed. The effect of HIS on the organizational structure is described: first, they tend to formalize rules and procedures; second, they centralize decision making at fairly high administrative levels; third, a new cadre of workers, specialists in the field, is introduced; fourth, there is an increased clarification of status differences, with a tendency to increase rigidity and reduce communication and interaction between levels of occupations and organizational units. Since low formalization, low centralization, high specialization, and low stratification are most conducive to employee acceptance of and accommodation to such technological change, tensions can arise if adjustments are not made.

The greatest impetus to the development of nursing information systems came about when Medicare-Medicaid coverage required nurses to provide data needed for reimbursement and to document the care given both in hospitals and in community health agencies. Effective use of computer systems in health care organizations requires that nurses be critical of the systems they evaluate and use, which means that they must learn about computers and what they can do. They must also help clarify and standardize the nursing data base. If not, nurses "will be left in the position of reacting to systems that other people design for us, systems designed to solve the problems as others perceive them."[17]

Other technology plays an important role in health care. Scientific and medical advances have gone beyond the imagination of science fiction. Theoretically, with the isolation of DNA and the process of cloning (production of genetically identical copies of an individual organism), a human being could be created by artificial means. Even the possibility is rather frightening and raises many ethical issues. In 1978, the birth of the first test-tube babies with the ovum fertilized outside the mother's body created a worldwide furor. The replacement of nonfunctioning human parts with artificial substitutes or human transplants has the potential of bringing a bionic era to reality. Already there have been implanted or attached titanium and polyethylene thigh bones; cords of woven Dacron for tendons; plastic, steel, and metal-alloy joints; orlon and Dacron blood vessels; plastic and titanium heart valves; artificial voice devices; and even, in 1982, the first artificial heart (although the patient died after some weeks). Moreover, progress has been made in electronic stimulation of the brain for hearing and seeing, and in developing miniaturized versions of the artificial kidney; versatile lasers can remove the cloudiness from the eyes of the visually impaired. Nuclear magnetic resonance (NMR), a new diagnostic imaging technique utilizing magnetic and radio frequencies to image body tissues and monitor body chemistry, is seen as a major breakthrough in both the diagnosis and treatment of a wide variety of conditions. It is also criticized because of its cost.

Use of such technology is also criticized for other reasons. Perhaps most controversial is the use of human parts from a dead or dying individual to maintain life in another person with nonfunctioning vital organs. Corneal transplants have been readily accepted, because the donor is already dead. The transplant of hearts, kidneys, and livers taken from an individual whose heart is still beating because of artificial life-maintenance techniques has produced not only ethical but legal problems (see Chapter 22). There are two major problems. First, the tremendous cost of using all of these transplant techniques means that, in almost all cases, someone must select those who will have surgery and a chance to live. Sometimes the poor risk or simply the poor have no access to these new techniques. Second is the question of whether it is morally right to precipitate the death of the person kept alive artificially by disconnection of machinery in order to use his vital parts for someone else.

Of increasing concern is the issue of when technology should be used to keep people alive. Only a few states and a few judges have chosen to make a definitive statement of when death occurs—at the cessation of brain functioning or heart functioning. The ability to prolong life artificially has been extremely disturbing to many in the health field and certainly to the families concerned. And the more sophisticated the techniques of survival, the more complex the decision. Legal aspects aside (Chapter 22), the decisions of when, or if, life-sustaining measures should be discontinued for a terminal patient and who should decide this (patient, family and/or physician, or court) are not easily made.

EDUCATION

Trends in education affect nursing in a number of ways: (1) the kind, number, and quality of students entering the nursing programs and the background they bring with them; (2) the development of educational technology, which frequently becomes a part of nursing education; and (3) the impact of social demands on education, which are eventually also extended to education in the professions, including nursing. Usually it is not just one social or economic condition that brings about change in education, nor is there only one kind of change. For instance, overexpansion by most institutions of higher education when the baby boom was at its height created a large pool of unemployed college graduates in the early 1970s. Some of these, as well as college students with a worried eye to the future, looked for educational programs that seemed to promise immediate jobs with a fu-

ture, among them nursing. Thus, what had once been a trickle of mature, second-degree students into nursing became a steady stream. As the baby boom group diminished, the overextended institutions of higher education and individual programs found it necessary to use marketing strategies of all kinds to attract enough students. They discovered the working adults in the community, who were a relatively untapped pool.

There were several definitive results. This diversity of age, background, education, and life experience in those seeking (or being sought for) advanced education has been an important factor in both social and political pressures for more flexibility in higher education. At the same time, providing such flexibility is one of the marketing strategies educational institutions are, after considerable resistance, relying on to attract the "older" prospective student. One focus is on liberalizing ways by which individuals can receive academic credit for what they know, regardless of when, where, or how they acquired that knowledge. Credentials are viable currency in the struggle for upward mobility, and those in the health field are as eager as others in society to be a part of this movement. In general education, the concepts of independent study and credit by examination have been explored by an increasing number of colleges, and a variety of testing mechanisms are being used to grant credit, including teacher-made tests and standardized tests, which have wide acceptance. One example of the latter is the College Level Examination Program (CLEP), which was developed some time ago by the Educational Testing Service and funded by the Carnegie Corporation. It includes tests of general education and numerous examinations in individual courses for which a number of colleges and universities award credit.

Pressure toward a more open curriculum has also been exerted on general and nursing education through recommendations in reports made by prestigious groups and foundations. For example, the Carnegie Commission on Higher Education conducted a series of studies that seemed to voice the complaints of the public about limitations imposed by higher education. In its special report, *Less Time, More Options: Education Beyond the High School* (1971), several recommendations were of particular importance to nursing education. In recommending that "professions, wherever possible, create alternate routes of entry other than full-time college attendance, and reduce the number of narrow, one-level professions which do not afford opportunities for advancement," the commission stated a particular concern with the "growth of horizontal professions in the health services that impede vertical mobility." It further recommended that "a degree (or other form of credit) be made available to students at least every two years in their careers (and in some cases every year.)"[18] An earlier report on medicine and dentistry had already recommended a health science core that could lead to training in a variety of health-related professions—a move toward horizontal mobility.[19] At the same time, two other national reports made recommendations in the same vein.[20,21]

That these pressures have had some results is clear when one sees the increased number of so-called external degree programs. Some are marginally legitimate operations that have given the whole concept a bad name with meaningless mail-order degrees, but more and more respected, accredited educational institutions have established external degree programs using various modes: weekend, evening, summer, or other time periods for concentrated classes; outreach programs for isolated areas or even the workplace; self-study courses with examinations; and a process of combining educational credentials and examination results. A particularly successful example of the last is the Regents College Degrees, previously the New York Regents External Degree Program, which includes both associate and baccalaureate degrees in nursing. (See Chapter 12 for more detailed information on this and other open curriculum practices in nursing.)

It was predicted that an aid to these new educational or flexible patterns was the use of all types of audiovisual media, computers, programmed learning, and other new techniques that can enhance the teaching-learning process. Although these methods appear to be generally successful, they are expensive, and there is some argument as to whether the learning acquired is superior to that gained by more traditional methods. One great asset appears to be that learning can be individualized more easily through use of these techniques and also that satisfactory learning can occur in places other than the classroom and in the teacher's presence—even to the point of checking out these learning tools as books are checked out from the library. The latter is particularly pertinent with a rising demand for continuing education in all professional fields, an aspect of the demand for current competence.

When Ronald Reagan became president in 1981, he made it very clear that he intended to dismantle the year-old Department of Education and limit federal spending for education. At the end of his first term, the department still existed, and while funding for certain educational programs had decreased, other funding had increased. In higher education, the major change was in federal assistance to college students, with, among other things, a means test being reinstituted for the Guaranteed Student Loan (GSL) program. What made education a major issue of the time was the report of the National Commission on Excellence in Education,[22] appointed by the Secretary of Education. The report began with the words, "Our nation is at risk." Warning that the United States was being overtaken by other countries in industry, science, and technological innovation, the report not only listed the indicators of the risk but made a number of strong recommendations. It concluded that the documented decline in educational performance was largely a result of "disturbing inadequacies" in the educational process at all levels. Among the recommendations were strengthened high school graduation requirements; a longer school year; higher standards for student performance and conduct, and higher admission requirements for colleges and universities; improvement of teacher preparation and improved working conditions for them; and demand by citizens for accountability of educators and officials holding leadership positions in the field, along with acceptance by the public of the fiscal support and stability needed to bring about these reforms.

Following this report were two others making equally strong recommendations for improvement in education, again with emphasis on leadership, teaching, higher standards, and federal support.[23,24]

There have also been serious faculty-related issues in the last several years. Although nursing still does not have sufficient numbers of appropriately prepared faculty in any of its educational programs, the economic pressures of the times affect these faculties as well as others in higher education. If there are not layoffs or oversupplies of doctorates, as in some disciplines, nursing faculties join the others in common concerns: heavier teaching loads; salary reductions; attacks on tenure; attacks on collective bargaining; and criticisms of the quality of teaching. In addition, there seems to have been an increase in court decisions regarding sexual harassment, sexual discrimination (in salaries, promotion, and retirement benefits), faculty rights, and civil rights.

It has been said that educational issues come in cycles, which may mean either that they are never resolved or that the passage of time brings different dimensions to them. Predictions about whether college enrollment will increase or decrease, whether the liberal arts or the professions and technologies will gain precedence, whether research or teaching will have priority, and whether graduates of certain programs will have a better future all fill the educational literature. It does appear, however that the criteria of excellence and pertinence may be the criteria in governmental and private support of research and education. How these trends, issues, and pressures affect nursing is specifically discussed in Chapter 12.

THE WOMEN'S RIGHTS MOVEMENT

Nursing, from its American beginning, was primarily made up of women, and some nurses have always been involved in the women's rights movement to some degree, but not nearly as much as one would expect. The suffragette route was not easy for women in the late nineteenth and early twentieth centuries, and often women did not support the movement. That reaction may have been caused, in part, by the negative, even vindictive, portrait newspapers painted of those in the movement, as illustrated by a few typical quotes:[25] "organized by divorced wives, childless women, and sour old maids," "unsexed women," "entirely devoid of personal attractions . . . these maiden ladies who perhaps have been disappointed, having found it utterly impossible to induce any young or old man into the matrimonial noose," "personally repulsive," "laboring on the heels of strong hatred towards men." Whether the opposition resulted from the fear of overthrowing "the most sacred of our institutions (marriage)" or "Are we to put the stamp of truth upon the feeling that men and women in the matrimonial relationship are to be equal?" is a moot point. Legal discrimination against women has not ended, even with the passage of women's suffrage in 1921. (See chapter 17.) There are also other manifestations of discrimination that are psychological rather than legal.

That many women in other occupations and professions, as well as housewives, have felt just as strongly is indicated by the resurgence of the "women's lib" movement, called by some one of the major phenomena of the last decade. As in any other movement, there have been extremists who have become famous (or infamous), but in general, the movement is becoming increasingly organized and powerful. Among the most active groups is the National Organization for Women (NOW), founded in 1966 and made up of women and men who support "full equality for women in truly equal partnership with men" and ask an end to discrimination and prejudice against women in government, industry, the professions, churches, the political parties, the judiciary, labor unions, education, science, medicine, law, religion, and every other field of importance in American society. NOW activities are directed toward legislative action to end discrimination, and it attempts to promote its views through demonstrations, research, litigation, and political pressure. Among actions taken are the development of a model rape law, endorsement of health education for women in self-help clinics, and support of women in training of health care personnel. Both NOW and other groups often organize consciousness-raising sessions for women to make them aware of their potential and aid them in achieving a better understanding of themselves and their role in society. The impact of the movement can be observed in newspaper reports, which show that both legal and social changes are occurring, slowly but surely, in relation to women's roles. A sudden, overwhelming about-face by men (and women) in terms of what women are, and can be, is not expected; attitudes are too deeply embedded. Forty years ago, psychoanalyst Karen Horney, who defied Freud's negative and degrading views on women, wrote, "The view that women are infantile and emotional creatures, incapable of responsibility and independence, is the work of the masculine tendency to lower women's self respect." The literature of psychiatry and, it is charged, the attitudes of many psychiatrists, are still influenced by Freud's notions. There is also insurmountable evidence that children are socialized into stereotyped male and female roles by books, use of toys and influence of parents,

teachers, and others—a problem being given special attention by feminists.*

Certainly these attitudes are not merely American. A 1974 UN report indicated that sexist attitudes were found around the world (and frequently held by UN delegates).

In 1975, the International Women's year culminated in a UN-sponsored conference in Mexico City, intended to develop a ten-year plan to improve the status of women, particularly stressing education and health care. More than 1,000 UN delegates and 5,000 other feminists and interested spectators attended, but at the end of the week, despite a document of official recommendations, the highly politicized meeting was not as successful as had been hoped. The UN allotted considerably less money to this conference than to others, and the preordained president of the conference was the male attorney general of Mexico. More serious was the division of interests of the women. The caucus of Third World women, for instance, showed little interest in the concerns of Western women. Equal pay and day-care centers were not issues in countries where most women have no voting or property rights. When 500 million of the 800 million illiterates in the world are women, they are not upset at the use of sexual stereotypes in books. The recommendations that emerged were a mixture and focused on encouraging governments to ensure equality in terms of educational opportunities, training and employment, to ameliorate the "hard work loads" falling on women in certain economic groups and in certain countries, to improve access to health services, better nutrition and other social services, to ensure that

---

*According to NOW, "A feminist is a person who believes women (even as men) are primarily people; that human rights are indivisible by any category of sex, race, class or other designation irrelevant to our common humanity; a feminist is committed to creating the equality (not sameness) of the sexes legally, socially, educationally, psychologically, politically, religiously, economically in all the rights and responsibilities of life." Wilma Scott Heide, "Nursing and Women's Liberation: A Parallel," *Am. J. Nurs.,* **73**:824 (May 1973).

women have equal rights with men in voting and participating in political life, and that both men and women have the right to determine the number and spacing of their children.

There was even greater anticipation by American women for the three-day National Women's Conference in Houston in 1977. Again, there was dissension on specific issues, particularly ratification of the Equal Rights Amendment (ERA), abortion rights, and sexual preference (lesbian) rights. It was said that the major breakthrough was the end of the psychological isolation constraining feminist activities.

The 1,442 delegates, elected at fifty-six state and territorial meetings that were open to the public, included just about all races and cultures in the United States (including four Eskimos) and a variety of the political and apolitical, rich and poor, housewives and career women. Their point of agreement was that they were tired of second-class citizenship and craved greater social and economic equality. It was an ebullient but tightly run proceeding. Said one news report,

> The conference was run with more efficiency and dispatch, more zest and panache than most conventions dominated by men. . . . No one could accuse the participants of being any less adroit, canny or Machiavellian than men. . . . What had not been clear was whether women who were eager to improve their lot, but had never been involved in the political process before, could be kept in order long enough even to discuss, let alone vote, on all these issues. Order was achieved by the kind of discipline any male politician would give his eyeteeth to attain.[26]

Although there were some protests that the majority ruled so firmly that the minority did not have full say, the final twenty-five-point National Plan for Action was passed by convincing majorities. Included in the final document were substantive resolutions calling for passage of the ERA, encouragement and re-

cruitment of women for political office and appointments, full and equal employment rights, support of human rights, peace and disarmament (the women's rights logo is a stylized dove), extension of Social Security benefits for housewives, federal rural plans to overcome problems of isolation, poverty, and underemployment, a strong focus on minority women, welfare and poverty as women's issues, and equal rights for lesbians (considered the most sensitive issue in terms of public acceptance). Included in the health-related area were protection of and support for battered women, children, and rape victims, a national health insurance plan with special provisions for women, expansion of research on contraceptive drugs, alcohol, and drug abuse, emphasis on safety of all drugs, participation of women in governmental health planning and policy groups, and funding to encourage women to enter the health professions.*

For all the high hopes, however, the next few years were a seesaw of win some, lose some. A bitter disappointment was the death of the proposed Equal Rights Amendment to the Constitution, three states short of the thirty-eight needed for ratification (see Chapter 17). Ten years after it was passed by Congress, and despite an extension of the deadline for ratification from 1979 to 1982, Indiana in 1977 was the last state to ratify. More than 450 national organizations endorsed the amendment, and polls showed that more than two-thirds of U.S. citizens supported it, but to no avail. The conservative opposition, including fundamentalist Christian churches, the so-called Moral Majority, the John Birch Society, the Mormon Church, and the American Farm Bureau, led a well-financed, smoothly organized, and politically astute campaign. Antiamendment forces assured state legislators that the Fourteenth Amendment offered sufficient protection to women, and claimed that the ERA would cause the death of the

---

*Details on these resolutions are in the March 1978 issue of *Ms.*, pp. 19–21, 81–84.

family by removing a man's obligation to support his wife and children, would legalize homosexual marriages, lead to unisex toilets, and most damaging, lead to the drafting of women for combat duty. Advocates of the ERA were later criticized as lacking political finesse and alienating women who were potential supporters—blacks, pink-collar (office) workers, and housewives. Amendment supporters lay heavy blame on men, particularly in legislatures and business.

After the defeat, the 50,000-member Eagle Forum, and its founder, Phyllis Schafly, the woman considered the leader of the anti-ERA forces, laid plans to campaign against sex education, the nuclear freeze, and "undesirable" textbooks.

Feminists determined to concentrate women's new consciousness and resources in building legislative strength to eventually pass the ERA and to mount a campaign for reproductive freedom, democratization of families, more respect for work done in the home, and comparable pay for the work done outside it. Once more, the results have varied. Another ERA bill introduced in Congress in 1983 was defeated by six votes in the House of Representatives, with a two-to-one Republican opposition. Yet both friends and foes of equal rights note that the feminist movement, along with other societal forces, has made a definite impact on American life. Some twenty years after Betty Friedan published *The Feminine Mystique* (called by the futurist Alvin Toffler "the book that pulled the trigger of history"), changes can be clearly identified. A 1983 poll of women showed attitudes quite different from those of 1970. More than twice as many cited general rights and freedom of career, jobs, and pay as the most enjoyable things about being a woman; 6, 8, and 26 percent, respectively, cited being a wife, homemaker, and mother.[27] Another poll, covering the same time span, noted that the goals of male and female college students regarding careers and family life were remarkably similar.[28] In the early 1960s, about 38 percent of the women were in the workforce; now over 50 percent

work. However, in 1984, it was reported that women working full time were still earning an average of sixty-two cents for every dollar paid to men.

Navarro attributes the traditionally low status of women in the workforce to the social role of the woman in the family, in which the wife has the job of taking care of the home and family at no salary. The employer of the husband, in essence, gets the work of two for the price of one. The wife has "emotional rewards," a concept carried over to other kinds of caring work. One of the ascribed virtues of womanhood is seen as being a good homemaker, and even now, to do something else may be criticized as neglecting home and family, woman's real work.[29]

Now there is a more militant attitude taken by women, and a new push to raise women's pay is evident. A growing number of lawsuits and union negotiations have challenged the male-female pay ratio based on the "comparable worth" theory. This theory, going beyond equal pay for equal work, calls for equal pay for different jobs of comparable worth. The intent is to revalue *all* jobs on the basis of the skills and responsibility they require. Neither the Equal Pay Act nor the Civil Rights Act brought about reform at any level of the workforce, but what might be a landmark case resulted in the state of Washington being ordered in 1984 to pay female workers up to $1 billion in back wages and increases because of such pay inequity. Many more suits are anticipated, and perhaps to forestall them, industry and business are becoming more interested in job evaluation studies (with, presumably, equal pay following). Just as important are a series of Supreme Court rulings that ban employers from offering retirement plans that provide men and women with unequal benefits. As one justice wrote, "An individual woman may not be paid lower monthly benefits simply because women as a class live longer than men."

Other calls for celebration were the appointment of the first woman to the Supreme Court (Sandra Day O'Connor), the first woman in space (Sally Kristin Ride, with a Ph.D. in physics), the first woman vice presidential candidate of a major political party (Geraldine Ferraro), and, perhaps more prosaically, an increase in the number of women in public and appointed offices at all political levels. Furthermore, the growing gender gap (a term used to identify the difference between men's and women's votes) is not being ignored by even the most conservative legislators, since women comprise more than 50 percent of the population.

The issue of women's rights is closely related to the problems, activities, and goals of women working in the health service industry. From 75 percent to 85 percent of all health service workers are women, and the largest health occupation, nursing, is almost totally female. These women-dominated occupations are also expanding most rapidly, but, as one writer indicated, "Health service is women's work but not women's power. . . . The health service industry is run by a small minority. It is run primarily by physicians, who have traditionally held the power, but also by the increasingly powerful hospital administrators, insurance company directors, government regulators, medical school educators, and corporation mangers. Most of these people are men."[30] According to Brown, the reasons for so many women in health care is that, first, they are an inexpensive source of labor; second, they are available; and third, they are safe, that is, no threat to physicians who, in order to expand their power and income, "must be assured of subordinates who will stay subordinate."[31]

One respected management consultant, appraising the power base in the booming health field, noted that power comes from influence with doctors and, to a lesser extent, administrators. "A respectful attitude toward doctors is essential."[32] Whether or not these points are valid, it is certainly accurate to say that for many women in the field today, these were once the best jobs available and the salaries were incredibly low for a long time.

Now it appears that women are looking to the health field for a career, not just a stopgap job. Breaking the barriers to advancement and recognition is one type of challenge, but it has also been noted that whether in the health field or elsewhere, women still have the major responsibility for the home as well. Most employed women, whatever their occupations, must struggle with conflicts between family obligations, personal desires and ambitions, and the demands and limitations of their work.[33]

This federal study also supported the conclusion of others about the role and the problems of women in health. Among the major issues cited were sex stereotyping and friction with male professionals. Virginia Cleland, an activist nurse, agrees. "Today, there is no doubt in my mind that our most fundamental problem in nursing is that we are members of a woman's occupation in a male-dominated culture."[34]

More than any other factor, the absence of professional autonomy for nurses (see Chapter 16) is considered a direct result of sex discrimination in nursing, with the end result that the patient/client ultimately suffers. The movement of nurses toward autonomy is seen partially as the result of the women's movement, and the struggles in achieving autonomy have certainly enhanced interest in the movement. The fight against sexual discrimination has gained new impetus in nursing, as well as in other segments of society, and has spilled over to include in the consumer movement the entire issue of women's health.

THE CONSUMER REVOLUTION

The consumer revolution, said to have begun when Theodore Roosevelt signed the first Pure Food and Drug Act in 1906, has been an accelerating phenomenon since the 1950s. Although various interpretations are put on the term, it might be broadly defined as the concerted action of the public in response to a lack of satisfaction with the products and/or services of various groups. The publics are, of course, different, but often overlapping: A woman unhappy about the cost and quality of auto repairs might be just as displeased by the services of her gynecologist, the cost of hospital care, or the use of dangerous food additives. One well-known health consumer advocate calls the increasing confrontations between consumer and provider just the "tip of the iceberg" of some major changes in American society. She says:

> The growth of "consumerism" has something to do with the transition from an economy of scarcity to one of abundance, with increasing education and income. It has a lot to do with television, faster communications, and rising levels of expectation. . . . Very importantly, consumerism involves, in one way or another, all income levels and all social groups, not just the poor, the blue collar workers, or the rich.[35]

There have probably always been dissatisfied consumers, but the major difference now is that many are organized in ad hoc or permanent organizations and have the power, through money, numbers, and influence, to force providers to be responsive to at least some of their demands. The methods vary but include lobbying for legislation, legal suits, boycotts, and media campaigns. One of the most noted, albeit highly criticized, consumer activists is Ralph Nader, whose Center for Study of Responsive Law produced a blitz of study group reports in the early 1970s that exposed abuses in a wide range of fields. Currently, his Health Research Group is one of the most influential in health consumerism. And there is an increasingly strong force moving in that direction. Consumers, who first concentrated their efforts against the shoddy workmanship and indifferent services offered in material goods, have now turned to the quality, quantity, and cost of other services, particularly in health care. Fewer patient/clients are accepting without protest the "I know best" attitudes of health care providers, whether physician, nurse, or any of the many others involved in health care. The self-help

phenomenon, in which people learn about health care and help each other ("stroke clubs" and Alcoholics Anonymous, for instance), has extended to self-examination—sometimes through classes sponsored by doctors, nurses, and health agencies. Interest in health promotion and illness prevention has also been manifested by the involvement of consumers in environmental concerns.

The dehumanization of patient care, which is contrary to all the stated beliefs of the professions involved, is repeatedly castigated in studies of health care. Although complaints often are directed at the care of the poor, too often it is a universal health care deficiency. The concerted action of organized minority groups led to the development of the American Hospital Association's Patient Bill of Rights,* which received widespread attention in 1973, followed by a rash of similar rights statements specifically directed to children, the mentally ill, the elderly, pregnant women, the dying, the handicapped, patients of various religions, and others. In some cases, presidential conferences and legislation have followed. The whole area of the rights of people in health care, which focuses to a great extent on patients' rights to full and accurate information so that they can make informed decisions about their care, has major implications for nurses (see Chapter 22).

An excellent example of the rise of a health consumer group is the Women's Health Movement, which emerged from women's disenchantment with their personal and institutional health relationships. Their complaints centered on physicians' attitudes toward women, which seem to be the result of both medical education and professional socialization. Not only are there the Freudian concepts but such recent gems as, "The traits which compose the core of the female personality are feminine narcissism, masochism, and passivity."[36] The fact that women's complaints of the health care system are neither isolated nor

---

*See Chapter 22.

trivial is attested to by the attention given by lay and professional media to such problems as unnecessary hysterectomies. However, the impetus toward organization is credited to the women's consciousness-raising groups of the 1960s, in which women shared their medical experiences and found support for taking action. The Women's Health Movement, identified as a grass-roots organization, came into existence around 1970 and by 1975 had increased to 1,200 identified groups providing direct services, and tens of thousands of women who considered themselves activists or participants. Groups are also active in Canada, Europe, South America, Australia, and New Zealand.[37] Their activities are centered on changing consciousness, providing health-related services, and working to change established health institutions. Specific and well-known (as well as controversial) entities are the various feminist health centers and their know-your-body and self-help courses and books. The organizations' scope of functions is increasing to include not only primary care, but nutritional, psychological, gerontologic, and pediatric services. Without doubt, those involved see the need for women to control their own essential femaleness as simultaneously related to the wider issues of female equality and liberation. "The health care system has been an agent of social control as equally restrictive as any political or economic system. Women seek to dissolve the power it exercises over them."[38]

Other consumers are also concerned with the power issue and are insisting on such rights as participation in governing boards of hospitals and other community health institutions, accrediting boards, health planning groups, and licensing boards. A revision of national legislation (PL93-641, National Health Planning and Resources Act of 1974, discussed in Chapter 19) and changes in licensure laws (discussed in Chapter 20) point out their increased success, in both the consumer revolution and the "rights" movement. What lies ahead in terms of more regulation, such as an overall federal consumer protection law, is not yet known.

OTHER FACTORS

The history of nursing makes clear the influence of socioeconomic factors on the profession. It is no different today. Double-digit inflation has already had an impact on the cost and support of nursing education, nurse supply and demand, and, perhaps, quality of care. Cost containment will probably be one of the leading health issues in the next decade.* Nurses who do not choose to make the effort to understand the hows and whys of health economics may find themselves at a loss to justify their utilization in a particular setting.

Also related to economics is the power of unions. Labor was said to be at a crossroads in 1978, with membership down to a forty-one-year low, with loss of bargaining elections at nearly 52 percent in 1977, its legislation repeatedly blocked by newly potent business lobbies and inflation-wary legislators; its aging leaders inspiring less public confidence than in any other American institution. In part, this was the result of an inability to adjust to postwar work patterns—a growth switch from industry to white collar, wholesale and retail trade, and service industries. In order to recoup their losses and regain their momentum of the 1940s and 1950s, unions are now turning to or beefing up other potential sources of union activity, such as the health care industries. This includes professionals and nonprofessionals, as demonstrated by the 1978 announcement of the American Federation of Teachers to concentrate efforts on organizing nurses and other health workers.

However, beginning with President Reagan's breaking of the air controllers' illegal strike in August 1981, by firing and subsequently replacing the air controllers, the un-

_____

*See Chapter 7.

ions have had special difficulties. Some employers simply threaten to file for bankruptcy, and the courts have supported their right to abrogate any existing union contract under those circumstances. Others, finding that they can withstand long strikes because the unemployed are willing to take the strikers' jobs, are demanding (and getting) paybacks of benefits and pay in new contracts, citing the poor economy and competition as the reason. Union leadership is blamed for not seeing the economic problems and being greedy earlier. Both unions and management have been warned to soften their adversarial approach.

Management is also trying a new technique to increase worker satisfaction. While far from widespread, there does seem to be growing interest in involving workers in decision making. A New York Stock Exchange survey found that 14 percent of American companies with more than 100 employees had reform programs, and a government study found that 44 percent of companies with more than 500 employees had groups in which workers and supervisors discussed plant operations, the so-called quality circles. Some labor experts say that these "reforms" (also known by such names as *job redesign, work humanization, employee participation, workplace democracy,* and *quality of work life*) are more cosmetic than real, since few workers participate in the companies' most important decisions, and that in a difficult situation most managers revert to an authoritarian stance. Others say that this new management style is necessary now that the nation is engaged in vigorous international competition. Similar techniques have been used in Europe and Japan for some time, and production success, particularly in Japan, has concerned American industry. Whether there will be backslidng when economic times are good is the question. Nevertheless, one long-standing hit on the bestseller list was a book that delineated the management style of America's best-run and most successful corporations.[39] Emphasized were a bias for action; satisfying the consumer;

fostering autonomy and entrepreneurship throughout the organization; showing respect for the individual; hands-on involvement (going to the workers); and clarity of company values. Many of these qualities seem to tie in with worker satisfaction and commitment to the job, and are also seen in the studies of the successful magnet hospitals described in Chapter 5.

FUTURE TRENDS

Preparing today for the future so that a profession, group, or individual will be in the forefront is often advised. Futurists have become popular writers and speakers, with their books often hitting the best-seller list. It has been noted that making predictions is a much more popular activity than evaluating their accuracy. One writer, surveying the fiction and nonfiction work of seers, concluded that most have "overestimated how much the world would be transformed by social and political change and underestimated the forces of technological change," and stated that scientists tended "to overestimate the chances for major scientific breakthroughs and underestimate the effects of straightforward development well within the boundaries of existing knowledge."[40]

Called a work of social analysis, Alvin Toffler's *The Third Wave*[41] received plaudits for at least raising thoughtful questions and criticisms for creating what some called pointless neologisms such as *indust-real* and *wave front analysis.* Toffler identified the First Wave as the period of agriculturalism, the Second Wave as that produced by the Industrial Revolution, and the Third Wave as created more or less by advances in science and electronics, with diversity replacing industrial uniformity. He predicted that the nature of work will be changed, becoming less repetitive and less fragmented, and with more employees working part-time or flexi-time by choice; that the "demassified" workforce and employees would want more responsibilities and more vital work, with a commitment worthy of their talents and skills; that people will, as part of a reunified family group, work in their "electronic cottage"; that the prosumer ethic already in existency (that is, the individual acting as both producer and consumer and producing for his or her own needs), will grow, with more interest in do-it-yourself and self-help activities.

There are now several companies in the prediction business and their executives tend to write books. One of the most successful identified "ten new directions transforming our lives."[42] These were derived from a content analysis of 6,000 local newspapers each month, which is part of the predicting methodology of the Naisbett group, as well as reviewing thousands of other newspaper and journal articles. To begin, Naisbett identified five bellwether states where most social invention was seen to occur: California, Florida, Washington, Colorado, and Connecticut. Briefly, the "megatrends" are as follows:

1. We are in a "megashift" from an industrial to an information-based society.
2. For every high-technology action, there is a "high-touch" reaction, or the technology will be rejected.
3. Our economy is becoming part of a global structure, moving away from isolation and national self-sufficiency. As a result, we will no longer be the world's dominant force.
4. U.S. corporate managers are beginning to think about the long term rather than the next quarter.
5. Our centralized structures are crumbling. We are decentralizing and growing stronger from the bottom up.
6. We are reclaiming our traditional sense of self-reliance after four decades of looking to institutions for help.
7. Citizens, workers, and consumers are demanding and getting a greater voice in government, business, and the marketplace.
8. We are moving from hierarchies to networking; the computer is smashing the pyramid.
9. The North–South shift in the United States is real and irreversible for the foreseeable future.
10. We no longer live in an either/or, chocolate-or-vanilla world; people have demanded and are getting a multitude of choices.

The accuracy of these megatrends, like that of other predictions, is yet to be determined. However, they were provocative enough to cause many (including nurses) to apply them to their own field.

REFERENCES

1. Alvin Toffler, *Future Shock* (New York: Random House, Inc., 1970), p.2.
2. "The World in 2000: Crowded, Unhealthy," *The Nation's Health,* Sept. 1980, pp 1, 12.
3. *The World Almanac and Book of Facts, 1984* (New York: Newspaper Enterprise Association, 1984), p. 596.
4. "The Wealth—and Poverty—of Nations," *New York Times,* Aug. 31, 1980, p. E3.
5. "Charting Global Childbearing," *World Health Forum,* 3:244 (1982).
6. Reid Reynolds, "Some Political and Ethical Problems in the Development of Family Planning," *International J. Health Serv.* 3:592 (1973).
7. Linda Atkinson et al., "Prospects for Improved Contraception," *Family Planning Persp.,* **12**:173–192 (July-Aug. 1980).
8. Larry Gordon, "The Awful Truth About Our Earth," *The Nation's Health,* Feb. 1981, p. 2.
9. "Census Totals Show Nation Is Diverse as Never Before," *The New York Times,* Sept. 6, 1981, p. E5.
10. Bruce Chapman, "United States Population: Changing Population Patterns," *The World Almanac and Book of Facts, 1984* (New York: Newspaper Enterprise

Association, 1984), p. 196.

11. Donald Grinberg. "The Abortion Activists," *Family Planning Persp.*, **13**:157–163 (July-Aug. 1981).

12. Lorraine Klerman, "Adolescent Pregnancy: A New Look at a Continuing Problem," *Am. J. Pub. Health,* **70**:776–778 (Aug. 1980).

13. Cathy Popescu, *America's Health: A Century of Progress But a Time of Despair* (Summit, N.J.: American Council on Science and Health, 1983).

14. Lewis Thomas, "Notes of a Biology-Watcher: The Health Care System, *New Eng. J. Med.,* **293**:1245 (1975).

15. "A Nation at Risk: The Imperative for Educational Reform," *Chronicle of Higher Ed.,* **26**:11–16 (May 4, 1983).

16. Coralee Farlee, "The Computer as a Focus of Organizational Change in the Hospital," *J. Nurs. Admin.,* **8**:20–26 (Feb. 1978).

17. Rita Zielstorff, "How Computer Systems Influence Nursing Activities in Hospitals," *Proceedings of the First National Conference on Computer Technology and Nursing* (Washington, D.C., 1983), p. 6.

18. Carnegie Commission on Higher Education, *Less Time, More Options: Education Beyond the High School* (New York: McGraw-Hill Book Company, 1971).

19. Carnegie Commission on Higher Education, *Higher Education and the Nation's Health* (New York: McGraw-Hill Book Company, 1970), p. 53.

20. Department of Health, Education, and Welfare, "Report on Licensing and Related Health Credentialing" (Washington, D.C., The Department, 1971).

21. Jerome Lysaught, *An Abstract for Action* (New York: McGraw-Hill Book Company, 1970).

22. "A Nation at Risk," op. cit.

23. "Federal Commitment to Excellence in Education Urged by Panel," *the Chronicle of Higher Ed.,* **26**: 5–8 (May 11, 1983).

24. "Summary of the National Science Board's Report on Education in Science and Technology," *Chronicle of Higher Ed.,* **26**: 10–16 (Sept. 21, 1983).

25. Teresa Christy, "Liberation Movement: Impact on Nursing," *AORN J.,* **15**:67–68 (Apr. 1972).

26. "What Next for U.S. Women," *Time,* **111**:21 (Dec. 5, 1977).

27. "Poll of U.S. Women Shows Jobs Rival Family Life," *The New York Times* Dec. 4, 1983, pp. 1, 66.

28. "For Students, a Dramatic Shift in Goals," *The New York Times,* Feb. 28, 1983, p. B5.

29. Vicente Navarro, "Women in Health Care," *New Eng. J. Med.,* **292**:400 (Feb. 20, 1975).

30. Carol A. Brown, "Women Workers in the Health Service Industry," *Int. J. Health Serv.,* **5**:173 (1975).

31. Ibid., p. 174.

32. Marilyn Moats Kennedy, "The Keys to the Kingdom," *Savvy,* **5**:53. (Feb. 1984).

33. Department of Health, Education and Welfare, *Executive Summary: A Story of the Participation of Women in the Health Care Industry Labor Force.* DHEW Publication No. (HRA)77–644, p.i.

34. Virginia Cleland, "Sex Discrimination: Nursing's Most Pervasive Problem" *Am. J. Nurs.,* **71**:1542 (Aug. 1971).

35. Nancy Quinn and Anne R. Somers, "The Patient's Bill of Rights: A Significant Aspect of the Consumer Revolution," *Nurs. Outlook,* **22**:243 (Apr. 1974).

36. J. R. Wilson et al., *Obstetrics and Gynecology* (St Louis: C. V. Mosby Company 1971), as quoted in Marieskind, "The Women's Health Movement," p. 219.

37. Helen Marieskind, ''The Women's Health Movement,'' *Int. J. Health Serv.* **5**(2): 218 (1975).

38. Ibid., p. 219.

39. Thomas J. Peters and Robert H. Waterman, Jr., *In Search of Excellence.* (New York: Harper & Row, Publishers, 1982).

40. Gerard K. O'Neill and Wayne Coffey, *2081: A Hopeful View of the Human Future* (New York: S and S/Touchstone, 1983).

41. Alvin Toffler, *The Third Wave* (New York: William Morrow Company, 1980).

42. John Naisbett, *Megatrends* (New York: Warner Books, Inc., 1982).

Health Care Delivery: Where?

Health care today is given in a variety of settings, such as hospitals, nursing homes, community health centers, state or city clinics, and the homes of patients/clients. Involved in this care are more than 3 million workers,* of which the majority are employed in hospitals. The size and complexity of the health care system alone create problems in the quality of service provided.

It is generally agreed that some of the essential elements of optimum health services in the community include a unified, cooperative team approach to care; a spectrum of services, including diagnosis, treatment, rehabilitation, education, and prevention; a coordinated community and/or regional system incorporating these services; continuity of care given by the hospital, community, physician, and other health agencies; a continuum of health services; and a program of evaluation and research concerning the adequacy of services in meeting patient and community needs. These elements are shown in Figure 7.1.

This chapter and the next are intended to present an overview of current health care delivery, its organization, and its workers. Spe-

cific details on how the nurse may function in these various settings are presented in Chapter 15.

DEFINITIONS

It has become popular to refer to health care delivery as being comprised of several levels: self-care, primary care, secondary care, and tertiary care. Another differentiation is primary, acute, and long-term care. Definitions vary and are somewhat hotly debated, but the following will provide a frame of reference.

Primary care: "(a) a person's first contact in any given episode of illness with the health care system that leads to a decision of what must be done to help resolve his problems; and (b) the responsibility for the continuum of care, i.e., maintenance of health, evaluation and management of symptoms, and appropriate referrals."[1] It is at this level that basic medical and other health care services are provided.

Millis, a layman who has had long-standing relationships with the health professions, puts

---

*Depending on who is included in the allied health category, the total may be as high as 8 million.

COMMUNITY HEALTH

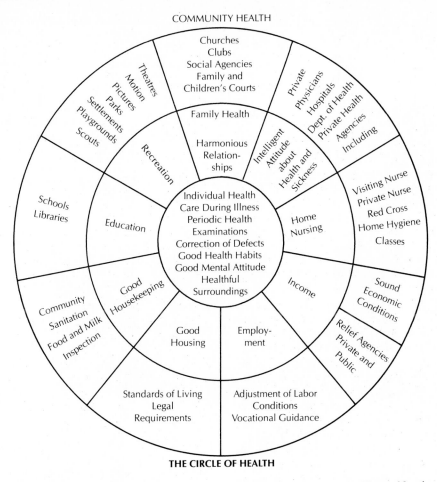

THE CIRCLE OF HEALTH

Figure 7-1. The circle of health. (Reprinted with permission from H. Frost: *Nursing in Sickness and Health*. New York: Macmillan, 1939, p. 86.)

it this way: "To me, primary care includes all the health services needed by a given population that are not provided by secondary and tertiary care. It includes health services as well as sickness services. It includes response to self-limiting disease, minor disability, and chronic and incurable disease. It includes prevention of disease, health maintenance, and public health. Most important, it includes self-care and thus addresses itself to those health problems that currently account for so much morbidity—automobile accidents, obe-sity, alcoholism, drug abuse, iatrogenic disease, and environmental hazards."[2]

Secondary care: the point at which consulting specialty and subspecialty services are provided in either an office (group practice) or community hospital inpatient setting.

Tertiary care: the point at which highly sophisticated diagnostic treatment or rehabilitation services are provided, frequently in university medical centers or equivalent institutions.

Acute care: "those services that treat the acute phase of illness or disability and has as its purpose the restoration of normal life processes and function."[3]

Long-term care: "those services designed to provide symptomatic treatment, maintenance, and rehabilitative services for patients of all age groups in a variety of health care settings."[4]

The definition of self-care, the first level of care, is self-explanatory. Its interpretation varies, chiefly in relation to whether it excludes all physician or other health professional involvement completely, even as a volunteer consultant to a self-help group.

SELF-CARE

Obviously, most people spend most of their lives in a relative state of health or at a level of self-care. The constitution of the World Health Organization (WHO) defines health as a "state of complete physical, mental, and social well-being, and not merely the absence of disease or infirmity," which, although it serves as a broad philosophical declaration, is more an optimum goal than a reality.

Also frequently quoted is Parson's definition: "a state of optimal capacity of an individual for effective performance of the roles and tasks for which he has been socialized."[5] On a practical level, the Public Health Service's National Center for Health Statistics defines health implicitly in its use of "disability days," when usual activities cannot be performed.

Self-care is not new and ranges from a simple matter of resting when tired to a more careful judgment of selecting or omitting certain foods or activities, or a semiprimary care activity of taking one or more medications self-prescribed or prescribed by a physician at some other point of care. Health care advice comes gratuitously from family, friends, neighbors, and the media (often with a product to sell). People also seek actively, although informally, information or advice from the same groups or a health professional acquaintance, but their self-care often becomes a matter of trial and error. Increasingly, a new consumer mentality has included in the public's self-care armamentarium the help of others with similar conditions or concerns (see Chapter 6), so that the individual has support and reinforcement as needed but can also detect at what point he/she needs professional help.

In some cases, a person may have had some level of professional care previously and may again, but a certain amount of informed self-diagnosis is not only less expensive for the public but may also serve a useful purpose for the individual. For instance, a mother who has been taught to take her child's temperature can give much more accurate information to a doctor or nurse practitioner, or avoid a call altogether if she also knows how temperature relates to a child's well-being. A blood pressure reading taken properly at home is more likely to identify a hypertension problem quickly than is a yearly physical examination. Dr. Kenneth Sehnert of Georgetown University developed an entire program for what he called the *activated patient,* teaching in an organized course format specific knowledge and skills that a lay person can learn and use. Included were such aspects as taking vital signs, use and abuse of medications, and when to call a doctor.[6] The program has aroused interest and is being used by others as well.

Norris has described seven areas of activity in self-care:

1. Monitoring, assessing, diagnosing—breast self-examination, and other monitoring for cancer, and diagnosing minor illnesses and communicable diseases.
2. Supporting life processes—teeth brushing, bathing, and other ritualistic habits.
3. Therapeutic and corrective self-care—care of minor and chronic illnesses, even serious conditions such as kidney disease, which requires dialysis.
4. Prevention of disease and maladjustment states—taking into consideration risk factors for certain illnesses such as cardiac

conditions; and methods of maintaining psychological well-being.

5. Specifying health needs and care requirements—youths demanding that their particular health needs be met as they perceive them.

6. Auditing and controlling the treatment program—women and minorities demanding better care.

7. Grass roots or self-initiated health care—using peers as therapists (Weight-watchers; smoking cessation programs).[7]

Because it has been determined in the last few years that life-style has a major influence on most serious illnesses, those who know what the risk factors are at least have the choice of making decisions leading to better health. Thus, health promotion and health education have a large part in maintenance of health.

One expert in the field defined these terms.

Health education [is] any combination of learning experiences designed to facilitate voluntary adaptations of behavior conducive to health in individuals, groups or communities. Health education strives to help people control their own health by predisposing, enabling and reinforcing decisions and actions consistent with their own values and goals. *Health promotion* is any combination of educational, organizational, economic, and environmental supports for behavior conducive to health. Health promotion is more aggressive than health education in that it preselects the behaviorist goals on the basis of epidemiological assessment. It also adds to the voluntary commitment of health education a dimension of economic and environmental intervention, sometimes through taxation, regulation of commerce, or legal enforcement, in order to support a specific behavior known to be conducive to health.[8]

Green notes that the role of parents as early models for children's health beliefs is undisputed, and that "early experiences and perceptions of the world around structure personal beliefs and shape attitudes."

Since this learned behavior may be deep-seated, it is often resistant to reeducation. Thus, changing undesirable eating patterns, smoking and drinking, and other aspects of life-style takes more than simple information. Other determinants influencing health attitudes and behavior are both cultural and socioeconomic.

Evaluative research on health education, health promotion, and self-care is being done, and is expected to provide helpful information on overcoming some of these obstacles. In eleven studies testing strategies for improving compliance of patients with blood pressure control, several factors seemed to be important: time for discussion between health care provider and patient; increased number of contacts; active patient participation; support by a significant other, and self-monitoring. This seems to reinforce the concept that a major condition of health education is self-determination, since any real change in behavior is at the level of individual decision making.

Given the choice of continued reliance on costly medical care and preventive care, what will the public decide? Various polls seem to indicate that the public in general believes that the health care system should give more emphasis to preventive rather than curative medicine.[9] The strongest support appears to come from business and union leaders (perhaps because of the increasing cost and overuse of health insurance that is often a job benefit). Still, in an experimental project in which comprehensive preventive and health maintenance services were offered free to an elderly population, only 7 percent chose to participate.[10] Moreover, reimbursement for health education is still not common, in either the public or the private sector, despite the rhetoric. What does seem to be catching on is at least a popular interest in a healthy life-style. Some employers have provided exercise periods and facilities, choices of food with low fat, salt, and cholesterol, and even health education programs. Schools are reemphasizing good health habits and are involving parents. Among the best-selling books are those on diet, exercise, and stress reduction; radio and television have also climbed on this popular bandwagon.

The role of government is equally evident. Cited as a positive example is Canada, which in 1974 proposed a plan to help people to keep healthy. Included were strategies for health promotion and regulation in its seventy-four points, as well as education campaigns, support of physical recreation activities, and regulation of advertising, food content, and pollution.[11] This is not an inexpensive undertaking and could not be implemented fully, but the philosophy and comprehensive efforts have been commended in the United States and elsewhere. In the United States, similar government interest was verbalized and the *Disease Control and Health Promotion Act* became law in 1976—but with little funding for health education.

In 1979, the U.S. Department of Health Education and Welfare (DHEW) published *Healthy People: The Surgeon General's Report on Health Promotion and Disease Prevention 1979,* which identified priority areas for the new decade. It also established broad national goals expressed in terms of lowering death rates or days of disability for five major life stage groups: infant, child, adolescent and young adult, adult, and older adult. *Promoting Health and Preventing Disease: Objectives for the Nation* followed in 1980, setting forth specific, quantifiable objectives necessary for the attainment of those goals. Included were family planning, pregnancy and infant health, immunization, blood pressure control, toxic agent control, occupational safety and health, surveillance and control of infectious disease, including venereal diseases, accident prevention and injury control, fluoridation and dental health, misuse of alcohol, tobacco, and drugs, control of stress and violent behavior, and physical fitness and exercise. Strategies included education, information, use of technology, health services, legislation and regulation, and specific economic measures.

The degree of governmental follow-through in these proposals has fluctuated with the vagaries of political pressures. Thus, some of the objectives set forth in the 1980 plan have been underfunded or neglected because they were not popular with a particular administration. Yet, because of rising health costs, the *idea* of health promotion and education continues to receive overt support.

A philosophical point is raised frequently is whether a government has the right to legislate individual choice. Attempts to mandate the use of seat belts and motorcycle helmets have not been successful. The more complex problems of smoking, drug use, and pollution control have not only personal but also economic ramifications. The bottom line is most often self-care or self-caring by the individual.

AMBULATORY CARE

It is not practical to discuss the institutions involved in the various types of health care delivery under the headings of primary care and so on, because there is considerable overlap of functions. For instance, hospitals and health maintenance organizations (HMOs) may deliver all levels and types of care, even encouraging or sponsoring self-care activities on the part of individuals and community groups. Therefore, institutions and agencies are presented as units.

Ambulatory care is generally defined as that care rendered to patients who come to physicians' offices, outpatient departments, and health centers of various kinds. Because it also includes a number of other noninpatient components such as emergency rooms and home care, the terms *community medicine* or *community health care* are also used.

Except for home care, most of these services currently involve physician–patient contact. Various sources indicate that the vast majority of care given by physicians is on an ambulatory basis; only about 10 percent of the people seen are admitted to a hospital. Most patient visits for health (or sick) care have been made to health care practitioners in solo, partnership, or private group practice on a fee-for-service basis. This is the major mode of organization for physicians and other health care providers generally acknowledged to be licensed to practice independently, such as dentists, chiropractors, podiatrists, and optometrists. Although there is a growing acceptance of nurses practicing independently, most people must be educated to that concept.

Physicians in private practice provide a range of health services and operate on a contractual basis (usually unwritten) with the patient—certain services for a certain fee. When a patient requires hospitalization, he or she pays the hospital for services provided there, except for the physician, who maintains an independent status and is paid directly on a separate fee basis. If a referral is made to specialists (secondary care), those specialists receive their fees, and the primary care physician sees the patient again when specialist services are no longer warranted. However, for various reasons, including the oversupply of physicians in some localities, more physicians are being employed full time by health care institutions, in which case patients do not pay physicians separately, and the office itself may be run and staffed by institutional personnel.

Nevertheless, about 60 percent of all active physicians are in private practice, and most patient visits to physicians are made in the office. If an emergency arises, the patient may be seen in a hospital emergency room where the physician has staff privileges. Few make house calls. A small percentage of physicians (usually in urban areas) do not have hospital staff privileges, in which case the patient may be seen in the hospital by a referred colleague. From a business and tax viewpoint, private practice may be a corporation or partnership or may have some other designation.

Little is known about how physicians distribute their time in office practice among history taking and examinations, diagnosing, therapy, teaching or counseling, supervising or teaching staff, and paper work; most appear reluctant to have outsiders look into their work. Nor is there much information on how doctors interact, what the doctor–patient relationship consists of, how decisions are made, how quality is monitored, or how much trav-

eling and meeting time is devoted to continuing education.[12] What is known is that approximately 75 percent of doctors in office practice classify themselves as being in some kind of specialty (not family practice), with the highest number in general internal medicine, general surgery, obstetrics and gynecology, and pediatrics.

Patients who can choose their own point of admission into the health care system usually start with a physician office visit, and there is increasing concern that, for all the importance of that choice, people do so on an unsophisticated and relatively uninformed basis—someone's recommendation, proximity to the home, or, at best, a blind choice from a list provided, at request, by the local medical society. Frequently, people do a preliminary diagnosis of their own symptoms and choose a specialist on the basis of the organ that seems to be involved. Because that physician may have no contact with the other specialists the individual has chosen at random, continuity and comprehensiveness of care are generally lacking.

A physician's private practice setting often consists of only the physician (solo practice) and some full-time or part-time clerical help and/or medical assistant, office nurse, and physician's assistant (PA), any of whom may also be a family member. Increasingly popular is group practice with one other physician in the same specialty or a multiple-physician specialty conglomerate with all of the workers previously cited plus x-ray and laboratory facilities with the appropriate personnel, and other supportive health professionals and services such as health education and physical therapy. More and more of these practice modes also include nurse practitioners (NPs) as employees or as full partners (see Chapter 15). Most private practitioners are paid by the patient or some form of third-party insurance. In recent years, offices serving primarily Medicaid patients in ghetto areas have been labeled "Medicaid mills," in part because of the poor quality of care and physician-encouraged overuse of services.

Prepaid group practices (PGP) are still relatively few but have received considerable attention. They are broadly defined as a medical care delivery system that accepts responsibility for the organizing, financing, and delivery of health care of a defined population.[13] At least 50 percent of the patients are covered by prepayment for as broad a range of services as possible. Two prominent PGPs are Kaiser-Permanente on the West Coast and the Health Insurance Plan (HIP) of Greater New York, both of which also operate in other areas of the country. Such prepaid groups are sometimes classified under the rubric of HMOs.

NURSE PRIVATE PRACTICE

Nurses have been in private practice since formal nursing programs were started (see Chapters 3 and 4). In a manner of speaking, private duty nursing was and is a professional practice for which the individual has professional and financial responsibility. However, at one time, fees and hours were set by hospitals, registries, or the professional associations, even though the nurse and patient or family essentially had a private contract with each other. Because of the Federal Trade Commission's tendency to consider fee setting as restraint of trade, the practitioner now has more control over the fee; however, to a great extent, the nursing care is given to a bed patient in the hospital or home for at least eight hours a day, with certain physician orders to be considered.

In an emerging concept of nurse private practice (see Chapter 15), the nurse has an office where patients are seen, although he or she may also make house calls. In this form of independent practice, nurses have the same economic and managerial requirements as physicians, with the added concern that reimbursement by third-party payers is still greatly limited. Some insurance companies reimburse, and some laws have been passed to allow for reimbursement of certain practitioners, particularly nurse-midwives and psychiatric clinical specialists. However, because much nurse reimbursement requires a physician's order or supervision, nurses are often dependent on patients' paying their own bills. Although some groups of nurses and a few individuals working in independent practice are surviving financially, frequently they also hold other positions, such as teaching posts. There are, of course, nursing faculty who carry a private practice to enhance their faculty role and are not dependent on that income. It should be noted that these nurses do not necessarily do what might be called medical diagnosis and treatment.

In a somewhat hybrid situation are the NPs who practice in an isolated area and are the sole source of health care for that population. These nurses are usually trained as family NPs (see Chapter 15). They may work under specified protocols, be in telephone contact with backup physicians, have arrangements with local pharmacists about prescriptions, have admitting privileges in some hospitals, or any combination of these. The nurses may be paid by the community or state, or by some other special arrangement. The primary care given is whatever is within the scope of that nurse's practice.[14]

HEALTH MAINTENANCE ORGANIZATIONS (HMOs)

The term *health maintenance organization (HMO)* may refer to a number of organizational entities. An early DHEW statement describes the HMO organizational base.

An HMO can be organized and sponsored by either a medical foundation (usually organized by physicians), by community groups who bring together various interested leaders or organizations, by labor unions, by a government unit, by a profit or nonprofit group allied with an insurance company or some other financing institution, or by some other arrangement. The HMO may be hospital-based, medical school-based, or be a free-standing outpatient facility or group of such facilities.[15]

According to the 1972 Social Security amendments, HMOs provide to enrollees, on the basis of a predetermined fixed cost or rate, comprehensive health services without regard to the extent or frequency of services. These services may be given directly or through arrangements with others, and include the services of primary care and specialty physicians and institutional services.

As of 1983, there were 178 operational HMOs of three basic types: the *group/staff HMOs,* delivering services at one or more locations through a group of physicians that have contracts with the HMO and are considered employees; the *individual practice association (IPA),* in which doctors have contractual arrangements but practice out of their own offices; and the *network HMO,* which contracts with two or more group practices to provide health services. When, in 1972–1973, some organizations received federal funding for HMO development, the AMA voiced strong opposition to what it called unwarranted federal competition in the practice of medicine. Nevertheless, the 1973 HMO Act was passed and authorized federal grants and loans over a five-year period. To be included were physician care, inpatient and outpatient care, medically necessary emergency health services, short-term evaluations and crisis intervention, mental health services, medical treatment and referral services for the abuse of or addiction to alcohol and drugs, diagnostic laboratory and diagnostic and therapeutic radiological services, and preventive services; dental care and prescription drugs could be contracted for. Services had to be available on a twenty-four-hour, seven-day-a-week basis, with subscribers paying nothing or only a minimum copayment at the time of service.[16]

Because some state licensure requirements differ from the federal criteria, some HMOs have chosen not to seek federal qualification. Luft lists essential characteristics of an HMO, regardless of whether it is federally qualified. The HMO:

1. assumes a *contractual responsibility* to provide or assure the delivery of a stated range of health services including at least physician and hospital services;
2. serves an *enrolled, defined* population;
3. has *voluntary enrollment* of subscribers;
4. requires a *fixed periodic payment* to the organization that is independent of use of its services (There may be small charges related to utilization, but these are relatively insignificant.);
5. assumes at least part of the *financial risk* and/or gain in the provision of services, *unlike* a fiscal intermediary.[17]

Care may be given at the HMO or at an institution with which it has an arrangement to cover what the HMO does not have. For instance, an HMO may have medical services and/or multiphasic diagnostic services, or it may actually function in a large hospital. However, a major emphasis is on prevention and health teaching, and nurse practitioners are involved in these as well as other aspects of primary care at HMOs.

For all their apparent benefits, HMO growth has been relatively slow. One reason is that physicians are still reluctant to change practice modes or oppose HMOs outright; another is that start-up and other costs of the comprehensive services are high, sometimes making HMOs noncompetitive with Blue Cross/Blue Shield; finally, the original DHEW regulations were so restrictive and complex as to create problems in implementation. Other problems are also cited: a scandal in California, where prepaid health plans contracting to provide comprehensive medical services for Medicaid patients were found to enroll subscribers without informed consent, to provide inadequate and depersonalized care, and to misuse funds; complaints about skimping on health services to cut costs; and some inaccessibility. The HMOs are working to overcome these problems and to develop marketing techniques to woo subscribers.

Research shows that the health outcomes for HMO subscribers are the same as or better than those in conventional settings, and consumer and provider satisfaction is generally good. Other research indicates that depending on the type of organization, HMOs may be more efficient and thus more cost-effective.

There is clear evidence that total medical costs for HMO enrollees are 10 to 40 percent lower than those of comparable individuals with health insurance.[18] To a great extent, that is due to a 30 percent lower hospitalization rate. It may also be due to the self-selection of enrollees. Because hospitalization is a major health care cost, HMOs also lower the national cost of health. This is undoubtedly a factor in congressional reauthorization for funding and loans for HMOs.

While there is no expectation that HMOs will replace private practice, the Bureau of Health Maintenance Organizations of DHHS has predicted that by 1990, 15 percent of the populace will be enrolled in HMOs. This is because the basis for growth (the number of HMOs) has increased significantly, the premiums are equal to or lower than those of other plans, and employees have recognized their value. Meanwhile, the competitiveness of the HMO presence in the community appears to have lowered some health care costs.

COMMUNITY HEALTH CENTERS (CHCs)

Out of the social unrest of the 1960s and early 1970s emerged the *neighborhood health center (NHC),* an ambulatory facility "based on the concepts of full-time, salaried physician staffing, multidisciplinary team health practice, and community involvement in both policy making and facility operations."[19] The NHC movement was stimulated by funding from the Office of Economic Opportunity (OEO) during the Johnson Administration. In many ways, NHCs were similar to the early charitable dispensaries, which were established because of the hospitals' lack of interest in ambulatory care and disappeared in the 1920s because of poor financing, poor staffing, and physician disapproval.

Now more commonly called *community health centers (CHCs),* they serve some 5 million people at about 800 primary care sites. They may be freestanding, with a back-up hospital for special services and hospital admissions, or legally part of a hospital or health department, functioning under that institution's governing board and license, but with a community advisory board.

CHCs are primarily found in medically underserved urban areas, where the minority poor and various ethnic groups rely on hospital ambulatory services for primary care. In many cases, the hospital clinic service and the emergency service, often expensive, overcrowded, fragmented, and disease-oriented, are inappropriately used. The emergency room, particularly, is found to be used more for nonemergency primary care than for emergencies because of its twenty-four-hour availability. Activist representatives of the poor complain that care is also disinterested and depersonalized. Although attending physicians are usually present at some point, much care is given by a rotating house staff, with no continuity of care. Even when NPs participate, care is usually episodic, and most do not carry a stable case load (although they could and want to). The reasons that hospital ambulatory care has not improved much, despite much visibility, are complex,[20] and there does seem to be some slow progress. However, their ineffectiveness is a major reason for the rise of the CNCs, called by some "one-stop health shopping" at acceptable, affordable prices, with interest in providing holistic health care. Often, they are at least partially staffed by the ethnic group served, so that communication is improved, and a real effort is made to provide services when and where patients/clients need them in an atmosphere of care and understanding. Use of nontraditional workers such as family health workers and an emphasis on using a health care team have been characteristic.

Although much of the health care given by CHCs is excellent, their problems have caused a drop in number from the peak development of the 1970s. Problems include tensions between community advisory boards and administrators of the center and/or the backup hospitals, and funding. Starting and maintaining CHCs is extremely expensive, and most patients can pay only through Medicare/Medicaid, if at all. There is still some federal support, but with the demise of OEO in the 1970s and other governmental cutbacks, CHCs have been forced to scramble for private foundation funds and to rely on Medicare/Medicaid funding. Few are self-supporting. When external funds are not available, severe program and personnel cuts are often necessary. The future of CHCs remains uncertain, in part because of a sociological question: Are they perpetuating a separate kind of care for the poor?

OTHER HEALTH CENTERS AND CLINICS

Variations of the CHCs are present in different parts of the country. *Rural health centers,* developed under federal financing such as regional health and the Appalachian projects or funded by communities or foundations, are the rural corollary to CHCs—existing to serve people, usually poor, in medically underserved areas (MUAs). Since few physicians are available, care is often given by NPs and PAs linked to physicians at other sites. In 1977, the Rural Health Clinic Services Act provided for reimbursement of NPs and PAs under certain circumstances.

Mental health centers or *community mental health centers* are intended to provide a wide range of mental health services to a particular geographic "catchment area." They may be sponsored by state mental health departments, psychiatric hospitals or departments of hospitals, or the federal government. Staffed by teams of mental health personnel, they may consist of single physical entities or networks, but are usually intended for short-term care, including "crisis intervention." The Community Mental Health Center Act (1963) and its later amendments facilitated the development of comprehensive services and stimulated the community mental health movement. It was intended, in part, to prevent the warehousing of mental patients and assist their reintroduction into the community. Unfortunately, deinstitutionalization moved faster than the available community services, and even today there are discharged mental patients living on the streets or in deplorable single-room occupancy hotels (SROs). While there are good halfway houses, day-care centers, and semisupervised living services, the services have not caught up with the demand.

Free clinics, often functioning in informal settings and sites, provide health care services to transient youths, minority groups, and students. They are usually staffed by volunteers. Their peak was reached in the early 1970s with the "flower child" generation; many of those that survived became more formally organized.

Women's clinics are usually owned and operated by women concerned about women's health problems and dissatisfied with the quality of care for women and the attitudes of many male health care providers. Most emerged out of the women's movement, along with the consumer and self-care movements. Services may include routine gynecological and maternity care and family planning, as well as some general health care. Emphasis is on self-help, mutual support, and noninstitutional personal care. Both nurse-midwives and lay midwives are used, as are supportive physicians, although many staff are lay people. In a number of cities and towns, the clinics have been harassed by conservative groups and medical societies, and some have had to become involved in lengthy and expensive legal suits.

Family-planning clinics, of which the 700 clinics of Planned Parenthood are most notable, provide a spectrum of birth control services and information. *Abortion clinics* have increased since the legalization of abortion and are sponsored by community and other groups, as well as proprietary organizations.

AMBULATORY CARE ALTERNATIVES
TO INSTITUTIONS

The 1980s brought increased complaints about the expense of health care, particularly in hospitals, and ushered in the "competitive model." The core of the model is that "consumer choice and market forces rather than regulation should be used to control health care costs. The hope is that competition would produce a 'competitive equilibrium,' that is, technically and economically efficient production along with efficient distribution of health services."[21]

As a result, alternative health care delivery modes, particularly in ambulatory care, developed and expanded. Among these are the *surgicenters,* independent proprietary facilities for surgery that does not require overnight hospitalization. The first was established in 1970 in Phoenix, Arizona, and their popularity has escalated. Some are specialized, such as the plastic surgery centers, but in general the centers can perform any surgery that does not require prolonged anesthesia. The more than 150 surgicenters are said to be able to perform up to 40 percent of all surgical procedures, including face lifts, cataract surgery, vasectomy, breast biopsy, dilation and curettage, knee arthroscopy, and tonsillectomy. Because of low overhead, surgicenters can charge as little as one-third of hospital costs for the same procedure, and patients like being able to return to home, or even work, the same day.

When it was evident that this new delivery mode was not only well accepted (some do as many as 6,000 procedures a year) but reimbursable by insurance plans, many hospitals joined the movement and set up "day surgery" centers.

Private, for profit, freestanding emergency centers (FECs) or emergicenters designed to treat episodic, nonurgent health problems, are considered among the fastest-growing facets of U.S. health care. Since the first opened its doors in 1976, 600 to 1,000 more have sprung up around the country. The term *freestanding* may refer either to an independent, physician-owned emergicenter or one that is hospital sponsored or affiliated. The sponsored emergicenter, sometimes referred to as the *hospital satellite emergicenter,* is hospital managed and owned; those affiliated or associated with hospitals have contracts for service. Typically, the emergicenters are in shopping centers or commercial and industrial areas, have a high patient turnover, a short (fifteen to twenty minutes) waiting period, and a cost that may be 30 to 40 percent lower than that of hospital emergency rooms. In 1981 they handled an estimated 85 million cases, 85 percent of which were not life- or limb-threatening emergencies; thus, emergicenters have the potential to be a lucrative business. Government regulation is still largely nonexistent, and a number of legal issues are bound to arise.[22] Other questions in relation to the emergicenters' impact on the more traditional health care facilities, such as who uses FECs, what problems are presented, and how they are treated, are part of a study funded by the National Center for Health Services Research (NCHSR).

Although some women are again turning to home births attended by midwives, a more popular and growing alternative to hospital births is the *childbearing center,* also called *birth center* or *childbirthing center.* These centers made their appearance in 1973, when the alienated and questioning middle class became disenchanted with hospital maternity care. The demonstration nurse-midwifery model was the Maternity Center of New York. Now about 125–150 out-of-hospital centers are operating in at least twenty-seven states. About one-third are operated by or utilize nurse-midwives; others are sponsored by physicians and/or lay midwives.[23]

There are both freestanding centers and a variation of the concept in hospitals. Both allow for more humane care in a high-quality, homelike setting with the father and other children present—all costing considerably less than hospital care. Lubic, the originator of the modern concept and the first center, estimates that if only one in four pregnant women had access to and used birthing centers, millions and perhaps billions of health care dollars would be saved.[24]

Although the birth centers have been extraordinarily safe, without the iatrogenic disease rate of hospitals, and consumers have expressed great satisfaction, it is generally agreed that standards should be set.

Nurse-managed centers (NMCs) were initiated about a decade ago when faculty in schools of nursing offered nursing services to the community and at the same time provided model teaching centers for their students. NPs in private practice, as described earlier, may also practice in such centers, whether or not they are university affiliated. Often the centers serve inner-city communities and, more rarely, middle-class clients. There are about sixty-three such centers in operation, with forty-four reported about to open. Most are sponsored by a school of nursing, with funding coming from a university, but there is a potential for support by private foundations, government or health care agencies, or any combination thereof. A bill was introduced into Congress in 1983, which, among other things, would directly reimburse care delivered by nurses in such centers (and also visiting nurse associations).

Patterns of practice for NMCs vary, but usually include health maintenance and health promotion services, such as risk factor screening, health education, and counseling for a variety of populations including the elderly, children, employees, and pregnant women. One that is licensed in Arizona offers adult and child health services, family planning, maternity care, immunizations, and referrals for serious conditions. Others report their services as health assessments (history, physical, and screening tests), mental health care, and chronic disease monitoring.[25]

Quality control, reimbursement, and organization are still issues in discussion, but the

prospect of this effective, humanized health care service controlled by nurses being a viable primary care alternative for the public is very exciting.

Another humanistically oriented as well as cost-saving mode of care is the *hospice*. The hospice movement was pioneered in Great Britain by Dr. Cicely Saunders at St. Christopher's Hospice in London. The first widely recognized hospice in the United States was Hospice, Inc., established in 1971 in New Haven, Connecticut. Modeled after St. Christopher's, its concentration was on improving the quality of patients' last days or months of life so that they could "live until they die." Two-thirds of the patients die at home, surrounded by their families, and free of technological, life-prolonging devices. The hospice functions on a twenty-four-hour, seven-day-a-week basis; backup medical, nursing, and counseling services are always available. Symptom control is a vital first step, and pain-relieving medications are not withheld.

Because third-party payers do not always cover such comprehensive care, increased public interest spurred experimental programs. DHEW regulations that funded demonstration projects in 1978 described the hospice concept:

> The goal of hospice care is to help terminally ill patients continue life with minimal disruption in routine activity, including working and remaining in the family environment. Hospice uses a multidisciplinary approach to delivering social, psychological, medical and spiritual services through the use of a broad spectrum of professional and voluntary care givers with a goal of making the patient as physically and emotionally comfortable as possible. Integral to the hospice concept is the philosophy that pain is preventable and can be controlled through the use of drugs.

The hospice experience in the United States has placed emphasis on home care. It offers physician services, specialized nursing services, and other forms of care in the home in order to enable the terminally ill patient to remain at home in the company of family and friends as long as possible. Inpatient hospice settings have been utilized primarily where there is no one in the patient's home to assist in the care of the patient, the patient's pain and symptoms must be closely monitored in order to be controlled, or the family needs a rest from the tedium and stress in caring for the patient (respite care).[26]

There has been a dramatic growth in hospices from 300 in 1980 to 1,200 in 1983. Hospices come in a variety of forms: "wholly volunteer programs, home services, free-standing buildings, in-hospital palliative care units or hospice teams, continuum-of-care subacute facilities and combinations of any two or three. Nursing functions may vary according to the organization form."[27] But whatever the setting, in reality it is a concept, an attitude, a belief that involves support of the family as well as the dying patient. It can be carried out in an ordinary hospital setting, with extraordinary perception.

As might be expected in this cost-conscious era of care, the policy question of reimbursement for hospice services has created considerable debate. A major victory was won when Congress enacted a law in 1982 which permitted Medicare reimbursement. However, the final regulations allowed a lower reimbursement rate than anticipated, and there was a feeling of distrust about the Reagan Administration's commitment to the program, so very few hospices enrolled in the program. One clear problem was the greatly varying costs of the different types of programs and the fear of escalating costs such as those that occurred with the renal dialysis program.

Renal dialysis centers were spurred into massive growth by their inclusion in the 1972 Medicare amendment. Once, the treatment of those with chronic kidney disease by using expensive artificial kidneys was a sensitive matter of "who shall live." When Congress decided that all should have that opportunity and funded it, the cost rose to unexpected millions of dollars. Many centers are freestanding, mostly physician owned or developed by proprietary organizations, but they also exist in hospitals. A whole new coterie of specialists at all levels has developed. The desired emphasis now is the less expensive home dialysis.

Another group of burgeoning facilities are those for rehabilitation of drug abusers. Most common are the *methadone maintenance programs* (substituting methadone for heroin, along with certain rehabilitative measures), which have had varying success. *Drug-free* programs include self-help and therapeutic resident programs, halfway houses, counseling centers, and "hot lines."

Adult day-care centers are agencies that provide health, social, psychiatric, and nutritional services to infirm individuals who are sufficiently ambulatory to be transported between home and center.[28] Psychogeriatric day-care centers were first opened in 1947 under the direction of the Menninger Clinic. Studies ordered by Congress in 1976 showed day-care centers to be cost effective, but no national policy on reimbursement followed. Funding now comes from uncoordinated disparate sources, and therefore some communities have set priorities as to who can use the services. Yet, day care has been shown to be superior to nursing homes for eligible individuals because of lesser cost, improved health and functional outcomes, and an increased quality of life. Unresolved issues are related to their use for young adults with debilitating diseases, the feasibility of rural centers, and the need for regulation and licensing.

Wholistic health care centers were so named by their founder as a protest against the fragmentation of care. These centers are actually described as primary care doctors' offices, generally located in a church, which offer pastoral counseling and health education as well as physical care. The health care team is made up of a physician, nurse, pastoral counselor, and client working together. A series of wholistic health centers were funded by a major foundation in a special project that seemed to have positive results. Granger Westberg, a prime mover of wholistic care, suggests that churches form "health cabinets" charged with improving the general health of the congregation, particularly through encouragement of health education and promotion.[29]

GOVERNMENT FACILITIES

In the federal government, at least twenty-five agencies have some involvement in delivering health services. Those with the largest expenditures in direct federal hospital and medical services are the Veteran's Administration, which operates the largest centrally directed hospital and clinic system in the United States, the Department of Defense (members of the military and dependents), and the Health Resources and Services Administration (HRSA) of DHHS.* HRSA operates one Public Health Service (PHS) hospital and the Indian Health Service hospitals, health centers, and field stations. (Because of costs, all PHS hospitals, with the exception of one devoted to Hansen's disease, have now been closed or turned over to non-federal owners.) The Bureau of Medical Services also provides services to the federal prison system and the U.S. Coast Guard. A variety of other DHHS agencies provide indirect funding or contracts for clinics, drug and alcohol rehabilitation centers, maternal-child and family planning, neighborhood health centers, and the National Health Service Corps. In direct federal hospital and medical services, DHHS spends the largest amount of money, primarily because of Social Security's Medicare/Medicaid and the Social and Rehabilitation Service.

State and local governments also have multiple functions and multiple services in health care delivery, directly through grants and funding to finance their own programs, and indirectly as third-party payers. Although most states have some version of a state health agency (SHA) or department of public health, health services are often provided through other state agencies, a situation that creates territorial battles, duplication, and gaps. In most states, operation of mental hospitals and the Medicaid program, two of the most important state health functions, is by departments other than the SHA. In direct services, some states operate mental, tuberculosis, or other hospitals and alcohol and drug abuse programs, provide noninstitutional mental health services, fund public health nursing programs and laboratories, and provide services for maternal and child health, family planning, crippled children, immunization, tuberculosis, chronic respiratory disease control, and venereal disease control. All are considered traditional public health services, in addition to environmental health activities.

On a local level, services offered by a health department depend a great deal on the size, needs, and demands of the constituency. There appears to be little information about local health departments or health officers. Those with considerable visibility are in large urban centers, where health problems are complex and generally unresolved.

Some large municipalities operate hospitals that provide for the indigent or working poor who are not covered by Medicaid or private insurance. Some health departments run school health services and screening programs. Some duplicate services offered by the state. There are little data on how much state and local agencies coordinate their services to avoid duplication or omission, but lack of coordination or cooperation is not uncommon. Although there is a great deal of criticism of most local health services in relation to high cost, waste, corruption, and poor quality, attempts to terminate any of them, particularly hospitals in medically underserved areas, become political conflicts, with representatives of the poor complaining that no other services

---

*The Department of Health, Education and Welfare (DHEW) became the Department of Health and Human Services (DHHS) in 1980.

are available and that the loss of local jobs will create other hardships. With all the politically sensitive issues involved, most health care experts are pessimistic about reorganization or major improvement of the health systems at any governmental level.[30]

HOME HEALTH CARE

Home health care is probably more of a nurse-oriented health service than any other, originating with Florence Nightingale's "health nurses"* and the pioneer efforts of such American nurses as Lillian Wald. Nevertheless, what Wald worked for in the late nineteenth century—comprehensive services for the patient and family that extend beyond simple care of the sick—is even more pertinent today.

Both short-term and long-term care are offered. The National Association for Home Care (NAHC) defines *home care* as "any or all of a full range of health care and social services offered to patients in their homes. From home birthings to hospice care, home care is for the ill, infirm, or disabled who elect to be treated at home rather than in an institutional setting." Two types are identified: comprehensive home health services, with a plan designed by a professional nurse in cooperation with a physician, and homemaker-home health aide services, required in addition to nursing and therapy and consisting of personal grooming needs, helping with the practice of self-help skills, and general housekeeping services. NAHC estimates that there are about 5,000 agencies each, not including hospices.

The National League for Nursing, which in cooperation with other groups accredits home health agencies, defines home health services as

an array of health care services provided to individuals and families in their places of resi-

dence or in ambulatory care settings for purposes of preventing disease and promoting, maintaining or restoring health, or minimizing the effects of illness and disability. Services appropriate to the needs of the individual and his family are planned, coordinated and made available by an organized health agency—through the use of agency-employed staff, contractual arrangements, or a combination of administrative patterns. Medical services are primarily provided by the individual's private or clinic physician, although in some instances agencies will employ or contract for physician's services.

These services must be available to the total population and must include all service components necessary to ensure the health and safety of those for whom such services are appropriate.[31]

The League gives particular attention to the types of services that make up home health care. Listed as basic, essential services are home health aide-homemaker, medical supplies and equipment (expendable and durable), nursing, nutrition, occupational therapy, physical therapy, speech pathology services, and social work. Other essential services, which may be provided through the combined, coordinated efforts of the agency and the community, include audiological services,* dental services, home-delivered meals, housekeeping services, information and referral services, laboratory services,* ophthalmological services,* patient transportation and escort services, physician's services,* podiatry services,* prescription drugs, prosthetic/orthotic services,* respiratory therapy services, and x-ray services.* In addition, environmental/social support services such as barber/cosmetology services, handyman services, heavy cleaning services, legal and protective services, pastoral services, personal contact services, recreation services, and translation services are highly desirable, and some might be developed as volunteer efforts.[32]

---

*Today the term *public health nurse* or *community health nurse* is used.

*Can be arranged for by the agency.

Agencies that provide home care have various organizational bases. As noted earlier, some cities, counties, and states provide home health care, but the general trend there is emphasis on services related to case finding, health teaching, and well-baby care, much of which is now clinic based. Visiting nurse associations (VNAs) of various names, which are voluntary agencies, have been the classic providers of home care. Depending on the location and resources, the spectrum of services varies greatly, but includes personal health services and patient/family teaching.

New entrants into the field are hospital-based home health services, the ''hospital without walls'' concept. A protoype program in Montefiore Hospital in New York City in the late 1940s provided nursing, medical, social, housekeeping, transportation, medication, occupational therapy, physical therapy, and diagnostic services. Since then, a large number of hospitals have initiated such programs, but the number of services may be limited. In some cases, most services, including nursing, are contracted for, by using established voluntary or proprietary agencies already in operation. At times, the program is little more than a coordination of services for continuity of care, which is nevertheless a vast improvement over what is still most common—discharge with no follow-up except for a clinic or physician appointment. In part because of the new prospective reimbursement system put into effect by the federal government in 1984 (described later) and the consequent pressure to discharge patients as soon as possible, more hospitals have become interested in setting up home care programs as a means of increasing income.

Most aggressive in providing services are the large number of proprietary agencies that are springing up throughout the country. Some offer comprehensive services; others concentrate their efforts on training and deploying home workers and home health aides. In these agencies, operated for profit, marketing is brisk and sophisticated. Although there have been complaints of poor-quality care, the readily available services on a twenty-four-hour-a-day, seven-day-a-week basis have proved to be highly competitive. One reason for the increase in interest is the financial support of Medicare/Medicaid. On the other hand, as in the HMOs, the complex restrictiveness of the regulations, particularly in relation to reimbursable services, leads to quality problems and severe financial burdens for the homebound patient and sometimes the agency. Determining the need for home care is not a simple matter and varies in terms of both the patient and the environment.

One VNA executive reported that in the early 1970s, when reimbursement for services became primarily Medicare based, large numbers of voluntary agencies across the United States closed because retroactive cost adjustment according to new Medicare rules caused severe losses. Some of those that survived best began to plan on a more businesslike basis, and new organizational patterns emerged. One includes the development of a holding company or major corporation with both a nonprofit (traditional VNA) and for-profit subsidiary, and others as necessary, somewhat similar to the new hospital models. The for-profit corporation may provide a variety of profitable services, such as home-health aides, chore services for the frail elderly, presurgery counseling before hospital admission, and vocational rehabilitation. The after-taxes profits from this corporation are then donated to the nonprofit corporation to provide the free services that have sometimes kept VNAs on the point of bankruptcy.

Both voluntary and official (governmental) agencies have been affected by the financial squeeze, and although total restructuring is not always possible, approaches have been used that were never even considered previously. One county agency, having lost its home-care certificate of need to a proprietary agency, successfully marketed its health teaching–health promotion services to industry and the public. Another developed a new market and gained increased economy by developing ''neighborhood nurse'' offices.[33] Other variations are block nursing[34] and nurses working out of the home.[35] Others have simply offered their traditionally high-quality services over a seven-day and twenty-four-hour span. Computers have become essential for keeping records and statistics and for case management.[36] Seen as the key was marketing of services.[37]

Comprehensive home health care is being hailed as both less expensive than institutional care and as a more effective, humane approach, especially for the elderly and chronically ill. Whether it is indeed cheaper may depend on what supportive services are needed. Is only health care needed, or a variety of social services? And what of the difficulty of coordinating the physician, agency, and patient, much less other entities? Consideration must also be given to the need for close planning and participation of the family; if the family or significant others are absent in a patient's life or unwilling to take on the necessary responsibility, home care may not be the most desirable approach for dependent individuals. On the other hand, with the participation of health professionals who have a commitment to this aspect of health care, reasonable assurance of quality, and adequate financing, home health care has tremendous potential for filling a health care gap.

EMERGENCY MEDICAL SERVICES

Ambulance services, originally a profit venture of funeral directors, are a vital link in transporting accident victims or those suffering acute overwhelming illnesses (such as myocardial infarctions) to a medical facility. In most cases, providing for such services, either directly or through contracts, has now become the responsibility of a community, a responsibility that is not consistently assumed. The unnecessary deaths due to delayed and/or inept care have received considerable attention, which was probably responsible for some important federal legislation. The Federal Highway Safety Act of 1966 contained performance criteria for emergency medical

services (EMS) and required states to submit EMS plans. The Emergency Medical Service Act of 1973 authorized three years of funding to states, counties, and other nonprofit agencies to plan, expand, and modernize EMSs, with special consideration to be given to rural areas. With continued federal and state funding and regulation, the previous diverse ambulance and rescue services of volunteers, firemen, police, and commercial companies are being coordinated with regional systems. Several hundred are now in place. Criteria include training of appropriate personnel, education of the public; appropriate communication systems, transportation vehicles, and facilities; adequate record keeping; and some participation by the public in policy making.[38]

Under these laws, emergency medical technicians (EMTs) have been trained and staff many ambulance services. Paramedics (advanced EMTs and EMTs II) have also been trained and staff the mobile intensive care units, which have very sophisticated equipment.

Between 1973 and 1978, the Robert Wood Johnson Foundation provided funds that allowed forty-four health departments and other entities to improve EMSs. An evaluation done at the end of that time concluded that both the quality and efficiency of the services had been upgraded. Considered responsible for some of the improvement was the training of paramedics, giving medical directions to ambulance teams by radio or protocol, centralizing emergency dispatch throughout a region, and setting up telephone numbers for all emergencies. The study also called for more support for such programs at all governmental levels.

HOSPITALS

There are some 7,000 hospitals in the United States. They are generally classified according to size (number of beds, exclusive of bassinets for newborns); type (general, mental, tuberculosis, or other specialty, such as maternity, orthopedic, eye and ear, rehabilitation, chronic disease, alcoholism, or narcotic addiction); ownership (public or private, including the for-profit, investor-owned proprietary hospital or not-for-profit voluntary hospital, which may be owned by religious, fraternity, or community groups); and length of stay (short-term, with an average stay less than thirty days, or long-term, thirty days or more). Hospitals vary from fewer than 25 to more than 2,000 beds. The most common type of hospital has been the voluntary, general, short-term hospital, followed by the local government, general, short-term hospital. The two major groups in terms of size are short-term general hospitals, averaging 160 beds, and long-term hospitals, averaging 900 beds. However, there are predictions that by 1990, 1,000 of the nation's 6,000 community hospitals may be forced to close. Causes pinpointed by the American Hospital Association (AHA) included financial cutbacks in federal funding, pressure by insurance companies and business to reduce health expenditures, and changing health care practices (such as those described earlier). If not closed, the small hospitals are likely to become part of a multi-institutional system, a major trend in health care delivery.

The term *teaching hospital* is applied to those hospitals in which medical students and/or residents and specialty fellows (house staff) are taught. It does not include those that provide educational programs or experiences for other health professionals or allied health workers. These hospitals (about 9 percent) usually have more than 400 beds and are in medical centers proximate to the medical school (in which case they are often tertiary care centers).

Because of all these variations, it is difficult to draw one picture of the hospital as an entity. Figure 7-2 shows a common organizational pattern of a general hospital, which illustrates both the lines of authority and the kinds of services available. Administrative organization of services varies greatly according to administrative philosophy and types of ser-

vice.[39] For instance, a hospital that has outreach facilities, home health services, or a long-term care facility differ greatly from a fifty-bed community hospital. Smaller hospitals may not have as many diverse clinical services and few, if any, education programs, but almost always there are business and finance departments, physical plant (maintenance of all kinds), laundry, supplies and storeroom, dietary and food services, clinical nursing units (inpatient and outpatient), and the other professional service units, such as laboratories, radiology, other diagnostic and treatment units, pharmacy, and perhaps social service. Some hospitals are now purchasing or sharing laundry and food services in the belief that this is less expensive in the long run. The physical layout of a hospital varies from one-story to high-rise, and may include large or small general or specialized patient units, special intensive-care units, operating rooms, recovery rooms, offices (sometimes including doctors' private offices), space for diagnostic and treatment facilities, storage rooms, kitchens and dining rooms, maintenance equipment, work rooms, meeting rooms, classrooms, chapel, waiting rooms, and gift and snack shops. Most hospitals have some form of emergency service, such as an emergency room, but many no longer maintain their own ambulance services. A great many have outpatient or ambulatory services, and perhaps an extended-care unit for patients who do not need major nursing service; some provide home care.

The nursing service has the largest number of personnel in the hospital, in part because of round-the-clock, seven-days-a-week staffing. Other departments, such as radiology and clinical laboratories, may maintain some services on evenings and weekends, and may be on call at nights. There is some trend toward having other clinical services available at least on weekends. For instance, a patient who needs rehabilitation exercises or other treatments in the physical therapy department lacks this necessary care in the evenings and weekends when that department follows the

ONE PATTERN OF HOSPITAL ORGANIZATION

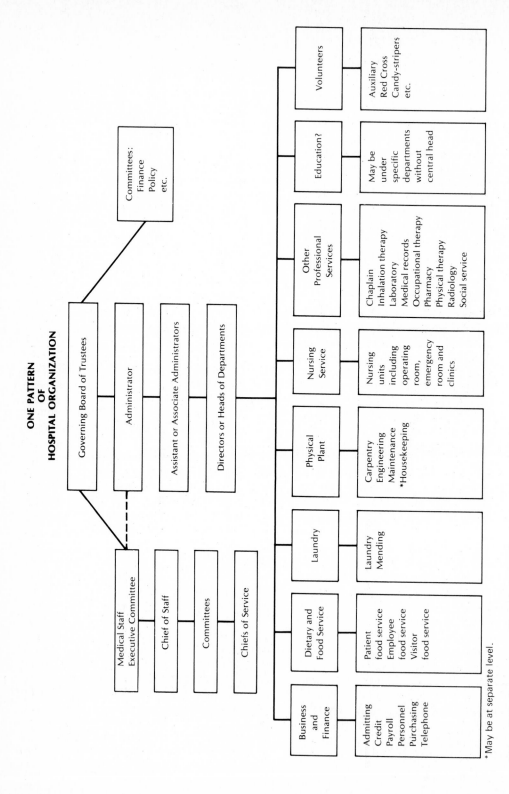

*May be at separate level.

Figure 7-2. One pattern of hospital organization.

usual eight-to-five, Monday-through-Friday staffing pattern.

The primary purpose of hospitals is to provide patient services. However, many also assume a major responsibility for education of health personnel in basic educational programs or in in-service programs, and participate in health research. Frequently, they are associated with schools of health professions and occupations, and provide the setting for health education and research, even though they do not finance such programs.

Hospitals are licensed by the state and presumably are not permitted to function unless they maintain the minimum standards prescribed by the licensing authority. ("Presumably" because the process of closing a hospital due to inadequate facilities and/or staff is long, difficult, and not always successful.) However, to be eligible for many federal grants, such as Medicare, and to be affiliated with educational programs, including medical residency programs, accreditation is necessary. Accreditation by the Joint Commission on Accreditation of Hospitals (JCAH) is voluntary and is intended to indicate excellence in patient care. Specific standards, usually more rigorous than those of the state, are set to measure hospital efficiency, professional performance, and facilities, and must be met in all facets of health care services (including nursing). Visits are made by an inspection team (that may or may not have a multidisciplinary makeup) that reviews various records and minutes of meetings, interviews key people, and generally scrutinizes the hospital. Reports are made that include criticisms and recommendations for action. Accreditation may be postponed, withheld, revoked, granted, or renewed on the basis of the inspection and review of the hospital's report and self-evaluation. Nurses are now usually included on the inspection team, and there is nursing input into the standards for nursing service. To be eligible for an accreditation survey by JCAH, the hospital must be registered or listed by the AHA, have a current unconditional license to operate as required by the state, and have a governing body, organized medical staff, nursing service, and other supporting services. JCAH is made up of key medical and hospital organizations, but not ANA or other health professional groups. Nor does it include consumers, a fact that has caused some anger among consumer groups. To placate these groups, some JCAH visitors have had open hearings to receive consumer input about the institution being inspected. Just how much weight is given to this evidence is not known. Again, change may be forthcoming, particularly because there has been public criticism that accreditation cannot be equated with excellence or even safety in patient care.

Voluntary hospitals are usually organized under a constitution and by-laws that invest the board of trustees with the responsibility for medical care. This governing board is generally made up of individuals representing various professional and business groups interested in the community. Although unsalaried and volunteer (except for proprietary hospitals, in which members are often stockholders), board members are usually extremely influential citizens and are often self-perpetuating on the board. This type of membership originated because at one time administrators of hospitals did not have a business background, and because of the still-present need to raise money to support hospitals. (Most trustees still see recovery of operating costs as their most crucial hospital problem.) Some consumer groups have complained that most members are businessmen, bankers, brokers, lawyers, and accountants, with almost nonexistent representation of women, consumers in general, and labor. Physicians also complain of lack of medical representation, although they work closely with the board and are subordinate to it only in certain matters. Because of these pressures, boards are gradually acquiring broader representation.

It is also possible that there will be some lessening of trustee power as hospitals adopt the corporate model, integrating the board of trustees and the administration of the hospital, with the board having full-time and salaried presidents and vice-presidents. The growth of mergers, consortia, and holding companies that are creating new business-oriented hospital systems may also change the role of trustees.

Public hospitals usually do not have boards of trustees. Hospital administrators are directly responsible to their administrative supervisors in the governmental hierarchy, which may be a state board of health, a commissioner, a department such as the Veterans Administration, or a public corporation with appointed officials. Presumably, all are ultimately responsible to the public.

Although *administrator* is still the generic term for the managerial head of a hospital, in recent years this title has included a variety of designations such as *president* and *chief executive officer,* usually called *CEO.* The hospital administrator, the direct agent of a governing board, implements its policies, advises on new policies, and is responsible for the day-to-day operations of the hospital. Some years ago, physicians and nurses frequently became hospital administrators, but increasingly this position is filled by a lay person with a management background and possibly a master's degree in hospital administration or business administration. Hospital or health administration, like any other, encompasses planning, organizing, directing, controlling, and evaluating the resources of an organization. In large institutions, the administrator (the vast majority of whom are men) has a staff of assistants or associates, each responsible for a division or group of departments. Forward-looking hospitals have recognized that the nurse administrator should hold one of these positions in order to participate in the policy-making decisions that inevitably affect the largest hospital department. Department heads or supervisors are next in the line of authority; these individuals are also gradually becoming specialists by education and experience in their area of responsibility.

The medical staff is an organized entity made up of selected physicians and dentists who are granted the privilege of using the hospital's facilities for their patients. They, in turn, evaluate the credentials of other physicians who wish to join the staff and recommend appointment to the hospital's governing board, which legally makes the appointments. A typical classification of medical staff includes honorary (not active), consulting (specialist), active (attending physicians), courtesy (those not wishing full status but wanting to attend private patients), and resident (house staff of residents and fellows). Through their committees, including the Credentials Committee, the medical staff is an impressive power in the hospital, for it is often in a position to control not only medical practice, but all patient care in the hospital. (The medical staff organization is parallel to and not subordinate to that of the hospital administration.)

Legal pressures, such as the *Darling* v. *Charleston Community Memorial Hospital* desision (see Chapter 21), increased malpractice suits, community pressures, and governmental pressures, through the Medicare amendments (see Chapter 19), are focusing on the responsibility of medical staffs to monitor carefully the medical care given and to institute immediately necessary improvements.

In hospitals where the medical staff is more progressive, there are nurses and other representatives on medical committees concerned with patient care, and decisions are made jointly. However, the idea of giving nurses and others admitting privileges has been generally resisted by medical staffs. In some institutions, nurse-midwives, NPs, and other health professionals such as podiatrists, have been given these admitting privileges with certain restrictions, usually under an "adjunct" rubric. Considered a breakthrough was the 1983 stand of the Federal Trade Commission that medical rules should permit participating hospitals to grant staff membership to nurse-midwives, NPs, and other nonphysician health professionals, and 1984 JCAH guidelines giving hospitals the option of granting such privileges.

There is some feeling among the nursing

leadership, however, that such approval should not come from the medical staff, but, if nurses are involved, from nursing administration. Although not widespread, in some hospitals, nursing staff bylaws enable nurses to be self-directed and self-governed, and allow for orderly change within nursing. With such a mechanism, adjunct nursing staff including community-based NPs could, after having been approved by the nurse credentialing committee, provide care to their hospitalized clients.[40]

The utilization review committee, required for Medicare reimbursement, reviews records to determine that the patient's admission is valid, treatment is appropriate, and discharge is in a reasonable time. Nurses have been participating in these committees and are even employed full time in some instances.

In the last several years, there have been dramatic changes in hospitals, and even more are expected. Much is due to health economics and the criticism hospitals have received for their part in causing costs to escalate. The precipitating factor was undoubtedly the government-mandated prospective payment system for hospitals, utilizing diagnostic-related groups (DRGs) to determine payment. The reactions have also been economically oriented. The "competitive model" advocated by the Reagan Administration accelerated the growth of for-profit corporations that bought, built, and leased hospitals and other facilities and operated them under a corporate mantle. Although the type of governance varies, the motive is profit. One executive reported his company's strategy as acquiring hospitals in areas with favorable business factors, creating sophisticated facilities that provide a broad base of services, and involving physicians in profit sharing. The services ranged from high-technology diagnostic and treatment centers to health clubs, including all varieties of ambulatory care facilities that acted as "feeders" to the hospital. Comprehensive long-term care facilities and psychiatric hospitals, as well as home care, were cited as increasingly profitable ventures.

Other hospitals joined in the corporate approach (as shown in Figure 7-3), requiring, in turn, well-prepared financial managers and business-oriented executive officers. The number of contract-managed hospitals, primarily investor owned, but also including church systems and other nonprofit systems, grew dramatically. In 1965, multi-institutional concepts were barely heard of, and only about 2 percent of the hospitals were so affiliated; by 1980, more than 30 percent of community hospitals were under some such arrangement, with more expected. As in community health, marketing became essential as fewer beds were filled because of the competition of other types of nonhospital health services (Figure 7-4). In addition, hospitals also added these and other services. (One institution has an air emergency service that helps to develop what has been called *captive distribution services.*) Shared buying and selling of equipment and supplies is another technique to save and make money. In projecting the future of the general hospital, some experts say that while remaining a pivotal component in health care, the system will shrink because of its cost. In the new reimbursement system, economics is and will continue to force hospitals into admitting and treating only the very sick, the case mix of fifty years ago. On an even more pessimistic note, it seems that "both patients and staff [will] become interchangeable parts of a 'curing and management machine.'"[41]

LONG-TERM CARE FACILITIES

Long-term care services for chronic diseases and conditions comprise one of the fastest-growing components of health care expenditures. In part this is due to the success of medical science in saving those who might have died of their condition at any stage of life, and in part to the fact that the nuclear family has no place for the incapacitated who, years ago, were simply cared for at home with no public help. As noted early, the use of ambulatory care facilities and a return to home care are

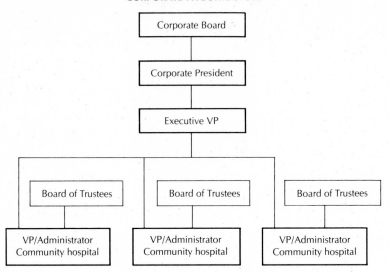

Figure 7-3. A multi-institutional model of corporate-type structure.

being advocated, but the fact remains that such care requires a considerable number of backup services, social and health related, that are neither easy to organize nor to coordinate and even less easy to be reimbursed for. Therefore, despite much rhetoric, institutional care for long-term patients, while considerably more expensive and often lessening the individual's quality of life, still appears to be necessary for part of the population. The fact that 21 percent of long-term care accounts for two-thirds of the long-term health care dollar makes institutional care an ongoing public concern.

There are two major categories of long-term care institutions: long-stay hospitals (for example, psychiatric, rehabilitation, chronic disease, and tuberculosis) and nursing homes. There are approximately 600 long-stay hospitals, mostly psychiatric and mostly government owned. Approximately 18,000 nursing homes, about 80 percent of which are proprietary, account for 70 percent of the institutionalized population.* Almost half have fewer than 50 beds, and 75 percent have fewer than 100 beds.[42] The largest number are in the Midwest and the fewest in the South.

Nursing homes can be classified according to the levels of care offered and whether they are certified for the Medicare and/or Medicaid programs. According to these regulations, a skilled nursing facility (SNF) which provides inpatient skilled nursing and restorative/rehabilitative services must provide twenty-four-hour nursing services, have transfer agreements with a hospital, and fulfill other specific requirements. An intermediate-care facility (ICF) provides inpatient health-related care and services to individuals not requiring SNF care. Nursing homes may be certified for either or both levels; about 25 percent are not certified at all. Some are also JCAH accredited.

---

*This does not refer to residential facilities that may provide some degree of nursing services over and above room, board, and personal care or "custodial" services.

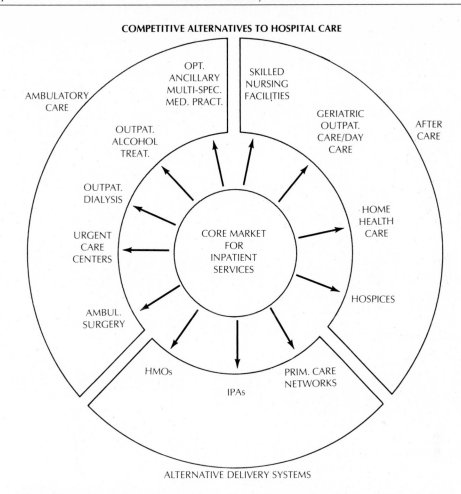

COMPETITIVE ALTERNATIVES TO HOSPITAL CARE

Figure 7-4. Competitive alternatives to hospital care. (Reprinted with permission from *Issues in Health Care*, Vol. 3 (no. 1), a publication of the International Accounting and Consulting Firm of Laventhol & Horwath, 1982, 13.)

The primary sources of payment for residents are Medicaid and personal or family income; at a much smaller level are welfare payments (about 6 percent) and Medicare (2 percent). The nursing home population is very old, with 85 percent over seventy-five and more than 10 percent over ninety. Patients usually have three to four chronic illnesses; half have psychiatric diagnoses. The majority are poor, white, unmarried women, whose sole significant source of income is a survivor (not retiree) Social Security check. The lack of Hispanics and blacks is seen as due to inequity in services, not cultural preferences. In almost all cases, residence in a nursing home is due to a lack of financial resources and/or family members to care for the patient outside.[43]

Most of the 1 million employees who care for nursing home residents are unskilled and untrained aides. Almost no direct hands-on care is given by licensed nurses, although at least one RN must be employed by every licensed nursing home. That one RN may also be the director of nursing and probably has no degree. For that matter, neither do most nursing home administrators. Medical care is also minimal, with fewer than 300 physicians employed by all the nursing homes. Over half of the patients stay less than six months, but after three years, discharge is usually to a terminal hospital stay or "discharged dead." Except in the best nursing homes, there is minimal social intercourse and activity.

In a 1974 government study, optimum nursing home care was described as preventive, protective, restorative, and supportive, meeting the medical, nursing, psychosocial, and rehabilitation needs of the individual. Unannounced visits that provided data for that report indicated that the degree of compliance varied a great deal, with particular laxity in adhering to safety standards, in meaningful participation of the physician, and in meeting the health care needs of patients and residents in the areas of rehabilitation and nutrition. Drug abuse and misuse and violation of patients' rights were also found. More regulations were promulgated to deal with these problems, and remedial projects were developed—among them training nursing home surveyors and upgrading the knowledge and skills of personnel, including doctors and nurses. One particularly hopeful step is the preparation of geriatric NPs, who have been found invaluable in providing the necessary long-term care for these patients.

There are still complaints about the quality of life, if not always the quality of physical care, in nursing homes. In some areas, voluntary ombudsmen regularly make checks to prevent or detect abuses. There are also a few adopt-a-grandparent or similar programs that give the residents caring social contacts outside the home.

The organizational structure of a nursing home is often much like that of a hospital, but the number of diagnostic and therapeutic departments is usually fewer, depending on the major purpose of the institution. The nursing home may or may not be associated with a particular hospital. Some extended-care facilities have expansive services providing a continuum of care from skilled nursing to home care. For those who can afford it, there are complexes in which older people can live in their own apartment for life; health care services, including skilled nursing, are made available when needed. Sometimes a nursing home and even a hospital are on site.

Experts disagree on the future of nursing homes. Nursing homes serve the socially isolated woman, a group that is increasing, but no one seems to want to expand the nursing home system because of concerns about cost and quality of care. Yet if *all* home care and support services were reimbursed, the "latent demand" might cause a financial catastrophe, since almost all of that care is now given without reimbursement by family and friends. As the older population increases, so does the need for a reasonable plan for their long-term care needs.

ISSUES AND PREDICTIONS

Today's $340 billion health care system is frequently condemned as a nonsystem focused on sick care.

Two critics described the medical care systems as follows:

> That great impersonal Hydra-headed technological monster clonking across the landscape, gobbling up the Gross National Product and excreting computerized bills, neither curing nor caring, growing two new hospital wings and a cobalt radiation unit for every general practitioner that is lopped off, engineered by greedy villans.[44]

> Today's health care crisis is a miasma of vested interests, obsolescence, malpractice, incompetence and questionable social concern. While some groups may be more guilty than others, few can properly throw the first stone.[45]

Three noted social scientists, in looking at today's medical care, held that:

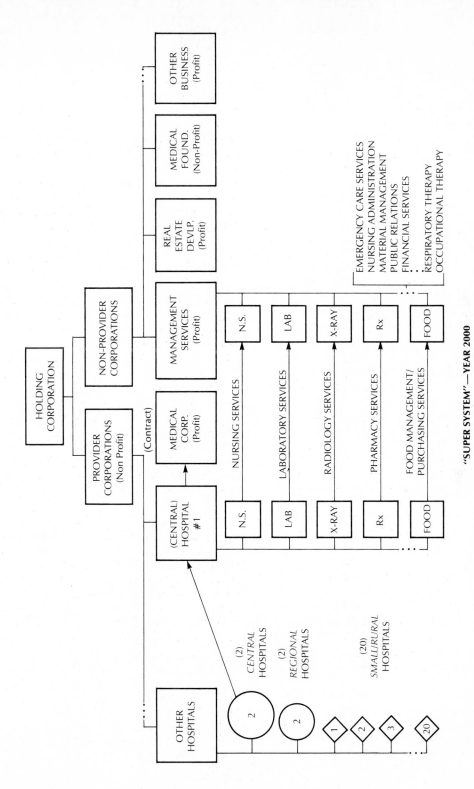

"SUPER SYSTEM"—YEAR 2000

Figure 7-5. "Super System"—Year 2000. (Reprinted with permission from John Coleman; Elizabeth Dayani; and Elsie Simms: Nursing careers in emerging systems. *Nursing Management*, 15 (Jan.), 1984, pp. 19–29.)

1. Public health measures, social conditions, and personal health behavior are the main determinants of health.

2. Our health system is too heavily weighted in the direction of hospital-based medicine and . . . there is need to give greater emphasis to community-based ambulatory care with a strong preventive component.

3. Many medical measures and interventions are not effective by any criterion. Those measures or interventions that are proved to be ineffective should be abandoned.

4. Many services now provided by physicians can be performed by other health personnel.

5. Iatrogenic illness is fairly extensive and is a very serious concern.

6. Costs in the health sector have risen disproportionately and economies and cost controls are warranted.

7. Some health and human services which presently are not available should be provided.

8. There is need for more humane health care.[46]

Few would argue those points, but one not mentioned is access to care. A 1983 report by the Robert Wood Johnson Foundation concluded that the American people have greater access to care than ever before, with the majority enjoying access to a personal physician or other regular source of general medical care. The chief complaints were out-of-pocket costs, waiting time to see a doctor, and the amount of information provided by doctors and nurses. The poor, the black, and the unemployed, some 12 percent of the population, had serious access problems. That this situation would probably worsen, given health economics, was acknowledged by a presidential commission on ethics, which concluded that "society has an ethical obligation to ensure equitable access to health care for all."[47]

Neither in the commission nor in the public is there total agreement on that statement, particularly in relation to the next step—access to all expensive high technology, the world of transplants and artificial parts. A survey of health policy leaders reported their general consensus that only a *minimum* level of health care is the right of *all* Americans and that uninsured persons without the ability to pay would experience a significant decline in the quality of their health service by 1995.[48] Even those who believe that health education and promotion could be the answer to high costs are not optimistic that there will be adequate commitment to the reality (not the concept) or that change will occur in any great hurry.

In the meantime, U.S. citizens spend more than 10 percent of their gross national product on health care—more than any other nation in the world. "Astronomical cost" were the watchwords, with the result that by 1984, most hospitals were forced by Medicare regulation and a new federal budget act into a whole new system of reimbursement. (See Chapter 19 for a longer discussion of TEFRA.) And the signs were clear that other health care facilities would soon fall under similar rules. Put simply, prospective reimbursement with DRGs meant that instead of being paid for the costs of a patient's stay after the fact, the *anticipated* cost of the patient's care according to the diagnosis or diagnoses and certain other factors was set, including the number of hospital days. If the hospital was able to provide the care at less than that cost, the excess could be kept; if the cost was greater, it had to be absorbed. This meant that care had to be effective and efficient. Also, whereas longer stays were once an advantage, the opposite was now true, indeed crucial. These shifts have brought about some of the changes noted earlier.

The public is somewhat ambivalent about these issues. People want cuts in costs, including taxes, which pay for many of these services, but they also want full, high-quality health care. Are both possible? They also have some ongoing complaints, besides high costs and access: fragmentation of services, maldistribution of health personnel, overspecialization of practitioners, inadequate quality, depersonalization, and loss of personal control within the system. It is clear that many of these issues are related to health manpower, which is discussed in Chapter 8.

Health care experts and policy makers have suggested remedies, but like the economic pundits, their "guestimates" of future trends are not totally reliable. Some place great faith in some sort of national health insurance, but the difficulty of assessing the cost and outcome of the assorted proposals has made the Congress slow to act, and with opposition in the administration, nothing will happen. Nevertheless, some predictions about the health care of the future from a number of "experts" are at least provocative.[49]

1. There will be a growing demand for geriatric services.
2. Successful organizations must be oriented to health, rather than medical care.
3. Hospitals will evolve into "human service" centers, including, besides the traditional acute care, fitness, counseling, employment services, personal care, nutrition, family planning, and other social services.
4. The patient will play a greater role in health care decision making.
5. Costs will increase, but the public will demand that health outcomes justify such expenditures.
6. The individual provider will be replaced to a large extent by the medic-computer.
7. The doctor glut will become greater, and many doctors will shift from private practice to group practice or a salaried partnership.
8. Increasingly, care will be delivered outside of the traditional hospital setting.
9. The number of hospitals will drop and multihospital systems will grow, to include possibly as much as 70 percent of the health care industry by 1986.
10. Home care will grow dramatically.
11. Workers will pay more of their health care expenses out of pocket, and thus will become more conservative users of health care.

12. For the urban poor there will be a deterioration in the quality of care. By the year 2000, a two-tier system of care will exist—unless there are major changes.
13. National health insurance is likely, with the probable form being a combination of public and private programs financed by the government, employers, and employees.

Some of these predictions are illustrated in Figure 7-5.

REFERENCES

1. U.S. Department of Health, Education, and Welfare, *Extending the Scope of Nursing Practice* (Washington, D.C.: The Department, 1971), p. 8.
2. John Millis, "Primary Care: Definitions of and Access to . . ." *Nurs. Outlook,* **25**:443 (July 1977).
3. US DHEW, op. cit., p. 10.
4. US DHEW, op. cit., p. 11.
5. Talcott Parsons, "Definition of Health and Illness in the Light of American Values and Social Structure," in E. G. Jaco, ed., *Patients, Physicians and Illness* (Glencoe, Ill.: Free Press, 1958), p. 176.
6. K. W. Sehnert, and J. T. Nocerino, *Activated Patient: A Course Guide* (Washington, D.C.: Center for Continuing Health Education, Georgetown University, 1974).
7. Catherine Norris, "Self-Care," *Am. J. Nurs.,* **79**:486–489 (Mar. 1979).
8. Lawrence Green and Katrina Johnson, "Health Education and Health Promotion," in David Mechanic, ed., *Handbook of Health, Health Care, and the Health Professions* (New York: Free Press, 1983), pp. 744–765.
9. Lester Breslow, "The Potential of Health Promotion" David Mechanic, ed., *Handbook of Health, Health Care and the Health Professions* (New York: (Free Press, 1983), pp. 50–66.
10. Anne Somers et al., "Preventive Health Services for the Elderly: The Rutgers Medical School Project," *Inquiry,* **19**:190–198 (Fall 1982).
11. Marc Lalonde, *A New Perspective on the*

Health of Canadians (Ottawa: Government of Canada), 1974.

12. Steven Jonas et al., *Health Care Delivery in the United States* (New York: Springer Publishing Co., Inc., 1977), pp. 122–123.

13. Ibid., p. 141.

14. Anne Warner, ed., *Innovations in Community Health Nursing* (St. Louis: C. V. Mosby Company, 1978).

15. USDHEW, *Health Maintenance Organizations: The Concept and Structure,* (Washington, D.C., 1971).

16. Jonas et al., op. cit., pp. 143–144.

17. Harold Luft, "Health-Maintenance Organizations," in Mechanic, op. cit., p. 319.

18. Harold S. Luft, "How Do Health Maintenance Organizations Achieve Their 'Savings'?" *New Eng. J. Med.,* **293**:1336–1343 (June 15, 1978).

19. Jonas et al., op. cit., p. 146.

20. Ibid., pp. 125–135.

21. Edward Ehlinger, "Implications of the Competition Model," *Nurs. Outlook* **30**:519 (Dec. 1982).

22. Miles Zaremski and Darryl Fohrman, "The Emergicenter: Has Its Time Arrived?", *Law, Medicine, and Health Care,* **11**:4–11 (Feb. 1983).

23. Ruth Lubic, "The Rise of the Birth Center Alternative," *The Nation's Health* **13**:7 (Jan. 1982).

24. Ruth Lubic, "Childbirthing Centers: Delivering More for Less," *Am. J. Nurs.,* **83**:1053–1056 (July 1983).

25. Norma Lang, "Nurse-Managed Centers—Will They Thrive?" *Am. J. Nurs.,* **83**:1290–1296 (Sept. 1983).

26. DHEW "Hospice Care." *Federal Register,* Vol. 43, 1978.

27. Virginia Thomas, "Hospice Nursing—Reaping the Rewards, Dealing with Stress," *Geriatric Nurs.,* **4**:22 (Jan.–Feb. 1983).

28. Kathryn Burris, "Recommending Adult Day Care Centers," *Nursing and Health Care,* **2**:437 (Oct. 1981).

29. Granger Westberg, "Multiplying Wholistic Health Centers," in Jack Lindquist, ed. *Increasing the Impact* (Battle Creek, Mich.: W. K. Kellogg Foundation, 1979).

30. Florence Wilson and Duncan Neuhauser, *Health Services in the United States,* 2nd ed. (Cambridge, Mass: Ballinger Publishing Co., 1982), pp. 229–238.

31. *Proposed Model for the Delivery of Home Health Services* (New York: National League for Nursing, 1974).

32. Ibid.

33. E. Eleanor Grimes, "Developing Neighborhood Nurse Offices," *Nurs. and Health Care,* **3**:138–141 (Mar. 1983).

34. Marge Jamieson and Ida Martinson, "Block Nursing: Neighbors Caring for Neighbors," *Nurs. Outlook,* **31**:270, 272 (Sept.–Oct. 1983).

35. Marybelle Smith, "A Team Approach to Health Care," *Nurs. Outlook,* **31**:271, 273 (Sept.–Oct. 1983).

36. Virginia Saba, "The Computer in Public Health: Today and Tomorrow," *Nurs. Outlook,* **30**:510–514 (Nov.–Dec. 1982).

37. Sarah Archer, "Marketing Public Health Nursing Services," *Nurs. Outlook,* **3**:304–311 (Nov.–Dec. 1983).

38. Barry Cooper, "As Emergency Medical Administrator," in Lowell Bellin and Lewis Weeks, ed., *The Challenge of Administering Health Services: Career Pathways* (Washington, D.C.: AUPHA Press, 1981), pp. 97–107.

39. Wilson and Neuhauser, op. cit., p. 23.

40. Frances Carson and Adrienne Ames, "Nursing Staff Bylaws," *Am. J. Nurs.,* **80**:1130–1134 (June 1980).

41. Odin Anderson and Norman Gevitz, "The General Hospital: A Social and Historical Perspective," in Mechanic, op. cit., pp. 305–317.

42. Diane Lawrence and Clifton Gaus, "Long-Term Care: Financing and Policy Issues," in Mechanic, op. cit., pp. 365–378.

43. Bruce Vladeck, "Nursing Homes," in Mechanic, op. cit., pp. 352–364.

44. H. Jack Geiger, "Who Shall Live?" (Book Review), *New York Times* Book Review Section, Mar. 2, 1972, p. 1.

45. Martha Rogers, "Nursing Is Coming of Age-Con," *Am. J. Nurs.,* **75**:1842 (Oct. 1975).

46. Sol Levine et al., "Does Medical Care Do Any Good?" in Mechanic, op. cit., pp. 394–404.

47. President's Commission for the Study of Ethical Problems in Medicine and Bio-

medical and Behavioral Research, *Securing Access to Health Care* (Washington, D.C.: U.S. Government Printing Office, March 1983).

48. *Health Care in the 1990s: Trends and Strategies* (Chicago, Ill.: Arthur Anderson and Company and the American College of Hospital Administrators, 1984).

49. Press release, American College of Hospital Administrators, Chicago, Ill., 1983.

8

Health Care Delivery: Who?

A hundred years ago, trained health manpower consisted of physicians, dentists, some pharmacists, and nurses. Now there are more than 250 acknowledged health occupations, with more being developed every day. Depending on whether the health care industry is defined narrowly or broadly, that is, whether all workers within the industry are included, the estimated number of workers ranges from almost 6 million to over 8 million. The latter figure might include certain supportive services. Health care facilities, like other places of business, employ secretaries, clerks, accountants, receptionists, messengers, and others to carry on business operations. In addition, institutions need laundry workers, dietary workers, cooks, plumbers, electricians, carpenters, maids, porters, and similar kinds of employees to function in the hotel-keeping aspect of their services.

Not included in any category are faith healers, root doctors, or certain untrained healers who rely on herbs, meditation, or other semi-self-care techniques of healing.

However, the overwhelming growth of personnel is in direct health services. Many of the health occupations and suboccupations have emerged because of inc.eased specialization in

health care, others on the peculiar assumption that several less-prepared workers can substitute for the scarcer professional. Some of these workers can be employed in almost any health setting—hospitals, nursing homes, clinics, doctors' offices, occupational health, and school health. Some work primarily in one setting. Most of these workers are not licensed; many are trained in on-the-job programs, and even more are trained in a variety of programs with no consistent standards. Others have standardized programs approved by the AMA and/or other health organizations. Generally, this entire group is categorized as *allied health manpower (AHM)* and is described later.

The most recent governmental figures on health manpower are presented in Tables 8-1 and 8-2. Their accuracy is acknowledged to be somewhat questionable, since the final figures came from a variety of sources, all of which have some problems in data collection. This is particularly true in relation to AHM because of discrepancies in definition, the great variety of work settings, the paucity of licensure data, lack of funding for AHM associations to invest in manpower research, and the fact that most of these workers belong to no association and, indeed, often come and go in the workforce depending on employer demand. Since AHM, defined broadly, could make up as much as 63 percent of all health manpower, the problems of accuracy are evident. Nevertheless, it is the periodic report to Congress by DHHS that is considered "official"; accordingly, the active health manpower supply was estimated as more than 3.8 million in 1982.

When health care is equated with medical care, a functional structure emerges, consisting of independent practitioners, dependent practitioners, and supporting staff. Jonas, although acknowledging that the lines separating the groups are unclear at times, describes the independent practitioners as those permitted by law to provide a delimited range of services (physicians, dentists, chiropractors, optometrists, and podiatrists); dependent practitioners as those permitted by law to provide a delimited range of services under the supervision and/or authorization of independent practitioners (nurses, social workers, pharmacists, dental hygienists, physicians' assistants, and various therapists); and supporting staff as those carrying out specific tasks authorized by and under the supervision of independent and dependent practitioners, frequently without specific legal delineation of tasks or authority.[1] As Jonas readily agrees, the scope of practice and autonomy of the dependent practitioners are a great source of conflict, particularly because many have an area of expertise not within the knowledge and skills of the independent practitioner. Moreover, the gray areas of overlapping practice are becoming greater; what a particular practitioner does may be legitimately within his/her scope of practice in certain circumstances and just as legitimately within that of another in other circumstances. The legal lines drawn also waver when it comes to supportive workers; there are tasks done by nurses' aides or practical nurses that are first of all part of a nurse's responsibility; in times and places of nurse shortages, they are often done with almost no supervision. With a rising acceptance

of medical care as a component of health care but not its totality, the independent-dependent status concept of health practitioners will undoubtedly undergo considerable revision.

Credentialing of the health care providers and their educational programs is under a variety of auspices: the state, a single professional organization, or a coalition of professional organizations. As of 1983, the educational programs of twenty-five allied health occupations were accredited by the Committee on Allied Health Education and Accreditation (CAHEA), a collaborative effort of national health organizations and medical specialty organizations with the American Medical Association (AMA). This accreditation process begins with acceptance of minimal requirements for entry into the occupation, labeled the "Essentials," which must be adopted both by the AMA Council on Medical Education and the particular collaborating organizations concerned. Other occupations follow other procedures with their accrediting group.

Practitioners who are not licensed may become certified or registered on a voluntary basis by the occupation's national organization or a parent medical group. The inconsistency of these various processes is the focus of some of the complaints about health care credentialing. In 1983, DHHS listed the following as health personnel licensed or certified in every state*: nursing home administrators, chiropractors, dentists, dental hygienists, practical nurses, professional nurses, optometrists, pharmacists, physical therapists, physicians (MD and DO), podiatrists, psychologists and veterinarians. This does not necessarily mean that licensure is required, only that it is available (see Chapter 20).

Compared to other nations, the United States has a more than ample supply of health workers, even in terms of the physician-popu-

---

*Not necessarily the territories or District of Columbia (D.C.).

TABLE 8-1
Estimated Active Supply of Selected Health Personnel and Provider-Population Ratios, 1970, 1975, 1980, and 1982

| Health Occupation | Estimated Active Supply | | | | Percent Change | | |
	1970	1975	1980	1982	1970–1982	1975–1982	1980–1982
Physicians	326,200	384,500	457,500	466,600[1]	43.0	21.4	2.0
Allopathic (MD)	314,200	370,400	440,400	448,660[1]	42.8	21.1	1.9
Osteopathic (DO)	12,000	14,100	17,140	17,970[1]	49.8	27.4	4.8
Podiatrists	7,100	7,300	8,900	9,600	35.2	31.5	7.9
Dentists	102,220	112,020	126,240	132,010	29.1	17.8	4.6
Optometrists	18,400	19,999	22,400	23,300	26.6	17.1	4.0
Pharmacists	113,700	122,800	143,800	151,400	33.2	23.3	5.3
Veterinarians	25,900	31,100	36,000	38,810	49.8	24.8	7.8
Registered nurses	750,000	961,000	1,272,900	1,372,300[2]	83.0	42.8	7.8
Rate per 100,000 population							
Physicians	156.0	174.4	197.0	198.8	27.4	14.0	0.9
Allopathic (MD)	150.0	167.9	189.5	191.0	27.3	13.8	0.8
Osteopathic (DO)	6.0	6.5	7.5	7.8	30.0	20.0	4.0
Podiatrists	3.5	3.4	4.0	4.1	17.1	20.6	2.5
Dentists	49.5	51.6	55.2	56.6	14.3	9.7	2.5
Optometrists	8.9	9.2	9.8	10.0	12.4	8.6	2.0
Pharmacists	54.4	56.6	63.0	65.0	19.5	14.8	3.2
Veterinarians	12.5	14.3	15.8	16.7	33.6	16.8	5.7
Registered nurses	319	366	560	590[1]	85.0	61.2	5.4

[1]Data are for 1981.
[2]Estimated from projections included in tables in the Chapter on Nursing.
Source: Report to the President and Congress on the Status of Health Personnel in the United States Vol. 1, (Washington, D.C.: U.S. Department of Health and Human Services, Bureau of Health and Professions, 1984), p. 16.

lation ratio. (In some countries, it is nurses who are in shortest supply). Types of American health workers are also considerably more diverse; other nations have experimented more with such physician substitutes as the Russian feldsher or Chinese barefoot doctor. The largest categories of health workers, in order, are nursing (all types, including aides), physicians, dentists and their allied services, clinical laboratory workers, pharmacists, and radiological technicians. As feminists are the first to point out, *manpower* is a misnomer; from 75 to 85 percent are women. However, they are, or have been, in the lower-paid and less powerful positions. Physicians, dentists, administrators, and others in policymaking positions are overwhelmingly male.

Except for the independent practitioners who are primarily self-employed, the mass of health workers are employed in institutions and agencies, with the greatest number concentrated in hospitals.

It would be unrealistic to attempt to describe all the professional and technical workers with whom nurses work or interact. However, an introduction to the most prevalent health occupations should provide a better understanding of the complex relationships in health care.

The organization of this chapter is primarily alphabetical, although on occasion two closely related groups may be described in logical succession. The education of RNs and practical nurses is described in Chapters 12 and 13 and the practice of nursing in Chapters 15 and 16.

Administration

Health services administrators manage organizations, agencies, institutions, programs, and services within the health care delivery system. They may work in any setting but are probably more visible in hospitals, nursing homes, neighborhood health centers, and community health agencies. The principles of management can be applied to any setting, and the role of the hospital administrator, described in Chapter 7, is a reasonable example of role and functions. Nurses are usually the administrators of nursing services, but a number also hold positions as top administrators, particularly in community health agencies. Although they may retain their nursing identity, they should be functioning as administrators and have the necessary educational background.

Usually, the appropriate credential is a master's degree in health services administration, hospital administration, or, recently, business administration. There are about 110 baccalaureate programs that prepare for beginning middle management positions.

Other positions in the operation of health facilities and plants are the usual business positions, finance, data processing, personnel, public relations, and admissions, with all types of jobs and educational levels.

An evolving issue in health administration education centers on the proper educational credentials. The need for such administrators has been debated, but growth of the field is indicated by the interest of educational institutions in initiating programs. Since the greatest increase in the number of programs has been at the baccalaureate level, experts in the field have raised the question of quality of education. This is seen as particularly pertinent because of the opposite educational trend— the demand for administrators prepared in business school. Although the latter is frequently recommended for administrators to deal with the serious economic pressures and concomitantly greater business orientation in health care delivery, especially hospitals, the need for a master's degree in business administration is also controversial. The question is raised as to whether

managers who are not familiar with, and sen-

sitive to, the sense of mission and the complexity of [a health care] organization's constituents will find it difficult to fulfill that mission or to satisfy those constituents. Any such failure will jeopardize the institution, regardless of the business knowledge and skills the manager may bring to the organization. . . . They can always lure statisticians and financial specialists to manage the day-to-day tracking of operations and cash flow, but they had better know enough about trends in the hospital environment and the imperatives of the hospital and its constituencies to properly anticipate change and position their institutions accordingly.[2]

The determination of the proper curriculum balance between managerial skills and knowledge of the health care delivery environment is also an issue because, at the same time that post-master's residencies in health care administration are being recommended, economic pressures in the field are lessening the opportunities for such employer-funded education.

Considered equally serious is the lack of appropriately prepared faculty, especially in financial management, since individuals with the proper background and education often choose to go into an industry where salaries are higher. Practitioner-teachers are considered one solution, but it has also been stated that it would not be a bad idea for some of the weaker programs that cannot afford the right kind of faculty to go out of business.

Allied Health Manpower

Allied health manpower (AHM) has been defined by the federal government to include

all those professional, technical, and supportive workers in the fields of patient care, public health, and health research who engage in activities that support, complement, or supplement the professional functions of physicians, dentists, and registered nurses, as well as personnel engaged in organized environmental health activities who are expected to have some expertise in environmental health.[3]

In a more recent report, it was noted that the services rendered by AHM range across the entire spectrum of service delivery and include every aspect of patient care, as well as services provided as part of community health promotion and protection. Examples given were emergency services; initial evaluation; treatment, therapy, and continued assessment; testing; acute care; long-term care; medical instrumentation; fabrication of devices; and record keeping.[4] AHM range from personnel with complex functions and the highest educational degrees, who have always had a great deal of autonomy, to those who function in relatively simple assisting roles and must be supervised, sometimes by others categorized as AHMs. Because of this diversity and changes in health care, there are many changes occurring within occupations/professions so identified. Since such a large percentage of health care personnel are AHM (see Table 8-2), it is ironic that there are so little fundamental data, but this is blamed on the elasticity of supply and the constant evaluation of the roles and responsibilities of certain occupations.

Role evaluation can be demonstrated in part by changes in education. At one time, most AHM were educated in almost apprentice-like programs in hospitals. In the 1960s, with the commitment of federal funds to AHM education, the growth of junior colleges, and increases in educational costs, many AHMs were transferred to a college setting, with the hospital remaining as a clinical practice site. Expansion of both junior and senior colleges was inevitable as the specialization needs grew and as more Americans wanted both a college education and a marketable skill. However, hospitals, vocational schools, and military institutions remained as sites of training programs.

The allied health occupations moved toward professionalism at various paces. Accreditation, certification, licensing, higher education, and demand for autonomy and increased scope of practice occurred in some; others turned to unionism. Ginzberg reports

that beginning salaries vary a great deal, even for the technically trained, but more shocking is the lack of opportunity for advancement and increased salary later. The salary and career prospects of AHMs are affected by the predominance of women in the field, which has a depressing influence on salary; the lack of significant long-term shortages; and the inability to bill on a fee-for-service basis, since most AHMs are employed by institutions or agencies, or by individual physicians and dentists, who set the qualifications, functions, and salaries. Moreover, since there is a potential oversupply of physicians and dentists, there is a greater tendency to control and limit the practice of certain AHMs.[5] Some of these issues will be explored further as specific occupations are discussed later.

Just what the future holds for the AHM contingent is difficult to say. Predictors of future employment opportunities are still citing the general health manpower field, and especially AHM, as good bets. There has also been some evidence that cheaper, less well prepared workers are being substituted for others, such as nurses.[6] On the other hand, health manpower experts predict a decline in AHM due to overexpansion, overpricing of services, "overprofessionalizing," a leveling off of modalities that require new types of technicians, their need for supervision, and, most important, the fact that most cannot be directly reimbursed and cannot show that they contribute to cost containment. There are predictions of internecine warfare for survival of competing AHMs and others. However, one expert also warns that all trends are cyclical, and that with social health problems and an aging population, a turnaround is inevitable.[7]

Chiropractic

Chiropractic is described by the American Chiropractic Association (ACA) as "a branch of the healing arts which is concerned with human health and disease processes. Doctors of chiropractic are physicians who consider man as an integrated being, but give special attention to spinal mechanics and neurological,

TABLE 8-2
Estimated Active Supply of Selected Allied Health Personnel, Selected Years, 1970–1982[1]

Allied Health Occupation	1970	1974	1978	1982
Total allied health personnel	658,000	828,000	1,026,000	1,166,000
Dental hygienists	12,000	23,000	34,000	43,000
Dental assistants	92,000	130,000	148,000	163,000
Dental laboratory technicians	26,000	39,000	47,000	55,000
Dietitians	12,000	31,000	28,000	35,000
Dietetic technicians	1,000	3,000	4,000	5,000
Medical records administrators	10,000	12,000	12,000	14,000
Medical records technicians	32,000	51,000	68,000	71,000
Laboratory workers	100,000	180,000	240,000	265,000
Occupational therapists	5,000	10,000	15,000	23,000
Physical therapists	11,000	18,000	28,000	34,000
Primary care physician's assistants	—	4,000	6,000	13,000
Radiologic service workers	75,000	95,000	108,000	125,000
Respiratory therapy workers	15,000	40,000	52,000	59,000
Speech pathologists/ audiologists	11,000	27,000	31,000	36,000
Other allied health[2]	40,000	175,000	200,000	225,000[3]

[1]Due to revisions and independent estimations, some numbers may differ from numbers that appear elsewhere.

[2]Includes such categories as dietetic assistant, genetic assistant, operating room technician, ophthalmic medical assistant, optometric assistant, and technician, orthoptic and prosthetic technologist, pharmacy assistant, occupational and physical therapy assistants, physician assistant, podiatric assistant, vocational rehabilitation counselor, other rehabilitation services, and other social and mental health services.

[3]Insufficient data for estimation; the 225,000 figure shown for other allied health personnel is an assumption based on general trends in health manpower employment.

Source: Report to the President and Congress on the Status of Health Personnel in the United States Vol. 2, (Washington, D.C.: U.S. Department of Health and Human Services, Bureau of Health and Professions, 1984), p. B–8–1.

muscular, and vascular relationships." Chiropractors use standard diagnostic measures, but treatment methods, determined by law, do not include prescription drugs and surgery. Essentially, treatment includes "the chiropractic adjustment, necessary dietary advice and nutritional supplementation, necessary physiotherapeutic measures, and necessary professional counsel."

By 1982, fourteen chiropractic colleges were either accredited or eligible for accreditation by the Council on Chiropractic Education (CCE), and enrollment was increasing. Successful completion of a minimum of four years of study in the sciences, public health, clinical disciplines, and chiropractic principles and practice, including clinical practice, preceded by two professional years of college, results in a Doctor of Chiropractic diploma. The practitioner may be designated *Doctor of Chiropractic, Chiropractic Physician,* or *Chiropractor.* Most are in private practice. They are licensed in all states, the majority of which require continuing education for relicensure. All fifty states and the District of Columbia and Puerto Rico recognize chiropractic as a health profession and authorize chiropractic services as part of their worker's compensation program, as do many federal health benefits programs; services are also reimbursable under Medicare and Medicaid.

In the past, both the AMA and the American Public Health Association (APHA) have passed resolutions in opposition to chiropractic, the AMA defining it as an unscientific cult. Referring patients to chiropractors or accepting referrals was considered unethical. However, in July 1980, after a series of legal actions and decisions against them, the AMA revised its rules governing medical (ethical) conduct to permit MDs to refer to Doctors of Chiropractic. This opened the door for improved interprofessional relationships.[8] There have always been some physicians who, noting the continual educational upgrading, see the eventual integration of chiropractic into the field of medicine, just as were homeopathy and osteopathy, also once considered unacceptable. Meanwhile, chiropractic is a portal to the health care system for thousands of people who prefer treatment that stresses personal counseling and attention and no use of drugs.

Clinical Laboratory Sciences

There are a number of technicians or technologists working in the clinical laboratories in such specialties as immunohematology, hematology, clinical chemistry, serology, microbiology, and histology. The physician in charge is a pathologist, although technologists may have specific responsibilities for technicians. *Medical technologists'* preparation includes three years of college science plus a year of professional course work in a CAHEA-accredited school covering all phases of clinical laboratory work. Certification is granted by the Board of Registry of Medical Technologists of the American Society of Clinical Pathologists, after successful completion of a board examination. The initials *MT (ASCP)* may then be used. Most states do not require licensure. Additional appropriate education and experience qualify a medical technologist for specialist certification in blood

banking, chemistry, microbiology, cytotechnology, or nuclear technology.

Bioanalysts are "multidisciplined clinical laboratory scientists who direct and/or supervise clinical laboratories. Trained in a variety of scientific disciplines, the bioanalyst is responsible for the overall technical and administrative functions of the clinical laboratory and is distinguished from many other clinical laboratory scientists by competency in several laboratory disciplines, as opposed to being a single specialty scientist."

Clinical Chemists "use complex chemical tests and procedures to analyze body tissues and fluids like urine and saliva. Through chemical analysis, they detect the presence and percentage of proteins, trace metals, hormones, drugs or other substances in the body to determine the patient's degree of health or the absence or presence of disease. Most clinical chemists work in hospitals or clinical laboratories. A master's degree in chemistry is generally the minimum preparation. Many clinical chemists hold the PhD or MD degree."[9]

Certified laboratory assistants, who perform routine laboratory tests, and *histologic technicians,* who prepare body tissues for microscopic examination by pathologists, are usually prepared in one-year hospital programs, also CAHEA-accredited. Certification is granted after passing as ASCP examination.

Dentistry

Dentists treat oral diseases and disorders. They may fill cavities, extract teeth, and provide dentures for patients. About thirteen percent of dentists specialize. The eight recognized dental specialties are oral surgery and orthodontics (correction of irregularities of teeth and jaws), which together make up 60 percent of specialist practice, endodontics (root canal therapy), pedodontics (children's dentistry), periodontology or periodontics (treatment of gums, bone and other surrounding tissue), prosthodontics (replacement of missing teeth), oral pathology (study of diseased oral tissues), and public health dentistry. These specialties usually require two or more additional years of training, and a specialty board examination. Dental school is preceded by two to four years of college with specific science courses; most entering students, however, are college graduates. The dental school curriculum is a three- to four-year course leading to a DDS (Doctor of Dental Surgery) or a DMD (Doctor of Dental Medicine) degree. All dental schools must be approved by the American Dental Association. Dentists are licensed in all states by taking a state board examination or a National Board of Dental Examiners exam. In some states, specialists must pass a special state examination. Nine out of ten dentists are in private practice; the others practice in institutions, the armed forces, and health agencies, teach, or do research. Most are located in large cities. An increasing number of minorites and women are entering the field.

In recent years, there has been concern about the increasing cost of dental education and a perceived oversupply of dentists. Some of the sixty dental schools are in severe financial difficulties and are threatened by closure. Legislators maintain that although there are many underserved areas of dental need, the production of more dentists does not solve the problem, since few dentists go to those areas; most prefer a more lucrative practice. The American Dental Association (ADA) is conducting a three-year project to develop a plan for the future of the profession. One distinguished professor of dentistry has suggested that the ADA and the private sector have set up a leadership cartel designed to restrict competition. His "areas for action" include training and using dental hygienists to give primary care in underserved areas, including simple preparation and filling of cavities, screening school children and the elderly, and teaching prevention. Utilization of comprehensive dental care of elementary school children, which is less than 25 percent in the United States as compared to 90 percent in some other industrialized countries and anticipation of the need for more periodontal and endodontic treatment, since more adults are keeping their teeth but are suffering from gum disease, are also suggested.[10]

One overall concern appears to be the fact that there *are* unmet oral health-care needs, but that it is almost impossible to project manpower needs for people who don't seek dental care.

Dental hygienists, almost all women, provide dental services under a dentist's supervision. They examine and clean teeth, give fluoride treatments, take x-rays, and educate patients about proper care of teeth and gums. In many states, hygienists' responsibilities have been expanded to include duties traditionally performed by dentists, such as giving local anesthetics, and it has been said that their training includes much more than they are permitted to do by most dentist employers. Hygienists are licensed in all states through the National Board of Dental Examiners examinations and are the only ancillary personnel permitted by law to clean teeth. An RDH is awarded after passing a written and practical certification examination.

Education may consist of two-, three-, or four-year programs leading to a certificate or an associate or bachelor's degree at vocational-technical institutes, community colleges, and universities. Those dental hygienists with master's degrees may be teachers or administrators. The vast majority of dental hygienists practice with dentists in offices. However, in recent years, a few have set up separate private practices, a move strongly opposed by dentists but approved in some states by court decision or attorney general rulings. A degree of resistance to dentist domination over their practice is emerging.

Dental assistants maintain supplies, keep dental records, schedule appointments, prepare patients for examinations, process x-rays, and assist the dentist at chairside, but their functions are also expanding. Most assistants complete a one- or two-year program at a community college or vocational-technical school. These programs award a certificate, diploma, or associate degree.

Dental technicians or *denturists* make and repair dentures, crowns, bridges, and other appliances, usually according to dentists' prescriptions. Denturists are lobbying to work directly with patients, saying that they not only charge less but are faster and better at fitting dentures. The ADA is fighting this move, insisting that dentists must have total jurisdiction over all oral disorders since they alone are trained to diagnose and treat them. However, five states have already licensed denturists to provide direct service, and the services are proliferating (if illegally) in other states. Most Canadian provinces have had licensed denturists for many years.

The education of denturists usually consists of a two-year certificate or associate degree program, although some prepare by working for three to four years as trainees in dental laboratories.

Dietetics and Nutrition

Nutritionist is a general occupational title for health professionals concerned with food science and human nutrition. They include dietitians, home economists, and food technologists. There is no required standard for use of the title, but a bachelor's degree in the area of home economics or nutrition is usual. A master's degree may be required for certain positions, especially in public health. Nutritionists may teach clients/patients, consult, engage in research, or teach in schools of the health professions.

Dietitians may have a general dietary background or preparation in medical dietetics. Medical or therapeutic dietitians are responsible for selection of appropriate foods for special diets, patient counseling, and sometimes management of the dietary service.

Clinical dietitians work with patients not only in the hospital, but in clinics, neighborhood health centers, or in the patient's own home. These patients include pregnant women, diabetics, and those with other nutritional problems.

A baccalaureate program with majors in food, nutrition, and food management is usually basic with the possible addition of a dietetic internship program approved by the American Dietetic Association. Certification is granted by the ADA.

A number of studies have been done on dietitians. Ninety-seven percent are females, and over half are over age thirty-six. These factors are seen as part of the reason for their poor self-image, their lack of emphasis on financial or hierarchical career mobility, and their tendency to function in a reactive or responsive manner. Although about 40 percent hold master's degrees, they do not compete for roles in emerging specialties and new markets.[11] To improve this situation, among the actions being considered by the ADA is third-party reimbursement and licensure. The latter is considered important in obtaining third-party reimbursement. In 1983, Texas became the first state to license dietitians albeit on a voluntary basis. Licensure does not protect the scope of practice of nutrition/dietetics to licensed or registered dietitians; it does protect those titles against unauthorized use.

Another concern is the delegation of functions to assisting personnel. *Dietetic technicians* graduate from one of two kinds of ADA-approved technical programs with an associate degree. A program with food service management emphasis allows the individual to serve as a technical assistant to a food service director and, with experience, to become a director. The program with nutritional care emphasis enables the individual to become a technical assistant to the clinical dietitian. Both programs require clinical practice.

A *dietetic assistant* is a graduate of an academic program in dietetics requiring a minimum of 90 hours of classroom instruction coordinated with 150 hours of clinical practice. Included are food preparation, basic nutrition, and menu planning; purchasing; storage, safety, and sanitation; personnel supervision; and cost control. These programs may also be

ADA approved. Most dietetic assistants serve as *food service supervisors* in hospitals, schools of nursing, schools, and nursing homes. However, a number of food service supervisors currently functioning in that position lack such preparation.

Health Educators

Community health educators help identify the health learning needs of the community, particularly in terms of prevention of disease and injury. They may then plan, organize, and implement appropriate programs, for example, screening devices, health fairs, classes, and self-help groups. Some health educators are employed by the state as consultants, others by insurance companies, voluntary health organizations such as the Heart Association, the school system (school health educators), and, occasionally, industry. Unfortunately, as governmental funding fluctuates, programs may expand or contract, and health educators may be eliminated or spread thin, as has happened in school health. A number of hospitals are employing *patient educators* or health educators to develop and direct programs of both patient education and community health education. Frequently, these people are nurses with or without training in health education and administration. Health eductors usually have baccalaureate or master's degrees in health education, public health, or community health education. Master's degrees may include an administration component.

Medical Records

Medical record administrators are responsible for preparation, collation, and organization of patient records, maintaining an efficient filing system, and making records available to those concerned with the patient's subsequent care. They may also classify and compile data for review committees and researchers. CAHEA accredits both four-year baccalaureate programs and one-year hospital-based programs preceded by a baccalaureate degree. After completion of these programs the candidate qualifies for certification administered by the American Association of Medical Record Librarians.

Medical record technicians assist the physician and the administrator in preparing reports and transcribing histories and physicals, and work closely with others using patient records. CAHEA-accredited programs are nine months in length and include theoretical instruction and practical hospital experience. *Medical record transcriptionists* have specialized courses in terminology in addition to typing and filing. Advances in computerization are creating major changes in the field, and a shortage in the field is predicted.

Medicine

Doctors of medicine and osteopathy practice prevention, diagnosis, and treatment of disease and injury. *Doctor of medicine degrees (MDs)* are awarded in 127 allopathic medical schools in the Unites States and are considered the first professional degree. Some physicians may later decide to acquire advanced degrees (master's or doctorates) in an advanced science or public health. Admission into medical schools after four, occasionally three, years of preprofessional college work is considered highly selective. Programs are usually four years in length, with required basic sciences and clinical studies. In the last two years students have clinical clerkships, usually in hospitals, but also in clinics or doctor's offices. In this first contact with patients, they are usually supervised and taught by attending physicians or residents as they apply their clinical and scientific knowledge. Generally, physicians and professors of science are the teachers in medical school, although others include ethicists, sociologists, and, occasionally, a nurse (not usually on a full-time basis). In some medical schools, nurse instructors have responsibility for teaching medical students in the clinical clerkship.[12] In most cases, medical education has little interdisciplinary focus, and contacts with other health profession students are seldom formalized, although sometimes students in a multidisciplinary setting develop interactional opportunities of their own.[13]

The number of women in medicine has increased to over 30 percent of the student body, but the percentage of minorities has remained at about 8 percent for several years. Mechanic predicts that medicine will remain disproportionately urban, white, male, and upper middle class.[14] Critics indicate that this is due to the cost of medical school and the lack of recruitment and support for minorities in particular. Other criticisms of medical education are: a reluctance to adapt programs to meet the challenges of new systems of health care; lack of interest in compassion and communication, with overemphasis on science and little emphasis on the psychosocial aspects of patient care.

The formalized program of education after the MD degree is titled *graduate medical education* and consists primarily of the residency, which is preparation for specialties, a period of two to five years. At one time, a one-year internship, usually rotating through the various clinical services, was the norm, but after years of debate and two major reports,[15] in the mid-1960s several changes occurred. Family practice was recognized as a specialty, both the rotating and the freestanding internship (almost a general working apprenticeship) were abolished, and residencies in hospitals with at least minimal university affiliations were developed. Almost all residency programs now are in such hospitals, but there is still a dichotomy—education on the one hand and a functional hospital apprenticeship on the other. Residencies seem to have three distinct components: acquisition of knowledge, skills, and professional behavior. On completion of the specified years of residency, the physician may take certification exams in the specialty and is board certified; if exams are not taken (or failed), he/she is board eligible. In some cases, continuing medical education is required for recertification.

For a number of years, there were more first-year residency positions than American medical school graduates, and graduates from foreign medical schools, including Americans, filled positions. In some states, the vast majority were foreign medical graduates (FMGs). Because of differences in the quality of education and language and cultural differences, problems often occurred. Now, however, it is anticipated that there will be so many American medical school graduates that they may have difficulty finding suitable residencies for the specialties desired, and legislation has cut drastically the number of FMG's (except for Americans trained abroad). An attempt by the Congress to force medical schools to save places for a certain number of Americans from foreign medical schools was not successful, even with the threat of withholding funds. As it is, DHHS regulations require alien FMGs to pass a stringent examination designed to test their knowledge of basic and clinical sciences before being admitted into accredited residency or fellowship programs. For students who have completed premedical education in the United States and have completed all but the internship or social service component, or both, of the foreign medical education, the "fifth pathway" provides another route to graduate medical education. After passing a screening examination and fulfilling other qualifications, these FMGs are given a year of supervised clinical training, usually with some didactic courses included. Successful completion gives them a better opportunity for residencies.

Although most American physicians choose specialties as their field of practice,* the need for more general practitioners is being met by designation of the field (thus the residency) as a specialty and heavy federal funding for those selecting that field. There is now some concern that soon there may be too many family practitioners as well.

Determination of what is too little or too much of a specialty seems to be unresolved

---

*The AMA recognizes thirty-four different specialties; the largest of the twenty-three boards are internal medicine, surgery, obstetrics and gynecology, psychiatry and neurology, pediatrics, radiology, and pathology.

whenever the issue arises. A recent example is the concern that there will not be enough physicians in preventive medicine (including public health), since there seems to be decreasing selection of that field. Yet certain experts say that with an excess of physicians in other specialties, inevitably some physicians will turn to those fields where there are openings.

In medical centers, a ''fellow'' is a postresidency physician who enters even more advanced, highly specialized, or research-oriented programs, although presumably still involved in teaching and patient care. Graduate medical education is under the direction of medical school faculty recognized as specialists or subspecialists. A relatively new issue in graduate education is the unionization of residents (with varied success) in order to obtain better conditions of work, especially reduction of the long hours that may threaten competence.

Physician licensure is mandatory in every state, some of which require continuing education for relicensure. Students may choose two routes to licensure, the National Board Examinations given by the National Board of Medical Examiners, for which they must be students or graduates of an American or Canadian medical school, or the Federal Licensing Examination (FLEX) given by the Federation of State Medical Boards. Part I and II of the Boards are given during the medical school years, with Part III given after the first year of graduate medical education; FLEX may be taken only after the first year of graduate medical education. The individual is not usually fully licensed until after one or the other of these exams is passed; before that, practice is covered by a temporary license or is on a student basis, just as it is with nurses until they have passed state boards. All but two states endorse the National Board certificate for licensure, and all now accept FLEX. Among the physicians not holding a license in any state, besides first-year residents, are the inactive and those engaged in medical teaching, research, or administration. About twenty-five states require continuing educa-

tion for relicensure (some state medical societies also demand it for membership).

The major modes of medical practice are described in the preceding chapter, but there are, of course, physicians in every setting where medical care is provided, as well as in medical or public health education, public health practice, and research. Some positions such as that of a medical director are primarily administrative and are beginning to be recognized as such.[16]

Although MDs are generally still held in high regard by the public, they have become the target of much criticism, and it appears that they often have difficulty coping with the radical changes in health care and society. For instance, while they have been blamed for the high cost of medical care, they say that one reason for the extensiveness of expensive diagnostic tests is the litigiousness of today's patient, which also drives up their malpractice insurance. At the same time, there are allegations of peer cover-up of incompetent practitioners instead of peer review and removal from practice. Now there are more deliberate efforts by medicine to identify ''impaired'' physicians and give them appropriate help until they are qualified to practice. Continuing medical education has also been strongly supported for maintaining competence.

With economic pressures, changes in health care delivery and reimbursement, and oversupply, some physicians are finding it necessary to market their services actively (advertising is now acceptable); others are moving into salaried positions that include bonuses for cost-effective practice. The projected oversupply may also be responsible for increased aggressiveness in trying to prevent nonphysician practitioners such as nurse-midwives and NPs from practicing and receiving direct reimbursement from clients. This can be interpreted as restraint of trade, and the Federal Trade Commission has ruled against the AMA several times on these issues—for example, in relation to advertising and referrals to chiropractors. However, MDs have also had some success in specific states in their attempts to restrain NPs, and the battle continues.

Still another issue is the maldistribution of physicians. National Health Corps physicians do seem to select rural areas for practice, but these areas, unattractive and isolated places and big city ghettoes still lack even a minimally satisfactory physician-population ratio, while more affluent areas have unnecessarily high ratios. Given the maldistribution and cost problems, and the new aggressiveness of other health professionals, there is a frequent reiteration of the question, "Why should the physician be the gatekeeper to health care?"

Doctors of osteopathy (DO) are qualified to be licensed as physicians and to practice all branches of medicine and surgery. DOs graduate from colleges of osteopathic medicine (now fifteen), accredited by the Bureau of Professional Education of the American Osteopathic Association (AOA). Admission to the colleges requires at least three years of preprofessional education at an accredited college or university. The DO degree usually requires four academic years of education; three of the nine accredited colleges have adopted an interdisciplinary approach, allowing for three years. Required basic sciences, anatomy, physiology, biochemistry, pathology, microbiology, and pharmacology, are much the same as those in medical schools, as are the clinical courses of medicine, surgery, pediatrics, obstetrics, gynecology, radiology, and preventive medicine. The major difference is the integration of osteopathic principles dealing with the interrelationship of all body systems in health and disease and special training in osteopathic palpatory diagnosis and manipulative therapy. After graduation, almost all DOs serve a twelve-month rotating internship, with primary emphasis on medicine, obstetrics/gynecology, and surgery, conducted in an approved osteopathic hospital. Those wishing to specialize must serve an additional three to five years of residency. Continuing education is required by the AOA for all DOs in practice.

Osteopathic physicians are considered sepa-rate but equal in American medicine; they are licensed in all states and have the same rights and obligations as allopathic (MD) physicians. The "something extra" they claim is emphasis on biological mechanisms by which the musculoskeletal system interacts with all body organs and systems in both health and disease. They prescribe drugs, use routine diagnostic measures, perform surgery, and selectively utilize accepted scientific modalities of care. DOs comprise about 4 percent of all physicians; most are general practitioners who provide primary care, usually in towns and cities of less than 50,000 population. The 213 osteopathic hospitals (155 accredited), located in 28 states, usually offer a full range of services. Nursing in osteopathic hospitals is comparable to that in any other hospital.

Physician's Assistants

In 1965, Dr. Eugene A. Stead, Jr. inaugurated a program for *physician's assistants (PAs)*, later called *physician's associates,* designed to assist physicians in their practice, either to enable them to expand that practice, or to give them time to pursue continuing education, or to have more time for themselves and their families. The students in the Duke University program came from a variety of backgrounds and included nurses and former military corpsmen. Shortly afterward, a series of programs, called MEDEX, developed specifically for ex-corpsmen, were funded by the federal government.

In the early years of these programs, there was a great deal of confusion about the education, role, legality, and scope of practice of the PA. Educational programs ran the gamut from a few months of on-the-job training to five years. Formalized programs prepared assistants to the primary care physician as well as specialists, particularly in urology and orthopedics.

In 1970, the National Academy of Sciences categorized the PA in three broad functional areas.

The Type A assistant is capable of approaching the patient, collecting historical and physical data, organizing these data, and presenting them in such a way that the physician can visualize the medical problem and determine appropriate diagnostic or therapeutic steps. He is also capable of assisting the physician by performing diagnostic and therapeutic procedures and coordinating the roles of other, more technical, assistants. While he functions under the general supervision and responsibility of the physician, he might, under special circumstances and under defined rules, perform without the immediate surveillance of the physician. He is, thus, distinguished by his ability to integrate and interpret findings on the basis of general medical knowledge and to exercise a degree of independent judgment.

The Type B assistant, while not equipped with general knowledge and skills relative to the whole range of medical care, possesses exceptional skill in one clinical specialty or more commonly, in certain procedures within such a specialty. In his area of specialty, he has a degree of skill beyond that normally possessed by a Type A assistant and perhaps beyond that normally possessed by physicians who are not engaged in the specialty. Because his knowledge and skill are limited to a particular specialty, he is less qualified for independent action. An example of this type of assistant might be one who is highly skilled in the physician's functions associated with a renal dialysis unit and who is capable of performing these functions as required.

The Type C assistant is capable of performing a variety of tasks over the whole range of medical care under the supervision of a physician, although he does not possess the level of medical knowledge necessary to integrate and interpret findings. He is similar to a Type A assistant in the number of areas in which he can perform, but he cannot exercise the degree of independent synthesis and judgment of which Type A is capable. This type of assistant would be to medicine what the practical nurse is to nursing.[17]

Differing levels of education were also recommended for the three groups, from short-term certificate programs to baccalaureate education.

The type A assistant gradually became today's PA; types B and C are in relatively limited categories and are considered assistants by various names, but not PAs. Although the AMA generally defines PAs as persons qualified by academic and clinical training to provide patient services under the supervision of a licensed doctor of medicine, a more comprehensive and legally oriented definition, once suggested by Nathan Hershey, is:

> An individual, not a physician, providing health services as an employee of a physician, or a health care institution such as a hospital or health center, who, under medical supervision and direction, engages in a range of activities and decision making that does not fall completely within the scope of activities of any of the traditional, currently licensed health professions or occupations, and whose range of health care activity includes some tasks and functions now reserved to physicians, and not recognized by laws as within the area of practice of any other health profession or occupation.

Continued federal funding after 1972 not only encouraged the growth of programs, but determined certain directions: training for delivery of primary care in ambulatory settings, placement of graduates in medically underserved areas, and recruitment of residents from these areas as well as minority groups and women. Several changes in programs occurred after that, primarily a concentration on assistants for primary care physicians (fifty-four AMA-CAHEA-accredited programs by 1983), and a disappearance of specialty programs. Only three prepare surgical assistants; there are no other formal accredited programs. Some seventy programs had been listed in 1974, up from twelve in 1972, but most of these probably did not meet standards for approval that the AMA had set in the early 1970s. The most recently accredited is the newly established (and only) program sponsored by an osteopathic medical school.

The institutional bases of the other programs are primarily schools of allied health, four-year colleges, and allopathic medical schools, with a few each in community colleges, teaching hospitals, and federal facilities. All these accredited programs have medical facilities and clinical medical teaching affiliations of some kind. Credentials given range from certificates and associate degrees to a Master of Science option. An increasing number of programs are offering baccalaureates.

The typical PA training program is two years in length and consists of six to twelve months of didactic study including anatomy, physiology, microbiology, pharmacology, psychology, medical science, and medical ethics, accompanied by nine to fifteen months of clinical training to develop practitioner skills. The clinical rotations or preceptorships introduce the student to potential areas of expertise, including family medicine, internal medicine, surgery, pediatrics, psychiatry, obstetrics/gynecology, and emergency medicine. This is intended to prepare the PA to:

1. Elicit a comprehensive health history
2. Perform a comprehensive physical examination
3. Order and interpret simple diagnostic laboratory tests
4. Develop diagnoses and management plans
5. Provide basic treatment for individuals with common illnesses
6. Provide clinical care for individuals with commonly encountered emergency needs

By law, all must be done under the supervision of a physician.

In recent years, PA residency programs ranging from nine to twelve months have been developed that provide further didactic and clinical education in various specialties. The twelve established or developing programs are in surgery, emergency medicine, pediatrics/neonatology, occupational medicine, and rehabilitation medicine. Some offer certificates,

two a master's degree. PA education is not seen as part of a career ladder leading to MD licensure, although some PAs may go to medical school later, just as they may turn to schools of public health or nursing in a career change. A certification mechanism was developed under the aegis of the National Board of Medical Examiners (NMBE), and the first exam was given in 1973. NMBE then cooperated with twelve other professional groups to form the freestanding independent National Commission on Certification of Physician's Assistant (NCCPA) in 1975, which has the responsibility for PA certification, including publishing yearly lists, by states, of certified PAs, and periodically recertifying PAs through continued demonstration of competency.[18] Most PAs are certified particularly because a number of states require certification for practice.

The most recent official report on PAs, made available in early 1984 by DHHS, noted a number of changes in the characteristics of PA students: an increase in women to 50.5 percent and in ethnic minorities to about 12 percent, and an increase in younger candidates. Only about 12 percent have served in the military (as opposed to the large number of corpsmen in the early years), and less than 10 percent lack college education or a degree before admission. The vast majority have had some kind of health care experience, primarily as orderlies or nurse's aides, various technicians, EMTs, and corpsmen; RNs, LPNs, and other health professionals are included. About half said that they prefer to work in communities of under 50,000, and about half are willing to work in medically underserved areas. The vast majority prefer family practice, with the next choice (about 12 percent) being emergency medicine. Preferred practice sites are physicians' offices, community-based or remote satellite clinics, and hospitals. Most PAs actually do practice in private offices and clinics, but there has been a noticeable increase in hospital placement to the point where two-thirds now practice in institutional settings compared to 43 percent in 1974. More employment in the prison system and in nursing homes is predicted.

About 16,000 PAs have graduated from approved programs or have obtained certification after completing informal programs or training; about 12,000 to 13,000 are estimated to be employed full time as clinical PAs. New York, California, Pennsylvania, and Texas have the largest number of PAs; about 23 percent practice in the Southeast. Approximately half practice in communities of under 50,000. Employment in medically underserved areas is not documented, but out of the twenty-three programs surveyed, roughly 33 percent of the graduates were deployed there.

The legality of PA practice was a particularly hot issue in the early 1970s, but by 1979, most states permitted PAs to practice. Most have specific statutes that authorize varied groups of nonphysicians to qualify as PAs and authorize qualified physicians to delegate medical tasks; a smaller number use the medical practice act's exemption clause, which allows physicians to delegate certain activities to selected others under their supervision. PAs are *not* licensed, but the state usually keeps a registration list. The major difference between a PA and an NP is that the PA, in all cases, *must* function under the supervision of a physician and cannot function independently. Physicians are legally responsible for their PAs and frequently must include the PAs in their own malpractice insurance.

There are still many unresolved issues related to PA practice, particularly in relation to role and functions. The American Hospital Association has published a statement on PAs in hospitals, which, overall, indicated that the medical staff and administration should formulate guidelines under which the PA can operate, with the request for the PA to be permitted to practice in the hospital being handled by the medical staff credentials committee. Emphasis is on medical supervision; however, current reality has shown that PAs go unsupervised in busy urban hospitals where they handle many emergency and other ambulatory patients. This has created a problem for

nurses, for the authority of the PA vis-a-vis the nurse is frequently not clear. Although the nurses' associations, some state boards, some courts, and attorneys general have indicated that nurses do not take PA orders, in other states the rulings are the reverse. Because the PA usually functions according to a protocol specified by the employer-physician, there may be an operational agreement reached similar to the basis on which a nurse carries out standing orders or some verbal orders from the physician. Nevertheless, there is frequently interdisciplinary conflict when roles are not clarified.

The future of PAs is uncertain. There is no upward mobility in the field, except for teaching; medical schools are not giving them any special advantages toward admission. It is freely admitted that federal support has been the major moving force in the establishment, direction, and maintenance of PA programs. This funding has been decreasing in the last few years and is expected to decrease even more. Costs are higher than for preparing master's degree NPs, and PAs have a much more limited scope of practice. To many people, however, including health professionals, the differences between PA and NP are minimal.

Although the expanded role of the nurse has been evolving for some time, it was not until about 1970 that it was clearly defined and that any reasonable number of NPs were functioning. This was particularly unfortunate in that the PA had, as a new health worker with considerable governmental support, received a great deal of public attention. The fact that both NPs and PAs performed some of the same medically oriented functions added to the confusion. At the end of 1971, the ANA issued a statement declaring that the term *physician's assistant* should not be applied to any of the NPs being prepared to function in expanded nursing roles.

Other key points that are still valid are:

Several types of assistants are being prepared and utilized to function under the medical direction to extend physicians' services. None of these assistants are prepared to be substitutes for nurses, because nursing practice is more than performance of delegated medical nursing activities. Neither are these assistants acceptable substitutes for physicians. This development is of concern to the nursing profession. Physician's assistants working in a setting where nursing practice is an essential element of health care present problems that flow from the legal and ethical relationships between physicians and nurses. Therefore, nurses and physicians together must clarify the situation. . . .

Because the economic status of each group involved in health care is part of the economic environment of every other group, the American Nurses' Association has a stake in the economic status of the emerging physician's assistant. The ANA reemphasizes that in establishing salary systems, recognition must be given to the character of responsibilities carried, and to requirements for education, experience and clinical expertise. In establishing the relationships between salaries of nurses and those of physician's assistants, the differences in their responsibilities, preparation and experience should be taken into account.

Concern about the economic status of nurses and PAs was, and is, realistic. Although NPs can offer services to the public beyond any that the PA can offer, frequently nurse and PA may be competing for the same job. For a number of reasons, the PA not only may be the one employed, but, as noted before, will also receive a higher salary than would be offered to the NP. Despite the fact that most physicians tend to say that they prefer nurses to PAs, the truth is that too often doctors have inadequate or no knowledge about the NP's capabilities. What they are talking about is a nurse as a PA. A number of nurses have made this choice, which is certainly theirs to make, although it has caused some negative reaction from other nurses and nursing associations. It is possible that the situation will be clarified as more NPs are prepared in standardized educational programs.

What impact the PA will have on nursing practice remains to be seen. It might be well to consider this early warning:

> If the physician's assistant becomes, in fact, a foreclosure on the development of increased, enhanced role functioning in nursing, then we think we are making a very serious mistake in terms of the long-run needs of the country. And we would hazard to suggest it will be a serious mistake for the profession of medicine as well as nursing and the health system generally.[19]

However, the crucial question lies in supply and demand. If MDs, NPs, and PAs all continue to be produced at the current rate and the predicted oversupply becomes reality in the next five years, who will survive?

Medical assistants (MAs) are usually employed in physicians' offices, where they perform a variety of administrative and clinical tasks to facilitate the work of the doctor; however, some do work in hospitals and clinics. They perform tasks required by the doctor, in accordance with specific state laws, and are supervised by the doctor. The medical assistant, among other things, answers the telephone; greets patients and other callers; makes appointments; handles correspondence and filing; arranges for diagnostic tests, hospital admissions, and surgery; handles patients' accounts and other billings; processes insurance claims, including Medicare; maintains patient records; prepares patients for examinations or treatment; takes temperatures, height, and weight; sterilizes instruments; assists the physician in examining or treating patients; and if trained, performs laboratory procedures. Most medical assistants train in one-year certificate or two-year associate degree programs given by community colleges, universities and vocational-technical schools.

Emergency Medical Care

Emergency medical technicians-ambulance (EMT-As) respond to medical emergencies and provide immediate care to the critically ill or injured. They may administer cardiac resuscitation, treat shock, provide initial care to poison or burn victims, and transport patients to a health facility. EMT-As do not determine the extent of illness, but set priorities in emergency care at the scene of the emergency, and monitor victims on the way to a hospital, often functioning under doctor or nurse voice directions or protocols. They are also responsible for the ambulance and supplies. Those with an EMT-intermediate (EMT-I) or EMT-paramedic (EMT-P) rating work at a more sophisticated level in emergency situations. They may defibrillate, administer intravenous fluids, do gastric lavage, and give medications by injection, also acting under physician/nurse voice direction when necessary. EMTs are trained in a U.S. Department of Transportation (USDOT) course, offered under various auspices (police, hospitals, health departments). The EMT-I and EMT-P credential requires 500 or more additional hours in conjunction with a hospital for clinical training. There is a National Registry of EMTs. Many serve as volunteers on ambulances, but, as noted in Chapter 7, paid EMT services are increasing. Some EMTs also have training as dispatchers.

Paramedics, a popular term that seems to encompass other allied health workers, is sometimes also applied to EMTs.

Nursing Support Personnel

Nursing assistants, nurses' aides, orderlies, and attendants functioning under the direction of nurses are all part of the group of ancillary workers prepared to assist in nursing care, performing many of the simple nursing tasks, as well as other helping activities besides nursing. Usually training has been on the job and geared to the needs of the particular employing institution, but there has been some increase in public school programs within vocational high school tracks or as outside public education services. The program may vary in length from six to eight weeks or more and costs little or nothing. Commercial programs usually cost the student an unrea-

sonable amount, make unrealistic promises of jobs, and frequently give no clinical experience; therefore these "graduates" are seldom employed. Sometimes students who drop out of certain practical nurse programs after six weeks receive a certificate as aides. In-service education during employment is relatively common. It should be remembered that the difference in training, patient care assignment, and ability may be enormous on both an individual and an institutional basis. These workers are not licensed or certified as a rule.

Community health aides of various kinds are found in ambulatory care settings. "Indigenous" health aides evolved because not enough physicians or public health nurses were available to help families described as disadvantaged to identify and correct their multiple, related medical and social problems. In addition, professionals do not always communicate effectively with disadvantaged minority clientele. Therefore, in those areas of service, community people are sometimes recruited and trained as health aides. Many are women not previously trained as vocational nurses or hospital aides. There is usually a limited didactic period with ongoing supervision and on-the-job instruction. Certain technical skills are learned, such as auditory and visual screening, but the primary purpose is to identify health problems or deficiencies, such as lack of immunization, poor oral hygiene, dermatological problems, and child development problems, and to assist and encourage families to seek and continue necessary medical, nursing, and other services. Although specific changes in the health status of the community are difficult to measure, on an anecdotal basis, evaluation seems to be positive. These workers may be based in a clinic, neighborhood health center, or other ambulatory care facility, and may also go into the community to do case finding rather than wait for the client to appear in the formal health facility.

As more attention is focused on keeping people at home rather than in institutions, the services of *homemaker/home health aides* have become reimbursable by Medicaid and Medicare under certain circumstances. The term *home health aide,* introduced in the Medicare Act in 1965, was added to the older term *homemaker.* The first homemaker services were made available in 1923 to substitute for a hospitalized mother. In the Depression, "housekeeping aides" were subsidized by the government to provide work for needy women. They were assigned to assist families with children, the aged, or the chronically ill.

The National Home Caring Council, which has developed a program of basic standards, defines today's worker as a trained, supervised person who works as a full-fledged member of a team of professional and allied workers providing health and/or social services. The aide is assigned to the home of a family or individual when home life is disrupted by illness, disability, or social disadvantage, or if the family unit is in danger of breakdown because of stress. Specific tasks include parenting, performing or helping in household tasks, providing personal care such as bed baths, or helping with prescribed exercises, and providing emotional support. Educational programs are usually developed by the employing agency, and a Council-approved program requires a minimum of sixty hours of classroom and laboratory instruction to prepare the individual for on-the-job functioning. Most are women who already have housekeeping skills; even so, there is some question as to how effectively they can really be prepared in the limited time suggested.

There is an increasing tendency for proprietary agencies to have homemaker/home health care services, and to contract these workers out to voluntary agencies. Although there is evidence that a well-trained, conscientious home/health aide can be extremely helpful to a sick person or disrupted family, there are also some serious problems in the selection of workers, the quality of training, and supervision. There are also some reimbursement problems when the homemaking part of the aide's function is reimbursable and the health part is not, or vice versa. However, the home-maker/home health aide is usually one person doing whichever aspect of the job is needed and is reimbursed in a particular situation. Most often, a combination of the services is needed by the client. Ongoing assessment of health professionals is intended to evaluate the need of the family/client for specific services.

The lack of reimbursement often prevents the use of homemaker/home health aides, for this can cost hundreds of dollars a month. Still, it is less costly health service than institutional care.

Operating room technicians (ORTs), or surgical technicians, or *surgical technologists* function in the the operating room and, sometimes, the delivery room. ORTs, under the direction of the operating room supervisor, an RN, perform required tasks, such as setting up for surgery, preparing instruments and other equipment before surgery, "scrubbing in" for surgery (assisting the surgeons by handing instruments, sutures, and so on), and otherwise assisting in the operating room.

Educational programs are most frequently offered by hospitals and some community colleges. It is recommended that they be at least a year in length, although some hospitals prepare ORTs in a short-term, intensive program plus on-the-job training. Teachers are usually operating room nurses, preferably with teaching background.

The *psychiatric technician* works in psychiatric and general hospitals, community mental health centers, and the home, working with the mentally disturbed, disabled, or retarded under the direction of a physician and/or nurse. In hospitals, he or she is concerned with the patient's daily life as it affects his physical, mental, and emotional well-being, including eating, sleeping, recreation, development of work skills, adjustment, and individual and social relations. In the community, focus is on social relationships and adjustments. In the hospital, psychiatric technicians are expected to give some routine and emergency physical nursing care, but their close contact with patients makes observation and reporting of the patient's behavior particularly important. In some institutions they function almost independently in group therapy and counseling, seeking consultation as necessary. They may be skilled in nursing, communication techniques, counseling, training techniques, and group therapy. The educational program has generally been one year long but an emerging standard seems to be a two-year associate degree program, which includes social and physical sciences, health education, laboratory work in group and interpersonal processes, and clinical experience. In some states psychiatric technicians have the opportunity to become licensed, sometimes under the Nursing Board.

Ward (unit) clerks or *ward (unit) secretaries* are usually trained on the job in an inservice program to assist in the clerical duties involved in the administration of a nursing unit. Ward clerks order supplies, keep certain records, answer telephones, take messages, attend to the massive amount of routine paper work and, in some cases, copy doctors' orders. This relieves the charge nurse to concentrate on administration of patient care instead of paper work. In the more progressive hospitals, unit clerks are on duty at least on the day and evening shifts and sometimes at night.

Unit managers take even broader responsibilities in the management of a patient unit (usually in a larger institution) and may report directly to hospital administration instead of nursing service administration. Unit clerks often function under the direction of unit managers. In some institutions, unit management is an early step in an administrative career, and managers have full administrative responsibilities.

Pharmacy

Pharmacists are specialists in the science of drugs and require a thorough knowledge of chemistry and physiology. They may dispense prescription and nonprescription drugs, compound special preparations or dosage forms, serve as consultants, and advise physicians on selection and effects of drugs.

With the increase of prepackaged drugs and the use of pharmacy assistants, pharmacists in hospitals and clinics are particularly interested in a more patient-oriented approach to their practice. They may be involved in patient rounds, patient teaching, and consultation with nurses and physicians. Pharmacists working in (or owning) drugstores have also been encouraged to increase their patient or client education efforts in terms of explaining medications. The educational program of pharmacists is usually a five-year baccalaureate program including two or more years of professional course work. Five-year programs give the bachelor's degree, six-year programs the Pharm D (Doctor of Pharmacy). The Pharm D is a relatively new development that occurred in part because of the complexity of today's drugs, their potential adverse reaction with each other as multiple drugs are prescribed (or taken), the increased use and abuse of drugs, the fact that physicians often do not have in-depth knowledge of drugs, and the successful implementation of clinical pharmacy services in the 1960s. Besides the traditional responsibilities of pharmacists, the Pharm D or clinical pharmacist provides consultation with the physician, maintains patient drug histories and reviews the total drug regimen of patients, monitors patient charts in ECFs and recommends drug therapy, makes patient rounds, and provides individualized dosage regimens.[20] In some states, such as California, clinical pharmacists may also prescribe (as do NPs and PAs), with certain limitations. This new role is well accepted by some physicians, usually those who have worked with Pharm Ds, and is considered an infringement on medical territory by others.

Trends in the field focus on the Pharm D. Enrollment for the first professional degree has been declining, although there has been an increase in women (to 50 percent) and a much smaller increase in minorities (to 14 percent). Arguments have been advanced that the Pharm D should be the first professional degree, eliminating the baccalaureate. Because they fear for their economic and professional status, a growing number of pharmacists are taking part-time and off-campus courses toward a Pharm D. Graduate education (Master of Science and Ph.D) has also increased, although slowly, because of the growing complexity of the field. Continuing education is emphasized for this reason, but also because more than twenty states require continuing education for relicensure. Pharmacists are licensed in all states.

What may or may not be a trend is the *pharmacist practitioner (PP),* who, much like the NP, is trained to give primary care: history and physical examinations and follow-through for common nonemergency conditions and chronic medical problems. The first program was initiated in 1973 for pharmacists serving in the Indian Health Services, and appears to work successfully.[21] *Pharmacologists* specialize in research and development of drugs to prevent or treat disease or prolong life. A medical degree or a four- to five-year Ph.D. program in pharmacology is usually required.

Podiatry

Podiatrists, doctors of podiatric medicine (DPM) (once called *chiropodists*), are professionally trained foot care specialists who diagnose, treat, and try to prevent diseases, injuries, and deformities of the feet. Treatment may include surgery, medication, physical therapy, setting fractures, and preparing orthoses (supporting devices which mechanically rearrange the weight-bearing structures of the foot). Podiatrists may note symptoms of diseases manifested in the feet and legs and refer the patient to a physician.

Podiatrists complete a four-year program of classroom and clinical work in a college of podiatry after a minimum of two years of college, but 85 percent have already had four years. Although they are permitted to practice immediately after graduation in almost all states, 95 percent apply for one or two years of residency training. The enrollment in the six colleges of podiatry has increased fivefold

in the last fifteen years, due largely to federal support. There has been an increase in women and minorities (each to 11 percent). A unique aspect of podiatric medical education is the attempt to develop a systemwide, competency-based curriculum. The National Board of Podiatry Examiners gives examinations that satisfy the requirements for licensure in more than forty states. Other states use their own examinations; seven require a residency, and an increasing number are requiring continuing education.

Most podiatrists are in private practice; others practice in institutions, agencies, the military, education, and research.

Podiatric assistants aid podiatrists in office management and patient care. Because of the increasing older population, the services of podiatrists may be needed more than ever. However, major federal cutbacks are putting severe financial pressures on the colleges, which are all private and get little or no state aid. Moreover, the medical profession is also fighting any attempt by podiatrists to expand their scope of practice, particularly in surgery. Yet podiatrists who have had surgical residencies and the requisite five years of practice, and have passed the exacting certification examination of the American Board of Podiatric Surgery, maintain that these physicians are unfamiliar with current podiatric education and practice or are protective of their own economic well-being

Psychology, Psychotherapy, and Mental Health

Psychology is the scientific study of mental processes and behavior, and *psychotherapy* refers generally to techniques for treating mental illness by psychological means, primarily through establishing communication between the therapist and the patient as a means of understanding ad modifying behavior. In the field of mental health, there is a great overlapping of therapists treating patients with various kinds of mental problems. Besides the physician (the psychiatrist), clinical psychologists, psychotherapists, nurses, social workers, and a variety of semiprofessionals trained in mental health participate in individual and group therapy. *Psychologists* may also give and interpret various personality and behavioral tests, as might a *psychometrician,* who is skilled in the testing and measuring of mental and psychological ability, efficiency, potentials, and functions. Education for psychologists and psychotherapists is often at the master's or doctoral level. Clinical psychologists have training in a clinical setting.

Public Health—Environment

Industrial hygienists deal with the effects of noise, dust, vapor radiation, and other hazards common to industry, on workers' health. They are usually employed by industry, laboratories, insurance companies, or government to detect and correct these hazards. Their education may include a baccalaureate in environmental health, engineering, or a physical or biological science.

Sanitarians, sometimes called *environmentalists,* apply technical knowledge to solve problems of sanitation in a community. They develop and implement methods to control those factors in the environment that affect health and safety, such as rodent control, sanitary conditions in schools, hotels, restaurants, areas of food production and sales. Most work in government, under the direction of a health officer or administrator. Education is generally a BS in public health or the physical or biological sciences.

Also educated in schools of public health, as well as elsewhere, are *biostatisticians,* who apply mathematics and statistics to research problems related to health, and *epidemiologists,* who study the factors that influence the occurrence and course of human health problems, including not only acute and chronic diseases, but also accidents, addictions, and suicides. Epidemiologists attempt to establish the courses of health problems by focusing on the biological, social, and behaviorial factors affecting health, illness, and premature death. They use investigative, analytical, and descriptive techniques. A specialized graduate degree is necessary for both biostatisticians and epidemiologists.

Radiology

Radiologists are physicians dealing with all forms of radiant energy, from x-rays to radioactive isotopes; they interpret radiographic studies and prescribe therapy for diseases, particularly malignancies. A number of technicians work under the direction of a radiologist in radiology departments.

The *radiologic technologist,* sometimes called *x-ray technician* or *radiology technician,* is concerned with the proper operation of x-ray equipment, preparation of patients for x-rays and therapy, developing of film, and some clerical work. Programs are usually two-year CAHEA-accredited hospital certificate programs, sometimes affiliated with a college or university. The graduate may become registered (AT) after passing an examination given by the American Registry of Radiologic Technicians. A few states license radiology technicians.

Radiation therapy technicians or *technologists* assist the radiologist in the treatment of disease by exposing affected areas of the patient's body to prescribed doses of radiation, operating and controlling complex equipment and devices, and maintaining records. A one- or two-year program in radiation therapy given by community colleges or hospitals is required. There are some baccalaureate programs.

A *nuclear medicine technologist* works with radioactive isotopes administered to patients for diagnosis and treatment. He or she positions and attends to patients, abstracts data from records, assists in the operation of scanning devices using isotopes, and has responsibility for safe storage of radioactive materials and disposal of wastes. CAHEA accredits both AD programs for technicians and baccalaureate programs for technologists. The latter must first be medical or radiological technologists or nurses.

Rehabilitation Services

Occupational therapy is concerned with the use of purposeful activity in the promotion and maintenance of health, prevention of disability, evaluation of behavior, and as treatment of persons with physical or psychosocial dysfunction, using a wide spectrum of treatment procedures based on activities of a creative, social, self-care, educational, and vocational nature. One important responsibility is helping patients with activities of daily living. Adaptive tools such as aids for eating or dressing may also be provided.

Occupational therapists, (OTs), the professional workers, and *occupational therapy assistants and aides* are usually employed in hospitals. However, OTs may also be in private practice or work for nursing homes or community agencies. Professional education for the occupational therapists is a baccalaureate program or a postbaccalaureate program and six to nine months of field experience leading to a certificate or master's degree. There are over fifty professional programs accredited by the CAHEA, out of eighty-one identified programs.

The American Occupational Therapy Association certifies for the professional entry-level occupational therapist registered (OTR) or certified occupational therapy assistant (COTA). In some institutions, professional occupational therapists are assisted by OT assistants or aides, who may be trained in one of the fifty-eight community college programs or on the job, which is now less common. They participate directly in the patient's activities.

Physical therapy is concerned with the restoration of function and the prevention of disability following disease, injury, or loss of body part; sometimes physical therapy is concerned with diagnosis. The goal is to improve circulation, strengthen muscles, encourage return of motion, and train or retrain the patient with the use of prosthetics, crutches, walkers, exercise, heat, cold, electricity, ultrasound, and massage. Most *physical therapists and PT aides* work in hospitals, but PTs may also work in private practice or for other agencies. The physical therapist designs the patient's program of treatment, based on the physician's stated prescription of objectives. He or she may participate in giving the therapy and/or evaluate the patient's needs and capacities and provide psychological support. The aides work directly under the physical therapist's supervision, with limited participation in the therapeutic program. As in occupational therapy, education for the PT is in a baccalaureate or postbaccalaureate program leading to a certificate or master's degree, which may be CAHEA accredited. Registration is possible through the American Registry of Physical Therapists, and all states now license PTs. There has been some limited effort to require licensure of physical therapist assistants, whose education is usually at the associate degree level.

Prosthetists make artificial limb substitutes. *Orthotists* make and fit braces. Both work with physicians and other therapists, and have direct patient contact to promote total rehabilitation services. A bachelor's degree in prosthetics or orthotics plus one year of clinical experience is usual; for those with a bachelor's degree, special four- to eight-month programs in hospitals or special university courses and clinical experience are available. *Orthotic/prosthetic technicians* make and repair devices but usually have no patient contact. Education is primarily in vocational/technical schools.

Rehabilitation counselors help people with physical, mental, or social disabilities begin or return to a satisfying life, including an appropriate job. They may counsel about job opportunities and training, assist in job placement, and help the person to adjust to a new work situation. The usual requirement is a two-year master's degree. Others assisting in patient rehabilitation include *art therapists, dance therapists,* and *music therapists* who work primarily with the emotionally disturbed, mentally retarded, or physically handicapped. *Recreational therapists* or *therapeutic recreationists* may plan and supervise recreation programs that include athletics, arts and crafts, parties, gardening, or camping. Professional status usually requires a master's degree, although some therapists have only a bachelor's degree; assistants are generally prepared at the associate degree level.

Respiratory Therapy

Respiratory (formerly *inhalation*) *therapy* personnel perform procedures essential in maintaining life in seriously ill patients with respiratory problems and assist in treatment of heart and lung ailments. Under medical supervision, the *respiratory therapy technician* administers various types of gas, aerosol, and breathing treatments, assists with long-term continuous artificial ventilation, cleans, sterilizes, and maintains equipment, and keeps patient records. The *respiratory therapist* may be engaged in similar tasks, but his or her more extensive knowledge of sciences and clinical medicine allows for the exercise of more judgment and acceptance of greater responsibility in performing therapeutic procedures. Respiratory therapy personnel usually work in hospitals and clinics.

A CAHEA-accredited program for technicians is one year long; certification is available. A therapist program, also CAHEA accredited, may culminate in an associate or baccalaureate degree, with a minimum of two years required. The baccalaureate programs sometimes build on the AD program and prepare for supervision and teaching. Respiratory therapists may be registered, but are not usually licensed.

Social Work

The *social worker* attempts to help individuals and their families resolve their social problems, utilizing community and governmental resources as necessary. Social workers are employed by community and governmental agencies as well as hospitals, clinics, and nursing homes. If the social worker's focus is on patients and families, he or she may be called a *medical* or *psychiatric social worker*. A master's degree is required for full professional status as a social worker, and membership in the National Association of Social Workers is open only to social workers graduated from, or students of, accredited schools of social work. Certification is granted by the Academy of Certified Social Workers after other criteria are met.

Social workers also have assistants and aides, who sometimes carry a client load in certain agencies. There may be only on-the-job training available for these workers, but in order to move upward they must acquire additional education. Some employers prefer a two-year associate degree in human or social services, even for this assisting level.

One professional issue cited by social workers is related to identity. Since social work was identified as a career only in the 1930s, there is still some preoccupation with defining the field. "Social workers . . . constantly struggle to identify the strands that hold social-work practitioners together despite the diverse populations they serve and the wide range of techniques they use."[22] A recent statement indicated that desirable goals "to improve the quality of life for everyone" were:

- help people enlarge their competence and increase their problem-solving ability
- help people obtain resources
- make organizations responsive to people
- facilitate interaction between individuals and others in their environment
- influence interactions between organizations and institutions
- influence social and environmental policy.[23]

It is interesting to note that nurses also may include such statements in their professional goals. Also, like nurses, social workers are concerned with the distribution, effectiveness, and cost of their service, as well as clarification of responsibilities of each educational level of practitioners. Some also admit to concern for their professional survival, particularly because of role overlap with other health professionals.

Speech Pathology and Audiology

Speech therapists and *audiologists* are specialists in communication disorders. Speech pathologists or therapists diagnose and treat speech and language disorders that may stem from a variety of causes. Speech therapists are particularly valuable in assisting patients whose speech has been affected by a cerebrovascular accident or patients with laryngectomies. Audiologists often work with children and may detect and assist with the hearing disorder of a child who has been mistakenly labeled retarded. Education for both specialties is at a master's level. There has been some attempt to require state licensure. The American Speech and Hearing Association offers a Certificate of Clinical Competence after specific criteria are fulfilled.

Vision Care

Ophthalmologists are physicians who treat diseases of the eye and perform surgery, but they may also examine eyes and prescribe corrective glasses and exercises. *Optometrists,* doctors of optometry (OD), are educated and clinically trained to examine, diagnose, and treat conditions of the vision system, but they refer clients with eye diseases and other health problems to physicians. After a variety of diagnostic tests, they may prescribe corrective lenses, contact lenses, and special optical aids as well as corrective eye exercises to provide maximum vision. Some may specialize in such areas as prescribing and fitting contact lenses.

A minimum of six years' education is required, with two years of college before optometry school, but most already have baccalaureates. About fifteen schools and colleges are accredited by the American Optometric Association Council. All states require licensure by state board examinations; most states accept the National Board of Optometry examinations.

The majority of optometrists are in private office practice; others are in group practice, hospitals, public health agencies, HMOs, research institutions, manufacturing organizations, the military, and other government agencies, or are teaching and doing research in colleges and universities. About 90 percent are involved in direct patient care activities.

Given the overlap in roles with ophthalmologists in the area of vision analysis, the increasing number of optometrists, and their complaint that their income is below acceptable levels, it is not unexpected to find conflict between the groups on their scope of practice. Optometrists are permitted to prescribe drugs in some states, but may not perform surgery. Both activities are strongly opposed by ophthalmologists. The Federal Trade Commission overturn of bans on professional advertising has also aided optometrists, since it made them more competitive in providing those services that can be rendered by both groups of professionals. However, it is predicted that optometrists will continue to fight for expansion of their scope of practice.

Optometric assistants assist optometrists by performing simple office and patient care duties. *Technicians* may also assist in office tasks, but usually assist in vision training and testing. Assistants complete a one-year certificate or diploma program; technicians, a two-year associate degree in paraoptometrics, given by vocational-technical institutes, two- and four-year colleges, colleges of optometry, and the military.

Opticians grind lenses, make eyeglasses, and fit and adjust them. Both AD programs and on-the-job apprenticeship qualify individuals for this job. *Optical laboratory technicians and mechanics* may be involved in polishing and grinding lenses.

Orthoptists, working under an ophthalmologists' supervision, correct crossed eyes in adults and children through special exercises. They may also aid with visual field and glaucoma testing. Two years of college or a bachelor's degree plus a twenty-four-month training program given in medical schools, vision clinics, or hospitals is required.

Other Health Workers

There are a number of other health workers not described in this chapter, such as those in science and engineering—anatomists, biologists, biomedical engineers (who design patient care equipment such as dialysis machines, pacemakers, heart-lung machines), and biomedical technicians (who maintain and repair the equipment); technicians dealing with instrumentation—diagnostic medical sonographers, electrocardiograph (EKG/ECG) technicians, electroencephalographic (EEG) technologists and technicians; specialists in dealing with the visually handicapped; biological photographers; medical illustrators; patient advocates (see Chapter 22); acupuncturists; health science librarians, and computer specialists, to name just a few. In addition, volunteers provide many useful services. That this list is not complete and is expanding may help to explain why, no matter how valuable individual services may be, the public often becomes angered by the fragmentation of services. Even health professionals may be unsure about who does what or when for the client's well-being. Yet, this list is not exaggerated; all of these specialties are part of what the federal government calls health manpower and allied health manpower, for which federal funds are often distributed for educational programs.

It is clear that if the public is to receive the services it requires, expects, and deserves, there must be direction given through the health care delivery maze.

ISSUES IN HEALTH MANPOWER

Many of the most serious issues in health manpower—numbers, distribution, proliferation, and especially quality of care—have become issues focused on credentialing. This multifaceted process, which has become a major concern of state and federal governments, is given full attention in Chapter 20.

However, the problem of health manpower planning transcends or, perhaps, precedes credentialing. The blame for proliferation of manpower is difficult to pinpoint. Is it the practitioners or administrators who see the

immediate need for quickly prepared assistants? Or is it the federal government that encourages proliferation through education and reimbursement support? The health care industry (and it *is* one of the largest industries in the United States) is labor-intensive. Health manpower frequently creates its own demands: if a certain type of practitioner is available, the availability of that service to the consumer expands—and, as the critics say, adds to the total cost of care.

Predicting demand and supply is no easy matter: development of health manpower resources may take as little as a few months or as long as ten years; in that time both demand and supply may shift rapidly; decisions on whether to expand or contract either education programs or health services frequently depend on uncontrollable external factors, such as the economy; current manpower data are inexact and usually out of date. Thus, it is not surprising that even the most educated guesses of demand and supply often err. What *is* left behind all too frequently is a mass of undereducated, poorly paid, non-cost-effective workers with little job mobility, poor motivation, and built-in anger. The result is increased union activity, and labor unions are accused of causing escalating costs.

It is true that in the 1960s improved salaries were a major budget item, and the need to move from what were often below-poverty wages to living wages was largely responsible for the jump. Since that catch-up period, the masses of workers have gained a new aggressiveness that affects not only monetary considerations, but power issues. Some are not necessarily in the best interests of the consumer. Nevertheless, one of the trends that was widely predicted is aggressive action by unions to organize every type of health worker—professional, technical, aide, clerical, maintenance, and housekeeping.

Whether this will be successful is now in doubt because of the tight economic constraints of health care institutions and their action in laying off workers of all kinds. Nurses are concerned because of the great tendency to substitute less prepared workers for nurses.

The issue of maldistribution is also not easily resolved. Maldistribution of professionals, toward attractive urban and suburban areas and away from isolated, poor, or ghetto areas, is a major problem. In some cases, nurses, PAs, physician-nurse, or physician-PA and/or nurse teams are giving care that is as good as or better than that provided by solo practitioners, but the service gap still exists. Even federal intervention, such as requiring service in medically underserved areas (about 30 percent of the United States) in return for supporting the practitioners' education, has had only short-term results—practitioners leave after their required service.

Health manpower education is a major issue. How many? What kind? Prepared where? Financed by whom? The education for all levels of health service practitioners is under scrutiny. Why is this education so costly? Could institutions develop more economical teaching-learning methods? Are minority groups being actively recruited? Are the types of workers in proper proportion? Should the government continue to subsidize the education of high-earning professionals? How much should any health profession be subsidized, and for whom—the programs or students? Are the practitioners appropriately prepared to give safe and effective care?

Another concern is the workability of the health care team. It is naive to expect that bringing together a highly diverse group of people and calling them a team will cause them to behave like a team. One obvious gap is their lack of communication and "practice" together, either as students or as full practitioners. Sports teams practice together intensively for long periods of time, both to develop a team spirit and to enhance and coordinate their individual skills to produce a functioning unit. Not only do health care teams not have (or take) time to practice together, but often there are serious territorial disputes as areas of responsibility overlap more and more. As for patients, who should

be members of the team, unless they are assertive, their only participation is as recipients of care.

Theoretically, legally clear distinctions of each profession would be helpful; practically, it is impossible. Successful coordination depends on collegial behavior and trust and full, frequent, open communication; otherwise, valuable participants in health care will continue to be underutilized. It has also been said that "society can no longer afford to use the physician as gatekeeper to control the flow of patients in and out of the health system."[24] Physician services should be saved to assist patients who need that level and domain of services. In other words, there must be other fully acknowledged practitioners in primary health care.

A review of the issues that each occupation sees as vital makes it clear that the struggle between medicine and other health care groups to expand or limit the scope of practice will continue and perhaps escalate. And, with the current economic pressures that are not expected to let up, various types and levels of workers may fight even harder to get and keep territory. The trend to increase educational criteria seems to permeate each occupational group, but almost all face the questions asked by the cost-conscious: "Will it cost the consumer more? Will it keep out the poor?"

One overriding issue is, who has power or should have power to make these decisions? The consumer? But who advises the consumer? All too often, the power figures in health care make policy, even if indirectly, by their input into legislation or major influential groups. For instance, a 1978 study report on manpower policy for primary health care by the prestigious Institute of Medicine of the National Academy of Sciences showed noticeable incongruities between the body of the report, based on numerous informational and analytical papers, and the recommendations. Although the data indicated a need for preventive care and health teaching, and the body of the report emphasized the importance of teamwork, equal reimbursement, and accountability of all professionals, there was no mention of prevention in the recommendations. Most related to physician education and reimbursement, and one specifically stated that NPs should be supervised by physicians if they provide any medical services. Physicians on the committee outnumbered by three to one any other represented group. However, one nurse on the committee pointed out the discrepancies in what was titled ''Comment'' at the end of the report.[25]

If there are any clear answers to these questions and issues, they have not been found or accepted. Consumers' restlessness with professional indecision and evasion of their concerns and complaints is reaching a critical stage. Even so, the action or nonaction of health planning groups, with major consumer input, shows that the politics of health care influence the behavior of both the practitioners and the consumers.

REFERENCES

1. Steven Jonas, *Health Care Delivery in the United States* (New York: Springer Publishing Co., Inc., 1977), p. 69.
2. Walter McNerney, ''The Evolution in Health Services Management,'' in David Mechanic, ed., *Handbook of Health, Health Care, and the Health Professions* (New York: Free Press, 1983), pp. 531–532.
3. Maryland Pennell and David Hoover, *Health Manpower Source Book 21: Allied Health Manpower Supply and Requirements 1950–1980* (Bethesda, Md.: U.S. Department of Health, Education and Welfare, 1970), p. 3.
4. *Report to the President and Congress in the Status of Health Personnel in the United States,* Vol. I (Bethesda, Md.: U.S. Department of Health and Human Services, Bureau of Health Professions, 1984), pp. B-8-2 and B-8-3.
5. Eli Ginzberg, ''Allied Health Resources,'' in Mechanic, *Handbook* op. cit., pp. 479–494.
6. Lucie Kelly, ''Nurse Clones for Sale,'' *Nurs. Outlook,* **31**:128 (Feb. 1981).

7. Emily Friedman, ''Ebb Tide for Allied Health,'' *Hospitals,* **57**:66–61 (Feb. 1, 1983).
8. M. Matters, ''Chiropractors and MDs: The Referral Doors Inch Wider,'' *Med. Economics,* **60**:157 (July 6, 1981).
9. ''200 Ways to Put Your Talent to Work in the Health Field'' (New York: National Health Council, Inc., 1983).
10. James Dunning, ''Dentistry at the Crossroads: A Study of Professionalism,'' *Am. J. Pub. Health,* **72**:651–652 (July 1982).
11. Susan Finn and Judith Gussler, ''Women's Issues and Dietetics: Implications for Professional Development,'' *Dietetic Currents,* **11**:1–4 (Jan–Feb. 1984).
12. Cathy Luginbill, ''Nurse Instructors for Medical Students,'' *Am. J. Nurs.,* **78**: 868–870 (May 1978).
13. Lynda Boyar et al., ''A Student-Run Course in Interprofessional Relations,'' *J. Med. Ed.,* **52**:183–189 (Mar. 1977).
14. David Mechanic, ''Physicians,'' in Mechanic, op. cit., p. 439.
15. Rosemary Stevens, ''Graduate Medical Education: A Continuing History,'' *J. Med. Ed.,* **53**:1–18 (Jan. 1978).
16. K. J. Williams, ''The Role of the Medical Director,'' *Hosp. Prog.,* **59**:50–57 (June 1978).
17. Report of the Ad Hoc Panel on New Members of the Physician's Health Team of the Board of Medicine of the National Academy of Sciences, *New Members of the Physician's Health Team: Physician's Assistants* (Washington, D.C.: National Academy of Sciences, 1970).
18. D. Glazer, ''National Commission on Certification of Physician's Assistants: A Precedent in Collaboration,'' in Ann Bliss and Eva Cohen, eds., *The New Health Professionals,* (Germantown, Md.: Aspen Systems Corp., 1977), pp. 86–92.
19. *Nurse Clinician and Physician's Assistant: The Relationship Between Two Emerging Practitioner Concepts* (Rochester, N.Y.: National Commission for the Study of Nursing and Nursing Education, 1971).
20. John Biles, ''The Doctor of Pharmacy,'' *J. Am. Med Assn,* **249**:1157–1160 (Mar. 4, 1983).

21. Gary Copeland and David Apgar, "The Pharmacist Practitioner Training Program," *Drug Intell. and Cl. Pharm.,* **14**:114–119 (Feb. 1980).
22. Rosalie Kane, "Social Work as a Health Profession," in Mechanic, op. cit., p. 496.
23. Ibid., p. 497
24. Virginia Cleland and Dawn Zagornik, "Appropriate Use of Health Professionals," *J. of Nurs. Admin.,* **1**:39 (Nov.–Dec. 1971).
25. Institute of Medicine, *A Report of a Study: A Manpower Policy for Primary Health Care* (Washington, D.C.: National Academy of Sciences, 1978), pp. 105–106.

NURSING IN THE HEALTH CARE SCENE

Nursing as a Profession

DEFINITIONS OF NURSING

Because the word *nurse* has certain connotations and because there are long-lived public images of nursing, concepts of the profession of nursing not only differ, but are contradictory and frequently inaccurate. Nursing implies a mother–child relationship, tending, watching over. Schulman notes that nursing's long historical orientation has been based upon a concept of "mother surrogate," a role "characterized by affection, intimacy, and physical proximity, with an orientation for meeting the needs of a dependent ward," providing for protection and identification. The other nursing role he sees as contradictory, even antagonistic—the "healer, change-oriented, dynamic, discontinuous, and fragmentary."[1]

There seems to be a public tendency to equate nursing with illness. Current dictionaries still define *nurse* as someone trained to care for sick people. Moreover, since the proliferation of nurses' aides and practical nurses after World War II, the public is even more confused as to who is the nurse. It is not unusual for patients to call anyone in a uniform who gives them personal care a nurse. Perhaps life was simpler when it was protocol for only the registered nurse to wear a white, long-sleeved uniform, white shoes and stockings, and, most important, the starched white cap and special pin of the nursing school, or, at least, the easily identified navy blue of the public health nurse. It was a symbol, a tradition, an image that came packaged with preconceived notions of what that uniformed figure could do. (Never mind that years ago, one key nursing figure described the uniform as a housedress and the cap as a dust cap).

Nurses tend to cherish a traditional image, even as they move into new roles and live uncomfortably with a blurred self-image. Kramer points out that nursing students enter schools with the concept that "real" nursing is bedside care, and that nursing programs can seldom remove that image, even if they try.[2] But, says one outspoken nurse, "real" nurses also engage in research, deliver babies, teach health, do psychotherapy, administer anesthesia, hang out a shingle, and diagnose patients and clients; "real" nurses work not only in hospitals, but in jails, homes, clinics, colleges, schools, industry, and in the most rural as well as urban areas. And most of all, "real" nurses use their brains as well as their hands and feet.[3]

There are many interpretations of nursing. Why not? There are many facets to nursing, and perhaps it isn't logical or accurate to settle on one point of view. All nurses must eventually determine their own philosophies of nursing, whether or not these are formalized. The public and others outside nursing will probably continue to adopt a concept or image that is nurtured by contact, hearsay, or education about the profession, and the first may be the most powerful determinant. This chapter seeks to present an overview of the components of nursing, examined in the light of professionalism, legal and other definitions, nursing process, nursing theory, nursing diagnosis, and nursing standards.

PROFESSIONS AND PROFESSIONALISM

Almost everyone talks about the *nursing profession* in the sense of an organized group of persons, all of whom are engaged in nursing (the phrase is used often throughout these pages). But another question discussed both within and without the ranks of nursing is whether or not nursing as a whole is an occupation, rather than a profession in the same sense that medicine, theology, and law have been called professions since the Middle Ages. (Crossword puzzles in a distinguished newspaper consistently used *hospital aide* for the crossword that spells out *nurse.*)

Professions have been historically linked with universities or other specialized institutions of learning, implying a certain high level of scholarly learning and study, including research. The specific criteria for a profession vary and are delineated more fully in some of the bibliography for this chapter. There is fairly general agreement, however, that professionalism centers on specialized expertise, autonomy, and service. Bixler and Bixler's characteristics of a profession modeled after Flexner's classic criteria[4] have achieved wide acceptance by many professionals:

1. A profession utilizes in its practice a well-defined and well-organized body of knowledge which is on the intellectual level of higher learning.
2. A profession constantly enlarges the body of knowledge it uses and improves its techniques of education and service by the use of the scientific method.
3. A profession entrusts the education of its practitioners to institutions of higher education.
4. A profession applies its body of knowledge in practical services which are vital to human and social welfare.
5. A profession functions autonomously in the formulation of professional policy and in the control of professional activity thereby.
6. A profession attracts individuals of intellectual and personal qualities who exalt service above personal gain and who recognize their chosen occupation as a life work.
7. A profession strives to compensate its practitioners by providing freedom of action, opportunity for continuous professional growth and economic security.[5]

Looking at these criteria objectively, it is clear that nursing does not totally fulfill all of them. It has been pointed out that nursing's theory base is still developing, that the public does not always see the nurse as a professional, that not all nurses are educated in institutions of higher learning, that not all nurses consider nursing a lifetime career, and that in many practice settings, nursing does not control its own policies and activities.[6] The last, a lack of autonomy, is considered the most serious weakness. Sociologists have long contended that an occupation has not become a profession unless the members of that occupation are "the ones who make the final decisions in the field of activity in which they are engaged."[7]

This issue is addressed in more depth in Chapter 16, and it can be seen that particularly in recent years, there has been progress both in achieving autonomy and, perhaps more important, nurses' recognition that this is important to both the profession and to themselves in terms of how they practice. This mental turnaround has something to do with the fact that more nurses are seeking higher education and that more are planning nursing careers as opposed to taking nursing jobs. And as intertwined as all of these professional threads are bound to be, more of the better-educated nurses are also involved in research and theory development.* If nursing is not considered a profession in the strictest sense of the word, it is certainly well on the way to becoming so. Viewing professionalism as a scale along which nursing may move, it can be said that "Nursing's present degree of profes-sionalism viewed in a negative way merits the title of semi-profession. Seen in the positive light, it may be called an emerging profes-sion."[8] Whether or not (and when) it will be-come a full profession depends on whether its practitioners choose this demanding status and continue to make progress.

It should be pointed out, however, that the term *profession* is essentially a social concept and has no meaning apart from society. Soci-ety decides that for its needs to be met in a cer-tain respect, a body undertaking to meet these particular needs will be given special consider-ation. (One philosopher maintains that society "owns" the professions.)[9] The contract is that the individuals of that favored group contin-ually use their best endeavor to meet those ob-ligations, constantly reexamining and scruti-nizing their functions for appropriateness and maintaining competence. When they fail to honor these obligations and/or slip into de-manding status, authority, and privilege that have no connection with carrying out their professional work satisfactorily, society may reconsider. A profession is seen as a body of individuals voluntarily subordinating them-selves to a standard of social morality more exacting than that of the community in gen-eral. "Only so far as this implicit contract is observed will a profession *as a profession* sur-vive."[10] That violation of this code eventually

brings retribution from society is evidenced today in the tightening of laws regulating pro-fessional practice and reimbursement. Certain behaviors, such as unprofessional conduct, may be specifically punished by removal of the practitioner's legal right to practice—li-censure. What comprises unprofessional con-duct may, again, vary from state to state, and also in time. This is discussed more fully in Chapter 20.

Because professionalism obviously brings with it certain real advantages, practitioners of all kinds seek professional status. Many seek it through licensure, which confers some of the privileges (and reponsibilities) of pro-fessionalism. An interesting model of profes-sionalism has been described as a "spectre" in which occupations are classified by degrees of professionalism, from unskilled employees to independent practitioners. In the "crown" of professionalism are the independent practi-tioners. Surrounding them are the employed professionals, and, holding a part of the pool or core of professional attributes, the semi-professional employees. Further down are skilled and unskilled employees. The lines be-tween all of these are broken to show the pos-sibility of mobility over time, both as individ-uals move upward and as occupations may move toward professional status. The further away from the crown the worker is, the less in-dependent he or she is of the organization or bureaucracy.[11]

On the other hand, despite the prestige of professionalism, many concepts that were tra-ditionally held are fading. For instance, col-lective bargaining, unionism, and strikes, once seen as the antithesis of professionalism, have been gradually accepted as legitimate ac-tivities by professionals who are employed. Physicians, nurses, teachers, social workers, and others have chosen that route as the only means left to gain certain concessions from employers. Obviously, the very fact that more professionals are employed, and thus lack a degree of autonomy, has precipitated this change.

In addition, there is an increasing tendency

---

*See Chapters 12, 13, 14.

to use the term *professional* in another context to describe one who has an assured competence in a particular field or occupation, such as a hairdresser, or someone who participates in an activity for pay as opposed to an amateur—a musician, artist, or baseball player. It is particularly interesting to note the changes in dictionary definitions over the years to include the last two concepts. Looking at it in the "pure" sense, however, the idea of professionalism has been called the most important and powerful in the belief system of nursing. But this ideology does not seem to provide all nurses with common beliefs and ideals about the profession.[12] Nurses themselves do not hold a common concept of professionalism. Six thousand nurses responding to a survey all felt that they were professional, but their concept varied from the majority view of professionalism as an "amalgam of competence, high ethical standards, medical knowledge, and compassion" to individual qualities such as sense of humor, well-groomed, cheerful, courteous, capable, and confident.[13]

In a scholarly but personalized treatise on her beliefs about nursing, Margretta Styles introduces new and challenging thoughts about professionalism. One provocative point is that professionalism is not, as perceived, rooted in a two-party arrangement between the professional and the client. Because today professions are practiced predominantly in some type of institutional setting, there are other factors to consider, such as multiple client systems. Faculty members, for instance, may have as clients students, the university, the health care agency, and the patient, to all of whom they have some accountability.[14] (What if their demands conflict?)

Styles' key point is that nurses should not set their sights on an external ideal—professionalism—and on externally applied qualifications, but rather should compete with themselves to be the best they can in accomplishing goals set by themselves—"self-actualized professionals forming an actualized profession." She summarizes the concept that she calls *professionhood:* "Our intent that nursing become

its utmost and that we as nurses become our utmost would be better served by a set of internal beliefs about nursing than a set of external criteria about professions."[15]

Professionalism, Styles maintains, emphasizes the *composite character of the profession* and "allows us to lose ourselves in the crowd; it permits the illusion of an 'I–they' relationship; it even encourages a nonproductive or counterproductive range of responses from passivism, escapism, and blamism. On the other hand, professionhood [focusing on the characteristics of the individual] . . . forces us to pay attention to our own image as the dominant figure in the mirror of nursing. It recognizes that the professionalism of nursing will be achieved only through the professionhood of its members."[16]

Therefore, we return again to the basic ingredient of professionalism—the individual nurse.

A scathing indictment of nurses who "want the name but not the game" might have some validity.

> Too small a percentage of nurses have "bought" professionalism as a way of life. The larger segment "mouth" the philosophy, go through the outward rituals, all the while digging deeper ruts from which to be extracted later by another "concerned" generation of truly professional nurses. These are the nurses who find status in the status quo. They are not progressive; they have just transferred their hard-core traditionalism to other setting, and labeled it progress. These are the nurses who demand professional recognition from others, but are reluctant to assume professional responsibilities. They may get caught up in the intellectual ferment around them, but they are not seriously engaged in the professional dialogue. They may be troubled about nursing's professional role, but for self-serving reasons. To the observer, there is serious imbalance between their professional commitment and their personal ambitions. They court professionalism but balk at the price. They command higher salaries, but avoid spending their own money on professional growth . . . if

they can use someone else's, namely, their employer's or the government's. Professionalism as a way of life implies responsibility and commitment.[17]

The Nature of Nursing: Some Definitions

In *Notes on Nursing: What It Is and What It is Not,* Florence Nightingale states in the most basic terms that nursing is to "put the patient in the best condition for nature to act upon him." Since that time, a number of other definitions have evolved, but the emphasis on care has not diminished, even in the scientific era. Definitions of nursing vary according to the philosophy of an individual or group, and interpretations of roles and functions vary accordingly.

One contemporary nurse said "Nursing is the art of helping people feel better—as simple and as complex as this."[18] Another included a spiritual component:

Nursing in its broadest sense may be defined as an art and science which involves the whole patient—body, mind, and spirit; promotes his spiritual, mental, and physical health by teaching and by example; stresses health education and health preservation as well as ministration to the sick; involves the care of the patient's environment—social and spiritual as well as physical; and gives health service to the family and the community as well as to the individual.[19]

A new graduate said that nursing means technical skill, but also caring, understanding, supporting, teaching, and, most of all, being there.[20]

A classic definition used by nurses internationally is that of Virginia Henderson, a distinguished American nursing educator and writer.

The unique function of the nurse is to assist the individual, sick or well, in the performance of those activities contributing to health or its recovery (or to peaceful death) that he would perform unaided if he had the necessary strength, will or knowledge. And to do

this in such a way as to help him gain independence as rapidly as possible. This aspect of her work, this part of her function, she initiates and controls; of this she is master. In addition she helps the patient to carry out the therapeutic plan as initiated by the physician. She also, as a member of a medical team, helps other members, as they in turn help her, to plan and carry out the total program whether it be for the improvement of health, or the recovery from illness or support in death. . . .[21]

Many other of today's nursing leaders hold similar concepts, worded somewhat differently or expanded into other configurations. Schlotfeldt states:

Nursing is an essential service to all of mankind. That service can be succinctly described in terms of its focus, goal, jurisdiction, and outcomes as that of assessing and enhancing the general health status, health assets, and health potentials of all human beings. It is a service provided for persons who are essentially well, those who are infirm, ill, or disabled, those who are developing, and those who are declining. Nurses serve all people—sometimes individuals and sometimes collectives. They appropriately provide primary, episodic, and long-term care and, as professionals, are independently accountable for the execution and consequences of all nursing services.[22]

Rogers noted that "nursing's first line of defense is promotion of health and prevention of illness. Care of the sick is resorted to when our first line of defense fails."[23] In the ANA position paper of 1965, the terms *care, cure,* and *coordination* were used as part of a definition of *professional practice* (see Chapter 12), and this phrase has been used numerous times, with individual interpretation of the components.

As nurses expand their functions into the new nurse practitioner role, *cure* has acquired a different meaning for some nurses, as management of the patient's care, which includes aspects of what has been medical diagnosis and treatment. Some nurses, like Rogers, feel that such medical (not nursing) diagnosis and treatment diminishes the role of the nurse as a nurse. (The same opponents also usually reject the term *nurse practitioner* or *NP*.) However, Ford, a pioneer of the NP movement, calls this "semantic roulette" and adds, "I'm not so concerned about the words. I'm convinced that nursing can take on that level of accountability of professional practice that involves the consumer in decision making in his care and also demands sophisticated clinical judgment to determine levels of illness and wellness and design a plan of management."[24] Ingeborg Mauksch voices similar sentiments,[25] as did the multidisciplinary group reporting to the Secretary of Health, Education and Welfare.[26]

This group considered the need to extend the scope of nursing practice in primary, acute, and long-term care. However, the role of nursing in primary care, with or without medically oriented skills, is receiving major attention. Fagin maintains that primary care has been the academic discipline of nursing, since its public health evolution in the early days of nursing.

> Nursing is defined as including the promotion and maintenance of health, prevention of illness, care of persons during acute phases of illness, and rehabilitation and restoration of health. Are these not also the functions of primary care as described by most writers . . . ?[27]

Although, over the years, nursing has been defined in specific situations according to the functions of nurses or the clinical fields in which they practice, or the specific job titles they may hold, there is a thread running throughout the definitions that indicates that the focus of nursing is the health of whole human beings in interaction with their environment—a wholistic,˙ humanistic focus. The

---

*The term *wholistic* seems to have been coined to refer to care related to the "whole" patient, physical and psychosocial. *Holistic* now generally refers to paranormal healing, an aspect of which is described by Dolores Krieger in the nursing literature. However, usage is not consistent and *holistic* is used by some authors in the sense of *wholistic*.

ANA 1973 *Standards of Practice* states, "Nursing practice is a direct service, goal-directed, and adaptable to the needs of the individual, family, and community during health and illness. Professional practitioners of nursing bear primary responsibility and accountability for the nursing care clients/patients receive."

An extremely significant step in the definition of nursing occurred in 1980 when ANA published *Nursing: A Social Policy Statement*. The work of a task force appointed by its Congress for Nursing Practice, the purpose was to answer the question, "What is nursing?" The introduction stated: "Trends well underway in nursing must now be reflected in a contemporary delineation of the nature and scope of nursing practice and a description of the characteristics of specialization in nursing. . . . This delineation of the nature and scope of nursing practice is tailored to the diversity, openness, and transition characteristic of the present, actual range of nursing practice."[28]

The definition was intended to maintain the historical orientation of the Nightingale and Henderson definitions, as well as reflecting the influence of nursing theory that is a part of nursing's evolution:

> Nursing is the diagnosis and treatment of human responses to actual or potential health problems.

Examples given of these human responses include self-care limitations; pain and discomfort; emotional problems; deficiencies in decision making and the ability to make personal choices; and self-image changes required by health status. The nurse can determine these responses through various forms of assessment. Diagnosis is seen as a beginning effort to conceptualize and name a perceived difficulty, and nurses use theory in the form of concepts, principles, and processes to understand these phenomena within the domain of nursing practice. The aims of nursing actions are to ameliorate, improve, or correct the problems and are intended to produce beneficial effects in relation to identified responses.[29]

Another component of the definition was the scope of nursing practice: "the contents of the nursing segment of health care." It was seen as having four defining characteristics:

- boundary—an external boundary that expands outward in response to changing needs, demands, and capacities of society.
- intersections—interprofessional interfacings that are meeting points at which nursing extends its practice into the domains of other professions.
- core—the basis of nursing care—"the phenomenon of concern to nurses are human responses to actual or potential health problems."
- dimensions—characteristics that fall within and further describe the scope of nursing, such as philosophy and ethics that guide nurses; responsibilities, functions, roles and skills that characterize their work.[30]

It was also noted that all nurses are responsible for including preventive nursing in their practice, that nurses provide care across the life span and in a variety of settings, and that they are ethically and legally accountable for actions taken in practice or delegated.

A separate section on specialization, which was called a mark of the advancement of the nursing profession, stated:

Specialization in nursing practice assists in clarifying, revising and strengthening existing practice. It also permits new applications of knowledge and refined nursing practice to flow from the specialist to the generalist in nursing practice and graduate to basic education, thus ensuring progress in the general practice in nursing.[31]

Criteria for specialists in nursing practice, roles and functions were delineated.

The social policy statement was intended to "assist nurses in conceptualizing their practice; to provide direction to educators, administrators and researchers within nursing; and to inform other health professionals, legislators, funding bodies, and the public about nursing's contribution to health care."[32]

Despite its somewhat obscure language at certain points (professions do have their own private jargon that, incidentally, can shut out others), which made it less than totally understandable to some nurses, much less non-nurses, the social policy statement was another major step in defining contemporary nursing.

Nursing Functions

Nursing functions can be described in broad or specific terms. For instance, classically, the common elements have included maintaining or restoring normal life function; observing and reporting signs of actual or potential change in a patient's status; assessing his or her physical and emotional state and immediate environment; formulating and carrying out a plan for the provision of nursing care based on a medical regimen, including administration of medications and treatments and interpretation of treatment and rehabilitative regimens; counseling families in relation to other health-related services; and teaching. Some of these are referred to in the social policy statement.

Of course, some nurses still see the nurse more as a manager of nursing care than as a face-to-face clinical practitioner—in other words, responsible for nursing care, supervising and coordinating the work of others, but not personally giving care. However, in recent years, there has been a return to a clinical emphasis.

The evolving role of the nurse is a particular focus of attention. One example is the description of functions delineated by a group of independent NPs, which specifically indicates differences between medical and nursing practice and stresses concern with the whole person and his reaction to illness rather than the disease itself.[33] In one study, nursing educators projected evolving functions as data gathering, including history taking and assessment; nursing diagnosis (and some aspects of medical diagnosis); nursing intervention; evaluation, including evaluation of nursing team performance and evaluation of community resources; and administration, including carrying twenty-four-hour responsibility for nursing care.[34] These have indeed evolved.

In defining functions that should be common to all nurses, Schlotfeldt identifies the following:

1. Interviewing to obtain accurate health histories.
2. Examining, with use of all senses and technological aids, to ascertain the health status of persons served.
3. Evaluating to draw valid inferences concerning individuals' health assets and potentials.
4. Referring to physicians and dentists those persons whose health status indicates the need for differential diagnoses and the institution of therapies.
5. Referring to other helping professionals those persons who need assistance with problems that fall within the province of clergymen, social workers, homemakers, lawyers, and others.
6. Caring for persons during periods of their dependence, to include:
   a. compensating for deficits of those unable to maintain normal functions and to execute their prescribed therapies;
   b. sustaining and supporting persons while reinforcing the natural, developmental, and reparative processes available to human beings in their quest for wholeness, function, comfort, and selffulfillment;
   c. teaching and guiding persons in their pursuit of optimal wellness;
   d. motivating persons toward active, knowledgeable involvement in seeking health and in executing their needed therapies.
7. Collaborating with other health professionals and with persons served in planning and executing programs of health care and diagnostic and treatment services.
8. Evaluating in concert with consumers, other providers, and policy-makers the efficacy of the health care system and planning for its continuous improvement.[35]

The degree of expertise with which a nurse carries out these functions depends on his or her level of knowledge and skills, but the profession has the responsibility of setting standards for its practitioners. In its *Standards of Nursing Practice,* the ANA incorporated and ordered standards in a nursing process sequence.

The Nursing Process

Yura and Walsh state that the term *nursing process* was not prevalent in the nursing literature until the mid-1960s, with limited mention in the 1950s.[36] Orlando was one of the earliest authors to use the term, but it was slow to be adopted. In the next few years, models of the activities in which nurses engaged were developed, and in 1967, a faculty group at the Catholic University of America specifically identified the phases of the nursing process as assessing, planning, implementing, and evaluating.[37] The nursing process is described as "an orderly, systematic manner of determining the client's problems, making plans to solve them, initiating the plan or assigning others to implement it, and evaluating the extent to which the plan was effective in resolving the problems identified."[38]

At this point, there is considerable information in the nursing literature about the use of the nursing process, and many schools of nursing use it as a framework for teaching. Yura and Walsh continue to develop their work on the concept.[39]

Nursing Theories, Concepts, and Models

As nursing has developed in professionalism, nursing scholars have developed theories of nursing, and the science of nursing is coming of age. A theoretical base of practice defines nursing's uniqueness; that is, it has a science of its own and is not simply an extension of another profession. In scientific inquiry, observations of seemingly unrelated phenomena are organized into intelligible systems that show relationships among the phenomena and a linking of truths.[40] Nursing research de-

scribes, understands, and predicts the life process of man, supporting the probability that
nursing can intervene effectively to promote
the maximum health of the well and ill in individuals and social groups.[41] Nursing theory is
the umbrella encompassing the concepts.

The shift in nursing education from the
practice setting of the hospital to the aca .emic
setting of the university brought with it a keen
interest in identifying and developing a scientific body of knowledge unique to nursing.
Theories were sought and formulated which
would distinguish nursing, first, from medicine, whose models of disease and dysfunction
historically had dominated nursing education
and practice, and second, from the common
caretaking principles and practices of helping,
protecting, and mothering found in the lay
public. Without research and theory building,
nursing scholars argued, nursing would be unable to carve out a role for itself in the future
health care system, and would thus allow itself
to be defined, instructed, and controlled by
other disciplines.

Although the 1950s and 1960s witnessed a
proliferation of nursing concepts and theories, the question of a body of knowledge specific to nursing probably began with Florence
Nightingale.[42] Among her other achievements,
she identified the relationship between patient
and environment as a major focus for nursing
intervention and provided ''hints'' which
would guide nurses in providing comfort,
speeding recovery, and preventing disease.
Like theories, her hints were derived from systematic observation of patients and their responses and, just as theory is used in education today, Nightingale submitted that by
using these hints, nurses could teach themselves. While her work was groundbreaking
for nursing science, the immaturity and transitional nature of nursing at that point in history is evident in her reference to the importance of precise observations, on the one
hand, and to ''common sense,'' for which she
had no clarifying definition, on the other. Accordingly, she explicitly distinguished nursing
knowledge from medical knowledge ''which

everyone ought to have.'' Nevertheless, the
seeds were sown for the development of a science of nursing which began to flower over
100 years later.

The question of the uniqueness of nursing
knowledge continues to be a thorny issue
among nursing theorists, particularly because
nursing is said to ''borrow'' so much of its
knowledge from other disciplines. While
many nursing scholars find this excessive bor-
rowing troublesome as they seek to identify
what is unique to nursing, others argue that
the uniqueness of nursing lies in its very reliance on many disciplines—that in fact, *because* it synthesizes knowledge from so many
disciplines, nursing provides a more comprehensive, holistic approach to patient care than
any of the other health professions.

Theory building in nursing takes several
forms and has several purposes. Mid-level theory, for example, has as its major goal the improvement of the technology of nursing, such
as the discovery of the most effective procedures for educating clients, managing post-
surgical patients, or helping families to deal
with death and dying. Since science and technology are linked in very important ways,
middle-range research is highly significant in
developing a body of specialized knowledge in
nursing. Grand theory, in comparison, takes a
more all-encompassing view of nursing, a
''world view'' that attempts to explain and define nursing—what it is, what it does, why it is
important, how it differs from other health
professions—and exposes to critical examination such concepts as *patient, nurse, illness,
health, support, care,* and *comfort.* A number
of grand theories have been proposed to guide
nursing research, education, and practice.

The *behavioral system model* is generally
credited to Dorothy Johnson. This theory
views nursing's client as one or more behavioral systems in interaction with the environment. Nursing's goal of action is to maintain
or restore the balance and stability of the person's behavioral system or to help the person
achieve a more optimum level of functioning
(balance) when this is possible and desirable.

Starting with nursing's traditional concern for the person who is ill, we have come to conceive of nursing's specific contribution to patient welfare as that of fostering efficient and effective behavioral functioning in the patient to prevent illness, and during and following illness.[43]

The *adaptation model* developed by Sister Callista Roy conceives of man in constant interaction with a changing environment, to which he must adapt. Man's adaptation is a function of the stimuli to which he is exposed and his adaptation level; man's adaptation level is such that it comprises a zone which indicates the range of stimulation that will lead to a positive response. (If the stimulus is within the zone, the person responds positively. If, however, the stimulus is outside the zone, the person cannot make a positive response.) Man has four modes of adaptation: physiological needs, self-concept, role function, and interdependence relations. After plotting the point on the health–illness continuum at which a patient currently rests, evaluating the factors which influence him, and judging the effectiveness of his coping mechanisms, the nurse intervenes by changing the person's response potential by bringing the stimuli within a zone where a positive response is possible.

> All nursing activity will be aimed at promoting man's adaptation in his physiological needs, his self-concept, his role function and his interdependence relations during health and illness.[44]

Martha Rogers' *Science of Unitary Man* includes a complex series of principles: helicy, resonancy, and complementarity, called *principles of homeodynamics.* Rogers depicts man, wholistically, as greater than the sum of his parts and moving through time and space as an integral part of an expanding universe, from the past to the future, which implies man's movement toward potential states of maximum well-being.

Nursing aims to assist people in achieving

their maximum health potential. Maintenance and promotion of health, prevention of disease, nursing diagnosis, intervention and rehabilitation encompass the scope of nursing's goals.[45]

The *general theory of nursing,* formulated by Dorothea Orem, is constituted from three related theories: the theory of self-care, as explanatory of the actions that individuals "personally initiate and perform on their own behalf in maintaining" their own human functioning, health, and well-being (the theory also extends to care of dependent family members); the theory of deficits for engagement in self-care or care of dependents when the deficit is attributed to the health state or health care requirements, as explanatory of why individuals or groups can be helped through nursing; and the theory that nursing systems are the end products created by nurses through their endeavors in nursing practice situations.

> Nursing is perhaps best described as giving of direct assistance to a person, as required, because of the person's specific inabilities in self-care resulting from a situation of personal health. Care as required may be continuous or periodic. Self-care means the care which all persons require each day. It is the personal care which adults give to themselves, including attention to ordinary health requirements, and the following of the medical directive of their physicians.[46]

Myra Levine lists four conservation *principles of nursing* that have as a postulate the unity and integrity of the individual. Nursing intervention is based on the principles of conservation of energy, structural integrity, personal integrity, and social integrity. Levine believes that the holistic approach to nursing care depends upon recognition of the integrated response of the individual arising from the internal environment and the interaction that occurs with the external environment.

> Nursing intervention means that the nurse interposes her skill and knowledge into the

course of events that affects the patient. . . .
When nursing intervention influences the adaptation favorably, or toward renewed social well-being, then the nurse is acting in a therapeutic sense. When the nursing intervention cannot alter the course of the adaptation—when her best efforts can only maintain the status quo or fail to halt a downward course—then the nurse is acting in a supportive sense.[47]

Finally, a special pioneer should be mentioned. Though seldom formally counted among nursing theorists, Lydia Hall is often considered to have inspired and profoundly influenced the concept of primary nursing. She contended that illness and rehabilitation are to be viewed as learning experiences in which the nurse's function is to guide and teach the patient through personal caregiving. According to Hall, this role is a response to the current societal need for long-term care of the chronically ill and is distinguished from the "curing" function of medicine.

> Our intent when we lay hands on the patient in bodily care is to comfort. While the patient is being comforted, he feels close to the comforting one. . . . If the individual who is in the comforting role has in her preparation all the services whose principles she can use to offer a teaching-learning experience around his concerns, the ones that are most effective in teaching and learning, then the comforter proceeds to something beyond [relief of anxiety and tension]—to what I call "nurturer"—someone who fosters learning, someone who fosters growing up emotionally, someone who even fosters healing.[48]

The main concepts upon which these and most other nursing theories are based are *man, nurse,* and *health.* Both Rogers and Levine, for example, use *man* as the organizing principle of their theories; Rogers views man in his entirety, while Levine focuses on the various components of structural, personal, and social integrity. Nurse-centered theories, on the other hand, take the nurse's actions and roles as their main theme but, like man-centered theories, vary in interpretation

of the concept. Thus, for Orem, the nurse is a substitute for the patient in the performance of self-care, while for Hall, the nurse is a teacher who assists the patient in making his illness or disability a learning experience.

Johnson's theory typifies those centered on health, which she views as a state of equilibrium which the nurse assists the patient to maintain. Roy also endorses a health-focused model but sees health as a continuum from wellness to illness.[49]

Most grand theories, including the ones presented here, are derived not from observation of empirical phenomena (what nursing is) but rather from a philosophical position on what nursing should be in the best of all possible worlds to be most effective or therapeutic. As such, they contain a significant value component which profoundly influences the acceptance and utility of the theory.

In contrast, a minority of nursing theorists suggest that nursing knowledge can be developed through scientific research, hypothesis testing, and empirical observation of what is. Leininger, for example, advocates the cross-cultural comparison of "caring" phenomena in which recurring themes and patterns, which are the essence of nursing as currently practiced, begin to "fall out" and allow us to construct a science of nursing, or, in Leininger's terms, a "science of caring."[50]

Certainly there is merit to both approaches. From the scientific perspective, nursing is an observational science, sharing with astronomy, zoology, anthropology, medicine, public health, and others a method for formulating its theories by chronicling and analyzing systematic observations. Unlike these other disciplines, however, nursing is still in the early stages of developing its taxonomy. Thus, from medical theory, we have a sophisticated set of classifications for describing disease, but we do not as yet have a very well-developed set of categories for describing sick *persons* (the focus of nursing) in terms of their responses to health and illness and developmental processes. All health sciences have much to gain by empirical observation of human responses to birth, death, illness, parenting, aging, stress, and other factors. Nursing, perhaps more than any other discipline, is in a position to observe and record these events and develop theories that shift clinical practice from being disease oriented to patient oriented.

However, the fact that most of the grand theories are based on the value orientations of the theorist rather than empirical observations does not mean that they are less functional or important for the development of nursing knowledge. Their value in generating new theories and hypotheses which are subsequently tested and refined in the real world of practice cannot be denied. In fact, theory does not even have to be scientific (capable of being refuted) to be useful. Historically, and even for some modern theorists, nursing has been guided by religious knowledge and theories which, while unscientific, may be very successful in providing a framework for effective clinical practice and education.

Indeed, it is becoming increasingly common to hear that in its rigid adherence to the scientific method in generating theory, nursing is trading its birthright of intuitiveness and humanism. Styles specifically calls for the reincorporation of human values and personal beliefs into nursing theory. Interestingly, Styles and her ancestor, Nightingale each make a strong case for nursing knowledge and practice based on *both* ideology and scientific theory, but a comparison of their positions on this issue provides a telling commentary on the direction of nursing theory over the last century. Florence Nightingale stressed that for nurses to best meet the need of patients, they could not solely rely on good intentions: "if you cannot get the habit of observation one way or another, you had better give up being a nurse, for it is not your calling however kind and anxious you may be."[51] Over 100 years later, Styles calls on the nursing community to be guided by ideology as well as science, to work toward what we *should be* and to include in professionalization such themes as commitment, personal motivation, and self-

actualization, as well as scientific discovery: "nursing, as a professional community, must have and hold a common, recitable ideology just as nations have their constitutional preambles and pledges of allegiance, fraternal societies have their oaths, religions have their creeds."[52]

Whether nursing emerges as a mature discipline as well as a profession in the next decade depends to a great extent on the direction that its theory building will take—for instance, constructing explanations of the relationship between nursing phenomena which can be tested against experience; developing its technological base, policies, and procedures; clarifying its concepts and categories; and reconfirming its philosophy and ideological base. Ultimately, the most important test of any theory is its applicability and utility in clinical practice.

Nursing Diagnosis

The ability to make a *nursing* diagnosis and to prescribe *nursing* actions are basic to the development of nursing science.

Provision of nursing care is a problem-solving process. The nurse first gathers data about her patient, then identifies the problem. An approach to the problem is selected and carried out. Finally, the results of this approach, in terms of consequences for the patient, are evaluated. By using this process the nurse can individualize her care and be accountable for providing a scientifically based service. Nursing diagnosis is the title given to the stage of identifying the problem.[53]

A diagnostic taxonomy (a set of classifications which are ordered and arranged on the basis of a single principle or set of principles) has been in the development stage for several years and may serve as a major communication tool among nurses. It could also facilitate public understanding of what nurses do; just as physicians can pinpoint what they do in relation to treating diseases, nurses can point out nursing diagnosis as the patient problems they try to resolve. However, interesting developments have occurred in recent years, with some argument about the usefulness and appropriateness of nursing diagnosis either as a concept or in practical application in the specialty fields.[54,55]

The growth of nursing diagnosis and nursing theories have been major developments in nursing in the last twenty years. Imperative now is continued and strengthened clinical research to develop and refine nursing theories that can serve as guides for nursing practice and as measurements of the extent to which nursing action attains its goals in terms of patient behavior.

WHAT IS NURSING?

It can easily be seen that there may not be a single definition of nursing. Perhaps there never will be, since nursing is a multifaceted profession. This is one problem legislators have had in writing a nurse practice act, which is, after all the legal definition of nursing. (These definitions, along with other aspects of licensure, are discussed in Chapter 20.) Nevertheless, at some point, every nurse has to decide what nursing is to him or her and how to interpret it to others. This chapter, its references, and its bibliography may provide a basis for such thinking, but the final determination is yours.

REFERENCES

1. Sam Schulman, "Basic Functional Roles in Nursing: Mother Surrogate and Healer," in E. G. Jaco, ed., *Patients, Physicians and Illness: Behavioral Sciences and Medicine* (Glencoe, Ill.: Free Press, 1963), p. 532.
2. Marlene Kramer, *Reality Shock: Why Nurses Leave Nursing* (St. Louis: C. V. Mosby Company, 1974), p. 21.
3. Carol Garant, "The Process of Effecting Change in Nursing," *Nurs. Forum,* **17**(2):158 (1978).
4. Abraham Flexner, "Is Social Work a Profession?" *Proceedings of the National Conference of Charities and Correction* (New York: New York School of Philanthropy, 1915), pp. 576–581.
5. Genevieve K. Bixler and Roy W. Bixler: "The Professional Status of Nursing," *Am. J. Nurs.,* **45**:730–735 (Sept. 1945).
6. Martha Sleicher, "Nursing *Is Not* a Profession," *Nurs. and Health Care,* **2**:186–191, 218 (Apr. 1981).
7. Robert Merton "Issues in the Growth of a Profession," Summary Proceedings, American Nurses' Association Convention, 1958 (New York: American Nurses' Association, 1958), p. 298.
8. Gail Stuart, "How Professionalized Is Nursing?" *Image,* **13**:18–23 (Feb. 1981).
9. B. B. Page, "Who Owns the Professions?" *Hastings Center Report,* **5**:7–8 (Oct. 1975).
10. Norah Mackenzie, "The Professional Ethic," *Int. Nurs. Rev.,* **13**:60–61 (July-Aug. 1966).
11. Byron Buick-Constable, "The Professionalism Spectre," *Int. Nurs. Rev.,* **16**(2):133–144 (1969).
12. Mary Gamer, "The Ideology of Professionalism," *Nurs. Outlook,* **27**:108 (Feb. 1979).
13. Robert Gulack, "'I'm a Professional'," *RN,* **46**:29–35 (Sept. 1983).
14. Margretta Styles, *On Nursing: Toward a New Endowment* (St. Louis: C. V. Mosby Company, 1982), pp. 19–20.
15. *Ibid.,* p. 76.
16. *Ibid.,* p. 8.
17. Alice Clarke, "Candidly Speaking: On *Nursing Forum* and Professionalism," *Nurs. Forum,* **7**(1):12 (1968).
18. Thelma Ingles, "What Is Good Nursing?" *Am. J. Nurs.,* **59**:1246 (Sept. 1959).
19. Sister M. Olivia Gowan, *Proceedings of the Workshop on Administration of College Programs in Nursing, June 12–24, 1944* (Washington, D.C.: Catholic University of American Press, 1946), p. 10.
20. Barbara MacDonald, "This I Believe . . . Nursing's Many Meanings," *Nurs. Outlook* **14**:56–57 (July 1966).
21. Virginia Henderson, *ICN Basic Principles of Nursing Care* (London: International Council of Nurses, 1961). Expanded in Virginia Henderson, *The Nature of Nursing* (New York: Macmillan Publishing Company, Inc., 1967).

22. Rozella Schlotfeldt, "The Professional Doctorate: Rationale and Characteristics," *Nurs. Outlook,* **26**:303 (May 1978).
23. Martha Rogers, "Doctoral Education in Nursing," *Nurs. Forum,* **5**:77 (1966).
24. "The Nurse Practitioner Question,' *Am. J. Nurs.,* **74**:2188 (Dec. 1974).
25. Ingeborg Mauksch, "Critical Issues of the Nurse Practitioner Movement," *Nurse Practitioner,* **3**:15 (Nov.–Dec. 1978).
26. "Extending the Scope of Nursing Practice," *Nurs. Outlook,* **20**:46–52 (Jan. 1972).
27. Claire Fagin, "Primary Care as an Academic Discipline," *Nurs. Outlook,* **26**:753 (Dec. 1978).
28. *Nursing: A Social Policy Statement* (Kansas City, Mo: American Nurses' Association, 1980), p. 1.
29. Ibid., pp. 9–12.
30. Ibid., pp. 13–18.
31. Ibid., p. 22.
32. Ibid., p. 30.
33. "Independent Practitioners Define Nursing Roles," *Am. Nurse,* **5**:2, 9 (Nov. 1973).
34. Gertrude Torres, "Educators' Perceptions of Evolving Nursing Functions," *Nurs. Outlook,* **22**:184–187 (Mar. 1974).
35. Schlotfeldt, op. cit.
36. Helen Yura and Mary Walsh, *The Nursing Process,* 2nd ed. (New York: Appleton-Century-Crofts, 1973), p. 19.
37. Ibid., p. 21.
38. Ibid., p. 23.
39. Helen Yura and Mary Walsh, *The Nursing Process: Assessing, Planning, Implementing, Evaluating* (Norwalk, Conn,.: Appleton-Century-Crofts, 1983).
40. Faye Abdellah, "The Nature of Nursing Science, Conference on the Nature of Science in Nursing," *Nurs. Res.,* **18**:390–393 (1969).
41. Kathleen Andreoli and Carol Thompson, "The Nature of Science in Nursing," *Image* **9**:30–36 (June 1977).
42. Florence Nightingale, *Notes on Nursing* (London: Harrison, 1859), reprinted by J. B. Lippincott, 1946.
43. Dorothy E. Johnson, "One Conceptual Model of Nursing," unpublished paper given at Vanderbilt University, 1968.
44. Sister Callista Roy, *Introduction to Nursing: An Adaptation Model* (Englewood Cliffs, N.J.: Prentice-Hall, Inc., 1976), p. 18.
45. Martha Rogers, *Educational Revolution in Nursing* (New York: Macmillan Publishing Company, 1961), p. 23.
46. Dorothea Orem, *Guides for Developing Curricula for the Education of Practical Nurses* (Washington, D.C.: U.S. Government Printing Office, 1959), pp. 5–6.
47. Myra E. Levine, *Introduction to Clinical Nursing* (Philadelphia: F. A. Davis, 1969), p. 10.
48. Lydia Hall, "The Loeb Center for Nursing and Rehabilitation," *Int. J. Nurs. Studies,* **6**: 81–95 (1969)
49. Barbara Stevens, *Nursing Theory* (Boston: Little, Brown and Company, 1979).
50. Madeline Leininger, "Caring: A Central Focus of Nursing and Health Care Services," *Nurs. Health Care,* **1**:135–143 (Oct. 1980).
51. Nightingale, op. cit., p. 63.
52. Styles, op. cit., p. 58.
53. Sister Callista Roy, "A Diagnostic Classification System for Nursing," *Nurs. Outlook,* **23**:91 (Feb. 1975).
54. Entire issue: *Topics Cl. Nurs.* (Jan. 5, 1984).
55. Elizabeth Hagey and Peggy McDonough, "The Problem of Professional Labeling," *Nurs. Outlook,* **32**:151–157 (May–June 1984).

10

Professional Ethics and Accountability

In earlier times, making ethical decisions in health care was probably not as simple as it appears in retrospect. But there were some givens: the physician was known to have the knowledge about the best course of treatment or action and was to be obeyed by the patient, the family, and certainly the nurse; there was a limit to that therapy, and when the heart stopped, the patient died; grossly malformed newborns and tiny prematures died too, with little expectation that they would live. The life span was considerably shorter, but if someone was dying of "old age," that was considered a natural, unstoppable process, and usually the dying occurred at home. Now, consider some not uncommon examples of ethical dilemmas today:

- A fragile man in his eighties, riddled with cancer, is admitted to the hospital. When his heart stops, he is resuscitated and awakens with tubes in every orifice. He begs to be allowed to die, but is repeatedly resuscitated.
- A twenty-six-year-old quadriplegic woman with cerebral palsy has herself admitted to a hospital and then asks to be kept comfortable, but allowed to die by starvation because she finds life unbearable. The hospital force-feeds her.

- An eighty-five-year-old man with many illnesses has been fasting in a nursing home to hasten his death. His daughter supports his decision, and he dies in a few days.
- Two physicians terminate intravenous feedings on a comatose man, with the consent of the family. They are reported by nurses and criminally prosecuted.
- A baby is born with Down's syndrome and various other congenital defects, one of which requires immediate surgery in order save the infant's life. The parents refuse permission because they believe that the child, if she survives, will not have a reasonable quality of life and they will not be able to care for her.
- Another baby with similar defects undergoes surgery, but the mother, an unwed teenager, cannot keep the child. It is in a public institution, requiring total care for all of its five years of life.

- A depressed patient admitted to a mental hospital refuses electroshock therapy after several treatments because he thinks it will kill him even though he is improving with treatment. He cannot care for himself at home, and his wife cannot manage his erratic behavior. He is committed, under that state's laws, given the treatment, and recovers.

- A retarded fifteen-year-old boy in a county home refuses kidney dialysis because he fears it. No effort is made to relieve his anxiety, and others on the hospital's waiting list are moved forward into therapy. The boy dies.

- Two men on the same hospital unit have a cardiac arrest within several minutes of each other. The first to arrest is an alcoholic street person with various other conditions: the other is a businessman with a wife and four children. There is one cardiopulmonary resuscitation cart. The resident says, "First come, first served" and resuscitates the alcoholic; the businessman dies.

- A young couple with two boys decide that they can only afford one more child and want a girl. If amniocentesis shows a boy, the mother wants an abortion.

- A couple had not been advised that they are carriers of a hereditary disease. Two of their teenage children have it, and one does not. When the mother becomes pregnant again, she decides on an abortion, but both parents decide not to "spoil the children's lives" by telling them that they may later manifest the disease.

- A well-liked nurse with many serious family problems seems to be under the influence of drugs or alcohol when she is on duty. The nurses are concerned that she will injure a patient and assume most of her assignments of very sick patients. They want to give her a chance to "straighten out her life" rather than reporting her and having her lose her job and perhaps her license.

- An older respected physician in a renowned hospital has been making mistakes in surgery. The residents have been able to catch and/or repair them thus far, but the scrub nurse thinks that he ought to be prevented from operating. No physician will report him officially.

- A patient about to undergo surgery clearly does not understand the risks or the available alternatives. The nurse tells the physician, but he replies that he did explain, that patients seldom understand these explanations, and that the patient should be prepared for surgery.

- A patient with cancer is on an experimental drug. Although hospital policy states that the physician must get an informed consent before the drug is administered, the patient's very prestigious physician calls in and tells the nurse to start the drug because it is important to begin at once; he will be in later to get the consent. When the nurse hesitates, her supervisor tells her to go ahead.

If you were the nurse involved in any of these situations, what would you do? Whose rights are or might be violated? The patient's? The family's? The nurse's? The doctor's? Society's? Nobody's? How much would you be affected by your own moral beliefs? If your action was contrary to what the hospital administrators, the physicians involved, or even some of your colleagues thought best (for whatever reason), would you be willing to face the consequences? What if your concept of "right" collided with a legal ruling? What if the patient or family asked you to help them?

All of these cases cited are real; a nurse somewhere faced one of these difficult situations (and probably others) and had to make a decision to act or not to act. How that decision was arrived at is the essence of ethics. As you read the sections on morality and the various theories of ethics, as well as the nursing code of ethics, consider the ethical problems given as examples, and note how your decisions depend on your ethical or, perhaps, moral beliefs.

MORALS AND ETHICS*:
A DIFFERENTIATION

There is a tendency to use the words *moral* and *ethical* interchangeably in the literature of the health professions. However, in the last few years, the need to differentiate between the two terms has become more evident, perhaps because the complexity of modern health care and the always-changing societal mores often create conflicting tensions in those who face a moral-ethical dilemma.

Kohlberg, structuring a theory of moral development, used the term *stages* for individual phases of moral thinking. In the 0, or Premoral, stage, the individual does not understand the rules or feel a sense of obligation to them, acting only to experience that which is pleasant (good) or avoiding that which is painful (bad). In the Preconventional Level, stages 1 and 2, the individual's moral reasoning is based on reward and punishment from those in authority. In the Conventional Level, stages 3 and 4, the expectations of the social group (family, community, nation) are supported and maintained. In the Postconventional Level, stages 5 and 6, the individual considers universal moral principles, which supersede the authority of groups. Kohlberg believes that most American adults function at stages 3 to 5, but moral maturity is gained at stage 6, when the individual makes up his/her own mind about what is right and wrong.[1] Although the term *moral* is used in this analysis, there are those who interpret stage 6 as a "universal, ethical principle orientation" because:

At this stage, morality is based on decisions of conscience, made in accordance with self-chosen principles of justice, which are comprehensive, universal, and consistent. These

principles are abstract and ethical, rather than concrete moral rules.[2]

Taking the viewpoint that moral values are usually based on religious beliefs, but also agreeing that an individual's ethics are based on self-examination, Maurice and Warrick state:

Ethical philosophy is the reflective analysis and evaluation of the goodness or badness of human conduct. Moral theology is the prescription decreed by divine authority regulating human conduct. Both ethics and morals indicate that goodness is that which leads to amity, wholesomeness, ease, peace, and well-being. Badness leads to the opposite. In short, goodness leads to happiness and order; badness to unhappiness and chaos. The difference, therefore, is the means to the end. Ethics deals with evaluation and responsibility whereas rules and obedience characterize morals.[3]

Churchill puts it more simply:

Morality is generally defined as behavior according to custom or tradition. Ethics, by contrast, is the free, rational assessment of courses of actions in relation to precepts, rules, conduct. . . . To be ethical a person must take the additional step of exercising critical, rational judgment in his decisions.[4]

The whole issue of ethics versus morals may seem to be a purely philosophical issue; however, given the differentiation described, the code of ethics of professional nurses may mandate action that goes beyond what their immediate associates see as necessary. It is also possible that individuals must struggle with what seems to be a conflict between ethical behavior and personal religious beliefs.

Approaches to Ethics

Curtin notes that not all health-care problems are ethical problems and gives the following characteristics of the latter: (1) they do not fall strictly within any one or all of the sciences; (2) they are inherently perplexing; (3)

---

*The term *ethics* will be used in this chapter, although *bioethics* is becoming popular in some of the literature. Frequently, *bioethics* seems to be used synonymously with *medical ethics,* and there are experts in the field of ethics who find its meaning unclear.

the answer reached will have profound relevance for several areas of human concern. She adds that some ethical problems are dilemmas, choices between equally undesirable alternatives. "A dilemma may not be solvable, but it is resolvable. Even though there is no right or wrong between two *equally* unfavorable actions, taking no action may be even worse than making the choice."[5] However, a true dilemma is relatively rare because often, if there is adequate information and time, there are clearer guidelines for action.

Three levels of decision making are described:[6] (1) the immediate level, in which there is no time for reflection, (the first deformed baby); (2) the intermediate level, in which there is some time for explanation and reflection (the individuals who want to die by fasting); and (3) the deliberate level, in which there is enough time to get information and to think and consult in order to make a rational decision (the parents with the hereditary disease). Curtin also indicates that the deliberate level of decision making is probably the most common, although people do not act in that manner because they find that difficult ethical decisions "are personally taxing, entail great responsibility and require a profound sensitivity to the human rights and values of others."[7]

The theories upon which ethical decisions are based are well described by Davis and Aroskar, two other noted nurse ethicists.[8] The *egoism* theory or position says that a decision is "right" because the doer or "agent," in this case the nurse, desires it; it is the most comfortable for that person, without consideration for how the decision might affect others. An example might be that the nurse simply prepares the patient for surgery, accepting the doctor's statement that the patient was given an adequate explanation.

The theory of *deontology* (formalism) asserts that rightness or wrongness must be considered in terms of its moral significance. *Act deontology* considers the agent's own moral values. *Rule deontology* suggests that there are rules or standards for judging morally, often a command by God. Thus, a nurse may

oppose abortion because of either personal moral beliefs or religious beliefs. *Utilitarianism* defines rights as the greatest good and the least amount of harm for the greatest number of people. For instance, deformed babies might be allowed to die rather than be a burden on society for many years.

More contemporary views have been offered by modern philosophers dissatisfied with the traditional choices. Frankena's *theory of obligation* focuses on the principle of beneficience and the principle of justice as equal treatment. However, the definition of these principles leads to some confusion. For instance, distributive justice is seen as treating people according to their merits or equally or according to their needs. The difficulty of deciding which criterion to use can be illustrated by considering this theory in the case of the two men with cardiac arrest.

Rawl's theory deals with *justice as fairness*—the distribution of benefits (good) or harm (evil) to society. The agents are supposed to function under a "veil of ignorance," not considering or knowing particular facts about themselves or others, such as sex, personal characteristics, or social class. The two principles of justice are equal rights for everyone and the greatest benefit given to the least advantaged. With this reasoning, the retarded boy would take precedence over others for the kidney dialysis, and efforts would be made to persuade him into therapy.

The *ideal observer* theory proposed by Firth requires that a decision be made from a disinterested, dispassionate consistent viewpoint, with full information available and consideration of future consequences. While this approach can theoretically be applied to any ethical situation, the probable impossibility of any one person being able to do so might necessitate the involvement of other people, perhaps an ethics committee.

These theories, which have been presented very briefly, are often complex and sometimes appear more philosophical than practical. However, they provide an interesting framework for the study of ethical decision making.

Such an analysis may help prepare you to deal better with real-life ethical situations. Not that they are always dramatic. As Levine wrote,

> Much of the emphasis on ethical issues in health care has been on life and death situations, dealing particularly with the definition of death and the distribution of limited life-sustaining resources. But there are overlooked ethical challenges in the mundane, everyday routine activities of professional practice, and these have gone largely unexamined.
>
> Ethical behavior is not the display of one's moral rectitude in times of crises. It is the day-by-day expression of one's commitment to other persons and the ways in which human beings relate to one another in their daily interactions.[9]

Another guide to ethical behavior is a professional code of ethics.

The Status of Ethical Codes

In the last several years, ethical behavior has been increasingly a topic of discussion in almost every field—business, politics, law, and, perhaps most of all, the health field. One symbol of this focus might be the new interest in codes of ethics. Codes of ethics, by whatever name, have been common in professions for some time. It is generally conceded that medicine was the first profession in the United States to adopt a code of ethics, but law, pharmacy, and veterinary medicine were also early comers. However, in the last decade or so, one interesting phenomenon has occurred: ethics has become fashionable, and codes have been newly adopted by organizations representing business and industry. In 1972, a survey revealed that the number of codes, although still few, had doubled in twenty-five years.[10] By 1982, 75 percent of individual membership organizations had codes, with 50 percent backed by an enforcement mechanism. Associations with company members are less inclined to have codes (less than 50 percent), and few are substantive and fewer policed.[11] This, some claim, is due to fear of antitrust problems. The example most frequently cited is that of

the American Medical Association (AMA), which spent vast amounts of money fighting the Federal Trade Commission's ruling that the AMA code of the time (pre-1980) that banned all advertising was restricting competition. The AMA lost on this and other restrictions that the code mandated.

Nevertheless, both business journals and the popular literature have been commenting on business and industry's burgeoning acceptance of the need for ethical behavior (code or no code). In fact, they are being advised to police themselves, before the government does it for them. Possibly the new outlook is at least partly a reaction to political and other scandals involving "respectable" people. Legislators, stimulated by public pressure, have increasingly incorporated aspects of ethical behavior into legislation, with legal penalties for violations. Indeed, in 1980, the United States Senate itself asked the Hasting's Center Institute of Society, Ethics and the Life Sciences to assist them in formulating a new Senate code of ethics. The process and results make fascinating reading.[12]

In the history of ethical codes, there is almost no theoretical literature on how they should be written. There are striking differences in both the format and the content of various codes, and even more dramatic changes in the revisions dictated by social changes. Not just the AMA code, but the ANA code, described later, are excellent examples of these contrasts. Moreover in some fields, the codes are a highly important document; in others, the practitioners seem unaware of them.

Many codes are strictly aspirational in tone, with no enforcement mechanism stated (such as that of the AMA). Others, like that of the American Bar Association (ABA), separate "ethical considerations" from "disciplinary rules." The first is nice; the second can entail punishment such as disbarment. Trying to do away with the distinction in a new code caused years of debate in the ABA, with no agreement.

One ethicist states that there is "no consensus across different fields and professions about the nature, function, and purpose of a code," or on whether there ought to be a code at all. He notes, "There is a fair degree of public and professional cynicism about codes and a wide range of complaints about them— that they are self-serving, pious, or public relation devices."

While he maintains that he has found little evidence to support the very negative charges, he notes that professional codes share a common dilemma: is there a reasonable balance between hard, tight, narrow, enforceable rules and stimuli to moral ideals, however hard to achieve in practice?[13]

Nevertheless, a code of ethics is considered an essential characteristic of a profession, providing one means whereby professional standards may be established, maintained, and improved. It indicates the profession's acceptance of the trust and responsibility with which society has invested it. The public has granted the professionals certain privileges, with certain expectations in return.

> The public expects ethical practice and conduct from professional men, and it is angered by violations of standards which it assumes ordinarily control practice. Each violation diminishes trust. Without trust, a profession would perish.[14]

In that context, professionals today need to look at their ethical codes in terms of whether they are focused on the consumer or are more inclined to emphasize professional etiquette— relationships within or across professional lines. For instance, in the previous AMA code, a statement about not associating professionally with anyone who does not practice a method of healing founded on a scientific basis was aimed at preventing, among other things, medical referrals to chiropractors. This, too, was deemed restraint of trade, and no such statement is found in the current code or, as it is called, "Principles of Medical Ethics" (Exhibit 10-1).

A similar point in the ethics/etiquette debate could be made about the ninth statement

in the Code for Nurses, which implies support of collective bargaining actions. Although improved conditions of employment might also improve nursing care, one does not necessarily follow the other in terms of protecting the patient. It *does* protect the nurse from charges of unethical conduct.

It is perhaps because of the influence of changing times that the self-serving aspects of ethical codes have diminished considerably over the last few years and recent revisions of most codes are beginning to show more concern for protecting society than for protecting the profession.

NURSING CODES OF ETHICS

Although Isabel Hampton Robb wrote a book on ethics and nursing practice at the turn of the century, and although there were columns on ethics in nursing journals, there was no formal code in early American nursing. In the early nursing literature, ethics appears to have been defined as *Christian morality*. There is some feeling that this was due in part to the authoritarian milieu in which nursing existed. Nursing education valued obedience, submission to rules, social etiquette, and loyalty to the physician, instead of judgment, responsibility, and humanitarianism. What might have been a substitute for an ethical code, Lystra Gretter's Florence Nightingale Pledge, quoted in Chapter 3, illustrates the mixture of contemporary morality, ethics, and loyalty expected in 1893.* It also appears to be based on the Hippocratic Oath associated with physicians and supposedly drawn up at the time of Hippocrates to express the commitments of the healing practitioners. You may be familiar with some of that oath's precepts:

---

*In 1935, Mrs. Gretter revised the last paragraph of the pledge to read, "With loyalty will I aid the physician in his work, and as a 'missioner of health' I will dedicate myself to devoted service to human welfare." The 1935 version is copyrighted by the Alumnae Association, Harper Hospital School of Nursing, Detroit, Mich.; the original is not copyrighted.

EXHIBIT 10-1

AMA Principles of Medical Ethics (1980)

PREAMBLE.

The medical profession has long subscribed to a body of ethical statements developed primarily for the benefit of the patient. As a member of this profession, a physician must recognize responsibility not only to patients, but also to society, to other health professionals. and to self. The following Principles adopted by the American Medical Association are not laws, but standards of conduct which define the essentials of honorable behavior for the physician.

[I.] A physician shall be dedicated to providing competent medical service with compassion and respect for human dignity.

[II.] A physician shall deal honestly with patients and colleagues, and strive to expose those physicians deficient in character or competence, or who engage in fraud or deception.

[III.] A physician shall respect the law and also recognize a responsibility to seek changes in those requirements which are contrary to the best interests of the patient.

[IV.] A physician shall respect the rights of patients, of colleagues, and of other health professionals, and shall safeguard patient confidences within the constraints of the law.

[V.] A physician shall continue to study, apply and advance scientific knowledge, make relevant information available to patients, colleagues, and the public, obtain consultation, and use the talents of other health professionals when indicated.

[VI.] A physician shall, in the provision of appropriate patient care, except in emergencies, be free to choose whom to serve, with whom to associate, and the environment in which to provide medical services.

[VII.] a physician shall recognize a responsibility to participate in activities contributing to an improved community.

Source: Reprinted with permission of the American Medical Association.

The regimen that I adopt shall be for the benefit of my patients according to my ability and judgment. . . . I will give no deadly drug to any. . . . Whatsoever things I see or hear concerning the life of men, in my attendance on the sick or even apart therefrom, which ought not be noised abroad, I will keep silence thereon, counting such things to be as sacred secrets.

The Nightingale Pledge is still recited or sung (as the Nightingale Hymn) by some graduating students of nursing as the Hippocratic Oath is recited by some graduating physicians.

After several years of trying to decide between a pledge of conduct and a statement on the ideals of the nursing profession, in 1926,

ANA's relatively new Committee on Ethical Standards presented to the ANA House of Delegates a suggested code of ethics (Exhibit 10-2). The purpose was not to provide specific rules of conduct, but to create an awareness of ethical considerations. The code is a realistic reflection of the times, and comparison with succeeding codes illustrates that although certain basic precepts of ethical behavior may persist, codes are altered by the demands of the times and changing concepts of an emerging profession by the professionals. For instance, in the next decade, nurses' ethical concerns encompassed such diverse topics as uniform requirements and outlining diabetic diets to a patient in the absence of a physician.[15] In 1940, a "Tentative Code," pub-

EXHIBIT 10-2

First ANA Suggested Code of Ethics (1926)

THE RELATION OF THE NURSE TO THE PATIENT

The nurse should bring to the care of the patient all of the knowledge, skill, and devotion which she may possess. To do this, she must appreciate the relationship of the patient to his family and to his community.

Therefore the nurse must broaden her thoughtful consideration of the patient so that it will include his whole family and his friends, for only in surroundings harmonious and peaceful for the patient can the nurse give her utmost of skill, devotion and knowledge, which shall include the safeguarding of the health of those about the patient and the protection of property.

THE RELATION OF THE NURSE TO THE MEDICAL PROFESSION

The term "medicine" should be understood to refer to scientific medicine and the desirable relationship between the two should be one of mutual respect. The nurse should be fully informed on the provisions of the medical practice act of her own state in order that she may not unconsciously support quackery and actual infringement of the law. The key to the situation lies in the mutuality of aim of medicine and nursing; the aims, to cure and prevent disease and promote positive health, are identical; the technics of the two are different and neither profession can secure complete results without the other. The nurse should respect the physician as the person legally and professionally responsible for the medical and surgical treatment of the sick. She should endeavor to give such intelligent and skilled nursing service that she will be looked upon as a co-worker of the doctor in the whole field of health.

Under no circumstances, except in emergency, is the nurse justified in instituting treatment.

THE RELATION OF THE NURSE TO THE ALLIED PROFESSIONS

The health of the public has come to demand many services other than nursing. Without the closest interrelation of workers and appreciation of the ethical standards of all groups, and a clear understanding of the limitations of her own group, the best results in building positive health in the community cannot be obtained.

RELATION OF NURSE TO NURSE

The "Golden Rule" embodies all that could be written in many pages on the relation of nurse to nurse. This should be one of fine loyalty, of appreciation for work conscientiously done, and of respect for positions of authority. On the other hand, loyalty to the motive which inspires nursing should make the nurse fearless to bring to light any serious violation to the ideals herein expressed; the larger loyalty is that to the community, for loyalty to an ideal is higher than any personal loyalty.

RELATION OF THE NURSE TO HER PROFESSION

The nurse has a definite responsibility to her profession as a whole. The contribution of individual service is not enough. She should, in addition, give a reasonable portion of her time to the furtherance of such advancements of the profession as are only possible through action of the group as a whole. This involves attendance at meetings and the acquisition of information, at least sufficient for intelligent participation in such matters as organization and legislation.

The supreme responsibility of the nurse in relation to her profession is to keep alight that spiritual flame which has illumined the work of the great nurses of all time.

Source: Lyndia Flanagan, *One Strong Voice.* Kansas City, Mo.: American Nurses' Association, 1976, pp. 89–91. Reprinted with permission.

lished in AJN, was not much different from the 1926 version. Even the more modern and first official Code for Nurses (1950) has been revised a number of times (1956, 1960, 1968, and 1976) and shows the influence of societal changes. For instance, the 1950 Code emphasized respect for the religious beliefs of patients; then, with the civil rights movement, the same statement was broadened to include "race, creed, color, or status"; and currently it stresses human dignity and the "uniqueness of the client unrestricted by considerations of social or economic status, personal attributes, or the nature of health problems." There is also decreasing emphasis on relationships with physicians and professional etiquette. The focus is on protection of the patient/client, and in this sense, represents a change to a real ethical code.

The 1976 version of the Code, with interpretive statements, was developed by an ad hoc committee of the ANA's Congress for Nursing Practice and is available from the American Nurses' Association (Exhibit 10-3). The interpretive statements are especially valuable because they not only enlarge upon and explain the code in more detail, but also provide more focus and direction on how the nurse can carry out the code. Particularly important is the first statement, which sets the tone of the nurse/client relationship as partners:

> Whenever possible, clients should be fully involved in the planning and implementation of their own health care. Each client has the moral right to determine what will be done with his/her person. . . .

Key areas in the interpretations deal with the nurse as patient advocate, nurse participation in political decision making and public affairs, and nurse involvement in advertising of products. Nurse accountability is a major issue and is considered important enough to require a separate statement; the code now has eleven instead of ten statements.

THE ICN CODE FOR NURSES

In 1933, the International Council of Nurses established an Ethics of Nursing Committee to study the method of teaching ethics in nursing, to survey activities by national organizations relative to ethics, and to collect data on ethical problems. From this evolved an ICN Code of Nursing Ethics which, after a long delay partially caused by World War II, was adopted in 1953 at a Grand Council meeting in Brazil. As might be expected, there was major emphasis on nurses, not the nursing profession. Nurses were expected to recognize the limitations as well as the responsibilities of their roles, especially when it came to obeying doctors' orders. With slight revisions in 1965 at Frankfurt, the code was retitled, the Code of Ethics as Applied to Nursing, underlining the commonalities in all codes. Finally, at the 1973 meeting in Mexico City, the Council of National Representatives accepted some drastic revisions (Exhibit 10-4). It was considerably shorter than the 1965 code, and many of the statements appeared to be combined and reworded. It was presented to the ICN congress as an effort to "enunciate concepts that would be clear, concise, universal, broad enough to be useful to nurses in many cultures but able also to stand the tests of time and social change." A striking change is one that makes explicit the nurse's responsibility and accountability for nursing care, deleting statements in the 1965 code that abrogated the nurse's judgment and personal responsibility and showed dependency on the physician that nurses worldwide no longer see as appropriate.

RESEARCH AND ETHICS

When the ANA Code was revised in 1968, the major change was the addition of a statement on the responsibilities of a nurse in research activities. Specific guidelines were delineated in the ANA publication *The Nurse in*

EXHIBIT 10-3

American Nurses' Association Code for Nurses (1976)

PREAMBLE

The Code for Nurses is based on belief about the nature of individuals, nursing, health, and society. Recipients and providers of nursing services are viewed as individuals and groups who possess basic rights and responsibilities, and whose values and circumstances command respect at all times. Nursing encompasses the promotion and restoration of health, the prevention of illness, and the alleviation of suffering. The statements of the Code and their interpretation provide guidance for conduct and relationships in carrying out nursing responsibilities consistent with the ethical obligations of the profession and quality in nursing care.

1. The nurse provides services with respect for human dignity and the uniqueness of the client unrestricted by considerations of social or economic status, personal attributes, or the nature of health problems.
2. The nurse safeguards the client's right to privacy by judiciously protecting information of a confidential nature.
3. The nurse acts to safeguard the client and the public when health care and safety are affected by the incompetent, unethical, or illegal practice of any person.
4. The nurse assumes responsibility and accountability for individual nursing judgments and actions.
5. The nurse maintains competence in nursing.
6. The nurse exercises informed judgment and uses individual competence and qualifications as criteria in seeking consultation, accepting responsibilities, and delegating nursing activities to others.
7. The nurse participates in activities that contribute to the ongoing development of the profession's body of knowledge.
8. The nurse participates in the profession's efforts to implement and improve standards of nursing.
9. The nurse participates in the profession's efforts to establish and maintain conditions of employment conducive to high quality nursing care.
10. The nurse participates in the profession's effort to protect the public from misinformation and misrepresentation and to maintain the integrity of nursing.
11. The nurse collaborates with members of the health professions and other citizens in promoting community and national efforts to meet the health needs of the public.

Source: Reprinted with permission of the American Nurses' Association.

Research: ANA Guidelines on Ethical Values.[16] The increasing participation of nurses in medical research as well as nurse-initiated research made this a timely statement. Certain points received emphasis: those implicit in the nurse's responsibility for rendering quality care, such as the protection of the individual's rights in relation to privacy, self-determination, conservation of personal resources, freedom from arbitrary hurt and intrinsic risk of injury, and the special rights of minors and incompetent persons. The nurse is expected to participate in a research or experimental activity only with the assurance that the project has the official sanction of a legally constituted research committee or other appropriate authority within the institutional or agency settings, and he or she must have sufficient

EXHIBIT 10-4

International Council of Nurses Code for Nurses (1973)
Ethical Concepts Applied to Nursing

The fundamental responsibility of the nurse is fourfold: to promote health, to prevent illness, to restore health and to alleviate suffering.

The need for nursing is universal. Inherent in nursing is respect for life, dignity and rights of man. It is unrestricted by considerations of nationality, race, creed, colour, age, sex, politics or social status.

Nurses render health services to the individual, the family and the community and coordinate their services with those of related groups.

NURSES AND PEOPLE

The nurse's primary responsibility is to those people who require nursing care.

The nurse, in providing care, promotes an environment in which the values, customs and spiritual beliefs of the individual are respected.

The nurse holds in confidence personal information and uses judgment in sharing this information.

NURSES AND PRACTICE

The nurse carries personal responsibility for nursing practice and for maintaining competence by continual learning.

The nurse maintains the highest standards of nursing care possible within the reality of a specific situation.

The nurse uses judgment in relation to individual competence when accepting and delegating responsibilities.

The nurse when acting in a professional capacity should at all times maintain standards of personal conduct that would reflect credit upon the profession.

NURSES AND SOCIETY

The nurse shares with other citizens the responsibility for initiating and supporting action to meet the health and social needs of the public.

NURSES AND CO-WORKERS

The nurse sustains a cooperative relationship with co-workers in nursing and other fields.

The nurse takes appropriate action to safeguard the individual when his care is endangered by a co-worker or any other person.

NURSES AND THE PROFESSION

The nurse plays the major role in determining and implementing desirable standards of nursing practice and nursing education.

The nurse is active in developing a core of professional knowledge.

The nurse, acting through the professional organization, participates in establishing and maintaining equitable social and economic working conditions in nursing.

Source: Reprinted with permission of the International Council of Nurses.

knowledge of the research design to allow participation in an informed, effective, and ethical fashion. If the nurse sees conflicts or questions related to the well-being and safety of the patient, this concern must be voiced to the appropriate person in the institution. At all times, nurses remain responsible for their own acts and judgments. These guidelines not only give specifics in research ethics, in which any nurse might be involved, but provide a basis for discussion on the whole issue of human research.

A more recent ANA statement on the ethical issues of research is *Human Rights Guidelines for Nurses in Clinical and Other Research* (1975), developed by two nurse researchers and accepted as a position statement on human rights for nurses engaged in various kinds of research.*

IMPLEMENTATION OF
THE NURSING CODE

The ANA Code of Ethics, like other professional codes, has no legal force, as opposed to the licensure laws, promulgated by State Boards of Nursing (not the nurses' associations). However, the requirements of the Code often exceed, but are never less than, the requirements of the law. Violations of the law may, of course, subject the nurse to civil or criminal penalties. Violations of the Code should be reported to constituent associations of ANA, which may reprimand, censure, suspend, or expel members. Most state associations (SNAs) have a procedure for considering reported violations that also gives the accused due process. Even if the nurse is not an SNA member, an ethical violation, at the least, results in the loss of respect of one's colleagues and the public, which is a serious sanction. All nurses, whether or not they are SNA members, should be familiar with the profession's ethical code, for they have a profes-

sional obligation to uphold and adhere to the Code and ensure that nursing colleagues do likewise.

Implementation of the Code is at two levels. Nurses may be involved in resolving ethical issues on a broad policy level, participating with other groups in decision making to formulate guidelines or laws. But the more common situation is ethical decision making in daily practice, on a one-to-one basis, on issues that are probably not a matter of life and death but must be resolved on the spot by the nurse who faces them.

The Code, and particularly its interpretations, are useful as guidelines here, but nurses must recognize that in specific incidents, the reaction will be both intellectual and emotional and strongly influenced by the nurse's cultural background, education, and experience. Bergman has presented a problem-solving format to help resolve ethical conflicts, but notes that the nurse must also weigh personal beliefs, the customs and mores of the persons involved, and legal aspects.[17]

A nine-step procedure, developed in a course on medical ethics, may also be useful in helping nurses to make ethical decisions and to think through their own ethical beliefs. These steps are as follows:

1. Identify the health problem. This clearly must be at least brought to light, if not agreed upon, before any decision can be made.
2. Identify the ethical problem.
3. State who's involved in making the decision (the nurse, the doctor, the patient, the patient's family).
4. Identify your role. (Quite possibly, your role may not require a decision at all.)
5. Consider as many possible alternative decisions as you can.
6. Consider the long- and short-range consequences of each alternative decision.
7. Reach your decision.
8. Consider how this decision fits in with your general philosophy of patient care.
9. Follow the situation until you can see the

---

*The legal/ethical rights of human subjects in research are discussed in more detail in Chapter 22.

actual results of your decision, and use this information to help in making future decisions.[18]

In using this system, it is helpful to refer to the ANA Code of Ethics so that the philosophical concept is more clearly related to the reality situation.

ETHICAL ISSUES AND DILEMMAS IN NURSING

The major ethical issues for those in the health professions today have been identified as the quality of life versus the sanctity of life; the right to live versus the right to die; informed consent; confidentiality; rights of children; unethical behavior of other practitioners; role conflict (who's responsible?); and the allocation of scarce resources (who shall live?). Increasingly, these issues have become subjects of legislation or court decisions (as discussed in Section 5), but even this does not lessen potential conflicts in which nurses may find themselves. Not only must they confront the distinct possibility that their personal value systems may be different from that of the profession, but they are also caught in the value systems of their employing institutions.

In the first situation, they must come to terms with their responsibility to the patient or client, regardless of their personal beliefs. For instance, nurses today are faced constantly with the need to make decisions about their roles in euthanasia or abortion. The decision for action may not be easy. When it comes to ending the life of a terminally ill patient or participating in an abortion, the nurse may choose not to participate if the action is against his or her moral principles. But what about caring for responding, reacting patients? There have been reports of health professionals neglecting or even abusing (mentally if not physically) patients about whom they have moral reservations, such as homosexuals, criminals, alcoholics, or women having abortions. Clearly, this situation is intoler-

able and violates any professional code of ethics. These actions, however, are taken on a personal level, and grossly unethical behavior is probably relatively rare. The conflicts nurses face often come from another source. Historically, nurses were seen as servants of physicians and were expected to be obedient and loyal to them. (Note the Nightingale Pledge.) As late as 1943, a book on nursing ethics flatly stated that an employed nurse was the servant of the hospital and that disobedience to the physician's orders was a violation of the employment contract. Certainly she was never to point out his mishandling of a case; it was better to resign. The nurse was seen as having "a duty of charity as a faithful servant to a master to protect the good name and reputation of the physician under whom she works."[19]

Even as times changed and ethical guides for nurses became less blatant in demanding loyalty at the price of harming the patient, the health care system still fostered the notion of loyalty to the employer and physician first. In fact, in 1973, one study found that many nurses, the majority of physicians, and even patients saw nurses as being accountable first to the physician or the employing agency. Of those nurses who did not agree, half felt that they were accountable to the profession of nursing, and others, first to themselves and then to the public.[20]

Since that time, the attitudes of many nurses have changed, although the nurses who were socialized to believe in loyalty first to the employer and doctor are still in the workforce. That there might be attitudinal differences based on age was shown in a survey on the ethics of nurses by a nursing magazine.[21,22] Most of the 5,000 respondents were employed below an administrative level in a hospital. Most were between the age of twenty-three and thirty-nine, and identified themselves as being in the moderate range in relation to general views and beliefs and "somewhat religious." The findings were interesting. Nurses over age fifty reported "very strong" ethical standards compared with an overall average of 34 percent voicing that opinion. Seventy-nine percent also reported being "perfectly conscientious" on the job all or most of the time, a considerably higher percentage than other groups. On the other hand, despite the feeling of the respondents that they and other colleagues were ethical (and equally so), 83 percent said that they had had to compromise their ethical values for some reason. Hospital policy, self-protection, a patient's request or demand, and a doctor's request were the chief reasons, although supervisor and peer pressures were also mentioned. Nurses over fifty tended to feel more pressured by hospital policy and younger nurses by doctors' requests. Nurses with master's degrees were more likely to carry out a patient's request than other nurses. (Several research studies have shown that nurses with advanced professional education have higher scores on moral reasoning,[23,24] but in this case, it may also be true that nurses with master's degrees have more status, influence, and security than others.) Nurses who compromised their ethical standards worried most about harming their patients or feeling ashamed, but one-fourth were also worried about getting into legal trouble. Nevertheless, the majority had either kept information from patients or had deceived them about their medications. They were more honest with doctors than with patients and their families.

Yet in another magazine survey in the same year,[25] nurses indicated that the nurse should give the patient full information if the doctor didn't. Male nurses, BSN nurses, and students were the most likely to support that statement. (Later, a working nurse noted that students might be less eager to do so once they were in the workforce and had to deal with job constraints.) It might be useful to remember that nurses have indicated that they would act in a certain ethical way when given a hypothetical situation, but under the pressure of a job situation, have succumbed to doing what they were told, obviously wrong though it was.[26] The nurses also felt that people should be allowed to die with dignity and seemed concerned about calling a code for a patient with an advanced terminal illness; however, most stated that they would call the code—often because of legal pressures.

In a follow-up survey which drew some national attention[27] fewer nurses were in favor of euthanasia than they had been about a decade earlier, but about 15 percent said that they had knowingly hastened a patient's death. "Hastening death" was not defined. Actually, a higher percentage had acknowledged doing this in 1974, but it was thought that now "legal paranoia" made nurses hesitate to aid dying.

The theme of loyalty to the doctor seems to have diminished, according to the ethics survey, although nurses expressed frustration because they felt they could not act against incompetent physicians. Younger nurses were more inclined to report them than older nurses, but a general response was that reporting at the hospital level was almost useless.

There are many other specific patient-related ethical issues with which nurses deal daily, but the law is becoming increasingly involved in one way or another.* At times, it is difficult to untangle ethical and legal responsibilities; indeed, there are times when the law or the legal decision in a case does not seem ethical in itself.

This situation only adds to the nurse's dilemma, but the dilemmas are not nursing's alone. The health professions, especially medicine, are equally concerned about ethics and about how the law fits in. Moreover, the issues are public concerns. In 1978, President Reagan appointed a commission to study ethical problems in medicine and biomedical and behavioral research. The commission's reports† covered such issues as informed consent, the right to die, whistle blowing in biomedical research, protecting human subjects, implementing human research regulations, genetic engineering, and access to health care. They were decidedly pro-public, pro-patient reports. Among other things, they

---

*See Chapters 20 and 22.
†See the Bibliography.

included results of polls and surveys taken on crucial ethical issues and did extensive searches of literature. The reports are discussed in Chapter 22.

There are also intraprofessional problems of ethics that nurses must face—problems not necessarily unique to the profession. A serious issue is the number of nurses impaired by dependence on drugs or other addictions. In the last few years, both state nurses' associations and individual employers have developed plans for helping these nurses, but also for protecting the public from them.[28] In addition, responsibility is being taken in dealing with incompetent nurses. However, much remains to be done.

Nurses as Patient Advocates

Over time, it appears that more and more often, nurses themselves, and others, have come to see nurses as natural patient advocates.[29,30] In a sense, this has been manifested by the fact that long before the American Hospital Association published its Patient's Bill of Rights,* the National League for Nursing (NLN) had drafted a statement on what the patient might expect from the nurse.[31] (This was done at a time when no one told patients what their caregivers should be doing.) The statement coincided closely with the statements in the ANA Code for Nurses.

Then in 1977, the NLN released a new document on patients' rights (Exhibit 10-5). Again, this clearly delineated nursing's support for patients' rights. It might be noted that many of these statements are now law.

Despite nurses' desire to search for ethical solutions and act accordingly, despite their desire to act as patient advocates, there are still some concerns. Suppose the nurse does carry out his or her ethical and legal responsibilities, such as being sure that a patient has given an informed consent before receiving a particular kind of treatment. What if this action comes into conflict with what the doctor or the hospital sees as a limit to the nurse's role? Will

the nurse's job be in jeopardy? Will he or she be subtly punished? What if the nurse reports unethical or illegal behavior on the part of another practitioner? Again, what happens? Who provides backup support? Nursing administration? Nursing peers? What of dealing with physicians who are incompetents, drug abusers, or alcoholics? Does the profession protect the co-professional or the public? Unlike personal ethical conflicts, these are real dilemmas that may have serious economic repercussions for the nurse, and it is quite possible that a nurse cannot resolve them alone. Instead, nursing must develop a support system for individual nurses who experience conflict in the employment setting with respect to implementation of the Code of Ethics, and the precepts of the Code must be widely publicized so that not only nurses, but also the public and others in health care, understand the ethical basis of nursing practice.

ACCOUNTABILITY

Accountability is a concept which has been discussed widely in nursing literature. Nursing students have been told that they must have it in order to be professional; practicing nurses are said to be accountable because they are licensed; and primary nursing, a system for delivering care, identifies it as a basic component of practice. Yet, despite all of the discussion, there is little evidence that accountability exists in nursing. Possibly the reason is that nursing has not yet structured accountability as an integral and nonoptional aspect of its practice. Feelings of accountability are much like feelings of patriotism; most of us have them but do not find means of expressing them on a day-to-day basis. Whether or not one feels accountable should not determine the level of accountability of a professional group, such as nursing; rather, the profession has an obligation to ensure accountability on the part of its members.

Accountability, as a professional characteristic and responsibility, is discussed by Par-

---

*See Chapter 22.

EXHIBIT 10-5

Nursing's Role in Patients' Rights (1977)

NLN believes the following are patients' rights which nurses have a responsibility to uphold:

- People have the right to health care that is accessible and that meets professional standards, regardless of the setting.
- Patients have the right to courteous and individualized health care that is equitable, humane, and given without discrimination as to race, color, creed, sex, national origin, source of payment, or ethical or political beliefs.
- Patients have the right to information about their diagnosis, prognosis, and treatment—including alternatives to care and risks involved—in terms they and their families can readily understand, so that they can give their informed consent.
- Patients have the legal right to informed participation in all decisions concerning their health care.
- Patients have the right to information about the qualifications, names, and titles of personnel responsible for providing their health care.
- Patients have the right to refuse observation by those not directly involved in their care.
- Patients have the right to privacy during interview, examination, and treatment.
- Patients have the right to privacy in communicating and visiting with persons of their choice.
- Patients have the right to refuse treatments, medications, or participation in research and experimentation, without punitive action being taken against them.
- Patients have the right to coordination and continuity of health care.
- Patients have the right to appropriate instruction or education from health care personnel so that they can achieve an optimal level of wellness and an understanding of their basic health needs.
- Patients have the right to confidentiality of all records (except as otherwise provided for by law or third-party payer contracts) and all communications, written or oral, between patients and health care providers.

Source: Reprinted with permission of the National League for Nursing.

sons.[32] "Professional groups must, to some essential degree, be self-regulating, taking responsibility for the technical standards of their profession and for their integrity in serving societal functions." He continues: "where a division of labor is involved . . . this will always have to include the legitimation of the functions of the groups and types of activity in question, of the ways in which the standards of performance of those functions are upheld, and of the protection or enhancement of the rights and interests of those outside the groups of performers of the functions on whom the actions of such groups impinge."

Although the feeling of accountability by individual nurses has been and is valuable in nursing practice, the profession needs to manifest its accountability. This objective cannot be accomplished only by continuing to discuss and foster feelings of accountability. Accountability must become a structural component of nursing practice which provides tangible evidence of evaluation and decision making in regard to nursing within health care.

Accountability, as defined by *Webster's* dictionary, means "subject to giving an account: answerable." There is a clear distinction between the reality of being answerable and feeling answerable, and being answerable is essential to nursing's professionalization and viability. Manifesting accountability in nursing practice provides the opportunity to evaluate nursing's contribution within health care and is a means of clarifying the significance of nursing to society. As accountability is discussed in relation to professional nursing, two questions consistently arise: Accountable for what? and Accountable to whom?

Accountable for What?

Accountability for what is perhaps the more important of the two questions. The history of nursing is filled with the need to answer for things for which it was not accountable, such as: why the medication prescribed by the physician was not received from the pharmacy; why the laboratory failed to draw blood for an ordered test; why the patient received the incorrect diet; why housekeeping did not clean a patient's room; and why the Radiology Department did not perform an ordered x-ray before noon. This type of answering is not accountability; rather, according to Lewis and Batey, it is "recounting."[33] One can only be accountable for that for which one is responsible, and one can only be responsible for those things which are clearly designated and accepted as one's responsibility. In addition, one must have authority to act and be expected to use judgment based on a body of knowledge in order to fulfill one's responsibilities as a professional. Then, and only then, can accountability be expressed. Accountability is not a vague feeling or an obscure concept. It is a clear obligation which must be manifested as a structural component of nursing practice, based on responsibility, authority, and autonomy.

Nursing is accountable for those professional responsibilities which are allocated and accepted. Those responsibilities change as knowledge expands and roles evolve; however, at any point in time nursing must clearly understand the scope and specificity of those responsibilities for which it is accountable. Responsibilities are delineated in nursing through practice acts of individual states, standards of care developed by recognized professional nursing groups, and position descriptions of organizations. Also, responsibilities may be individually negotiated between a nurse and a client. Responsibilities in nursing should be consistent with and reflective of current knowledge and role definitions. Clearly defined responsibility is a component and the basis of professional accountability. Although the terms *responsibility* and *accountability* are often used interchangeably, they are not the same. Batey and Lewis define responsibility as "a charge for which one is answerable," whereas accountability consists of answering in relation to the fulfillment of defined responsibility.[34]

Accountability is defined by Mundinger as "answerable, which is, so to speak, after the fact. It also has the sense of outcome accomplishment rather than process. People are likely to say accountable when they are looking for justification of an outcome, whereas responsible is used more often when describing an action to be carried out."[35]

Mundinger cites the following interaction. "Two different professionals (a nurse and a physician) with the same client (or different clients) can be responsible for the same things (in terms of initiation and methodology), but because of different and unique theory and therapy, they will be accountable for different results."[36]

In order to fulfill a responsibility effectively and to answer subsequently for outcomes in relation to its fulfillment, one must have authority which is commensurate with the responsibility. Authority is the "freedom granted by one in authority" or the right to act. Basic authority in nursing is granted by licensure which recognizes knowledge required for minimal competency. Additional authority is derived from expert knowledge and the authority of a position. The nursing profession has established credentialing mechanisms which are recognized in some practice settings as validation of expert knowledge and are used as a prerequisite for increased responsibility and authority. Certification through the ANA specialty groups is one example of such credentialing. The important issue for nursing is that the potential for accountability is dependent on having appropriate authority to fulfill responsibilities. Such authority cannot be assumed but must be specifically allocated in order to have legitimacy for nursing action.

In nursing, the delineation of responsibilities and the allocation of authority to fulfill those responsibilities alone do not characterize professional practice. As discussed by Batey and Lewis, it is essential that nurses be expected to exercise autonomy and independent judgment, and that both independent and interdependent decisions which are binding be made in the fulfillment of responsibilities. Autonomy in nursing has traditionally referred only to those aspects of practice which were totally within the control of nursing. Today's health care environment precludes, to a large extent, a totally independent domain or practice; but autonomy as interdependent decision making is no less valuable and is essential to nurses' meaningful participation in activities (accountability). The expectation of others of autonomy in fulfilling responsibilities must be accompanied by the willingness of nurses to take the risks involved in decision making and implementation. Such actions can be defended only when they are based on theoretical foundations and not on intuition. Mundinger describes autonomy as the basis for collaborative practice, which is "equal cooperation in goal setting and in action."

Accountability in nursing means answering for those things that have been defined and accepted as responsibilities of nursing. Responsibilities must be consistent with and derived from nursing's knowledge base. Legitimate and commensurate authority acquired by expert knowledge and acknowledged by positional authority is essential to the effective fulfillment of responsibility. Professional nurses must be expected to exercise autonomy and must be willing to make independent and interdependent decisions as part of every phase of their practice. Answering in relation to responsibilities is the process whereby nursing can be evaluated and its significance rec-

ognized. The lack of clarity regarding accountability in the past has resulted from addressing the issue as a perception or a feeling, not a structural component of practice.

The American Nurses' Association (ANA) Social Policy Statement[37] defines nursing, points to defining characteristics of nursing, and discusses the scope of nursing practice. Broad responsibilities of nursing are contained within this document, and it is these responsibilities for which nursing as a profession must answer. In addition, nurses are licensed within each state to practice nursing, and nurse practice acts describe responsibilities for which all licensed nurses in each state are answerable. Individual educational preparation and varying degrees of expertise and experience determine the responsibilities of individual nurses in multiple settings. Each licensed nurse is accountable not only for the responsibilities defined by a nurse practice act, but also for the responsibilities of a job description which are contractually offered and accepted as expectations of employment.

Accountable to Whom?

ANA's Social Policy Statement states that "nursing can be said to be owned by society, in the sense that nursing's professional interest must be, and must be perceived as, serving the interests of the larger whole of which it is a part."[38] Because traditional nursing practice has evolved primarily within the hierarchical structure of organizations such as hospitals, it has often been unclear to nurses to whom they were answerable. Nurses have frequently interpreted the object of accountability as being the physician or the institution in which they are employed. These perceptions have contributed to the slow growth of the professionalization of nursing. In reality, the traditional role of the nurse consisted of performing delegated tasks or carrying out policies of the institution. In this sense, nurses were answerable to physicians and institutions for these functions. As nursing's body of knowledge has expanded and its roles have been delineated, the traditional object of answerability has changed. Nurses, physicians, and institutions are equally accountable for their specific functions within health care delivery, and there is now a sharing of accountability to society and the recipients of care. An increasing number of malpractice suits recognize this difference as physicians, nurses, and administrative personnel, as well as other providers of care, are listed as defendants. Ultimate accountability for nursing practice and its outcomes must be provided to its recipients within society. Nurses cannot claim immunity or justification for inadequate or inappropriate nursing care because they followed a physician's orders or an institution's policies. Consumers are demanding individual and collective accountability. These extrinsic factors in society provide support for the development of structures of accountability within nursing practice which will strengthen the professionalization of nursing and clarify nursing's role within health care. They also demand that nursing critically evaluate the quality and quantity of its contribution.

Some of the mechanisms employed by nursing to answer for its practice include licensure, credentialing, peer review, and quality assurance. The nursing profession has established a minimum level of knowledge which must be demonstrated by examination in order to receive a license to practice nursing. Many states have developed more specific standards of practice which are used as a guide by which to judge questionable practice. Several states also have criteria stipulating that additional education is required to perform specific nursing functions. Evidence of continuing education as a requirement for the renewal of licensure is a part of some states' standards. The purpose of these mechanisms of accountability is to protect the public from incompetent caregivers and to assure minimal competency as a requirement for the privilege of practicing nursing and advanced competency for expanded roles.

Credentialing through certification is a voluntary mechanism whereby individual nurses validate specialized or advanced knowledge in a given area of practice. This growing trend provides a method of demonstrating to consumers differing levels of knowledge and competence. It may, in some cases, be a prerequisite stipulated by an employer for specific positions or roles.

Peer review is another tool used for evaluation and accountability. The ANA has defined *peer review* as "the process by which registered nurses, actively engaged in the practice of nursing, appraise the quality of nursing care in a given situation in accordance with established standards of nursing practice." Four major purposes for peer review are given: (1) to evaluate the quality and quantity of nursing care; (2) to determine the strengths and weaknesses of nursing care; (3) to provide evidence to utilize as the basis of recommendations for new or altered policies and procedures to improve nursing care; and (4) to identify those areas where practice patterns indicate more knowledge is needed.[39]

There are two types of peer review. The first is a system which focuses on clients and recipients of care. Most peer reviews which focus on clients are done as a nursing audit. The Joint Commission on Accreditation of Hospitals requires the existence of such a structure in hospitals. This type of peer review includes both retrospective and process audits. Committees and subcommittees develop criteria against which past or present documentation of care is compared. Although the standards set for peer review are generally those determined by nursing in the setting where the evaluation is done, the ANA Standards of Practice,[40] made more explicit for evaluation purposes, are frequently considered a logical starting point.

The second type of peer review focuses on individual practitioners and theoretically gets to the essence of individual and collective accountability. Unfortunately, it is almost nonexistent in nursing or, for that matter, in other health care disciplines. Passos lists some of the problems associated with the acceptance and utilization of the total concept of peer evaluation.

1. Facing the issue of trust.
2. Relating professional standards, developed by peers, to the policies and procedures which govern settings where nurses practice.
3. Closing the gap between actual practice and the boundaries of practice as defined in nursing practice acts.
4. The confidentiality of recipient data, which must be dealt with in peer review in any type of "audit" procedure.
5. Helping nurses to accept the lack of anonymity of their performance—individuals must be identifiable if one of the uses to which we must put evaluation is the judgment of the level of accountability of nurse practitioners in the setting.
6. Cost analyzing nursing contributions at different levels of quality.[41]

She concludes:

If we cannot find solutions for the problems of how accountability is to be manifested, monitored, regulated and controlled, how will we know that a nurse behaving in a particular way in a given situation is performing with the professionalism for which she is accountable? If we fail to concern ourselves with the means by which manifest nurse behavior can be monitored and regulated, then there is no point in talking about the attribute. . . . [42]

Some recent efforts have been made within clinical career ladder review procedures to incorporate peer review as a component of consideration for promotion. However, most nursing care delivery systems are designed in such a way that individual excellence or incompetence is masked by collective responsibility.

Quality assurance programs within some practice settings are manifestations of accountability. Criteria are developed which identify the standards which must be met for specific practice privileges within nursing in a particular setting. These standards address requirements beyond minimal preparation and may be used for the initial granting of privileges or credentialing of current staff for ex-

panded roles. This activity is related to the responsibility of nursing to monitor its members and to ensure that standards set by nursing organizations are consistently met. In order to meet accreditation standards by the Joint Commission, most hospitals have established multidisciplinary quality assurance activities which provide a forum for interdependent decision making and evaluation of overall outcomes of care. Nursing must seize such opportunities to articulate its role and to make visible its documented contribution to and significance in patient care.

Some nursing organizations have structured their practice setting's governance in such a way that nurses involved in clinical practice have the right and responsibility to participate in its governance activities. Such activities include the development of policies and procedures, evaluation and selection of equipment and supplies used in patient care, recruitment and retention activities, and quality assurance and primary nursing committees. All of these activities have a role to play in the fulfillment of responsibilities to clients and offer a means of demonstrating accountability for nursing practice.

Societal forces now manifest an "era of accountability" which demands that one be answerable for those things for which one assumes responsibility. Nursing as a profession and nurses as individuals must justify outcomes of nursing care in relation to their defined responsibilities with regard to the quality, appropriateness, and affordability of care. In order to fulfill this professional obligation, each nurse must understand and operationalize the concept and structural components of accountability.

Avoid taking on responsibilities that are not clearly within the domain of nursing. Be sure that actions are documented at all levels of practice. Acquire the authority of knowledge and position for each responsibility. Be sure that it is understood that professional nurses exercise independent judgment and participate in interdependent decision making based on a specific body of knowledge. Be willing to take the risks of collaboration. Then evaluate the outcomes in relation to responsibilities in individual practice and within the profession, and answer to society for nursing practice. Then and only then will the questions subside as to whether or not nursing is a profession or what its significance is within society. Accountability in every aspect of practice is the challenge facing nursing.

REFERENCES

1. Lawrence Kohlberg and Elliot Turiel, "Moral Development and Moral Education," in G. Lesser, ed., *Psychology and Education* (Chcago: Scott, Foresman and Company, 1971), as described in Ruth Bindler, "Moral Development in Nursing Education," *Image,* **9**:18–20 (Feb. 1977).
2. Rosemary Krowczyk and Elizabeth Kudzma, "Ethics: A Matter of Moral Development," *Nurs. Outlook,* **26**:255 (Apr. 1978).
3. Shirley Maurice and Louise Warrick, "Ethics and Morals in Nursing," *MCN,* **2**:343 (Nov.–Dec. 1977).
4. Larry Churchill, "Ethical Issues of a Profession in Transition," *Am. J. Nurs.,* **77**:873 (May 1977).
5. Leah Curtin, "Human Problems: Human Beings," in Leah Curtin and M. Josephine Flaherty, eds., *Nursing Ethics: Theories and Pragmatics* (Bowie, Md.: Robert J. Brady Company, 1982), p. 39.
6. Ibid., p. 40
7. Ibid.
8. Anne Davis and Mila Aroskar, *Ethical Dilemmas and Nursing Practice* (New York: Appleton-Century-Crofts, Inc., 1978), pp. 19–29.
9. Myra Levine, "Nursing Ethics and the Ethical Nurse," *Am. J. Nurs.,* **77**:846 (May 1977).
10. Robert H. Smith, "New Directions for Ethical Codes," *Assoc. and Society Manager,* **7**:124 (Dec.–Jan. 1974).
11. Jonathan Walters, "Uphold a Code of Ethics in the Eighties?" *Assn. Mgt.,* **35**:63 (Oct. 1983).
12. "Revising the United States Senate Code of Ethics," Special Supplement, *Hasting's Center Rep.,* **11**:1–28 (Feb. 1981).
13. Ibid., pp. 3–4.
14. William McGlothlin, *Patterns of Professional Education* (New York: G. P. Putnam's Sons, 1960), p. 211.
15. Lyndia Flanagan, *One Strong Voice* (Kansas City, Mo.: American Nurses' Association, 1976), pp. 88–91.
16. "The Nurse in Research: ANA Guidelines on Ethical Values," *Am. J. Nurs.,* **68**:1504–1507 (July 1968).
17. Rebecca Bergman, "Ethics—Concepts and Practice," *Int. Nurs. Rev.,* **20**(5):141 (1973).
18. Mary Murphy and James Murphy, "Making Ethical Decisions Systematically," *Nurs. 76,* **6**:CG13 (May 1976).
19. D. T. V. Moore, *Principles of Ethics,* 4th ed. (Philadelphia: J. B. Lippincott Company, 1943), Chapter 13.
20. Minerva Applegate, "A Pilot Study for Determining Relationships Between Members of the Medical and Nursing Profession," unpublished paper, Teachers College, Columbia University, May 1973.
21. "How Ethical Are You?" Part 1. *Nurs. Life,* **3**:25–33 (Jan.–Feb. 1983).
22. "How Ethical Are You?" Part 2. *Nurs. Life,* **3**:46–56 (Mar.–Apr. 1983).
23. Patricia Chishan, "Measuring Moral Judgment in Nursing Dilemmas," *Nurs. Res.,* **30**:104–109 (Mar.–Apr. 1981).
24. Shake Ketefian, "Critical Thinking, Educational Preparation, and Development of Moral Judgment Among Selected Groups of Practicing Nurses," *Nurs. Res.,* **30**:98–103 (Mar.–Apr. 1981).
25. Ronni Sandraff, "Is It Right? Protect the M.D . . . or the Patient?" *R.N,* **44**:28–33 (Feb. 1981).
26. C. K.Hofling et al., "An Experimental Study in Nurse–Patient Relationships," *J. Nerv. Ment. Dis.,* **143**:171–180 (1966).
27. "The Right to Die," *Nurs. Life,* **4**:47–53 (May–June 1984).
28. "Help for the Helper," Special Section, *Am. J. Nurs.,* **82**:57–587 (Apr.1982).
29. Mary Kohnke, "The Nurse as Advocate," *Am. J. Nurs.* **80**:2038–2040 (Nov. 1980).
30. Gerald Winslow, "From Loyalty to Advocacy: A New Metaphor for Nursing,"

Hastings Center Rep., 14:32–39 (June 1984).

31. National League for Nursing, *What People Can Expect of Modern Nursing Service* (New York: National League for Nursing, 1959). Also found in Lucie Kelly, *Dimensions of Professional Nursing,* 4th ed. (New York: Macmillan Publishing Company, 1981), p. 181.

32. Talcott Parsons, *Action Theory and the Human Condition* (New York: Free Press, 1978), pp. 39–40.

33. Frances Lewis and Marjorie Batey, "Clarifying Autonomy and Accountability in Nursing Service: Part II," *Nurs. Admin.,* **12**:10–15 (Oct. 1982).

34. Marjorie Batey and Frances Lewis, "Clarifying Autonomy and Accountability in Nursing Service: Part I," *Nurs. Admin.,* **12**:14 (Sept. 1982).

35. Mary Mundinger, *Autonomy in Nursing* (Germantown, Md.: Aspen Systems Corp., 1980), p. 24.

36. Ibid.

37. American Nurses' Association, *Nursing: a Social Policy Statement* (Kansas City, Mo.: The Association, 1980).

38. Ibid. p. 3.

39. American Nurses' Association, "Peer Review Guidelines Proposed," *Am. Nurse,* **5**:1, 5 (July 1973).

40. American Nurses' Association, *Standards of Nursing Practice* (Kansas City, Mo.: The Association, 1973).

41. Joyce Passos, "Accountability: Myth or Mandate," *Nurs. Admin.,* **3**:16 (May–June 1973).

42. Ibid., p. 21.

CHAPTER 11

Profile of the Modern Nurse

Who are today's nurses? How do they differ from the nurses of ten or twenty years ago? Or do they? A study of the actual and perceived characteristics of nurses was part of the vocational image research done by social scientists in the 1940s and 1950s, and a great deal of data are available from that period. Later, these kinds of studies were carried out by nurses, particularly in relation to personality characteristics and attitudes. Unfortunately, most of the latter have been small studies by graduate students, with considerable limitations in scope. Thus, comparisons are difficult, particularly in the personality studies for which a large number of instruments are available.

The small studies on these topics continue, usually at the master's level, but national studies are limited. The best-known deal with nurse satisfaction/dissatisfaction (cited in Chapter 5) and with contemporary nursing leaders (to be discussed in Chapter 16).

A popular source of information about nursing attitudes is the nursing magazine poll. A number of magazines have found the poll to be a way of stimulating reader interest and maybe even attracting new subscribers. There is no question that they *are* usually interesting, but they must be considered with an objective

eye (some would say a jaundiced eye). There are, of course, some obvious caveats. First, usually only readers of that magazine are the sample. Second, only those who feel strongly about the particular topic are apt to respond. A more subtle problem may be less apparent to a casual reader. The orientation of a magazine and/or its desire to elicit answers that can be interpreted dramatically or that support a particular viewpoint may result in the wording of questions that could be read several ways. The further interpretation of the author or editor, and the points that are highlighted, can, intentionally or not, mislead the reader.

One example is a survey done by a journal whose editorial stance has been directed toward the nondegree staff nurse. The survey was presumably aimed at finding out how nurses felt about the entry into practice issue.[1] Unfortunately, the questions tended to be slanted toward expected answers—that most nurses in that readership did not agree with the ANA position that entry into professional practice should be at the baccalaureate level. In general, this was the answer that emerged; however, because of the unclear questions, the poll cannot be viewed as definitive, despite the editor's insistence. For instance, to the question "What would make you professional?"

47.8 percent answered bachelor's degree, 42.8 percent diploma degree, 16.8 percent associate degree, and 19.1 percent equivalency exam. It appeared that almost everyone supported his or her own program, and a few more opted for the baccalaureate. Yet, at another point, most agreed that advanced education was desirable. In the long run, the only clear result of the poll was that it showed that many of the nurses who responded had a somewhat confused picture of what the ANA position really was—a situation that caused considerable emotionalism, because their inaccurate interpretation was that nurses without baccalaureate degrees would find both their status and their jobs threatened. That alone, of course, does present one aspect of nursing attitudes at the time. The same magazine had readers respond, by coupon, to a single question, "Have you ever thought of giving it [nursing] up?" Although only 500 answered out of the over 300,000 readers the magazine claimed to have, the editors insisted that the respondents were representative. Perhaps they were, since the reasons given for wanting to leave were almost identical to the complaints of most staff nurses—poor salaries and working conditions, lack of status, and lack of respect by administrators. But few people in any field could say that they *never* thought of giving up their work, so the question was more dramatic than useful. An interesting point is that listed among the jobs nurses took "when they left *nursing*" were industrial, home care, office, and public health *nursing*![2] Some of these surveys will be reported, with some warnings about perceptions and interpretation. It may or may not be significant that the number of respondents is dropping considerably.

For demographic data, there is a greater likelihood of obtaining national samples, and in these the difficulty lies in the inconsistency of study components from year to year. Overall, however, the studies and surveys are rather provocative and present an interesting overview of the practitioners of nursing today. The heterogeneity of nursing is quickly evident, for today's nursing workforce in-

cludes men and women who might have graduated forty-five years ago, as well as new graduates. Therefore, their attitudes and perhaps their behavior have been affected by concepts that span that time period.

There are also differences between the image and the reality. This has always been true. When Dickens wrote about the slovenly Sairey Gamp, dedicated women were functioning as nurses. Even the British newspapers' glowing reports of Florence Nightingale as the gentle lady with the lamp overlooked her tough and efficient administrative stance, which had a large part in providing better care for soldiers in the Crimea. Nevertheless, Simmons, who has summarized a large number of these studies, notes that these role images operate as forces in the social milieu to promote or impede progress in nursing.[3] Indeed, the American Academy of Nursing found the public image of nursing so detrimental that changing the image was made a priority for the 1980s.

This chapter, in building a profile of the modern nurse (and student), will deal with four major entities: demographic data, personality characteristics of nurses, nursing attitudes, and the nurse as seen by the public. Comparisons to previous data are made when useful. Obviously, it is necessary to present only a synopsis of the available data, but both the references and the bibliography will provide useful follow-up. Additional data about today's nurses are also incorporated in other chapters, such as 9, 10, 13, and 15.

GENERAL DEMOGRAPHIC DATA

The most current, general, comprehensive demographic data about nurses comes out of the Division of Nursing of the Department of Health and Human Services. The most recent (as of early 1985) is the 1980 report.[4] There are later data (1982) indicating an increase in numbers, but they provide no detailed information. Where possible, comparisons will be made with the 1977 survey[5] (Table 11-1).

There are easily discerned trends, even in

TABLE 11-1
Who Are the Nurses?

	1980	1977
Total RN population	1.7 million	1.4 million
Employed in nursing*	76.6%	69.8%
	(about 32% part time)	(about 30% part time)
Sex		
Female	96.1%	98.0%
Male	3.0%	2.0%
Ethnic-racial background		
White/non-Hispanic	90.4%	92.0%
Black	4.3%	2.5%
Asian/Islander	2.4%	2.1%
Hispanic	1.4%	1.4%
American Indian/Alaskan Native	0.28%	0.20%
Age		
Under 25	9.6%	6.0%
25–34	36.2%	30.3%
35–44	23.3%	24.1%
45–54	17.2%	19.8%
55–64	15.7%	15.8%
65 or over	4.5%	5.8%
Marital status		
Married	70.6%	68.9%
Divorced, separated, widowed	13.8%	12.0%
Never married	14.8%	14.0%
Places of employment		
Hospital	65.6%	61.4%
Nursing home	8.0%	8.1%
Community health	6.6%	7.9%
Physician's office	5.7%	7.1%
Nursing education	3.7%	3.9%
Student health service	3.5%	4.2%
Occupational health	2.3%	2.5%
Private duty nursing	1.6%	2.9%
Other	1.7%	1.0%
Type of position		
Staff nurse	65.0%	63.6%
Head nurse and supervisor	13.1%	15.5%
Administration (service and education)	4.8%	4.9%
Instructor	4.7%	4.9%
Clinical specialist/clinician	2.1%	2.0%
Nurse practitioner/midwife	1.3%	1.0%
Nurse anesthetist	1.1%	1.3%
Other	6.8%	8.6%
Higher educational preparation		
Doctorate	0.2%	0.2%
Master's	5.1%	3.9%
Baccalaureate in nursing	20.7%	15.9%
Other baccalaureate	2.6%	1.6%
Diploma	50.7%	67.0%
Associate degree	20.1%	11.3%

*Data refer to *employed* nurses. Some figures do not total 100% because of no response.
Source: U.S. Department of Health and Human Services, Health Resources and Services Administration.

this short period, and even more when earlier data are reviewed. For instance, there is a slow but perceptible increase in men and ethnic minorities. Also, the average age of the working nurse is dropping somewhat, and fewer nurses over sixty-five are working (possibly because of the availability of pensions including Social Security, a relatively recent development). The younger nurse appears to be staying in the workforce longer. There is still a decline during the prime childbearing ages, but an increase from forty-five to forty-nine. Married nurses tend to work part time, but are increasingly more inclined to work. An interesting phenomenon is that about one out of seven nurses now holds a second job, usually with a temporary nurse agency. While the *percentage* of nurses in nurse clinician/nurse practitioner positions has not increased, this category hardly existed a decade ago because of the few nurses involved. In terms of education, the decline of the diploma as the most common educational credential is clear; undoubtedly, a number of nurses have now added a baccalaureate. Something that is not evident in the statistics has been reported by educational programs, particularly at the baccalaureate and higher levels—an increase in the number of second careerists into nursing. The fact that these people already hold degrees and are therefore older when they enter nursing will change the statistics and, perhaps, the face of nursing.

THE NURSING CAREER PATTERN STUDY

Probably the most comprehensive current study of nurses, which includes more specific details, is the longitudinal NLN Nursing Career Pattern Study, begun in 1962. It was designed to obtain definitive biographical characteristics of nursing students, their occupational goals, and their reasons for their choice of nursing as a career. Later, the Department of Health, Education and Welfare (DHEW) supported extension of the study to include students who entered associate degree, diploma, and baccalaureate RN programs in 1965 and 1967. The 6,893 students who graduated from the 259 basic nursing programs in the 1962 group became part of the cohort that was surveyed one, five, ten, and fifteen years after graduation.* Although declining over that period, from 96 percent the first year, the response rate for the 15 year segment was still at 70 percent. The study was completed in 1981, and the reports in total probably supply the most comprehensive data on nurses practicing today.[6]

Almost all students admitted to the three programs were women. The highest percentage of men (4.5 percent) occurred in an associate degree program in 1967. Most students were native born. Most entering students were eighteen or nineteen, but those in associate degree programs were usually older, only a little more than 50 percent being under twenty. Approximately one fourth of the AD students were or had been married, compared to 4 percent in the other programs. More than a third of the married students in AD programs reported having three or more children, compared to one fifth of the married diploma students.

More than 95 percent of all students entering diploma programs, 92 percent in baccalaureate, and 90 percent in AD programs were white. The number of blacks entering baccalaureate programs increased slightly in 1967, but decreased in AD programs. Never was there the proportional ethnic distribution of white and black equal to the United States census data (around 11 percent black). Most students indicated affiliation with a Christian religion. Higher proportions of students entering diploma programs were Catholic, possibly because a number of Catholic groups continue to operate diploma schools, so that if a student wishes a religiously affiliated school, the diploma program would be readily available. The oldest child, usually a daughter, en-

---

*The original number of entering students was 11,439.

tered nursing in all programs in higher proportion than other siblings.

More than 60 percent of entering baccalaureate students were in the top fourth of their high school class; almost half of the diploma students, and more than a third of the AD. The great majority of all students came from communities of less than 50,000, and more than 75 percent were attending nursing schools in their home state. The only geographic mobility was seen in baccalaureate students, of whom one-fifth left their home state.

Some of the students in all programs had attended a nursing school before, this being most prevalent (about 17 percent) in AD programs. Between 30 and 40 percent of these had attended a practical nursing school or were already practical nurses; a smaller percentage had gone into diploma and baccalaureate programs.

Generally, both parents were living and native born. Fathers of AD and diploma students were predominantly sales or clerical workers or had a skilled trade. For baccalaureate students, "sales or clerical worker" was also a frequent category, but professional or semiprofessional ranked second, followed by skilled workers. Only among diploma students did semiskilled or unskilled make up 12 percent or more of the total group.

Fathers of baccalaureate students had twelve and "sixteen or more" years of education most frequently; diploma and AD students twelve years, but a considerable number reported eight years or less education. Most employed mothers in all groups were sales or clerical workers; only in the baccalaureate group were service-type positions, usually schoolteachers, recorded. About 4 to 9 percent of the students' mothers were nurses, the most in the baccalaureate group. Essentially, students came from families within the $5,000 to $9,999 or $10,000 to $14,999 category. Students in all three programs received some financial assistance, those in baccalaureate programs requiring most (up to 41 percent).

The predominant reason for entering nurs-

ing, given by all students, was "to help others." About a third of each group said that they had chosen nursing because it is a good, desirable, respected, worthwhile, or rewarding profession. Around 15 percent thought nursing would provide good economic security, and a number felt that it was one field in which a woman could always find employment. Previous employment or volunteer work in the health field influenced a small percentage of students, and a slightly smaller percentage (between 5 and 10 percent) mentioned nursing as a calling or vocation, or implied some religious influence. Up to 20 percent simply stated that they had "always wanted to be a nurse." Most frequently mentioned as having influenced the student to enter nursing were members of the family, a friend, or an acquaintance, whose occupation was not mentioned. If the occupation of the helpful person was mentioned, it most frequently was nursing. These factors are quite similar to those found in a smaller study.[7]

Students also answered open-ended questions about the nursing program they had elected to enter. Of the baccalaureate students, most wanted both college and nursing and also felt that with baccalaureate educations they would have a better nursing career. Associate degree students selected their programs primarily because of the program length, and secondly for financial reasons. Reasons for selecting the diploma program were evenly divided between the belief that it would give them a better education and the length. In all cases, most students chose their specific school because they believed it was a good school and the location was convenient.

Essentially all students felt that they would do general nursing in hospitals after graduation, and almost all planned to work after marriage. Approximately 40 to 50 percent of the AD and diploma students were planning more education after graduation; the baccalaureate students were almost equally divided among "yes," "no," and "undecided" answers.[8]

A follow-up of the Nurse Career Pattern

Study (1975) focused on graduation and withdrawal from nursing programs.[9] A comparison of the AD, diploma, and BS graduates ten years after graduation presents some interesting similarities and differences.[10] At that point, only 9 to 11 percent had remained single. Of the married or formerly married (about 6 percent), only 11 to 13 percent reported having no children; between 65 and 68 percent had two or more children. Evidently, having small children affected the nurses' working patterns. Whereas about 90 percent were working one year after graduation, this dropped at the five-year and again at the ten-year mark to 60 percent (BS), 64 percent (diploma), 67.5 percent (AD). The reasons most frequently given were home responsibilities, children, and no financial need to work, as well as difficulty in getting suitable hours. The older married AD student, who had been the most likely to complete the program, also tended to remain in the workforce longer. The numbers of the married women working part time increased with the years and appeared to be directly related to child care. Most of the single and formerly married were still working full time in nursing. Only a little more than 3 percent of the diploma nurses were working in nonnursing positions, but double that number of baccalaureate nurses had changed fields, about half to other professions. Positions held by the nurses ten years after graduation covered almost every field of nursing, but more than 60 percent of the AD and diploma nurses remained in hospital nursing, as opposed to 42 percent of the baccalaureate nurses. The next largest percentage of AD nurses (7 percent and under) were employed in doctors' or dentists' offices, public health agencies, and nursing homes; baccalaureate nurses (15 to 16 percent) in schools of nursing, community health agencies, and public or private schools. Except for those who were working part time, only about 30 percent of AD and diploma and 24 percent of BS nurses remained in staff positions. In each group there were teachers, head nurses, and supervisors. In contrast to both AD and diploma graduates, baccalaureate nurses were most likely to be teachers and least likely to be head nurses.

AD nurses were most likely (84.6 percent) to have worked in two or more states, diploma nurses least likely (43 percent). All groups found it easier to get the type of position they wanted prior to 1970. The two major reasons cited concerning difficulty after that period were unavailability of either desired hours or the clinical field.

The final phase of the study showed some interesting trends in career patterns.[11] Six out of ten of the nurses reported working for ten or more years, with 27 percent having worked the entire time. The most likely worker was the older married female AD graduate whose children were beyond school age (or who had learned to manage school and children during her education). Because the others tended to marry within five years of graduation, they often showed a gap in service, but it appeared that there was an increase in return to the labor force after ten years. Except for the last five years, there was a decrease in full-time work.

As the time from graduation lengthened, fewer nurses worked in hospitals (down from 80 to 52 percent). Instead, they turned to positions in public health, nursing education, doctors' offices, and nursing homes. The first two choices may have been related to educational progress. Twenty-three percent of the associate degree graduates and 16 percent of the diploma graduates earned baccalaureates; 25 percent of the baccalaureate graduates earned master's degrees, usually in a clinical specialty. About 59 percent had made no further attempt at formal education. The percentage who continued their education is larger than that of the general nursing population, and Knopf states that this may have to do with the fact that they entered nursing during the "entry into practice" issue and recognized the need for further education—or that the better-educated might be more likely to answer the questionnaire. Those who had continued their education were more likely to be in the nurse labor force at the fifteen-year interval, but they were also slightly more likely to be working in nonnursing positions.

Knopf noted several disturbing findings. Three out of ten stated that they would not choose nursing again as a career. Whether that was due to dissatisfaction, the availability of other career opportunities today, or some other reason was not determined. (A similar attitude was found in some of the magazine polls.) However, baccalaureate nurses who would elect nursing again voted for entering the same type of program; about 43 percent of both AD and diploma graduates opted for their original program. Slightly more diploma and AD graduates than baccalaureate graduates stated that they would not choose nursing again. This may also account for the fact that over the years, an increasing number of all graduates, particularly baccalaureate ones, chose to leave nursing for other careers.

MINORITY GROUPS IN NURSING

Studies on the general population of nursing students and graduates are inevitably influenced by the fact that the majority of nurses are both women and white. There is increasing interest in the minority groups in nursing, such as blacks, American Indians, and Hispanics, but also including the male minority. In the studies now existing, there is some concentration on blacks, and questions usually focus on why they do or do not enter nursing, why such a large proportion do not complete nursing education programs, and possible answers to these problems. Reasons given that explain why many of the racial and ethnic minorities, who are often also considered socioeconomically deprived, do not enter nursing include lack of role models, lack of understanding of what nursing is, lack of proper counseling, and inability to qualify because of poor academic records.[12] A summary of some of these studies and others as they relate to blacks is presented in one study that concentrates on methods of retaining these students.[13] A specific group of disadvantaged black baccalaureate students given special pre-

nursing counseling and guidance, academic help, and orientation to nursing were compared to all disadvantaged students in the NLN Career Pattern Study (all programs) who did not have such concentrated attention. (Actually most of the latter were white.) It was found that the first group had a lower dropout rate, and fewer of those who did withdraw did so because of disenchantment with nursing or academic failure. It was concluded that such help is a key factor in retention, although most of the students did not need all aspects of the remediation programs. It was considered meaningful that underachievers in high school who successfully completed the nursing programs had been given academic, personal, and financial assistance, a fact that might have implications for student selection on the basis of test scores and high school grades. An interesting fact emerged concerning students who became RNs: both study groups indicated dissatisfaction with their working conditions—not their salary. It was recommended that a follow-up study determine the reasons for dissatisfaction.

A 1977 DHEW study on health manpower presented additional information on black women entering collegiate nursing.[14] (Almost no black men showed interest in the field.) About one in ten aspiring nurses in 1974 was a black woman, frequently from a severely disadvantaged background in terms of both education and economics. Black women students tended to be older than white students, and almost two in five were financially independent of their parents, more than any other group of females interested in health careers. They also expressed major concern about their ability to pay for their college education, but few received scholarship aid or sought loans. Therefore, it is not surprising that most enrolled in two-year colleges. Although unsure of their academic and mathematical ability, black women who planned to become nurses, like their white counterparts, rated themselves high on public speaking, writing, leadership, popularity, intellectual and social self-confidence, motivation, and physical attractiveness, and they set a high priority on helping others. They seemed to have a wider range of interests and were more concerned with future financial success and less in raising a family.

Nursing recruitment for all ethnic minorities has gradually increased, stimulated particularly by federal grants available since 1965. By 1980,[15] RNs with minority racial-ethnic backgrounds accounted for about 7.2 percent of the nurse population; about 14.1 percent of the total U.S. resident population consists of these minorities. In 1981, over 10 percent of the enrollments in schools of nursing were minority students, with baccalaureate programs having the largest percentage (12.8 percent). In an NLN survey, 77 percent of the responding programs reported having admitted at least one minority student; 65 percent reported graduating at least one. Both seem surprisingly low.* As it now stands, a little more than one-third of the minority nurses in the workforce hold a diploma, and slightly fewer a baccalaureate. Seven percent have earned master's or doctoral degrees. Thus, a higher percentage of minority nurses hold baccalaureate or higher degrees than their white counterparts. Those most likely to have a baccalaureate are Asians (45.7 percent); blacks are more likely to have ADs, and the others diplomas. The American Indian/Alaskan Native group is the most likely minority to have a master's degree, but the number is very small. A very positive factor in the increase in doctoral minority nurses has been the American Nurses' Association (ANA) Minority Fellowship Program that began in 1974. It provided stipends and other forms of support to ethnic-minority students seeking doctoral education.[16]

Minority nurses at all educational levels continue to exhibit higher employment patterns, with about 89 percent employed in nursing. Those employed in nursing are younger than those not employed; most are married, but over 20 percent have never married. Other demographic data available are similar to those of the general nursing population.

Men have been neglected as potential sources of nurse power, although male nurses have existed almost as long as female nurses in the United States. By 1910, about 7 percent of all student and graduate nurses were men, but in succeeding years the percentage declined, until by 1940 it had dropped to 2 percent. Most men were graduates of hospital schools connected with mental institutions; not many schools (for men) were affiliated with general hospitals, and few coeducational ones existed.*

Men suffered the same discrimination in nursing that women encountered in male-dominated fields, although this was not always the fault of nursing. For instance, male nurses were kept in the enlisted ranks in the regular armed services until 1966, when, with the continuous pressure of the ANA, commissions were finally available to them in the Regular Nurse Corps. During World War II, male nursing students were not exempt from the draft, although the need for nurses was critical. Therefore, nursing enrollment for men dropped drastically to fewer than 200. After the war, enrollment began to climb slowly until in the 1971–1972 academic year, a total of 5,170 men, about 6 percent, were admitted to basic RN programs, nearly twice the proportion enrolling over the previous three years, and 2,751 to PN programs (more than in any other type of program). Of the RN programs, most men were enrolled in associate degree programs and the fewest in diploma programs. Graduation figures for men were also higher: in the next years, the percentage of men enrolled remained at about 5 percent in RN programs and 4 percent in PN programs, as did the percentage in the workforce (2 percent). By 1981, there was still about a 5 percent enrollment in both RN and PN programs, although the percentage in the workforce rose (Table 11-1).

---

*Practical nurse (PN) programs report 91 percent.

*See Chapter 3.

The increase in enrollment may be attributed in part to the Nurse Training Act of 1971, which called for identification and recruitment of "individuals with a potential for education or training in the nursing profession." Two interesting programs that developed at that time were an AD program in Texas aimed at discharged medical corpsmen and an evening diploma program in New York for retiring policemen and firemen. Completion rates have been considerably higher than those for other types of nursing schools, but then the major reasons given by many men for entering the field were job availability, security, and mobility, as well as working conditions and salary. (Interest in people is also a factor.)

Although the 1980 survey did not select men for in-depth study, it had previously been reported that in comparison with women, more are employed in nursing after graduation, and of these, some 60 percent work full time. Like women, they are most likely to be employed in hospitals; their second choice (11 percent) is the military. Only one-third hold staff-level positions in hospitals, which may be related to their greater tendency to work full time and also their desire to move into better-paying administrative positions. Some female nurses, particularly those who are younger, perceive employer discrimination in favor of males, but although male salaries were found to be higher, this may have had to do with the selection of positions. Also, as with the black nurses, there may be some relationship to job choice in large urban centers.

Some surveys and studies show that overall, female nurses recognize that male nurses are accepted by both patients and physicians and believe that they can make a valuable contribution to nursing.[17] Discrimination has been highlighted primarily in assignment of private duty nurses and in the care of women in obstetrics and gynecology[18,19] and in nursing homes. Some have gone to court, with negative results for men.* The opposite belief, that

men nurses will dominate the higher echelons of nursing, is also voiced, even in other countries.[20-22] Studies (many using small samples) of the attitudes, values, personality characteristics, and concerns of men who choose nursing as a career show varied results, often related to geography and the time of the study.[23-27]

Comparison of several studies seemed to indicate that men are now less likely to come into nursing to increase their social and economic status, because their parents are already at a middle-class or higher socioeconomic level. It seems that men are influenced into nursing through previous contacts or work in the health field. Their families seldom encourage them, but usually do not object. Men report that although friends are generally supportive, they get negative reactions from other classmates and strangers, who show a tendency to view them as homosexuals. These attitudes have created some role strain for the men, as did women in authority. Students voiced opposing opinions that they were spoiled and favored by women in these positions or that they were discriminated against or at least treated differently from women students; some noted no differences. Small studies in personality have reported such varying data as: men nurses have more empathy than women nurses or any nonnursing college student; men and women in nursing are more likely to have similar attitudes and personalities than those outside nursing; and men maintain the high social values necessary to the nursing profession, at the same time bringing their own critical, rational, and empirical interests to the field.

PERSONALITY CHARACTERISTICS OF NURSES

Studies of the personality characteristics of nurses vary a great deal and therefore are probably more interesting than useful. Most involve only a small sample and are probably not applicable to the total population. Which

---

*See Chapter 22.

personality traits are studied depends both on the overall purpose of the researcher and the type of test used.

A much-quoted study using the Edwards Personal Preference Schedule (EPPS) focused on the personality characteristics of heterogeneous groups of nursing students as compared to female college students.[28] Considered most striking was that these studies indicated that nurses had a greater need for deference (need to conform to custom) and a smaller need for dominance (need to supervise and direct action of others) than the college students. Six of the seven studies indicated that nursing students have a greater need for endurance (need to complete a job undertaken) and a smaller need for autonomy (need to be independent of others in making decisions). Also generally indicated was a greater need for order (need to have things organized). There was some further indication that nurses had more need for abasement (need to give in and avoid fights) and nurturance (need to help others) and a smaller need for exhibition (need to be the center of attraction), affiliation (need to form strong attachments), and change (need to do new things). One interpretation made by the author was that these personality characteristics were encouraged by head nurses and supervisors and were perhaps acquired as a matter of survival on the future work scene. He questioned whether the more aggressive, independent, dominant, original thinkers had been forced out of nursing programs. There was some objection to Costello's report by nurses who felt it was extremely negative,[29] but he defended it strongly.[30] One of the critics of the study later summarized updated data, and some variations were found.[31]

In essence, it was found that over the years, neither those entering nursing nor those in the field were as likely to have these characteristics at all, or as definitively. However, although personality characteristics might be changing both because of self-selection into the profession and because of the changing environment in and out of nursing, the "old" personality is still present to an extent and is probably a factor in nursing's delayed progress toward autonomy.

Small studies have also been done on the personalities of nurses in various specialty areas, with inconsistent findings. All of these studies, although of interest, should be regarded with some caution. The lack of consistent findings creates some questions of overall usefulness, although the heterogeneity of nurses is undoubtedly a key factor in their diverse results.[32]

ATTITUDES OF NURSES

One kind of research on nurses that has been done continually explores their attitudes about nursing in general, work situations, and reactions toward certain kinds of patients. The finding of the NLN study previously cited, indicating that individuals entered nursing because they "wanted to help others," has been consistent over the years. Therefore, because it is evident that a number of students left nursing before completing the program, or did not work in nursing after graduation, and because nurses have also been accused of some indifference to quality care, the basic question arises: why? A number of writers have cited "disillusionment with nursing" as a major reason why nurses leave jobs or nursing itself. Yet, further investigation seems to show that the disillusionment, for graduates as for students, is related more to the practice setting than to the practice. Whether the study is almost twenty years old[33] or one of the many new studies,* nurses still appear to find their greatest satisfaction in relation to patient care. Many are discouraged because they cannot give the comprehensive care that they believe in, but are forced into functional and bureaucratic work patterns and nonnursing tasks that do not give primary attention to the patient's total care.[34,35] In nursing, as in any profession, there are some who are primarily interested in nursing as a job or in earning

---

*See Chapter 5.

money—the so-called utilizer, migrant, or appliance nurse (one who works only long enough to buy a new home appliance). However, the majority of nurses still apparently have some of the same motivations with which they entered nursing.

How nurses felt about nursing and how nursing could be made more attractive to the disillusioned was a particularly "hot" topic in the late 1970s and early 1980s, when the nursing shortage became alarming. A favorite gimmick of some of the journals aimed at the "average" RN was to run reader polls to determine nurses' attitudes, particularly about themselves and their work setting. Often the response was quite good, in part because, as many nurses said, "Nobody listens to us," and as the experts said, those being asked about what ailed nurses consisted of everyone but the staff nurse. As might be expected, the complaints (quite justified as a rule) followed a similar pattern and related more to working conditions than to patient care. In the more formal studies done later, such as those reported in Chapter 5, the findings were similar. One example might be seen as fairly typical.[36-38]

In this study on job satisfaction, the three major dissatisfactions were unsafe practices, which included incompetent nurses and doctors; overcrowding and dangerous understaffing; poor leadership, with ineffective nursing service administrators and indifferent authoritarian hospital administrators; and communication breakdown both to and from administration. Nevertheles, 79 percent of nurses found their jobs satisfying (about the same as those in the NLN study). Nurses in administration, education, community health, industry, and schools of nursing were most satisfied. (Studies of NPs show that they are also very satisfied with their jobs.) In terms of clinical areas, the most satisfied were emergency room nurses and the least satisfied were psychiatric nurses. Four out of five nurses in hospitals believed that they worked in situations in which they were unable to take care of patients as well as they could or should.

A number of other interesting findings related to opinions about working hours, physical working conditions, and morale. Cited overwhelmingly as the most important consideration of both men and women in looking for a job was opportunity for professional growth; supportive nursing administration was also high on the list. The least important factors for women were fringe benefits, and for men, choice of hours or shifts. The fact that a 1974 study listed both salary and fringe benefits as high on the list of influential factors in seeking a workplace[39] may indicate that in the few intervening years these had improved enough to be generally satisfactory or that in any one region they tended to be competitive in like agencies.

The ambivalence of nurses in relation to job satisfaction and dissatisfaction may also be reflected in another magazine sample taken among subscribers.[40] The "average nurse" answering this questionnaire was a married staff nurse in her mid-twenties, working in a community hospital in an urban center, and earning $8,000 to $12,000 a year. She was not a union member but did belong to her professional organization. These nurses were ambivalent about joining unions, but the majority either approved or agreed that "someone should represent nurses, but not unions." Their major reasons for the need to organize were to make management listen, gain increased wages, gain more fringe benefits, and gain more say in the quality of patient care.

In a similar survey six years later,[41] nurses were about evenly split about the desirability or necessity of unions and whether professionalism and unionism were compatible. The strongest support came from younger nurses, the greatest opposition from nurses over forty-five and nurse managers. Reasons for a union centered on a "no other way" feeling about dealing with the administration. Opposition focused on the negative reputation of unions and their lack of real interest in or knowledge about nurses' concerns other than economic and similar job issues. Some preferred representation by the state nurses' associations, apparently not considering them "real" unions, but others found them inadequate. Generally, it was felt that unions were helpful in improving working conditions and economic benefits, but relatively useless in improving quality of patient care.

That the quality of care is important to nurses was indicated by another survey, first done in 1976 and repeated in 1983.[42-45] An interesting point is that in 1976, 10,000 nurses responded to the poll and about 2,300 responded in 1983. Why? Are nurses tired of polls, tired of the subject, or more wary? (The magazine released the first poll to the popular press, which created a temporary media furor about nurses and their jobs.) A comparison between the two polls shows that generally nurses are a little more pleased with the quality of health care (60 percent say it is good or excellent), although 15 percent still would not choose to go to the hospital where they work, for a serious illness. This view is probably not as negative as it seems, since it has been shown that both doctors and nurses tend to turn to a medical center for a serious illness, and most nurses do not work in medical centers. As might be expected, in the highly rated hospitals, nursing morale was high, physicians were considered competent, and there were patient care conferences and committees and peer review. Nurses in both polls rated doctors and nurses highly in providing physical care, but much lower in providing psychological care and family support. Nurses had firm opinions on the causes of poor patient care—primarily inadequate staffing, too many nondirect nursing activities, inadequate budgets, inadequate support from nursing administration, and interdepartmental hospital politics as well as nursing politics. This still held true for the later poll, but indifferent treatment of patients by doctors was also in the upper third of complaints. Rated as the "worst" departments were dietetics and housekeeping; nursing was considered by far the best (63 percent). Nurses receiving the poorest rating were foreign-trained nurses, agency nurses, and nurses returning after an absence of several years. Rated highly were LPNs, part-time and recent nurses, and nursing assistants. Floating nurses and recent graduates fell in the middle. Nurses also rated practices that improved care. Topping the list were nursing histories, peer review (nursing audit), and nursing care plans, followed by nursing diagnoses and patient care conferences. In the list of ways to improve health care, a major point was nurse autonomy and participation; also important was promotion of interdisciplinary teamwork.

Both in this survey and in the one on ethics, which was referred to in Chapter 10, nurses admitted to physician and nurse errors and incompetence, the reasons for these errors, and the action needed (see Chapter 20). Even more strongly, they expressed real concern about the life–death issues emerging from the use of technology—treating severely handicapped infants and the terminally ill, comatose, or brain-dead. This survey resulted in a larger response than usual and, if nothing else, brought some pragmatic realism to a philosophical topic.

Finally, a word should be said about nurses' attitudes toward certain types of patients. There has been some evidence that nurses do not view all types of patients equally favorably; for example, they tend to be more negative toward the elderly, alcoholic, criminal, mentally ill, or those with certain kinds of conditions. A number of studies, usually small, have been done on these topics. The purpose is primarily to determine what these attitudes are and why, how they affect patient care, and how to encourage or change particular attitudes. Actually, nurses do not react very differently from middle-class, white lay people, and that is what nurses are today. Apparently, nurses have not moderated their attitudes significantly.

THE IMAGE OF NURSING

As might be expected, people derived their image of the nurse from a variety of sources: personal acquaintance, contact during their own or someone else's illness, or the media—books, magazines, newspapers, radio, and television.

Personal acquaintance almost always introduces the factors of like or dislike with little relation to, or knowledge of, professional performance. The emotionalism involved in contacts during illness is inevitable, because neither patient nor family and friends can be objective then. The media vary the image according to whether an article is intended as a sensational exposé, a factual review, or entertainment. There is also some indication that an individual's social status has an effect on his perception of the nurse. The public has traditionally held two extreme images of the nurse (whom they tend to see as female). One portrays her as humanitarian, altruistic, more or less competent, and endowed with sympathy, compassion, and an exceptional ability to gain rapport. The other portrays her as a professional, well-trained, technically efficient, cool-headed and able, and relatively independent.[46] In the last twenty-five years, the concept of the nurse as a manager, removed from patient care has been added, and more recently, the nurse as supernurse.

In Birdwhistell's 1947 study[47] and Deutscher's 1955 study,[48] both in the Midwest, the upper class looked down on nursing, whereas the lower class considered it "the noblest of professions," and both men and women agreed that they would like their daughters to be nurses, in part because they could make good marriages and give their husbands and children the advantage of their acquired knowledge. In terms of social status (Birdwhistell), the upper class saw the nurse as somewhat higher than the hairdresser but considerably lower than the social worker—a skilled menial who would be tipped. The middle class placed the nurse higher than the stenographer but lower than the secretary, someone who works before marriage, a widow, divorcee, or career woman (someone who cannot get a husband or is a neglectful wife). Middle-class women felt that their own daughters should go to college, where they

would meet "people of their own class." All three classes considered the nurse "faster" or "freer" in sexual matters than women in other occupations. Surprisingly, a later study of nurse self-images showed that nurses' recognition of the last image was common, but they also felt that the public saw them as hardworking women with considerable technical knowledge and skill and generally devoted to their patients.

In 1961 Friedson presented somewhat similar findings. The nurse was considered most helpful by the lower class and praised for her teaching, counseling, and knowledge, but the upper class felt that she had little to offer.[49] Other social scientists agreed that, in general, the public did not see the nurse as a professional.

Although the early studies may appear totally out of date, remnants of these attitudes persist. One sociologist reports that the public is generally favorable toward nursing as an institution or profession within the general society and considers it prestigious and altruistic, but that in the hospital setting the image of the nurse is still associated with the performance of menial tasks; the nurse is an efficient and competent drudge who is an extension of the doctor's right hand. This sociologist feels that, in general, the image may be static, rooted in conditions existing five, ten, or twenty years ago, and that the nursing profession should make a serious effort to correct the image.[50] Others agree.[51]

At best, as one survey indicates, considerable confusion about nursing exists.[52] Although a vast majority of the public surveyed identified nursing as a profession, there was almost no support for nursing autonomy, and most thought nurses functioned best as assistants, not colleagues, of the doctor. The better-educated, more affluent respondents were more inclined to support nurses' expanded role, collegiality, and autonomy (although the latter percentage was quite low). On the other hand, they were least likely to want a daughter to become a nurse, and very few in any category, especially men, wanted a son to do so. Yet the adjectives used most often about nurses were: responsible, knowledgeable, caring, competent, skilled, efficient, neat, dedicated, and kind.

An examination of differences in occupational prestige as seen by physicians, graduate business students, and patients presents still another insight. Compared with a variety of physician specialists and others in the health field, patients rated RNs above some physicians, the director of nursing, the hospital administrator, and all other health professionals; physicians rated all nurses above other health professions or occupations except dentistry, as did graduate students. The most important criterion stated by all three groups was "degree of skill." A number of questions were raised as to how much the prestige rating was influenced by personal contact and how much by reputation or image.[53] In Maryland, for instance, where a 1979 poll to determine how citizens rated the various professions placed nursing at the top of the list, nurses were active in political and community affairs and quite visible as productive, respected professionals.*

There is no doubt that some misconceptions result from contact with various uniformed health workers in hospitals, who are not always clearly identified as aides, PNs, or RNs. (In the 1979 *RN* magazine survey, most people identified a nurse by the white cap and uniform.) But another major influence is the media. Interviews and research articles or programs generally portray the nurse in a reasonably accurate way. As a rule, however, in fiction, the media have not,† and still do not, correct a distorted image. Comic strips, novels, and television tend to portray the nurse (almost always female) either as a very sweet and/or sexy young girl, playing obedient handmaiden to the doctors, or as a tough,

starched older woman, efficient and brusque. The popularity of medically oriented television series in the 1970s was supposedly a reflection of the public's intense interest in the field. But the images of the nurses portrayed have been no more accurate, and even nursing advisers to the shows seldom get the script changed. On the screen, Nurse Rached in the award-winning movie *One Flew Over the Cuckoo's Nest,* which was also a book and a play, was probably thoroughly hated by millions of people. An equal number may have leered at the nurses in the British hospital comedy series or *MASH,* or even in the various pornographic films where nurses are portrayed primarily as sex objects.[54]

Even literature is not immune.[55] Still, in the last few years, one of the best-selling nonfiction books was *Nurse,* which gives an accurate description of nursing practice in a hospital. A Broadway hit focused on the struggle of a woman overcoming a stroke, and the critics commented repeatedly on the sensitivity and support of the nurse as an important ingredient in the patient's improvement. With the president's veto of the Nurse Training Act in late 1978, newspapers across the country ran articles, columns, and political cartoons indicating disapproval of the veto. There are also an increasing number of newspaper and magazine articles on the changing role of the nurse,[56] particularly in relation to the nurse-midwife and NP. It is a fact that a number of the latter were suggested or encouraged by nurses who recognized the importance of nurses' visibility as professionals.

Accuracy in the portrayal of nurses in the entertainment media will probably always be difficult, because the concern is entertainment, not truth. Inaccurate portrayal could probably be claimed by most occupations. Yet, some minority groups, through concerted action, have had some impact, as have women's groups, through complaints or boycotts. At the least, the inaccuracies have been brought to light. However, nurses will also recognize some of the nurse figures in the media, even if they are exaggerated. Are there

---

*As reported by *AJN,* December, 1979.

†Kalisch and Kalisch, funded by the federal government, have published a fascinating series of articles on nurses in the media. A number are listed in the bibliography.

not nurses, like Rached, who are dominating, prejudiced, rigid, even cruel in their practice? Eliminating them might be important in changing the public image, for then fiction will not imitate fact. It would also help if nurses themselves did not tarnish the image of nursing, as when they pose nude in pornographic magazines or show contempt for nursing.[57]

One concern of nurses is how physicians perceive them and their profession. Historically, the perception is of an inferior, with some interesting ramifications. The Deutscher study revealed that physicians tended to place nurses slightly below teachers but above social workers in occupational ratings (but thought nurses more humanitarian than teachers). On a scale of saint, Sunday school teacher, housewife, waitress, or "loose woman," to choose the term which to them most resembled a nurse, the majority chose the morally neutral category of housewife. (The next highest categories were saint and Sunday school teacher.) Another interesting point is that older physicians generally rated nurses more favorably on all questions than did younger physicians. This was also true of another study, where, in addition, physicians objected to professionalization of nurses.[58]

If physicians' current image of the nursing *profession* can be equated with their image of the nurse, it is clear that their perceptions are as confused as they were 100 years ago. (See Chapters 3 and 4.) Now, as then, there are physicians and leaders in organized medicine who see and applaud the changes in nursing toward full professionalism; others find this trend either threatening, incongruent with what they think a nurse's role should be, or not as desirable as the "good old days."[59]

Supporting this contention is another survey by a nursing journal.[60] The vast majority of physicians surveyed saw nurses as their assistants and gave extremely limited definitions of nursing. Younger physicians were more inclined to think that nurses needed BSNs, encouraged expanded roles, and favored (to a minor degree) giving nurses more responsibil-

ity. The clinical expertise of nurses, as defined by physicians, was praised by most. Although this survey presents some interesting viewpoints, it should be remembered that the kinds of questions asked frequently create a particular slant to such polls. For instance, another physician survey published in another journal within the same time frame seemed to contradict not only the findings of the other survey but nurses' concepts of physicians' attitudes.[61]

A final comment should be made about the patient's image of an ideal nurse. Individuals, particularly when writing as former patients, have indicated that they wanted to be treated as human beings—wanted the nurse to be kind, friendly, pleasant, courteous, considerate, smiling, concerned, and reassuring. They are often not concerned with her competence but simply trust her to be safe. In one study, "tender touch" was cited as the nurse's most important trait. A composite picture of the ideal nurse image as described in interviews with patients and nonpatients in a 1960 study revealed:

> She is qualified to the degree of being proficient. That is to say, she really knows her job. It's most important for her to understand me; that is, she can put herself into my shoes, experience some of my problems. While she is performing her work she expresses a sort of gentleness and friendliness. She is well-informed in other than her major role responsibilities. She is congenial with others, even though I am her primary concern. She appears to be happy. I don't mean that she is "bubbling over," but she is a person who seems to be enjoying life. Whenever I need her most, she is right there supporting me. I want to be able to really talk to her, and I expect her to be able to express herself well. Sometimes, even before I become uncomfortable, she will anticipate my needs and make me comfortable. When she performs a function she takes time to explain the "whys" and "hows" of it. She is always clean and well-groomed; and finally, I guess I do want her to feel sorry for me at certain times.[62]

The magazine surveys and other public feedback give some evidence that patients may not feel too differently today, especially older people.[63,64]

Obviously, there is no one profile of the modern nurse, particularly in these dynamic times. However, the information obtained from these various studies tells us a great deal about the practitioners of nursing. An oft-quoted but unidentified statement defines nurses as a "migrating mass of maidens mediating matrimony." That may still be true in some cases, but it tells only a small part of the nursing story.

REFERENCES

1. Anthony Lee, "No!" *RN,* **42**:83–93 (Jan. 1979).
2. "Getting Fed Up?" *RN,* **44**:18–25 (Jan. 1981).
3. Leo Simmons and Virginia Henderson, *Nursing Research—A Survey and Assessment* (New York: Appleton-Century-Crofts, 1964), p. 172.
4. "The Registered Nurse Population, an Overview," *National Sample Survey of Registered Nurses, November 1980* (revised Nov. 1982) (U.S. Department of Health and Human Services, PHS, HRSA, BHP, DHHS), Publication No. HRS-P-OD-83-1.
5. Aleda Roth et al., *1977 National Survey of Registered Nurses* (Kansas City, Mo: American Nurses' Association, 1979).
6. Lucille Knopf, *From Student to RN* (Bethesda, Md.: Department of Health, Education, and Welfare, 1972).
7. Joe Taylor and Frances Richter, "What Motivates Students Into Nursing?" *Hospitals,* **213**:59–61 (Jan. 1, 1969).
8. Knopf, op. cit., pp. 7–17.
9. Lucille Knopf, *Graduation and Withdrawal from RN Programs* (Bethesda Md.: Department of Health, Education and Welfare, 1975).
10. "Nurse Career Pattern Study: Baccalaureate Degree Nurses Ten Years After Graduation," *NLN Data Digest* (Mar. 1979).
11. Lucille Knopf, "Registered Nurses Fifteen Years After Graduation: Findings from the Nurse Career-Pattern Study," *Nurs. Health Care,* **4**:72–76 (Feb. 1983).
12. Michael Miller, "On Blacks Entering Nursing," *Nurs. Forum*, **11**:248–263 (Summer, 1972).
13. M. Elizabeth Carnegie, *Disadvantaged Students in RN Programs* (New York: National League for Nursing, 1974).
14. *Freshmen Interested in Nursing and Allied Health Professions: A Summary Report,* DHEW Publication No. HRA 77-46, 1977.
15. *Facts About Nursing 82–83* (Kansas City, Mo.: American Nurses' Association, 1983), pp. 24, 122.
16. Hattie Bessent, *Future Nurse Researchers,* Vols. I and II (Kansas City, Mo.: American Nurses Association, 1983).
17. Myron D. Fottles, "Attitudes of Female Nurses Toward Male Nurses," *J. Health Soc. Behav.,* **17**:98–110 (June 1976).
18. Bruce Nortell, "Leading Cases—Male Nurse and Sex Discrimination," *JAMA,* **237**:1610–1611 (Apr. 11, 1977).
19. Robert Foote, "Double Standards?" *Am. J. Nurs.,* **80**:1610 (Sept. 1980).
20. Rita Austin, "Sex and Gender in the Future of Nursing, Part 1," *Nurs. Times,* **73**:113–116 (Aug. 1977).
21. Rita Austin, "Sex and Gender in the Future of Nursing, Part 2," *Nurs. Times,* **73**:117–119 (Sept. 1977).
22. Peggy Nuttall, "British Nursing—Beginning of a Power Struggle?" *Nurs. Outlook,* **31**:184–187 (May–June 1983).
23. Bonnie J. Garvin, "Values of Male Nursing Students," *Nurs. Res,* **25**:352–357 (Sept–Oct. 1976).
24. Malcolm Macdonald, "How Do Men and Women Students Rate in Empathy?" *Am. J. Nurs.,* **77**:998 (June 1977).
25. Ben Groff, "The Trouble with Male Nursing," *Am. J. Nurs.,* **84**:62–63 (Jan. 1984).
26. "Male Nurses: What They Think of Themselves—and Others," *RN,* **44**:61–64 (Oct. 1983).
27. "Nursing Is Still Considered Woman's Work," *RN,* **45**:70–75 (June 1984).
28. C. G. Costello, "Attitudes of Nurses to Nursing," *Can. Nurse,* **63**:42–44 (June 1969).
29. E. Kemp and J. Peitchinis, "Nurses' Atti-

tudes: Fact or Fallacy,'' *Can. Nurse,* **64**:51–53 (Feb. 1968).

30. "Dr. Costello Answers His Critics," *Can. Nurse,* **64**:54 (Feb. 1968).

31. Jacquelyn Peitchinis, "Therapeutic Effectiveness of Counseling by Nursing Personnel," *Nurs. Res.,* **21**:138–148 (Mar.–Apr. 1972).

32. Barbara Lewis and Cary Cooper, "Personality Measurement Among Nurses: A Review," *Int. J. Nurs. Stud.,* **13**:209–229 (1976).

33. Simmons, and Henderson, op. cit., pp. 182–196.

34. Marlene Kramer, *Reality Shock: Why Nurses Leave Nursing* (St. Louis: C. V. Mosby Company, 1974).

35. "Non-Nursing Functions: Our Readers Respond," *Am. J. Nurs.,* **82**:1857–1860 (Dec. 1982).

36. Marjorie Godfrey, "Job Satisfaction, Part I," *Nurs. 78,* **8**:89–102 (Apr. 1978).

37. Marjorie Godfrey, "Job Satisfaction, Part 2," *Nurs. 78,* **8**:105–120 (May 1978).

38. Majorie Godfrey, "Job Satisfaction, Part 3," *Nurs. 78,* **8**:81–95 (June 1978).

39. Marjorie Godfrey, "Your Fringe Benefits: How Much Are They Really Worth?" *Nurs. 75,* **5**:73–75ff. (Jan. 1975).

40. Marjorie Godfrey, "Someone Should Represent Nurses," *Nurs. 76,* **2**:73–90 (June 1976).

41. Anthony Lee, "A Wary New Welcome for Unions," *RN* **45**:35–40 (Nov. 1982).

42. G. Ray Funkhouser, "Quality of Care, Part I," *Nurs. 76,* **6**:22–31 (Dec. 1976).

43. G. Ray Funkhouser, "Quality of Care, Part II," *Nurs. 77,* **7**:27–33 (Jan. 1977).

44. "How Good Is Health Care Today?, Part 1," *Nurs. Life,* **3**:24–31 (July–Aug. 1983).

45. "How Good Is Health Care Today?, Part 2," *Nurs. Life,* **3**:42–49 (Sept.–Oct. 1983).

46. Lucie Young, "A Frame of Reference for Nursing Education," unpublished Ph.D. dissertation, School of Education, University of Pittsburgh, 1965, p. 127.

47. Simmons and Henderson, op. cit., pp. 175–181.

48. Irwin Deutscher, *A Study of the Registered Nurse in a Metropolitan Commu-* *nity* (Kansas City, Mo.: Community Studies Inc., 1957), as reported in Simmons and Henderson, op. cit., pp. 179–184.

49. Eliot Friedson, *Patients' Views of Medical Practice* (New York: Russell Sage Foundation, 1961).

50. Hansi Pollak, "Community Attitudes," *Int. Nurs. Rev.,* **14**:37–38 (Jan.–Feb. 1967).

51. Linda Hughes "The Public Image of the Nurse," *Adv. Nurs. Sci.,* **2**:55–72 (Apr. 1980).

52. Anthony Lee, "How Nurses Rate with the Public," *RN,* **42**:25–39 (June 1979).

53. Stephen Shortell, "Occupational Prestige Differences within the Medical and Allied Health Professions," *Soc. Sci. Med,* **8**:1–9 (1974).

54. Alan Wheelock, "The Tarnished Image," *Nurs. Outlook,* **24**:509–510 (Aug. 1976).

55. Lucy Ham, "Reflections of Nursing: Portrait or Caricature?" *Image,* **13**:9–12 (Feb. 1981).

56. Patricia Moccia and Kate Pfordresher, "Health Care Revolution: If Nurses Had Their Way," *Ms.,* May 1983, pp. 104–106, 146.

57. Alice Ream, "Our Undertrained Nurses," *Newsweek,* Oct. 25, 1983, p. 17.

58. Thomas Ford and Diane Stephenson, *Institutional Nurses: Roles Relationships and Attitudes in Three Alabama Hospitals* ((University of Alabama Press, 1954), as reported in Simmons and Henderson, op. cit., pp. 176–177.

59. David Ambrose, "Physicians and Nurses Rank Importance of Nursing Activities," *Hospitals,* **51**:115–118 (Nov. 1977).

60. Anthony Lee, "How Nurses Rate with MDs: Still the Handmaiden" *RN,* **42**:20–30 (July, 1979).

61. Loy Wiley, "What Doctors *Really* Think of Nursing—and Nurses," *Nurs. 79,* **9**:73–77 (Aug. 1979).

62. Jane Holliday, "An Ideal Image of the Professional Nurse with a Method for Formulating a Composite Ideal Image," unpublished Ed.D. dissertation, Teachers College, Columbia University, 1960.

63. Cynthia Kelly, "GN's Sparkling Older Authors," *Ger. Nurs.,* **4**:153–157 (May–June 1983).

64. Lois Grau, "What Older Adults Expect From the Nurse," *Ger. Nurs.*, **5**:14–18 (Jan.–Feb. 1984).

NURSING EDUCATION
AND
RESEARCH

Major Issues and Trends in Nursing Education

Unlike most professions, nursing has a variety of programs for entry into the profession (also called *basic, preservice,* or *generic education*). This situation confuses the public, some nurses, and employers. The three major educational routes that lead to RN licensure are the diploma programs operated by hospitals, the baccalaureate degree programs offered by four-year colleges and universities, and the associate degree programs usually offered by junior (or community) colleges. A master's degree program for beginning practitioners is also available at a few colleges, and a professional doctorate in one. These programs admit students with baccalaureate or higher degrees in fields other than nursing.

Although at one time diploma schools educated the largest number of nurses (more than 72 percent of the total number of schools in 1964 were diploma), the movement of nursing programs into institutions of higher learning has been consistent. Between 1964 and 1983, associate degree (AD) programs expanded from 130 to 764. In this period, BSN programs grew from 187 to 421. At the same time, diploma programs decreased from 833 to 281. In 1983 the National League for Nursing reported 1,432 schools and 1,466 basic RN programs.[1]

The pattern, then, has been an increase in all collegiate programs and a decrease in diploma programs. A zero growth rate in admissions, which had been predicted, occurred in 1977; however, by 1980, all basic RN programs had admitted an increasing number of students. The change in the admission rate reflects the closing of diploma programs and the diminished growth of new collegiate programs. However, such unpredictable factors as the sudden shortage of practicing nurses, as occurred in 1979, or the decreased amount of federal aid to schools, in the 1980s, often change the picture.

There are certain similarities that all basic nursing programs share, in part because all are affected by the same societal changes.

1. Nursing education is becoming more expensive, and financial support is less available for schools and students. The inflationary costs affecting society and education also affect nursing programs and the institutions in which they are located. Moreover, the better the preparation of the teachers and the quality of other resources and facilities, the more costly the program. Both state and federal governments have been tightening the financial

reins on programs, apparently indifferent to the effect on quality or student needs. Therefore, although there is verbal encouragement for faculty to develop innovative programs, funds are seldom available for this purpose. Tuition seldom covers the cost of the program, but, even so, it has been rising consistently. Students are finding it more and more difficult to receive scholarships, loans, and grants, particularly with the great cutback in federal funds beginning in 1972. Also, because of both costs and social trends, fewer students live in dormitories, and those who do pay for room and board.

2. The student population is more heterogeneous. Few, if any, schools refuse admission or matriculation to married students with or without families. Often, leave is granted for childbirth. It is not unusual to have a grandparent in a class, as more mature individuals look for a new or better career. The tight job market in many fields brings to nursing individuals with degrees and sometimes careers in related or unrelated fields. As noted in Chapter 11, in the last decade, all programs have included more men and other minority groups, in a small but definite percentage. In all cases, the diploma programs admit the lowest percentage of these groups.

3. Educational programs are generally more flexible. Educational trends in this direction, plus the admission of a very mixed student body, including aides, LPNs, and RNs seeking advanced education, have required a second look at proficiency and equivalency testing, self-paced learning, and new techniques in teaching. The popularity of the external degree program indicates this trend.[2]

4. Educational programs copy from each other or are subject to the same waves of educational faddism and jargon. For instance, where once curricula were based on the same standard clinical and supportive courses, the "integrated" curriculum became popular in the 1950s. Today most faculty subscribe to models and theoretical frameworks as the basis for curriculum development.

5. State approval is required and national accreditation is available for all basic programs. Every school of professional nursing, in all three categories as well as practical nurse programs, must meet the standards of the legally constituted body in each state authorized to regulate nursing education and practice within that state. These agencies are usually called *state boards of nursing* or some similar title. Without the approval of these boards, a school cannot really operate, because the graduates would not be eligible to take the licensing examination. In addition, many schools of nursing also seek accreditation by the National League for Nursing. Accreditation by the League is a voluntary matter, not required by law. Increasing numbers of schools seek it, however, because it represents nationally determined standards of excellence and non-accreditation may affect the school's eligibility for outside funding or retard the graduates' entrance into BSN or graduate programs.

6. Faculty and clinical facilities are scarce resources. Faculty with the recommended doctoral degree for baccalaureate and graduate programs and the master's degree for other programs are increasing in number, but the total need has not been met. Today about 0.2 percent of the 1.3 million employed nurses hold doctorates.[3] Clinical facilities are at a premium. Most schools, including diploma programs, use a variety of facilities. In large cities, several schools may be using one specialty hospital or clinical area (particularly obstetrics and pediatrics) for student experience. In rural areas, distance, small hospitals, and fewer patients are problems. Community health resources are very limited. Schools are also searching for new types of clinical experiences with various ethnic groups and in new settings such as hospices.

7. There is a slow but perceptible trend

toward involving students in curriculum development, policymaking, and program evaluation. Social trends and the maturity of students, with their demands to have a part in the educational program, are making some inroads on faculty and administrative control of schools.

8. All nursing students have learning experiences in clinical settings. Somewhere a myth arose that only practical nurse and diploma students gave "real" patient care in their educational programs, that AD students barely saw patients, and that baccalaureate students prepared only for teaching and administration. In fact, the time spent in the clinical area differs among programs within a particular credential as much as it does among various types of programs. In all good programs, students care for selected patients in order to gain certain skills and knowledge.

9. It is generally agreed that the standards by which nursing education programs are judged should include criteria involving the organization and administration of the *institution* itself (financial support, other support services, a review process for quality); *students* (selection, retention, evaluation, participation in identifying and evaluating program goals); *faculty* (preparation, research and publication efforts, development and evaluation of programs, participation in governance); *programs* (objectives, theoretical framework, curriculum of study, satisfactory learning opportunities, relationships with service institutions, and evaluation); *facilities and resources* (funds, support services, library, facilities specific to the program).

EXTERNAL CONSTRAINTS ON NURSING EDUCATION

Nursing education, like other educational fields, is strongly affected by external constraints over which it has limited or no control.[4] To constrain means to compel, oblige,

force, or restrain. Nursing education is the object of multiple constraints: those imposed as a part of the system of higher education, those imposed by the responsibilities of a health profession to the public, and those imposed by a more or less cohesive group of practitioners who are, in essence, employers, employees, colleagues, change agents, and even critical consumers. That the constraints imposed by these groups may conflict with each other only adds pressure. Nevertheless, it should not be assumed that the results of these constraints are necessarily bad.

The effects of the national economy are not limited to increased costs of the program and increased tuition. Nursing, viewed as a profession "where you can always get a job," is attractive not only to other careerists whose fields are in decline, but also to second-career housewives. On the other hand, the fact that more temporarily retired nurses are likely to work, coupled with the general inability of anyone to guess accurately nurse manpower needs, leaves schools in a quandary as to how many students they should admit. New limitations to federal and state funding for both schools and students put more constraints on expansion, or perhaps more accurately, indicate the direction of new programs. For instance, NP programs increased, in part, because they were funded. Any specialty, such as oncology, psychiatry, even preparation for administration or teaching, seems to expand or contract according to available funding. Moreover, the content of the curriculum may be influenced by the federal guidelines required if federal funds are accepted.

Changing student bodies reflect a changed economy and financial incentives to admit certain students. Federal programs have increased minority representation in schools of nursing. Nursing schools have been closed because a board of directors decided that they were not economically feasible to operate. Nevertheless, a tight money market has also resulted in a creative sharing of resources and in regional planning for nursing education.

Naturally, professional education is influenced by the knowledge explosion and technological advances. For nursing, this demands that practitioners keep up-to-date and raises multiple questions of curriculum content. Should nurses be educated as generalists or specialists? At what educational level? For primary, secondary, or tertiary care? For acute or long-term care? At what level? If new graduates are expected to practice at a minimum safe and effective level, what is the minimum content that should be in all curricula? If something new is added, should something be deleted, or should less be taught about everything? Are there more effective ways for students to learn, such as independent, self-paced learning? The increase in knowledge also puts more pressure on the profession to create and/or expand a knowledge base for nursing. How then to enlarge the miniscule number of nurses with doctoral education and research interests? These questions are being answered in a variety of ways by nurse educators, and are being raised in the halls of Congress as the various nursing bills are debated.

There are a number of social movements that affect nursing education. One noted previously is the recognition of students' rights. Another is renewed emphasis on the American belief in upward mobility. Moving to advanced education in nursing for either PNs or RNs has generally not been easy; most returning students believe that unnecessary obstacles have been placed in their way. Pressure by organized minority groups and unions, as well as the studies and edicts of national commissions and state and federal governments, have all been important factors in developing more flexible educational patterns. The public's legitimate demand for competent practitioners has also focused more attention on continuing education. In addition, changes in the delivery of health care services, which may involve both new techniques (space medicine, organ transplants) and new or newly emphasized settings (maternity centers, neighborhood health centers and surgicenters), clients (teenagers, the elderly), health attitudes (prevention, self-care), or other concerns (environmental

health, iatrogenic disease), as well as the changing role of other professionals and paraprofessional health workers, all affect nursing education.

Finally, there are the constraints placed on nursing education by the profession, the organizations that represent it, and its various practitioners. These pressures can create more strain than external forces because, unfortunately, there is no common nursing tradition, so that the demands often conflict. One key example is the lack of agreement between nursing education and nursing service about the utilization of the graduates of the three kinds of programs. Anther conflict addresses the difference in philosophy as to whether professional nursing education can be a series of steps that build on previous experience and education, or whether professional education is so different from technical education that it requires a fresh start. Nurses also question whether graduate education must be primarily clinical. Even though both state board approval and accreditation are fairly well controlled by nurses and affect educational programs, there is no agreement at state or national levels. Most devastating of all is the bitter divisiveness caused by the issue of entry into practice.

ENTRY INTO PRACTICE

With at least three types of basic educational programs evolving in nursing, the uncertainty of both the public and the profession as to the differences among these practitioners has appeared to escalate. To add to the confusion, graduates of all programs are eligible to take the same licensing examination and have the same passing score. There have been arguments that no one could expect the public and employers to differentiate among nursing graduates when all are designated as RNs on licensure. Often, RNs are employed in the same capacity, with the same assignments, same expectations, and same salary. Are they all professional nurses? If so, what justification is there for three separate educational programs?

An important function of ANA is that of setting standards and policies for nursing education. A major action, taken in 1965, by the Committee on Education, resulted in the ANA position that nursing education should take place within the general educational system. Reaction to the position paper* was decidedly mixed. Although the concept underlying the paper had been enunciated by leaders in nursing since the profession's inception, reiterated through the years, and accepted as a goal by the 1960 House of Delegates, many nurses misunderstood the paper's intent and considered it a threat. Probably the greatest area of misinterpretation lay in the separation of nursing education and practice into professional, technical, and assisting components. Minimum preparation for professional nursing practice was designated at the baccalaureate level, technical nursing practice at the associate degree level, and education for assistants in health service occupations was to be in short, intensive preservice programs in vocational education settings, rather than in on-the-job training. An obvious omission in the position paper was the place of diploma ad practical nurse education. A large number of hospital-based diploma graduates, students, faculty, and hospital administrators were angered by the omission. A major source of resentment was that the term *professional nurse* was to be reserved for the baccalaureate graduate.

Even in this period of confusion, it was recognized that the largest system of nursing education, the hospital school, could not be overlooked or eliminated by the writing of a position paper. Later, both the ANA and NLN prepared statements which advocated careful community planning for phasing diploma programs into institutions of higher learning. It was also pointed out that as practical nursing programs improved and increased their course content, their length became close to that of the associate degree program. Nevertheless, the storm raged for more than fifteen years, although repeated attempts were made to clarify the content and intent of the position paper. It was felt that ANA suffered a membership loss through the alienation of some diploma nurses. As expected, social and economic trends gradually brought about many of the changes suggested by the position paper, and the definitions of *professional nurse* and *technical nurse* were widely used in the literature (although there was no major indication that employers were assigning nurses according to technical or professional responsibilities). In June 1973, in what some considered a belated effort to placate diploma nurses, assure them of their importance to ANA, and encourage unity in the profession, a "Statement on Diploma Graduates" was issued. In essence, the statement asked all units of ANA to give special attention to the needs and interests of diploma graduates, particularly in relation to continuing education and upward mobility. In addition, a task force was appointed "to examine the contemporary relevance of the terms 'professional' and 'technical' to distinguish basic preparation for nursing practice and to recognize all registered nurses as professionals."[5] Although there appeared to be no major reaction from diploma nurses to this statement, some nurses considered it a step backward, because it appeared to reject the concept that professional nursing was different from technical nursing.[6]

In February 1974, the Commission on Nursing Education approved a report on the contemporary relevance of the terms *professional* and *technical*. Meanwhile, the NLN's associate degree group rejected the term *technical,* but others continued to use it.

In 1976, the New York State Nurses' Association's voting body overwhelmingly approved introduction of a "1985 Proposal" in the 1977 legislative session. Although variations of the proposal evolved over the next

*Correctly titled: "Educational Preparation for Nurse Practitioners and Assistants to Nurses—A Position Paper."

few years, the basic purpose of the legislation was to establish licensure for two kinds of nursing. The professional nurse would require a baccalaureate degree, and the other, whose title changed with various objections, would require an associate degree. The target date for full implementation was 1985; currently licensed nurses would be covered by the traditional grandfather clause, which would allow them to retain their current title and status (RN). The bill did not pass but was consistently reintroduced during each legislative session. Some time later, the Ohio Nurses' Association introduced similar legislation without success. Immediately, the 1985 Proposal became both a term symbolizing baccalaureate education as the entry level into *professional* nursing and a rallying point for nurses who opposed this change. There was, and is, considerable opposition from some diploma and AD nurses and faculty, some hospital administrators, and some physicians. Nursing organizations were formed whose major focus was opposition to such proposals. Nevertheless, an increasing number of state nurses' organizations, primarily made up of diploma nurses, voted in convention to work toward the goal of baccalaureate education for professional nursing. In 1978, the ANA House of Delegates passed such a resolution, as did the National Student Nurses' Association. The ANA resolution had emerged from an ANA-sponsored "Entry into Practice" conference held earlier that year. The 400 or so participants included representatives from various nurses' associations, the federal government, all types of schools of nursing, as well as administrators and staff nurses from all types of employment settings. The paper and the recommendations of group discussions have been published.[7] The major recommendations supported the concept of two categories or types of practitioners in nursing (although they could not agree on titles), that competencies be developed for those levels, and that career mobility opportunities be increased, including the use of innovative and flexible educational programs. All these recommendations were

incorporated into resolutions that the ANA House of Delegates also approved in 1978.

Entry into practice and its inevitable corollary, changes in nurse licensure, continue to be a major issue in nursing. Most nursing organizations, and, of course, state nurses' associations (SNAs), have taken a stand or are in the process of doing so. Although most state nurses' associations favor the 1985 proposal as a necessary and inevitable step in the development of nursing, the California Nurses' Association was the first to support a clear career ladder plan.

The NLN has played an interesting role in the entry into practice debate. In 1979, it supported all pathways (baccalaureate, associate, diploma and practical nursing). Given the structure of the NLN and its historic position as the accrediting body for each level of nursing education, this statement is understandable. In 1982, however, the Board of Directors endorsed the baccalaureate degree as the criterion for professional practice.[8] This position was affirmed when the voting body met in Philadelphia in June 1983.*

In the long debate about the nature of education for practice, it is not surprising that there are those who think that the system should stay as it is,[9,10] others who opt for changing the baccalaureate nurse's title and license to indicate advanced preparation,[11] and a few who are anticipating the time when a professional nurse doctorate, like the MD and DDS of physicians and dentists, will be the entry level to the profession.[12]

Some natural fears of nonbaccalaureate nurses are to be expected: that they will lose status and job opportunities despite the grandfather clause and that those who desire baccalaureate education will find it too expensive, unavailable, or rigidly repetitive. As to the first, there is already some selectiveness and has been; in the latter, there is slow, but definite progress. These issues will not be quickly resolved, but inevitable societal and

---

*See the convention reports published in *Nursing Outlook* in the odd years.

professional changes, such as the decrease in diploma schools and the expectations of professional practice (nursing is the only health profession for which entry is less than a baccalaureate) will be major factors in the final outcome. There are problems that must be resolved and data obtained (for example, will costs limit access to professional nursing? Will such a plan improve patient care?).[13] Because nursing loses power every time its practitioners battle internally it is imperative that nurses work together toward a satisfactory conclusion, one that includes appreciation and respect for all competent nurses and focuses on providing the best possible nursing care to the public.[14]

In the meantime, there has been a quiet revolution, one that may end the recurrence of the entry into practice issue that has followed nursing throughout its history.[15,16] Where once ANA conventions were consumed with entry into practice debates, now the question in education is: how do we facilitate the transition?* The 1980 Social Policy Statement,[17] which clearly stated that baccalaureate education was the basis of professional nursing practice, was accepted with praise, and the Cabinet on Nursing Education continued to work toward this goal.[18] In the next biennium, ANA provided grants to several SNAs to implement their plans to establish the baccalaureate as the minimum educational qualification for professional nursing and set its timetable for implementation in all states before the end of the century. The final report of the interdisciplinary National Commission for Nursing (Chapter 5) saw pursuit of the baccalaureate as an "achievable goal."[19] A three year project funded by the W. K. Kellogg Foundation in late 1984 to carry out selected Commission recommendations included the objective: ". . . to outline the common body of knowledge and skills essential for basic nursing practice, the curriculum content that supports

*See the reports of ANA conventions in *Nursing Outlook* and the *American Journal of Nursing* in the even years.

it, and a credentialing process that reinforces it." (See Chapter 5.) For the time being "entry into practice" still evokes controversial actions. Diploma programs led an attempt to rescind the NLN statement in 1983, but were defeated.[20] Some nurses in some states that still have many diploma programs occasionally use successful political tactics (often hospital association funded) to prevent acceptance of a 1985 Proposal-type statement at SNA conventions,[21] but at the next year's meeting, the baccalaureate support statement may be approved and the two opposing groups work together to help RNs get their baccalaureates. Although many RNs are not convinced that baccalaureate education necessarily means professionalism,[22] others have been, and back to school they went.[23]

OPEN CURRICULUM PRACTICES

One of the key developments in nursing education is the implementation of the open curriculum concept, which the NLN defines as a system "which incorporates an educational approach designed to accommodate the learning needs and career goals of students by providing flexible opportunities for entry into and exit from the educational program, and by capitalizing on their previous relevant education and experiences."[24]

This concept has emerged only gradually. Nurse educators who were most aware of social and economic trends and sympathetic to the goals of those struggling for upward mobility began to plan and implement programs. Others ignored the signs of disillusionment among those seeking further education in nursing. Both the poor and ethnic minorities, often guided into lower-level nursing positions, and the middle-class nurses who had chosen diploma or associate degree education, as well as service corpsmen returning from active duty, became irritated at the difficulty of moving into other levels of nursing. All became increasingly hostile toward a system that offered no credit for previous study and experience, or, at most, recognized a few liberal arts courses. Unions included in their contracts provisions for organized programs of education for nonprofessionals. Other health workers turned to the legislatures. The result was evident in such states as California, which enacted laws to force schools of nursing to give credit to prospective students with previous health experience,[25] and in recommendations of the federal government.[26,27]

Soon it became evident that nursing programs were responding to the mandate for more flexibility. An NLN survey in 1971 showed that approximately 1,500 of the approximately 2,700 practical, diploma, associate degree, and baccalaureate programs in nursing provided some aspect of educational mobility. A 1976 report provided valuable information about the types of practices, planning methods, special resources, benefits and difficulties, evaluation methods, and self-estimates of program success from the respondents (34 percent) of the 1765 programs that had designated themselves as offering some sort of open curriculum practice.[28]

Today, there are many more.[29] At the least, they accept transfer credit as a means of advanced placement. Innovative programs have designed new methods for measurement of knowledge and competency or have developed entirely new programs. There are a variety of approaches for providing flexibility in nursing education. The ladder approach, which provides direct articulation between programs, is used to move from nursing assistant to practical nurse to AD or diploma nurse to baccalaureate nurse, with any combination in between. For some, this means the ability to begin at a basic level and move one step at a time to the highest achievable level. For others, it means that one can aim at a particular level but be able to exit at distinct points, become licensed, and earn a living if necessity or circumstances dictate. An increasing number of baccalaureate programs are also being developed that enroll only RNs into the upper division, accepting past nursing education as the lower division to be built on.[30]

There are, of course, those nurse educators who do not agree that the ladder is a viable concept. They believe that each program in nursing has its own basis, content, and goals, that one cannot be based on another, and that the ladder tends to denigrate the role of workers at each level, implying the necessity to move upward. One solution seems to be the utilization of standardized and teacher-made tests to measure the individual's knowledge, according to a clear delineation of the achievement expectations of the program. There are a number of standardized tests available in both the liberal arts and nursing, but there is still some question as to how to test for clinical competency. Methods used include the use of videotapes, simulated experiences, practicums, and minicourses in the clinical setting. Also being used are the performance assessment centers of the Regent's College Degree program, as well as their paper-and-pencil exams.[31]

An exciting approach is to allow students to proceed through a course at their own pace through testing, self-study, and the use of media. A number of schools are experimenting with self-pacing and self-learning, and reports indicate that students find it stimulating and satisfying.

Other ways of giving more opportunities for students are to offer courses more frequently, during evening hours, weekends, and in summer, to allow part-time study, and to have class sessions off the main campus in areas convenient to students living in communities not easily accessible to the main campus. The last is sometimes considered a form of external degree or "university without walls."[32]

The Regents College Degree, formerly called the *New York State Regents External Degree,* is an example of an open curriculum that moves far beyond this simple concept. The purpose of the program is to meet the needs of those individuals who choose to learn on their own, whether through individual study, job experience, travel, coursework, or other forms of life experience. It is open to all applicants, without regard to age, residence, or methods of preparation. The program's philosophy is that what a person knows is more important than where or how he learned it. The entire program is based on testing.

In 1971 an associate degree in nursing was included in the program, developed by a committee of noted associate degree educators.[33] In late 1974, work on this first external degree in nursing was completed, including tests for clinical competency. Applicants are not eligible to take the clinical performance examination, given in actual patient care settings, until all the clinical paper-and-pencil exams are passed.

The baccalaureate program for the external degree, completed in 1979, provides additional opportunity for nurses seeking a bachelor's degree in nursing. Both programs are accredited by the NLN. The outreach of this program is reflected in its statistics. By 1983, 2,200 candidates had earned associate degrees and 600 had earned baccalaureate degrees. Approximately 9,000 persons are enrolled in the program.[34] Information may be obtained by writing to Regents College Degrees, Nursing Office, Cultural Education Center, Albany, New York 12230.

Although there are some educators who oppose the external degree on philosophical grounds[35] and others who fear the competition in the tight market for students, studies conducted relative to the program are providing data of significance to other states contemplating external degree programs that include nursing. Cooperative ventures with various colleges, service institutions, and service systems (such as the Air Force Nurse Corps) are part of the extensive Regents outreach.[36] The data have also helped educational programs seeking more effective techniques for proficiency and equivalency testing. There is evidence that the examinations to measure clinical proficiency developed in the external degree program are helpful tools in traditional educational settings. The availability of performance assessment centers in five regions has made the validation of nursing performance more accessible. Before September 1983,

candidates had to travel to New York to complete their clinical proficiency examinations.[37]

If the 1985 Proposal becomes a reality, the necessity for upward mobility becomes even more essential, but RN students must beware of diploma mills.[38] Of greatest importance in these changes in education is the fact that individuals will have greater opportunities to continue formal education that is of good quality, if they desire, and both nursing and society will benefit.

DOES NURSING EDUCATION PREPARE COMPETENT PRACTITIONERS?

From the time that the last diploma program gave up the apprenticeship approach to nursing education, there have been accusations that the new graduates of modern nursing programs are not competent. Further investigation usually shows that new graduates are not as technically skillful or as able to assume responsibility for a large group of patients as the nurses with whom they are compared—the diploma graduates of yesterday. Nevertheless, the criticisms are understandable. For the director of nursing with fiscal constraints, a lengthy orientation and in-service program is a strain on the budget; for the staff nurse and supervisor, someone who requires extra help or supervision on a usually short-staffed unit is a temporary impediment.

For some unknown reason, useful communication between nursing education and nursing service is erratic at best and nonexistent at worst. In some areas, joint appointments of faculty and clinicians enables each to contribute to the goals of the other, but this practice is largely limited to medical centers and university programs.[39] Other productive steps are joint planning for experiences during the student's educational program or an externship[40] or internship[41] and opportunities for faculty to practice during weekends, summers, or sabbaticals. Unfortunately, however, although there seems to be little disagreement on the qualities, knowledge, and skills nurses need, there is almost no agreement on how much of each and what level of competency is needed at graduation.

Although graduates from all three types of programs are the targets of employer disapproval,[42] the diploma graduate, whose program is focused on the hospital and who frequently stays at the hospital, may find adjustment a little easier. Associate degree graduates who have been practical nurses and have had experience in caring for many patients are also somewhat immune from criticisms about slow adjustment. However, because most graduates today do not have these backgrounds, how justified are the criticisms? How differently do the graduates of the RN programs perform?

There is a question, first of all, as to whether the various kinds of programs actually prepare different kinds of practitioners. Nurse educators say they do, but often the statements of philosophy and objectives or the NLN competency statements, described in Chapter 13, have obvious areas of overlap. Moreover, some believe that there is a lack of clarity in how heads of AD and BS programs see their type of program as differing from the other. Specifically, most programs do not seem to adhere to the differences spelled out in the literature. For instance, some AD program directors think their graduates have as broad a judgment base as the baccalaureate nurse, and many prepare these nurses for administrative functions without the necessary educational base. On the other hand, this is probably a matter of catching up with reality, because many employers give AD nurses responsibilities for which they are not prepared. But should the teacher then educate the employer instead of reeducating the student?

The nursing literature abounds with articles on content and methods; nurse educators are most certainly concerned about preparing the best possible practitioner. There is concern that new graduates be competent to give both physical and psychological/emotional care. Just how much of this is best taught in a clinical setting is a point of controversy. How

much of what kind of clinical experience prepares nurses best? It has been suggested that additional emphasis be given to the physical care needed because of the patients' pathophysiological problems. There is also some indication that students need practice in basic technical skills, which some schools deal with by encouraging additional self-study in labs. In others, a concentrated period of time in one or two clinical areas at the end of the program eases students into the work situation and allows them to integrate their clinical knowledge and skills over a continuum of time and to learn to organize the care of larger groups of patients, setting appropriate priorities. Certain programs also have cooperative arrangements with clinical facilities to allow students a paid work-study period in the summer, or specific academic terms in which they work full time while supervised in practice.[43] Clerkships, preceptorships, field placements, or clinical electives are other options. There are mixed feelings about whether working as an aide or ward clerk is helpful because of the limited legal scope of practice and the possibility that students are subtly forced into assuming more responsibility than is legal.

If success in state boards is considered to be a criterion for competency, the results are no more definitive; differences within each type of program are greater than those among the programs.[44] As to differences in practice among diploma, AD, and BSN nurses, this has been difficult to determine because most studies have been done by graduate students. Not only are the numbers small and the studies seldom replicated, but what is being measured is usually different from study to study. However, one study of nurses, with a national sample of 2,000, did find significant differences in the clinical practice of diploma, AD, and BSN nurses. Almost 10,000 critical incidents (self-reports or reports of observed behavior) were classified and analyzed. The report noted:

Baccalaureate nurses were most often involved in incidents concerning leadership and professional responsibility; patient teaching and promotion of psychological well-being; exchanging and recording information about the patient; and planning patient care. They were least often reported in activities involving intrusive procedures, medications, treatments and other routine patient care activities. The fewest associate degree nurse incidents were about patient teaching and psychological care, clinical assessment and judgment, exchanging information and planning patient care. Diploma nurses were most involved in incidents about clinical assessment and judgment as well as responding to emergencies; and least involved in exercising professional prerogatives.[45]

The data used by this study were gathered in the late 1970s.

In 1979, the members of an NLN Task Force on Competencies of Graduates of Nursing Programs, after reviewing the literature and analyzing statements of the NLN educational councils abut each of their programs,* concluded that there *were* differences in the competencies (defined as minimal expectations of new graduates) in education, practice, and accountability. The common core of all was seen as nursing theory and the nursing process, although the latter varied in depth and breadth. A chart comparing the expectations of the graduates clearly showed the ambiguity of the statements of competency and some amazing omissions. For instance, specific competencies as communicator, patient teacher, and manager of patient care were identified only by the AD statement. It was also noted that other differences occurred in the practice role in terms of structured/unstructured settings and focus of care. Another difference was in accountability, which increased with the amount and type of education and experience.[46]

One of the most bitter arguments in nursing education is whether baccalaureate or diploma nursing provides the "best" education

for professional nursing. In a thought-provoking article, Ramphal maintains that a potentially profession-destroying tragedy is that the strengths traditionally characteristic of diploma education and the strengths of collegiate education are so often seen as either/or propositions.[47] At times, clinical competence is misequated with "sheer technical competence that is fundamentally anti-intellectual, anti-conceptual and anti-theoretical." But emphasis on the conceptual part of nursing "divorced from a base in practice, runs the risk of triviality, at best, and solipsistic pseudointellectualism, at worst." Another option was suggested.

An ideal professional nursing education program seems conceivable which would combine strengths characteristic of each type of program at its best: 1) a program in which the talents of faculty combine the capabilities of clinicians who either are continuing in practice or frequently return to practice and who are not content with current practice but are actively engaged in improving it; 2) a program in which the faculty as a group is also endowed, not only with intellectual command of relevant theories and concepts, but in which some, at least, are actively engaged in theory development through research, particularly clinical research; 3) a program in which students' understanding of theories and concepts is enriched through clinical teaching by instructors able to help them gain intellectual command of theory through practice; and 4) a program in which at least some clinical practice provides an opportunity for students to experience continuity and accountability in order to develop clinical judgment—that is, the weighing of alternatives in decision making necessary for responsible professional practice.[48]

One could add to this a vital ingredient that is possibly best taught by role models if it is not already a part of the individual nurse's makeup—the quality of human kindness, the caring aspect of nursing, which, although it cannot substitute for knowledge, skills, and

*See Chapter 13.

competency, is indispensable. Without it, there is no nursing care.

Arguments about which type of graduate is best prepared to work in hospitals have been intensified by high-technology health care. Recent changes in federal payment for hospital care for Medicare patients has put restrictions on the use of the acute care hospital, and emphasis on clinic and home care compounds the dilemmas of educators and nurse administrators. To orient new graduates, most hospitals have launched major staff development efforts to prepare new or returning nurses for specialty care. But as the health care economy becomes more restrictive under prospective payment plans and flat-rate reimbursement under the diagnostic related group (DRG) method,* there will be less money to retrain nurses for hospital practice. This trend will intensify the debate about the content of basic nursing education.

PREPARATION OF FACULTY AND EDUCATIONAL ADMINISTRATORS

The quality of teachers in any educational program and the leadership of the program's director are key factors in the overall quality of the program. They develop and implement the curriculum, usually select the students and provide a milieu in which learning is either a chore or a joy, or something in between.

Teaching a clinical subject is not the same as teaching a course in liberal arts; teachers must not only know the theoretical concepts, but should also be competent practitioners and role models. Should they also know how to teach? How to evaluate? These questions are arising in other practice disciplines because for years practicing clinicians have been the teachers, whether or not they were able to communicate their knowledge to students. The problem in nursing is twofold. Because of trends and opportunities in graduate education, there are nursing faculty who have

*See Chapters 7 and 19.

learned curriculum and teaching skills, but shy away from actual patient care because they feel inadequate, and there are newly minted clinicians with graduate degrees who have difficulty communicating their know-how. Expanding knowledge and new nursing roles also combine to create a situation in which experienced teachers who have been competent in their field must continually acquire new skills, such as physical assessment skills.

Currently, graduate education seems to be focused on both a clinical major and a functional minor (teaching or administration, primarily). However, the programs also seem to be geared to specialty areas or separated into acute care (episodic) or primary care. How well are these teachers prepared for integrated curricula or for the AD programs in which teaching at a specialty level is a luxury? And is there a place for a teacher whose graduate degree is not in nursing?

A serious problem is that some teachers of nursing do not yet meet the academic requirements for their positions. This means that a large number of students are being taught by faculty with approximately the same level of formal education as the students.

The lack of qualified faculty also tends to lead to academic inbreeding, which has serious implications for high-quality education.[49] In 1982 abut 20 percent of full-time nurse faculty in RN programs had less than a master's degree. Most taught in diploma programs. (Practical nurse faculty have very few master's-prepared faculty). About 8 percent had doctorates, 90 percent of whom taught in baccalaureate or graduate programs. These figures show an ongoing improvement in educational preparation.[50] Yet, the education for *all* university faculty is usually a minimum of a doctorate, and it is generally agreed that all other teachers of nursing programs should have at least a master's. The lack of appropriate credentials, regardless of the teacher's individual qualifications, puts nursing faculty at a distinct disadvantage in a university setting. Frequently, they are not considered true colleagues (a problem they also have when dealing with physicians in the clinical setting), and they have difficulty in competing for higher rank, tenure, or appointment on committees. Some believe that these factors help create problems in faculty relationships with students, causing an inclination to be repressive.[51]

Currently, most faculty have doctorates from programs other than nursing, usually education. This does not seem inappropriate. However, if faculty also do research in their field, how does such a doctorate prepare one for clinical research? Is a doctorate in a related science preferable? With the scarcity of doctoral nurses, the type of degree has not yet become a serious issue, but it is tending in that direction. On the other hand, even those faculty with doctoral education in nursing face problems they had not anticipated. It appears that nursing doctoral programs are designed to prepare graduates as researchers and scholars rather than as experts in teaching, clinical practice, or even administration.[52] And yet, the reality is that they spend most of their time teaching—probably at the undergraduate level. They complain that heavy clinical loads prevent them from taking time for research.[53] Yet they are chastised for being less scholarly and less productive than their other university colleagues.[54] Deans are advised to give them short-term contracts unless they make scholarly contributions to the program; probably they will not survive in the promotion-tenure race anyhow. They may then seek to concentrate on research and writing, and students have low priority. Students resent it, and in truth, teaching may suffer. But what kind of role model should the teacher be to the student? Scholar? Clinician? Teacher? In a time of economic retrenchment with heavier teaching assignments, can the faculty member be all three—adequately?[55] It should be noted that these are primarily problems of university or college faculty. In AD and diploma programs, there is not yet such an emphasis on scholarly productivity. How these issues affect doctoral education is discussed in Chapter 13.

The issue of preparation for the decanal role has received some attention in the last few years. Usually, the dean of a baccalaureate and a higher-degree program is expected to hold a doctoral degree. However, research-oriented doctoral study does not prepare a person to assume the academic and administrative role that is mandated. One national survey shows that the doctoral degrees held by deans include PhDs in nursing and other disciplines, as well as professional degrees in education and health administration.[56] Very few deans have had educational programs specifically designed to prepare them for the decanal role; few are available. In recent years, the American Association of Colleges of Nursing (AACN), in concert with the NLN, has presented a continuing education program for deans. AACN has also developed a program for prospective deans and has inaugurated a mentor system, matching the novice with a senior academic administrator.

ACCREDITATION

The major accrediting organization for all nursing programs is the NLN.* The issues involved relate in part to the accrediting process and in part to who should do the accrediting.[57] In the first major DHEW report (1971) that examined all forms of health manpower credentialing, accreditation is defined as "the process by which an agency or organization evaluates and recognizes an institution or program of study as meeting certain predetermined criteria or standards."[58] As noted previously, educational accreditation is a voluntary process, but it presumably indicates excellence in program and resources and therefore attracts students and faculty.

Concern about the accreditation of health education programs led to a major Study of Accreditation of Selected Health Education Programs (SASHEP), the report of which was released in 1972. Sponsored by the American

---

*The history and process is described in Chapter 26.

Medical Association, the Association of Schools of Allied Health Professions, and the National Commission on Accreditation, the SASHEP report proved as controversial as the accrediting system. In essence, it concluded that

> Problems of accountability, structural deficiencies, pressures for expansion and increased levels of financial support, and the absence of objective scientific validation of accrediting standards and procedures have converged to undermine the potential effectiveness, social value, and public credibility in many health fields. Heavy social reliance on accreditation as a manpower credentialing mechanism has tended to focus increased public attention on the shortcomings of accreditation. . . .[59]

The SASHEP working papers and reports thoroughly explore such issues as the expense of accreditation to colleges and universities with multiple health profession or occupation programs, particularly indirect costs in faculty and administrative time for preparation and materials; the inconsistency in the criteria and approach of each discipline; the rigidity of some accreditation boards that discourage innovation; the discontent of allied health groups controlled by the "parent discipline"; the lack of public representation on accrediting bodies; and, most of all, the lack of scientific development and validation of accreditation criteria. Although nursing was obviously not one of the groups for whom the report was directly intended, some of SASHEP's criticisms of the accreditation system apply just as much to the long-established NLN accreditation process.

In addition, there has been increased governmental activity on the accreditation issue. The Federal Trade Commission (FTC) has raised a "restraint of trade" question when an organization both accredits the educational programs and then provides a certification mechanism for the graduates of that program. Two long-standing examples are the American College of Nurse Midwives and the American Association of Nurse Anesthetists, both of which have been the sole accreditors of the educational programs in their respective specialties and also the sole certifiers of the practitioners.* Because in many states a nurse cannot practice that specialty without certification and certification exams are not open to those who did not attend an accredited program (except in rare special circumstances), the FTC maintains that such total control over practice may lead to restraint of trade. As ANA accredits short-term nurse practitioner programs and also increases its certification programs for entry into the specialty, the same charge may be leveled.

Perhaps the new manifestation of an old disagreement is the most important issue to be resolved in nursing. Should ANA, NLN, AACN, or a new credentialing center control the accreditation of all nursing education programs? Although most nursing leaders are members of both ANA and NLN, and most deans belong to AACN, there is significant disagreement about this question. There are philosophical and power issues: should the "real" all-nurse professional organization set educational standards and accredit programs, or should the NLN, which was given that responsibility at the reorganization of the major nursing organizations in 1952, continue? Should the AACN, which represents the interests of the academic deans and directors, direct accrediting activities? Should all accreditation activity be handled by a new credentialing center? There is also an obvious matter of control and income. Considerable income is derived from activities related to accreditation: agency membership, consulting, and the accreditation process. These resources provide attractive incentives to enter the business of accreditation. Another factor, which is not to be discounted, is the bias or belief system of the accreditation agency. Rejection of programs or denial of accreditation can be attributed to organizational or reviewer bias rather

---

*Both organizations have now separated these activities from overt association control (see Chapter 27).

than application of criteria or standards. Responses to decisions about accreditation have also stimulated the who-shall-accredit debate.

The summary statement on accreditation from the Credentialing Study, briefly described in Chapter 5, is:

> Accreditation is the process by which a voluntary, non-governmental agency or organization appraises and grants accredited status to institutions and/or programs or services which meet predetermined structure, process, and outcome criteria. Its purposes are to evaluate the performance of a service or educational program and to provide to various publics information upon which to base decisions about the utilization of the institutions, programs, services, and/or graduates. Periodic assessment is an integral part of the accreditation process in order to ensure continual acceptable performance. Accreditation is conducted by agencies which have been recognized or approved by an organized peer group of agencies as having integrity and consistency in their practices.[60]

At the same time, the committee recommended that all education programs and organized nursing services seek accreditation and that definitions and standards be established by the professional society (ANA). The process of accreditation was to be one of the functions of a credentialing center, seen as a federation of organizations that could conceivably include the NLN and other organizations that accredit nursing programs. However, the NLN, which refused to participate in the credentialing study, also rejected the final report. Nevertheless, the ANA started its own credentialing center. Just what impact all of this will have on nursing credentialing is still to be determined.

Other Issues

There are a number of other issues in nursing education, such as those related to continuing education. What kind of continuing education do nurses need? Who decides? Who is best qualified to provide it? Who should pay?

Should it be mandatory for relicensure? Who is responsible for seeing that it is available to all nurses? Will it improve practice?*

Other issues relate to recruitment and retention of minority students who may or may not fall into the "disadvantaged" category; legal aspects of admission and student and faculty rights (Chapter 22); what kind and how much preparation is needed for specific clinical areas, such as operating room nursing, public health nursing, and occupational health nursing; the kind of education for RNs entering baccalaureate programs (basically the same as for the generic student? advanced? specialized?), and intradisciplinary education (should PN and various RN students learn together?). Interdisciplinary education has also been a point of discussion for some time, with relatively little action taken. There has been minimal experimentation with the concept of core courses from which individual students could move to various health professional programs, as well as certain shared courses when students are already enrolled in separate programs. One approach that takes considerable planning but has shown some good results places professional students in working teams to provide coordinated care for patients (usually in a home or a clinic).

In 1978, in a survey of all types of nursing education programs, the directors listed their "most difficult problems to solve":

1. Financial problems
2. Professional leadership, direction, and cohesion
3. More qualified faculty
4. Career mobility and articulation
5. Production of more competent graduates
6. Role confusion and changes
7. Conflict between nursing education and service
8. Determination of appropriate competency levels
9. Adequate clinical facilities[61]

---

*See Chapter 13 for further discussion.

These almost match issues in nursing education, identified by others as well.

As nursing education, like the society in which it exists, continues to be more complex, new issues will emerge as others are resolved. The danger lies in nonresolution of long-term issues that are professionally divisive and potentially detrimental to the public's welfare.

REFERENCES

1. *Nursing Student Census with Policy Implications, 1984* (New York: National League for Nursing, 1984), p. 3.
2. Carrie Lenburg, "Preparation for Professionalism Through Regents External Degrees," *Nurs. and Health Care,* **5**:318–325 (June 1984).
3. "The Registered Nurse Sample: An Overview," in *National Sample Survey of Registered Nurses* (Washington, D.C.: Department of Health and Human Services, Bureau of Health Professions, 1982).
4. Lucie Kelly, "External Constraints on Nursing Education," in Janet Williamson, ed. *Current Perspectives in Nursing Education: The Changing Scene* (St. Louis: C. V. Mosby Company, 1978), pp. 9–19.
5. "Statement on Diploma Graduates," *Am. Nurse, 5:*5 (June 1973).
6. Dorothy Sheahan, "The Hospital School Graduate—Can the Birthright Be Restored?" *Nurs. Forum,* **12**:260–279 (Fall 1973).
7. American Nurses' Association, *Entry Into Practice: Proceedings of the National Conference,* Feb. 13–14, 1978 (Kansas City, Mo.: The Association, 1978).
8. "Position Statement on Nursing Roles—Scope and Preparation," *Nurs. and Health Care,* **3**:212–213 (Apr. 1982).
9. See the survey reported in *RN* in 1979: January, pp. 83–93; February, pp. 39–46; March, pp. 52–58 present arguments against the 1985 Proposal. The April issue, pp. 64–76, concludes that it is inevitable and necessary but requires careful planning. See also the 1980 survey: "Surprising New 'Mandatory BSN' Findings," May 1981. (Begins on the front cover.)
10. Jane Woodward, "Must We Downgrade Nurses to Upgrade Nursing?" *RN,* **43**:90–96 (May, 1980).
11. Margaret McClure, "Entry Into Professional Practice: The New York Proposal," *J. Nurs. Admin.,* **6**:12–17 (June 1976).
12. Rozella Schlotfeldt, "The Professional Doctorate: Rationale and Characteristics," *Nurs. Outlook,* **26**:302–311 (May 1978).
13. Andrew Dolan, "The New York State Nurses' Association 1985 Proposal: Who Needs It?" *J. of Health, Politics, Policy and Law,* **2**(4):508–530 (Winter 1978).
14. Lucie Kelly, "End Paper: Me-Politics and Nursing," *Nurs. Outlook,* **27**:303 (Apr. 1979).
15. Joan Lynaugh, "The 'Entry Into Practice' Conflict—How We Got Where We Are and What Will Happen Next," *Am. J. Nurs.,* **80**:266–270 (Feb. 1980).
16. Teresa Christy, "Entry Into Practice: A Recurring Issue in Nursing History," *Am. J. Nurs.,* **80**:485–488 (Mar. 1980).
17. American Nurses' Association, *Nursing: A Social Policy Statement* (Kansas City, Mo.: The Association, 1980).
18. American Nurses' Association, *Education for Nursing Practice in the Context of the 1980s* (Kansas City, Mo.: The Association, , 1983).
19. National Commission on Nursing, *Summary Report and Recommendations* (Chicago: The Commission, 1983).
20. Edith Lewis, "Special Report on the NLN Convention," *Nurs. Outlook,* **31**:246–247 (Sept.–Oct. 1983).
21. Lucie Kelly, "End Paper: The Day Nobody Listened: October, 1979," *Nurs. Outlook,* **27**:809 (Dec. 1979).
22. Delores Schoen, "A Study of Nurses' Attitudes Toward the BSN Requirement," *Nurs. and Health Care,* **3**:382–387 (Sept. 1982).
23. Barbara Smullen, "Second-Step Education for RNs: The Quiet Revolution," *Nurs. and Health Care,* **3**:369–373 (Sept. 1982).
24. Carrie Lenburg and Walter Johnson, "Career Mobility Through Nursing Education," *Nurs. Outlook,* **22**:266 (Apr. 1974).

25. Lucie Kelly, "Nursing Practice Acts," *Am. J. Nurs.,* **74**:1312–1313 (July 1974).

26. Department of Health, Education, and Welfare, *Report on Licensure and Related Health Personnel Credentialing* (Washington, D.C.: The Department, 1971), pp. 74–75.

27. Department of Health, Education, and Welfare, *Credentialing Health Manpower* (Washington, D.C.: The Department, 1977), pp. 16–17.

28. Lucille Notter and Marguerite Robey, "Open Curriculum Practices," *Nurs. Outlook,* **27**:116–121 (Feb. 1979).

29. Lois Deleruyelle, and Pam Chally, "Credit Where Credit Is Due," *Am. J. Nurs.,* **84**:105–106 (Jan. 1984).

30. Jean Kintgen-Andrews, "The Development of an Articulation Model," *Nurs. and Health Care,* **3**:181–188 (Apr. 1982).

31. Carrie Lenburg, "Regents External Degrees: An Update," *Nurs. Outlook,* **32**:250–254 (Sept.–Oct. 1984).

32. Almost the entire issue of *Nursing Outlook,* Sept.–Oct. 1984, is devoted to a description of alternate educational patterns for RNs.

33. Dolores Wozniak, "External Degrees in Nursing," *Am. J. Nurs.,* **73**:1014–1018 (June 1973).

34. Lenburg, "Preparation for Professionalism," op. cit., p. 321.

35. Sister Dorothy Sheahan, "Degree, Yes—Education, No," *Nurs. Outlook,* **22**:22–26 (Jan. 1974).

36. Lenburg, "Preparation for Professionalism," op. cit., pp. 323–325.

37. Ibid., p. 321.

38. Fay Carol Reed, "Education or Exploitation?" *Am. J. Nurs.,* **79**:1259–1261 (July 1979).

39. Ann Marriner, "Unification of Nursing Education and Service," *Nurs. Admin. Q,* **8**:58–64 (Fall 1983).

40. Nancy Fire et al, "Externship Programs: The Presbyterian Hospital Model" *Nurs. Outlook,* **32**:209–211 (July–Aug. 1984).

41. Carol Strauser, "An Internship with Academic Credit," *Am. J. Nurs.,* **79**:1071–1072 (June 1979).

42. Doris Wagner, "Nursing Administrators' Assessment of Nursing Education," *Nurs. Outlook,* **28**:557–561 (Sept. 1980).

43. Susan Harkins et al., "Summer Externs: Easing the Transition," *Nurs. Mgt.,* **14**:37–39 (July 1983).

44. Eileen A. McQuaid and Michael Kane, "How Do Graduates of Different Types of Programs Perform on State Boards?" *Am. J. Nurs.,* **79**:305–308 (Feb. 1979).

45. Angeline Jacobs, "Clinical Competencies of Baccalaureate, AD and Diploma Nurses—Are They Different?" *Issues,* **1**:1–3, 6 (Winter 1980).

46. *Working Paper of the NLN Task Force on Competencies of Graduates of Nursing Programs* (New York: National League for Nursing, 1979).

47. Marjorie Ramphal, "Rethinking Diploma School and Collegiate Education," *Nurs. Outlook,* **26**:768–771 (Dec. 1978).

48. Ibid., p. 770.

49. Michael Miller, "Academic Inbreeding in Nursing," *Nurs. Outlook,* **25**:172–177 (Mar. 1977).

50. National League for Nursing, *NLN Nursing Data Book* (New York: The League, 1984), p. 92.

51. Thetis Group and Joan Roberts, "Exorcising the Ghosts of the Crimea," *Nurs. Outlook,* **22**:368–372 (June 1974).

52. Patricia Beare et al., "Doctoral Curricula in Nursing," *Nurs. Outlook,* **29**:311–316 (May 1981).

53. Frances Taira and Suellen Reed, "Is That Doctorate Necessary?" *Nurs. Outlook,* **31**:12–15 (Jan.–Feb. 1983).

54. Shannon Perry, "A Doctorate—Necessary But Not Sufficient," *Nurs. Outlook,* **30**:95–114 (Feb. 1982).

55. Dorothy Kellmer, "The Lack of Effective Faculty Role Models within Professional Schools," *Nurs. and Health Care,* **3**:44–45 (Jan. 1982).

56. Sister Bernadette Armiger, "The Educational Crisis in the Preparation of Deans," *Nurs. Outlook,* **24**:164–168 (Mar. 1976).

57. Lucie Young Kelly, "Credentialing of Health Care Personnel," *Nurs. Outlook* **25**:568 (Sept. 1977).

58. Department of Health, Education, and Welfare, *Report on Licensure and Related Health Personnel Credentialing* (Washington, D.C.: U.S. Government Printing Office, 1971), p. 7.

59. National Commission on Accreditation, *Study of Accreditation of Selected Health Educational Programs Commission Report* (Washington, D.C.: The mission, 1972), pp. 15–16.

60. American Nurses' Association, *The Study of Credentialing in Nursing: A New Approach, The Report of the Committee* (Kansas City, Mo.: The Association, Jan. 1979), p. 89.

61. Jerome Lysaught, *Action in Affirmation: Toward an Unambiguous Profession of Nursing* (New York: McGraw Hill Book Company, 1981), p. 111.

13

Programs in Nursing Education

Educational preparation for licensure as a registered nurse takes place primarily in diploma programs, associate degree (AD) programs, and baccalaureate (BSN) programs. As noted in Chapter 12, the numbers have been shifting, with a decrease in diploma programs and an increase in AD and BSN programs. This chapter gives an overview of these educational modes, as well as graduate education and continuing education. The open curriculum is discussed in Chapter 12.

DIPLOMA PROGRAMS

The diploma, or hospital, school of nursing was the first type of nursing school in this country. Prior to the opening of the first hospital schools in the late 1800s, there was no formal preparation for nursing. But after Florence Nightingale established the first school of nursing at St. Thomas's Hospital, England, in 1860, the idea spread quickly to the United States.

Hospitals, of course, welcomed the idea of training schools because, in the early years, such schools represented an almost free supply of nursepower. With some outstanding exceptions, the education offered was largely of the apprenticeship type; there was some theory and formal classroom work, but for the most part students learned by doing, providing the majority of the nursing care for the hospitals' patients in the process.

This is no longer true. Today, in order to meet standards set in each state for operation of a nursing school and to prepare students to pass the licensing examinations, diploma schools must offer their student a truly educational program, not just an apprenticeship. Hospitals conducting such schools employ a full-time nurse faculty, offer students a balanced mixture of coursework (in nursing and related subjects in the physical and social sciences) and supervised practice, and look to their graduate nursing staff, not their students, to provide the nursing service needed by patients. The educational program has been generally three years in length, although most diploma schools have now adopted a shortened program. Upon satisfactory completion of the program, the student is awarded a diploma by the school. This diploma, it should be understood, is not an academic degree. Because most hospitals operating schools of nursing are not chartered to grant degrees, *no* academic credit can be given for courses taught by the school's faculty. For this and economic and educational reasons, large numbers of diploma schools enter into cooperative relations with colleges or universities for educational courses and/or services. It is not uncommon for diploma students to take physical and social science courses and, occasionally, liberal arts courses at a college. If these courses are part of the general offerings of the college, college credit is granted. Credit is usually transferable if the nursing student decides to transfer to a college or continue in advanced education. (If the course is tailored to nursing only, it is often not transferable to an advanced nursing program, but is sometimes counted as an elective.) Hospital schools usually provide other necessary educational resources, facilities, and services to students and faculty, such as libraries, classrooms, audiovisual materials, and practice laboratories. At one time, it was taken for granted that students would be housed, and the school had dormitory and recreational space, as well as educational facilities, in a separate building. Although the physical setup may still be thus arranged, such housing must now be paid for and may also be used by others educated in or involved with the hospital. The primary clinical facility is the hospital, although the school may contract with other hospitals or agencies for additional educational experiences. Advocates of diploma education usually say that early and substantial experiences with patients seem to foster a strong identification with nursing, particularly hospital nursing, and thus graduates are expected to adjust to the employee role without difficulty.

Admission requirements to diploma schools usually call for a college preparatory curriculum in high school, with standing in the upper half, third, or quarter (depending on the school) of the graduating class. Personal characteristics and health are also assessed.

There are a variety of concepts of what the diploma graduate is or should be. A statement approved by the NLN Council of Diploma Programs in 1978 is found in Exhibit 13-1.

Diploma school graduates still constitute the largest number of practicing nurses. In 1964, more than 88 percent of the 582,000 employed nurses were diploma school graduates. However, with the drop in the number of diploma schools, this percentage is also decreasing. In the 1982–1983 academic year, 11,704 students completed a diploma program as compared to 23,855 with BSNs and 41,849 with ADs.[1]

The perceptible shift away from diploma school preparation for nursing can be explained (in an oversimplified way) by three factors: (1) some hospitals are terminating their schools, either because of the expense involved in maintaining a quality program and the objections of third-party payers, such as insurance companies and the government, to having the cost of nursing education absorbed in the patient's bill, or because of difficulty in meeting professional standards, particularly in employing qualified faculty; (2) increasing numbers of high school graduates are seeking some kind of collegiate education; and (3) the nursing profession is more and more committed to the belief that preparation for nursing, as for all other professions, should take place in institutions of higher education.

These social and educational trends will probably continue, but it is expected that diploma programs will be on the scene for some time and that quality programs will continue to prepare quality graduates. The vast majority of current diploma programs are NLN accredited, and many of the schools that dissolved or were "phased into" associate degree or baccalaureate programs were also accredited. The 1970 National Commission study recommended that strong, vital schools be encouraged to seek regional accreditation and degree-granting status, but only a few have done so. Another recommendation, that other hospital schools move to effect interinstitutional arrangements with collegiate institutions, has been acted upon more readily.[2]

Although hospitals are less likely to operate schools, they continue as the clinical laboratories for nursing education programs. In the communities where new associate or baccalaureate degree programs are opening, there is of-

EXHIBIT 13-1

Role and Competencies of Graduates of Diploma Programs in Nursing

NURSING

The graduate of the diploma program in nursing is eligible to seek licensure as a registered nurse and to function as a beginning practitioner in acute, intermediate, long-term, and ambulatory health care facilities. In order to fulfill such roles, graduates should demonstrate the following competencies:*

ASSESSMENT

- Establishes a data base through a nursing history, including a psychosocial and physical assessment.
- Utilizes knowledge of the etiology, patho-physiology, usual course, and prognosis for the prevalent illnesses and health problems.
- Establishes priorities when providing nursing care for one or more patients.
- Recognizes the significance of nonverbal communications.

PLANNING

- Formulates a written plan of nursing care based on the assessment of patient needs.
- Includes in the nursing care plan the effects of the family or significant others, life experiences, and social-cultural background.
- Involves the patient, family, and significant others in the development of the nursing plan of care.
- Incorporates the learning needs of the patient and family into an individualized plan of care.
- Applies principles of organization and management in utilizing the knowledge and skills of other nursing personnel.

IMPLEMENTATION

- Meets the health needs of individuals and families.
- Utilizes concepts, scientific facts and principles when providing nursing care.
- Performs technical nursing procedures.
- Initiates appropriate intervention when environmental and safety hazards exist.
- Initiates preventive, habilitative, and rehabilitative nursing measures, according to the needs demonstrated by patients and families.
- Performs independent nursing measures and/or seeks assistance from other members of the health team in response to the changing needs of patients.
- Collaborates with physicians and members of other disciplines to provide health care.
- Documents nursing interventions and patient responses.
- Utilizes effective verbal and written communication.
- Communicates pertinent information related to the patient through established channels.
- Assists the physician in implementing the medical plan of care.
- Applies knowledge of individual and group behavior in establishing interpersonal relationships.
- Teaches individuals and groups to achieve and maintain an optimum level of wellness.
- Utilizes the services of community agencies for continuity of patient care.
- Protects the rights of patients and families.

EVALUATION

- Evaluates the effectiveness of nursing care and takes appropriate action.

• Initiates and cooperates in efforts to improve nursing practice.

*Competency, as used in this document, is the ability to apply in practice situations the essential principles and techniques of nursing and to apply those concepts, skills, and attitudes required of all nurses to fulfill their role, regardless of specific position or responsibility.

Source: Reprinted with permission of the National League for Nursing, 1977.

ten planning for new programs to evolve as diploma programs close—a phasing-in process. This cooperation enables prospective candidates for the diploma program to be directed to the new program, qualified diploma faculty to be employed by the college, and arrangements to be made to use space in the hospital previously occupied by the diploma school. Cooperative planning provides for continuity in the output of nurses to meet the needs of the community. Good diploma schools have met these needs well for many years.

ASSOCIATE DEGREE PROGRAMS

By far the greatest increase in programs and students has been in associate degree programs in nursing that are two years in length and offered by junior or community colleges, and occasionally by four-year colleges (about 25 percent). Associate degree education for nursing is a relative newcomer on the education scene. The first three programs were started in 1952; by 1965 there were more than 130 such programs, and in 1983 there were 764 AD programs graduating more than 41,000 students each year. More than half of these schools are NLN accredited, and most of the others are accredited by regional accrediting groups as part of their college's accreditation.

The associate degree program is the first nursing education program to be developed under a systematic plan and with carefully controlled experimentation. In her doctoral dissertation, published as a book in 1951, Mildred Montag conceived of a nursing tech-

nician able to perform nursing functions smaller in scope than those of the professional nurse and broader than those of the practical nurse. This nurse was intended to be a "bedside nurse" who was not burdened with administrative responsibilities. Montag listed the functions as (1) assisting in the planning of nursing care for patients, (2) giving general nursing care with supervision, and (3) assisting in the evaluation of the nursing care given.[3] The emerging community college was seen as a suitable setting for this education. Nursing education would be in the mainstream of education, and the burden of cost would be on the public in general, not on patients. The curriculum was to be an integrated one, half general education and half nursing, with careful selection of educational and clinical experiences.[4] An associate degree would be awarded at the end of the two years. The program was considered to be terminal and not a first step toward the baccalaureate.

At the end of 1951, the five-year Cooperative Research Project in Junior and Community College Education for Nursing was funded, and seven junior colleges and one hospital school were selected to participate in the project; each had complete autonomy in the development and conduct of its pilot program, but had free access to consultation from the project staff (see Chapter 5).

The results of the project showed that AD nursing technicians could carry on the intended nursing functions, that the program could be suitably set up in community colleges, with the use of clinical facilities in the community without charge or student service, and that the program attracted students. The success of the experiment plus the rapid growth of community colleges combined to give impetus to these new programs.*

Over the years, as Montag predicted, the AD curricula have varied and changed: for instance, when college policies permit, there is a tendency to put a heavier emphasis and more time on the nursing subjects and clinical experiences, sometimes through the addition of summer sessions. Some programs are also adding team leadership and managerial principles because their graduates are put in positions requiring these skills.

There are changes in philosophy as to what the technical nurse is and does. In one study, AD deans agreed that the knowledge base of the AD program was narrow in scope, the judgment area was as broad as that of the professional nurse, and the responsibilities were similar. They agreed that the technical nurse worked under the supervision of the professional nurse but should be considered a collaborator with professionals. Some did not see the program as terminal, seeing a difference in amount rather than kind of *professional* education.[5] The entire concept of the AD nursing program as terminal has changed over the last twenty years, along with general societal and educational concepts of *terminal*. Obviously, no educational program should be terminal in the sense that graduates cannot continue their education toward another degree. Whether or not they get full or only partial credit for their previous education depends on the philosophy and policies of the baccalaureate program they select. The growth of articulation models, (PN to RN) is impressive. Often these consist of a consortium of programs of each type, and the student may progress through the various programs in an immediate continuum or break at each licensure level, returning later if desired.† One survey of AD students in such a consortium indicated that less than

one-fourth saw the degree as terminal.[6] Nevertheless, what should be emphasized is that the AD nurse need not continue *formal* education to hold a valuable place in the health care system.

Because the catalogs of most AD nursing programs declare that they are preparing for technical nursing practice, the description of technical practice as differentiated from professional practice in the controversial ANA position paper on nursing education may be helpful:

> Technical nursing practice is carrying out nursing measures as well as medically delegated techniques with a high degree of skill, using principles from an ever-expanding body of science. It is understanding the physics of machines as well as the physiologic reactions of patients. It is using all treatment modalities with knowledge and precision.
>
> Technical nursing practice is evaluating patients' immediate physical and emotional reactions to therapy and taking measures to alleviate distress. It is knowing when to act and when to seek more expert guidance.
>
> Technical nursing practice involves working with professional nurse practitioners and others in planning the day-to-day care of patients. It is supervising other workers in the technical aspects of care.
>
> Technical nursing practice is unlimited in depth but limited in scope. Its complexity and extent are tremendous. It must be rendered under the direction of professional nurse practitioners, by persons who are selected with care and educated within the system of higher education; only thus can the safety of patients be assured. Education for this practice requires attention to scientific laws and principles with emphasis on skill. It is education which is technically oriented and scientifically founded, but not primarily concerned with evolving theory.[7]

Whether the term *technical* will continue to be used is not clear. The concept of a technical worker, honored in other fields, has not been fully accepted in nursing, possibly because it is considered a step down from the *professional*

---

*For an excellent, brief overview of the history, development, and achievements of the AD programs, see Alice Rines, "Associate Degree Education: History, Development, and Rationale," *Nurs. Outlook*, 25:496–501 (Aug. 1977).

†See Chapter 12.

label that has been attached to all nurses through licensing definitions and common usage over the years. Montag, noting the difficulty of choosing an appropriate term for the new type of proposed nurse, said, "It is also probable that the term 'nursing technician' will not satisfy forever, but it is proposed as one which indicates more accurately the person who has semi-professional preparation and whose functions are predominantly technical."[8]

The use of the term was rejected by the NLN Council of Associate Degree Programs in a 1974 action which noted that *technical* as applied to nursing practice was not fully understood or accepted. It was also rejected by the National Student Nurses' Association as connoting a less qualified nonprofessional. Even ANA sometimes seems to shy away from specifically designating the other-than-professional nurse as technical, although the 1979 model practice act does use term. The term *associate nurse* seems to be more acceptable.

More important than the name are the role and functions of the associate degree nurse. Because of nursing shortages, lack of understanding of the abilities and preparation of technical nurses, a tendency to use the diploma nurse of previous years as a standard, and general traditionalized concepts of nursing roles, employers have often not used AD nurses in the manner that best utilized their preparation. Like nurses through the centuries, AD nurses have been placed quickly as team leaders and charge nurses, positions in which they were not intended to function.*

In 1978, the NLN Council of Associate Degree Programs published a statement on the "Competencies of the Associate Degree Nurse on Entry into Practice" (see Exhibit 13-2). The "Assumptions Basic to the Scope of Practice" are particularly interesting because they clarify the kind of client and setting in which the AD nurse can function:

---

*The diary of Linda Richards, first "trained" nurse to be educated in America, has a familiar ring. See Linda Richards, *Reminiscensces of Linda Richards* (Boston: M. Barrows and Co., 1929).

The practice of graduates of associate degree nursing programs:

- Is directed toward clients who need information or support to maintain health.
- Is directed toward clients who are in need of medical diagnostic evaluation and/or are experiencing acute or chronic illness.
- Is directed toward clients' responses to common, well-defined health problems.
- Consists of nursing interventions selected from established nursing protocols where probable outcomes are predictable.
- Is concerned with individual clients and is given with consideration of the person's relationship within a family, group, and community.
- Includes the safe performance of nursing skills that require cognitive, psychomotor, and affective capabilities.
- May be in any structured care setting but primarily occurs within acute- and extended-care facilities.
- Is guided directly or indirectly by a more experienced registered nurse.
- Includes the direction of peers or other workers in nursing in selected aspects of care within the scope of practice of associate degree nursing.
- Involves an understanding of the roles and responsibilities of self and other workers within the employment setting.

Like other RNs, AD nurses are accountable for their own practice and are expected to function ethically and legally. In addition, the NLN Council made a point of saying that although these nurses work within the policies of an employing institution, they would also work within the organizational framework to initiate change in policies or nursing protocols.

There has been some complaint that AD nurses are not proficient in some technical skills, cannot handle large patient loads, and are slow to assume full staff nurse responsibilities and activities.[9,10] The reaction of some AD educators to these complaints, which has been to lengthen the program by adding clinical time or pseudointernships, has, in turn,

EXHIBIT 13-2

Competencies of the Associate Degree Nurse on Entry into Practice

ROLES OF PRACTICE

Five interrelated roles have been defined for graduates of the associate degree nursing program based upon the above assumptions underlying the scope of practice. These roles are: provider of care, client teacher, communicator, manager of client care, and member within the profession of nursing. In each of these roles, decisions and practice are determined on the basis of knowledge and skills, the nursing process, and established protocols of the setting.

Role as a Provider of Care. As a provider of nursing care, the associate degree nursing graduate uses the nursing process to formulate and maintain individualized nursing care plans by:

Assessing

• Collects and contributes to a data base (physiological, emotional, sociological, cultural, psychological, and spiritual needs) from available resources (e.g., client, family, medical records, and other health team members.)
• Identifies and documents changes in health status which interfere with the client's ability to meet basic needs (e.g., oxygen, nutrition, elimination, activity, safety, rest and sleep, and psychosocial well-being).
• Establishes a nursing diagnosis based on client needs.

Planning

• Develops individualized nursing care plans based upon the nursing diagnosis and plans intervention that follows established nursing protocols.
• Identifies needs and establishes priorities for care with recognition of client's level of development and needs, and with consideration of client's relationship within a family, group, and community.
• Participates with clients, families, significant others, and members of the nursing team to establish long- and short-range client goals.
• Identifies criteria for evaluation of individualized nursing care plans.

Implementing

• Carries out individualized plans of care according to priority of needs and established nursing protocols.
• Participates in the prescribed medical regime by preparing, assisting, and providing follow-up care to clients undergoing diagnostic and/or therapeutic procedures.
• Uses nursing knowledge and skills and protocols to assure an environment conducive to optimum restoration and maintenance of the client's normal abilities to meet basic needs.

   Maintains and promotes respiratory function (e.g., oxygen therapy, positioning, etc.).
   Maintains and promotes nutritional status (e.g., dietary regimes, supplemental therapy, intravenous infusions, etc.).
   Maintains and promotes elimination (e.g., bowel and bladder regimes, forcing fluids, enemas, etc.).
   Maintains and promotes a balance of activity, rest, and sleep (e.g., planned activities of daily living, environmental adjustment, exercises, sensory stimuli, assistive devices, etc.).
   Maintains an environment which supports physiological functioning, comfort, and relief of pain.

Maintains and promotes all aspects of hygiene.

Maintains and promotes physical safety (e.g., implementation of medical and surgical aseptic techniques, etc.).

Maintains and promotes psychological safety through consideration of each individual's worth and dignity and applies nursing measures which assist in reducing common developmental and situational stress.

Measures basic physiological functioning and reports significant findings (e.g., vital signs, fluid intake and output).

Administers prescribed medications safely.

• intervenes in situations where:

Basic life support systems are threatened (e.g., cardiopulmonary resuscitation, obstructive airway maneuver).

Untoward physiological or psychological reactions are probable.

Changes in normal behavior patterns have occurred.

• Participates in established institutional emergency plans.

Evaluating

• Uses established criteria for evaluation of individualized nursing care.
• Participates with clients, families, significant others, and members of the nursing team in the evaluation of established long- and short-range client goals.
• Identifies alternate methods of meeting client's needs, modifies plans of care as necessary, and documents changes.

Role as a Communicator.   As a communicator, the associate degree nursing graduate:

• Assesses verbal and non-verbal communication of clients, families, and significant others based upon knowledge and techniques of interpersonal communication.
• Use lines of authority and communication within the work setting.
• Uses communication skills as a method of data collection, nursing intervention, and evaluation of care.
• Communicates and records assessments, nursing care plans, interventions, and evaluations accurately and promptly.
• Establishes and maintains effective communication with clients, families, significant others, and health team members.
• Communicates client's needs through the appropriate use of referrals.
• Evaluates effectiveness of one's own communication with clients, colleagues, and others.

Role as a Client Teacher.   As a teacher of clients who need information or support to maintain health, the associate degree nursing graduate:

• Assesses situations in which clients need information or support to maintain health.
• Develops short-range teaching plans based upon long- and short-range goals for individual clients.
• Implements teaching plans that are specific to the client's level of development and knowledge.
• Supports and reinforces the teaching plans of other health professionals.
• Evaluates the effectiveness of client's learning.

Role as a Manager of Client Care.   As a manager of nursing care for a group of clients with common, well-defined health problems in structured settings, the associate degree nursing graduate:

EXHIBIT 13-2 (*Continued*)

- Assesses and sets nursing care priorities.
- With guidance, provides client care utilizing resources and other nursing personnel commensurate with their educational preparation and experience.
- Seeks guidance to assist other nursing personnel to develop skills in giving nursing care.

Role as a Member within the Profession of Nursing.   As a member within the profession of nursing, the associate degree nursing graduate:

- Is accountable for his or her nursing practice.
- Practices within the profession's ethical and legal framework.
- Assumes responsibility for self-development and uses resources for continued learning.
- Consults with a more experienced registered nurse when client's problems are not within the scope of practice.
- Participates within a structured role in research (e.g., data collection).
- Works within the policies of the employee or employing institution.
- Recognizes policies and nursing protocols that may impede client care and works within the organizational framework to initiate change.

Source: Reprinted with permission of the National League for Nursing, 1978.

been criticized by others who say this perverts the AD educational philosophy, which emphasizes an integrated curriculum and carefully selected learning experiences, enhanced by backup practice laboratories and student conferences.[11,12] Many educators, also believe that the AD students' request for additional clinical experience is probably no more frequent than that of other students, reacting to criticisms that new graduates are not instant, seasoned practitioners. Almost everyone agrees that AD graduates have a good grasp of basic nursing theory, have inquiring minds, and are self-directed in finding out what they don't know. It is also generally agreed that a good orientation program is the key to satisfactory acclimation to the work setting. However, 1983 changes in the federal Medicare programs (PL 98–21) may limit the scope of orientation programs that hospitals can provide. Certainly there are nurse administrators who see the AD graduate, properly utilized, as an asset to nursing service.[13] One point on which nursing in general agrees is that the AD nurse is here to stay and makes a vital contribution to health care.

BACCALAUREATE DEGREE PROGRAMS

The first baccalaureate program in nursing was established in 1909 under the control of the University of Minnesota, through the efforts of Dr. Richard Olding Beard. Since then, these programs have become an increasingly important part of nursing education.

The individual enrolled in a baccalaureate degree program in nursing obtains both a college education culminating in a bachelor's degree and preparation for licensure and practice as a registered professional nurse.

The program considered by the ANA as minimum preparation for professional nursing is usually four academic years in length. Unless the college is tax supported, with minimal tuition fees, baccalaureate nursing education is usually more expensive for students than other basic programs.

The baccalaureate degree program includes courses in general education and the liberal arts, the sciences germane to and related to nursing, and in nursing. In some programs, the student is not admitted to the nursing major (nursing courses) until the conclusion of the first two years of college study. In other programs, nursing content is integrated throughout the four years.

As in the other nursing programs, the baccalaureate program has both theoretical content and clinical experience. The baccalaureate student, who studies courses in the physical and social sciences will have greater depth and breadth, because students majoring in nursing take the college courses in the sciences and humanities with students majoring in biology or English literature. Nursing majors meet the same admission requirements and are held to the same academic standards as all other students. The nursing program is an integral part of the college or university as a whole.

A statement on the "Characteristics of Baccalaureate Education in Nursing" was developed by the NLN Council of Baccalaureate and Higher Degree Programs in 1979. It is found in Exhibit 13-3.

The most notable differences between baccalaureate education and that of the other basic nursing programs are related to liberal education, development of intellectual skills, and the addition of public health, teaching, and management concepts. Baccalaureate nurses have the opportunity to become liberally educated. Almost all programs allow free electives in the humanities, and many allow electives in the sciences and nursing courses. Nursing students are able to participate in cultural and social activities throughout their whole program and develop relationships with professors and students in other disciplines. Although technical skills are essential to nursing, learning activities that assist students to develop skills in recognizing and solving problems, applying general principles to particular situations, and establishing a basis for making sound clinical judgments are also given emphasis. This enables the nurse to function more easily when a familiar situation takes an unexpected turn or when it is necessary to deal with an unfamiliar situation. The baccalaureate program is the only basic program offering both theory and practice in public health nursing. There are also courses in health assessment and administrative and teaching principles. These skills are clearly necessary when the baccalaureate nurse functions as a primary nurse or as team leader, coordinating, planning, and directing the activities of other nursing personnel. It is on the basis of such backgrounds that the roles of a baccalaureate nurse are sometimes described as those of a practitioner engaged in direct patient care, teacher, leader, collaborator, and student (an inquiring person).[14] Of great impact is the early preparation of the baccalaureate nurse as nurse practitioner in primary care (see Chapter 15), which is a newer manifestation of these roles.

On completion of the program, most BSN graduates select hospitals as their place of employment, but then often turn to public health nursing. The changing pattern of health care delivery described in Chapter 7 has made home care and ambulatory care centers attractive employment sites for new baccalaureate graduates. However, those hospitals that have primary nursing, which gives nurses individual responsibility for a group of patients also seem to attract and retain baccalaureate nurses. Graduates with long-term plans for teaching, administration, or clinical specialization continue into graduate study. As noted in Chapter 11, BSN graduates are more likely to complete a graduate degree than their diploma or AD counterparts.

The number of RNs enrolled in baccalaureate programs has increased steadily. In 1982–1983, 48 percent of the almost 9,000 RNs graduating from baccalaureate programs held nursing diplomas; 55 percent held associate degrees.[15] In most nursing programs, RNs receive some credit and/or advanced standing for their previous education through challenge examinations. Frequently, courses and clinical experiences are individualized to meet RNs' needs and goals. However, RN students pursue the baccalaureate curriculum and earn the

EXHIBIT 13-3

Characteristics of Baccalaureate Education in Nursing

The baccalaureate program in nursing, which is offered by a senior college or university, provides students with an opportunity to acquire: (1) knowledge of the theory* and practice of nursing; (2) competency in selecting, synthesizing, and applying relevant information from various disciplines; (3) ability to assess client needs and provide nursing interventions; (4) ability to provide care for groups of clients; (5) ability to work with and through others; (6) ability to evaluate current practices and try new approaches; (7) competency in collaborating with members of other health disciplines and with consumers; (8) an understanding of the research process and its contribution to nursing practice; (9) knowledge of the broad function the nursing profession is expected to perform in society; and (10) a foundation for graduate study in nursing.

Nurses are prepared as generalists at the baccalaureate level to provide within the health care system** a comprehensive service of assessing, promoting, and maintaining the health of individuals and groups. These nurses are prepared to: (1) be accountable for their own nursing practice; (2) accept responsibility for the provision of nursing care through others; (3) accept the advocacy role in relation to clients; and (4) develop methods of working collaboratively with other health professionals. They will practice in a variety of health care settings—hospital, home, and community—and emphasize comprehensive health care, including prevention, health promotion, and rehabilitation services; health counseling and education; and care in acute and long-term illness.

Baccalaureate nursing programs are conceptually organized to be consistent with the stated philosophy and objectives of the parent institution and the unit in nursing. These programs provide the general and professional education essential for understanding and respecting people, various cultures, and environments; for acquiring and utilizing nursing theory upon which nursing practice is based; and for promoting self-understanding, personal fulfillment, and motivation for continued learning. The structure of the baccalaureate degree program in nursing follows the same pattern as that of baccalaureate education in general. It is characterized by a liberal education at the lower division level, on which is built the upper division major. In baccalaureate nursing education, the lower division consists of foundational courses drawn primarily from the scientific and humanistic disciplines inherent in liberal learning. The major in nursing is built upon this lower division general education base and is concentrated at the upper division level. Upper division studies include courses that complement the nursing component or increase the depth of general education.

Consistent with the foregoing characteristics and directly related to the "Criteria for the Appraisal of Baccalaureate and Higher Degree Programs in Nursing," the graduate of the baccalaureate program in nursing is able to:

• Utilize nursing theory in making decisions on nursing practice.
• Use nursing practice as a means of gathering data for refining and extending that practice.
• Synthesize theoretical and empirical knowledge from the physical and behavioral sciences and humanities with nursing theory and practice.
• Assess health status and health potential; plan, implement, and evaluate nursing care of individuals, families and communities.
• Improve service to the client by continually evaluating the effectiveness of nursing intervention and revising it accordingly.
• Accept individual responsibility and accountability for the choice of nursing intervention and its outcome.
• Evaluate research for the applicability of its findings to nursing actions.
• Utilize leadership skills through involvement with others in meeting health needs and nursing goals.

• Collaborate with colleagues and citizens on the interdisciplinary health team to promote the health and welfare of people.
• Participate in identifying and effecting needed change to improve delivery within specific health care systems.
• Participate in identifying community and societal health needs and in designing nursing roles to meet these needs.

*Throughout this statement, theory is used in the universal sense as it applies to all disciplines.

**The health care system includes social, cultural, economic, and political components. It can be conceptualized from an individual perspective of nurse and client/family to the broad, national health care scene. For the most part, the graduates of baccalaureate programs in nursing work within the local health care system although fully aware of the regional and national health care scenes. The master's graduates in nursing are proficient in working within the local health care system and have learned to extend their influence and effectiveness to and through the regional and national levels.

Source: Reprinted with permission of the National League for Nursing, 1979.

same degree as generic students. Although many more educational opportunities now exist for RNs,* some, because of circumstances, desire, or lack of counseling, choose nonnursing majors, which generally precludes their acceptance in a graduate program in nursing.[16] A noticeable trend is admission of students with baccalaureate or advanced degrees in fields other than nursing. These students, of course, receive a second baccalaureate. Depending on how many of their previous courses satisfy the BSN requirements, their program may consist primarily of the upper-division major nursing courses. A few baccalaureate programs have been especially designed for the baccalaureate graduate. However, there are other alternatives for these second careerists.

OTHER GENERIC EDUCATIONAL PROGRAMS FOR RN LICENSURE

A number of years ago, several nursing education programs, such as those at Yale and Western Reserve University, admitted only baccalaureate graduates and granted a master's degree in nursing as the basic educational credential. Today, there is a resurgence of interest in such programs. Some prepare for a generalist role, others for a specialty as clini-

---

*The Regents External Degree and other programs for RNs are discussed in Chapter 12.

cal specialist or nurse practitioner. Depending on the school's philosophy and state law, the student may take the licensing examination before completion of the master's.[17,18] (Not included in this discussion is the ladder concept, in which a student may get a license after completion of an AD or baccalaureate and then continue directly to the master's degree.)

The first program for a professional doctorate (ND) for college graduates was established at Case-Western Reserve in 1979. It was designed for "liberally educated men and women who are gifted intellectually, willing to invest themselves in a rigorous, demanding, rewarding program of study, and committed to a sustained professional career."[19] As described, the program, if adopted by others, should be located only in universities with health science centers preparing several types of health professionals. Because such universities also offer advanced graduate education, ND students are prepared in an academic climate of scholarship and research. Faculty are prepared at the highest level of scholarship, with some engaged in teaching and research and others, jointly appointed, master's-prepared clinicians engaged in clinical practice, teaching, and some aspect of research. The curriculum prepares the ND graduates to become proficient in the delivery of primary, episodic, and long-term nursing care, and to evaluate their own practices, and that of their assistants, since they are accountable for the outcomes of all nursing practice. Graduates of this program would continue graduate study in a specialization and/or a functional area such as teaching or administration. As is true of medical students whose professional degree is a doctorate, they might also obtain a master's or PhD concurrently with the first doctorate. This innovative approach, seen as a major step toward the emergence of nursing as a full-fledged profession, will be under close scrutiny for some years to come.

GRADUATE EDUCATION

Graduate education in nursing, of a kind, can be traced back to the first decades of the twentieth century. However, there was considerable confusion in those early years in that what was called graduate education was actually education *for graduate nurses* beyond their basic diploma program. The first program concentrated on public health nursing and preparation for teaching and supervision. As late as 1951, it was finally recognized that there was little differentiation between the programs leading to a baccalaureate degree and those leading to a master's; the master's was found to be little more than a symbol that the nurse had previously earned a bachelor's degree. This led to a series of recommendations to place graduate education for nurses on the same basis as that in other disciplines.[20] In the following years, graduate programs *for practice* in public health nursing, teaching, and education were developed, but in 1952 only 1,449 nurses had completed programs for advanced nursing practice, teaching, supervision, and administration, a figure aptly described by the League as "microscopic" compared with the nation's needs.[21] By 1962, nurses with graduate preparation had increased to 11,500 out of the 550,000 nurses in practice at that time. The Surgeon General's Report, citing the need for teachers, nurse administrators, and others requiring advanced education, called for a doubling of baccalaureate graduates and a tripling of master's and doctor's degrees by 1970.[22]

Even with the federal traineeships, scholarships, and loans that followed the report, that goal was not achieved. In 1972, there were approximately 25,000 nurses (out of 778,470) with master's degrees (not all in nursing).[23] About 1,000 had doctoral degrees. By 1980, the number of nurses holding master's degrees or doctorates had increased to about 5 percent of the total number of nurses, as opposed to 3.3 percent in 1972.[24] About 4,000 held doctoral degrees, most of which were not from a school of nursing.

Today, the purpose of master's education is to prepare professional nursing leaders in the areas of clinical specialization, teaching, and administration. Nurses with these special skills and knowledge are desperately required now and will be for the foreseeable future.

Perhaps because so much of the emphasis in graduate programs over the years had been on attaining functional skills in teaching and administration, with little attention given to clinical knowledge and skills, a 1969 ANA statement on graduate education proclaimed that the "major purpose of graduate education should be the preparation of nurse clinicians capable of improving nursing care through the advancement of nursing service and theory."[25] However, it soon became evident that nurses in education and administration did indeed need the functional skills required in these fields. Almost ten years later, a new statement focused on "the preparation of highly competent individuals who can function in diverse roles, such as clinical nurse generalists or specialists, researchers, theoreticians, teachers, administrators, consultants, public policy makers, system managers, and colleagues on multidisciplinary teams . . . prepared through master's, doctoral, and postdoctoral programs in nursing that subscribe to clearly defined standards of scholarship."[26] Nontraditional graduate programs, such as those previously described, were also encouraged because they "can provide for significant contributions to the advancement of scholarship in nursing."[27] Other nontraditional approaches, such as interinstitutional exchange programs, consortium arrangements, and satellite and off-campus programs, were also cited as innovative and approved ''in concert with beliefs about pluralism, diversity, and flexibility in graduate education.''[28]

It is interesting to note that programs in *nursing* are specified, presumably signaling that master's and doctoral degrees in other fields, without a nursing component, are not encouraged. A 1979 NLN statement also emphasizes expansion of nursing knowledge: ''Individuals prepared at the master's level in nursing improve nursing and health care through their expert practice, and through the advancement of theory in nursing.'' Acquisition of research methods is considered essential. In general, master's education in nursing includes concentrated study of a specific area of nursing, introduction to research methods, and independent study of a nursing problem, using research techniques. The latter is called a *master's thesis, project,* or *study.*

Most NLN-accredited master's programs offer study of a clinical area, such as medical-surgical nursing, maternal-child nursing, community health nursing, or psychiatric nursing with advanced experience, based on a theoretical framework developed by that faculty and including relevant advanced courses in the natural and social sciences. The depth of clinical study varies in relation to whether the nurse plans to become a clinical specialist or nurse practitioner or wishes to concentrate on a functional area such as teaching, administration, or consultation, for which other appropriate courses will also be offered. Increasingly, a practicum (planned, guided learning experiences in a practice setting that allow a student to function within the role) is being recommended for the functional as well as the clinical areas. These practices vary from program to program, from one day a week for a semester to almost a year's full-time residency.

Master's degree education in nursing has been described as providing students with an opportunity to:

(1) acquire advanced knowledge from the

sciences and the humanities to support advanced nursing practice and role development; (2) expand their knowledge of nursing theory as a basis for advanced nursing practice; (3) develop expertise in a specialized area of clinical nursing practice; (4) acquire the knowledge and skills related to a specific functional role in nursing; (5) acquire initial competence in conducting research; (6) plan and initiate change in the health care system and in the practice and delivery of health care; (7) further develop and implement leadership strategies for the betterment of health care; (8) actively engage in collaborative relationships with others for the purpose of improving health care; and (9) acquire a foundation for doctoral study.[29]

Graduate programs in nursing vary in admission requirements, organization of curriculum, length of program, and costs. Admission usually requires RN licensure, graduation from an approved (or accredited) baccalaureate program with an upper-division major in nursing,* a satisfactory grade point average, achievement on selected tests, and sometimes nursing experience. Part-time study is available in some programs, but often certain courses must be taken in sequence, and at least some full-time study may be required. Reduced federal support and fewer traineeships have stimulated faculty to develop more part-time study options. It should be remembered that not all graduate programs offer all possible majors. An NLN pamphlet, ''Master's Education in Nursing, Route to Opportunities in Contemporary Nursing,'' presents an overall view of all accredited nursing master's programs, including curricula, clinical and functional majors, and admission requirements, availability of part-time study, length of program, approximate cost, and availability of housing.

Although some nurses obtain graduate degrees outside the field of nursing, advanced positions in nursing usually require a nursing

---

*Some programs will admit a few nurses without BSNs and assist them in making up deficiencies.

degree, preferably with advanced clinical content and experience.* Currently, there are some 120 universities with accredited nursing master's programs in the United States, (about 112 with clinical majors). Obviously a suitable nursing program is not necessarily accessible to all nurses who seek graduate education. Nevertheless, selection of a suitable graduate program is essential, and nurses should carefully review catalogs to determine which programs meet their career goals.

Nurses with master's degrees are expected to assume leadership positions in one way or another, in terms of both the profession and public service. A renewed recognition of the importance of interdisciplinary collaboration is also worth noting:

> The leadership strategies developed and implemented for the betterment of health care encompass the range of activities needed to influence both nursing education and nursing practice constructively. Furthermore, these strategies are designed to promote the personal and professional investment of self and to employ professional standards and ethical conduct. The leadership strategies emanate from a broad theoretical base and enable the leader to prescribe, decide, influence, and facilitate changes for nursing and health. The direction and scope of leadership are directly related to one's field of operation and to the publics served. The roles of change agent and consumer advocate are also affected through the selection and implementation of a broad range of appropriate strategies.

The interdisciplinary collaboration role of the graduate of a master's program is characterized by initiation and interpretation. Master's-prepared nurses utilize newly acquired functional role skills to design, initiate, and assume a leadership role as well as a collaborative role. They take an active part in deline-

---

*The exception may be graduates from schools of public health, who have had programs in public health nursing and/or administration that do not include clinical components per se.

ating the goals and standards of the group and in designing the mode and terms of operation. One of the major responsibilities of a master's graduate in nursing is to interpret the role and function of nurses to others.[30]

The first American nurse to earn a doctorate received her PhD in psychology and counseling in 1927. Until 1946, when two of the forty-six colleges and universities offering advanced programs in nursing also initiated doctoral education for nurses, nurses who desired doctoral studies had to attend programs outside of nursing. By 1969, some twenty-five different doctoral degrees were being awarded to nurses, including the Doctor of Nursing (DN), Doctor of Nursing Science (DNS or DNSc), Doctor of Nursing Education (DNEd), and Doctor of Public Health Nursing (DPHN), as well as Doctor of Philosophy (PhD), and Doctor of Education (EdD). There is still disagreement, and some confusion, in nursing circles as to the kind of education and degree a nurse should get in a doctoral program. The first definitive statement on doctoral education in nursing was made by the NLN in 1955, the same year that the DHEW Division of Nursing activated the Predoctoral and Postdoctoral Nursing Research Fellowship Program in order to assist nurses to qualify for doctoral study in a discipline outside nursing and to encourage the preparation of research personnel. At that time, the NLN committee considering graduate programs made certain assumptions about the doctoral degree:

> (1) the doctorate should not be a third professional degree in nursing but should be based upon a second professional degree and constitute new and enlarged experience in relevant intellectual disciplines and scholarly research in the application of such disciplines to nursing; (2) the degree could be interdisciplinary, possibly in the social sciences, biological sciences, and education; (3) in those institutions not permitting interdisciplinary doctor-

ates, the degree should be awarded in a single discipline such as sociology, biology, and the like.[31]

By 1960, the major activity in doctoral education for nurses focused on establishing collaborative arrangements with other disciplines in a university through which nurses could receive doctoral degrees. Only four institutions offered doctoral programs in which an area of nursing, teaching, or administration in nursing was the focus of study.[32] In 1963, the Nurse Scientist Graduate Training Grants Program was initiated by DHEW and new attention was given to doctoral study. The national nursing organizations and universities held a number of programs and conferences to discuss philosophical bases and explore trends affecting doctoral study.

The "appropriate" doctoral degree for nurses has been a matter of debate. Some nursing leaders favor granting a PhD in nursing with a minor in a relevant discipline. Others have felt that although the nursing PhD is an ultimate goal, nursing science is not sufficiently developed to made this practical immediately. Instead they suggest either a PhD in some other discipline with a minor in nursing or a strictly professional degree such as the DNS. It is believed that a nurse with an academic degree (PhD) in a cognate discipline could help to generate knowledge, and the nurse with the professional degree (EdD or DNSc) would apply this new knowledge.

The following varied principles concerning doctoral education for nursing are most often stated:

1. The doctoral program should be pursued in an established discipline such as the natural, biological, or behavioral sciences with or without a minor in nursing.
2. A program culminating in a PhD with a major in nursing should give candidates a theoretical base of pure research in nursing.
3. Programs leading to a professional degree, e.g., DNSc should prepare the graduate for

scholarly practice of nursing as a clinical specialist or nurse therapist.
4. Doctoral programs in health care administration, public health, and education should be open to nurses who wish to prepare for such relevant fields of practice.[33]

The Nurse Scientist Program, federally funded, gave considerable impetus to the first principle, and in 1973 there were nine institutions with formal programs for the nurse-scientist. With discontinuation of federal funds, these programs were essentially nonexistent a few years later. However, they served an important role in preparing teachers and researchers. There are also strong proponents of the second principle by those who firmly believe that "nursing is characterized by an organized body of abstract knowledge specific to nursing . . . not a summation of facts and principles drawn from other sources," and who feel that nursing's future as a learned profession and its yet unrealized potential for human service are dependent largely to the extent that scholarly education through doctoral study is made explicit.[34] The concern of others is that practitioners of nursing use concepts from related disciplines to develop, test and apply nursing theory and conduct research contributing to nursing knowledge and practice. And finally, there are those who feel that administrators in education and nursing services would find degrees in relevant fields most valuable.

The ANA statement on doctoral programs takes a relatively broad view:

> Doctoral programs of study are designed to prepare nurses as theoreticians, scholars, researchers, administrators, health policy teachers, planners, and clinicians. Now and in the future, doctoral programs should be directed toward the formulation and testing of theories; the creation of research designs, methods, and tools to study nursing and health problems; and the development of scientific and humanistic knowledge appropriate to the care of man in health and illness.[35]

Although there are still many nurses enrolled in nonnursing doctoral programs, the pendulum may have swung toward doctoral degrees in nursing in the last few years. By 1983, twenty-seven doctoral programs in nursing were established, and a number of other schools were in the planning process. The specific degrees included EdD, PhD, DNS, DNSc, and ND, with areas of study in all major specialties in nursing as well as nursing education and administration. The growth is phenomenal, considering that in 1970 there were only six programs.[36] The major area of development has been within state universities. It is anticipated that by 1990, doctoral education in nursing will be available in every state. While this may be a desirable goal, there is a great deal of concern about quality.[37]

The characteristics of high-quality nursing doctoral programs have been described as follows:

1. Well-prepared faculty holding earned doctorates, with the majority holding a doctoral degree in nursing.
2. Evidence of research and scholarly productivity of faculty.
3. Maintenance of a learning climate conducive to intellectual curiosity, advancement of clinical knowledge, and identification of researchable problems.
4. Evidence of continuous, active, productive, quality-based research in the parent institution.
5. Selection of students who are intellectually capable and professionally committed to nursing and the health care of all people.
6. Philosophical and financial accountability of the parent institution to support a doctoral program in nursing and make university resources available for the conduct of the program.
7. Consideration of regional and national resources to enhance program offerings, assure quality, and augment areas of faculty expertise.
8. Provision for evaluation of the doctoral program and the impact of graduates.[38]

These make clear the need for appropriate faculty and resources.*

Although the role of doctoral nurses is still not clearly understood by many lay people and even some other disciplines, nursing leaders see an urgency in increasing this too small pool of scholars, because the shortage is expected to remain acute into at least the late 1980s. Their role is well described by one:

> . . . doctoral programs in nursing must be designed to prepare highly knowledgeable and competent researchers, clinicians, teachers, and administrators for academic and service settings. As doctoral programs increase in number, it is important that they maintain commitments to highly disciplined modes of thought, quality research work, and demonstrated skills in writing and leadership. If doctoral education for nurses maintains such commitments, the critical leadership crises in nursing would be mitigated; leadership, new scientific and humanistic thrusts will take their place in nursing history. Nurses who are graduates of doctoral programs should have a scientific and humanistic grasp of general and special problems of nursing, and should be prepared to challenge past modes of thought and to risk new kinds of nursing practices.[39]

To determine the characteristics of doctoral nurses and what they are doing, the American Nurses' Foundation has done two surveys, one published in 1973† and the other in 1981.[40] Some interesting data can be summarized from the second survey. The typical doctoral nurse was a forty-nine year-old married white female who earned her doctorate at age forty-one. (Males are slightly more likely to be married.) The geographic distribution was uneven, with the majority of the group living in

---

*A relatively recent phenomenom is the external doctorate described by H. Terri Brower, "The External Doctorate," *Nurs. Outlook*, **27**:594–599 (Sept. 1979).

†This can be found in the fourth edition of Lucie Young Kelly *Dimensions of Professional Nursing*, New York: Macmillan Publishing Co. 1981.

the South Atlantic and Middle Atlantic states. Most of the nurses had been educated in a diploma program; there was about a nineteen year time lapse between the time of first graduation and the doctorate. With the baccalaureate nurses (one-third of the group), there was about a seven-year time lapse until the master's, and an average eight-year lapse between the master's and the doctorate. It takes both men and women about four and a half years from entry to completion of a doctorate. These figures do not relate to doctorates in other fields, which may take longer. The federal government was the most frequent source of educational funds. Of the participants in the study (1,956), an average of 10 earned their doctorates each year from 1932 to 1957; about 15 from 1958 to 1967; 30 from 1963 to 1969 and, beginning in 1970, about 100 (except for 1977, when the figure was 200). Fifty-three percent of the nurses held a PhD, and about 34 percent held an EdD, the most popular degree prior to the 1970s. The DNS/DNSc was first awarded in the 1960s, and the percentage holding the degree, although still small (about 5 percent), is increasing rapidly. The JD has also increased over the years and is held primarily by younger nurses. Men are more likely to hold a PhD or DNS/DNSc. Education was the most common field of study; nursing was the field for about one-fifth. The majority of these nurses were employed (90.6 percent); most worked fulltime. Only 1 percent were unemployed and seeking employment. Work settings included primarily educational institutions, but also hospitals, community health agencies, and governmental agencies; some nurses were self-employed in the private practice of law, medicine, counseling, or nursing. Teaching was the primary function cited, but many listed a combination of functions. About 25 percent were in administration. Research as a major function was listed by only 7 percent. About 6 percent reported holding or having held a postdoctoral appointment,[41] primarily to obtain research experience; most of the others chose to study in a specific area or to gain experience in health service or educational administration.

This report was part of the data submitted to the Institute of Medicine (IOM) in the study of nursing and nursing education.* The fact that a projected need for nurses with masters and doctorates in 1990 (256,000 and 14,000, respectively) was clearly not going to be met was undoubtedly a major factor in their recommendation to increase and expand graduate programs. Certainly, the availability of federal funds for programs and students will facilitate such expansion, but it will be the responsibility of nursing to see that the quality of each is good and serves the American public.

PROGRAMS FOR PRACTICAL NURSES

Professional nurses work closely with practical nurses (PNs) in all branches of hospital and public health nursing. Moreover, in the last few years, an increasing number of PNs have been entering RN programs at either a beginning or an advanced level. It is helpful, therefore, to be informed about the educational preparation of a PN, as well as the basic RN programs.

Practical nurses (called *vocational nurses* in Texas and California) fall into four general groups: (1) those whose only teacher has been experience and who are not licensed to practice (this type of PN is gradually disappearing from the scene); (2) those with experience but no formal education who have taken state-approved courses to qualify them to take state board examinations and become licensed; (3) those who have been licensed through a grandfather clause; and (4) those who have graduated from approved schools of practical nursing and, by passing state board examinations, have become licensed in the state or states in which they practice. There are also a few who were enrolled in RN programs and

---

*See Chapter 5.

were permitted by their state law to take the PN examination after a certain number of courses. The large majority of LPNs are licensed by examination. Although PNs in the third catagory can be legally employed, employers with a choice usually prefer graduates from an approved school who have been licensed by examination.

PNs are usually educated in one-year programs in vocational, trade, or technical schools (53 percent), hospitals, or community colleges. Academic credits are awarded by the colleges. In 1982, there were 1,319 PN programs, which admitted about 60,000 students, a slight increase from the previous academic year. Graduations declined.[42] The growth rate of both programs and numbers of students had been increasing steadily over the years, but appears to have leveled off and perhaps decrease. PN education has been heavily supported by the federal government for some time. The desire for LPNs to reach RN status is manifested by their increased admission to (and graduation from) RN programs. For some years, PN programs have seemed to attract more blacks, more men, and more older students than any other type of nursing program. However, many of these potential students, if qualified, now seem to choose AD or baccalaureate programs.

Legitimate PN programs must be approved by the appropriate state nursing authority and may also be accredited by either NLN or the National Association for Practical Nurse Education and Service (NAPNES). The latter accredits only about 26 programs. Upon graduation, the student is eligible to take the licensing examination (NCLEX-PN)* to become a licensed practical nurse (LPN) or a licensed vocational nurse (LVN). The licensing law is not mandatory in all states but all nursing organizations support mandatory licensure. NAPNES does an annual survey of all licensing boards which helps pinpoint trends (such as the increase in the requirement for a high school diploma or its equivalent for admission).

*See Chapter 20.

PN programs emphasize technical skills and direct patient care, but a (usually) simple background of the physical and social sciences is often integrated in the program. Clinical experience is provided in one or more hospitals and other agencies. The number of skills that are taught increases each year, probably because of employers' demands.

There is some trend to make a PN program the first year of a two-year associate degree program. A student may exit at the end of the year, become licensed and work, or become licensed and not work and continue into the second year, becoming eligible for the RN examination. Some RN programs, particularly for the associate degree, give partial or total credit for the PN program (often only if the PN has also passed the licensing examination). In PN programs, most teachers have a baccalaureate degree or less, but NLN recommends preparation for the broad scope of nursing and preparation in teaching. As in all areas of health care, there is a need for continuing education programs. Employers frequently offer courses, reviews, or inservice programs for giving medications and performing new treatments, but the two PN organizations and NLN have provided programs on care of geriatric patients, psychiatric patients, and others. There are also numerous continuing education programs geared particularly toward the LPN licensed by waiver.

LPNs work in hospitals (73 percent), extended care facilities (18 percent), nursing homes, doctors' offices, private homes, and other health facilities, including to some extent, community health agencies. They care for patients of all ages, but mostly adults. According to a survey done by the National Council of State Bords, entry-level PNs are primarily involved in the following activities:

- admitting clients;
- helping clients with personal hygiene, bathing, ambulation, and meals;
- helping clients with body alignment, including range-of-motion exercises and maintaining traction;
- care of dying clients, including providing

time for them to talk and emotional support to the family;

- skin care, cast care, ostomy care, enemas, and urinary catheterizations;
- such respiratory care as monitoring oxygen therapy, supervising coughing and deep breathing exercises, doing postural drainage, and nasopharyngeal and endotracheal suctioning, but not suctioning the tracheo-bronchial tree;
- obtaining culture specimens from all areas except the cervix;
- performing CPR and checking emergency supplies and equipment;
- cleaning furniture and equipment;
- administering compresses, sitz baths, and alcohol baths for local temperature modification;
- using ice, baths, and heating pads, but not hypo/hyperthermia machines for systemic temperature modification;
- measuring all vital signs except CVP and mean arterial pressure; and
- administering medications by most standard routes except IV.[43]

They are least likely to be involved in activities that require technological skills.

Both NLN and NAPNES have published statements on LPN entry-level competencies. The NLN statement is found in Exhibit 13-4. The NAPNES statement is almost identical.[44]

Because PNs are often pressed to perform functions beyond the level of their education (such as charge nursing and certain specialty practice), there has been an increasing movement of PNs to "be paid for what we do, not what we are." However health economics and LPN layoffs have brought new concerns. In August 1984, citing "concern for job safety" the National Federation of Licensed Practical Nurses (NFLPN) House of Delegates endorsed two levels of nursing (RN and LP/VN) and the expansion of the LP/VN curriculum program to at least 18 months. An implementation date of 10 years was set.

Continuing Education

Professional practitioners of any kind must continue to learn because they are accountable to the public for a high quality of service—a service impossible to maintain if pertinent aspects of the tremendous flow of new knowledge are not integrated and used.

A thought-provoking model of the fleeting hold professionals have on what they learn was described some years ago in a journal:

Assuming that the professional life of an individual (in this example, a physician) is forty years, the amount of clinically applicable knowledge available in mid-career should be 100 percent. However, the body of knowledge available at the time of the educational program is only about half, leaving 50 percent useful. It is only possible to teach a fraction of this knowledge in any educational program, leaving 20 percent useful. Of this, a small part is erroneous, leaving 19 percent useful. Not all that is taught is learned, leaving 16 percent useful. Much of what is learned is forgotten within a few years, leaving 8 percent useful; some of what is learned is never used because of specialization, leaving 5 percent useful. Much of what is learned becomes obsolete in 20 years, leaving 3 percent of useful knowledge gained in the professional's basic educational program.[45]

While the precision of the figures can obviously by challenged, the message is clear, even in nonquantitative terms: ongoing learning (continuing education) is necessary if a professional is to function effectively.

For nurses, specifically, the need for continuing education is primarily to keep them abreast of changes in nursing roles and functions, acquire new knowledge and skills (and/or renew that which has been lost), and modify attitudes and understanding. To achieve these goals, various approaches to continuing education can be utilized, such as formal academic studies that might lead to a degree; short-term courses or programs given by institutions of higher learning that do not necessarily provide academic credit; and independent or informal study carried on by the practitioner, utilizing opportunities made available through professional organizations and employing agencies. It should be made clear that continuing one's education does not

EXHIBIT 13-4

Competencies of Graduates of Educational Programs in Practical Nursing.

Competencies are the minimal expectations of the new graduates of an educational program in practical nursing.

Introduction

Licensed practical nurses (LPNs), in some areas called licensed vocational nurses (LVNs) are prepared to function under the definition and framework of the role specified by the nurse practice acts of the states where they are employed. LPNs/LVNs are prepared to function under the guidance of a registered nurse or licensed physician as responsible members of the health care team. LPNs/LVNs are concerned with basic therapeutic, rehabilitative, and preventive care for people of all ages and different cultures in various stages of dependency.

Practical nursing students are prepared in educational programs that stress clinical experiences primarily in structured care settings such as hospitals and nursing homes. Clinical practice is correlated with basic therapeutic knowledge and introductory content from the biological and behavioral sciences. Planned and supervised experiences are directed toward teaching students to perform nursing measures with precision, safety, and efficiency consistent with current nursing concepts and practices. Communication skills and mental health concepts are integrated into the total curriculum. Qualified nurse educators guide students in the nursing process and care planning.

Graduates of Practical Nursing Education Programs can be expected to have the following competencies:

Assessing

- Contributes to the identification of basic physical, emotional, and cultural needs of the health care client.
- Identifies basic communication techniques in a structured care setting.
- Interviews health care clients to obtain specified information.
- Identifies overt learning needs of the health care client.
- Observes the health care client and communicates significant findings to the health care team.
- Identifies appropriate resources in some other agencies within the health care delivery system.

Planning

- Contributes to the development of basic nursing care plans in an institutional setting.
- Contributes, with assistance, to the development of health plans for health care clients and/or families.

Implementing

- Safely performs basic therapeutic and preventive nursing procedures, incorporating fundamental biological and psychological principles in giving individualized care.
- Shows respect for the dignity of individuals.
- Applies basic communication techniques in a structured care setting.
- Demonstrates the ability to do incidental teaching during routine care.
- Shares assigned responsibility for health care delivery in structured situations.

Evaluating

• Seeks guidance as needed in evaluating the care given and making necessary adjustments.
• Identifies own strengths and weaknesses and seeks assistance for improvement of performance.

Role as a Member within the Profession of Nursing

• Recognizes own role as an LPN/LVN in the health care delivery system.
• Seeks out and takes advantage of learning situations and opportunities for own continuing education.

Source: Reprinted with permission of the National League for Nursing, 1979.

mean that enrollment in a formal academic, degree-granting program is necessary, although it might well be a reasonable route for a nurse who has specific career goals. On the other hand, neither does achievement of the highest academic degree mean an end to continued learning.

One statement of philosophy, probably not too different from that developed by other groups, is useful in delineating the scope of continuing education:

Continuing education in nursing consists of planned, organized learning experiences designed to augment the knowledge, skills, and attitudes of registered nurses for the enhancement of nursing practice, education, administration, and research, to the end of improving health care to the public. Defined broadly, continuing education is a lifelong learning process that builds on and modifies previously acquired knowledge, skills, and attitudes. The structure and content of continuing education must be flexible in order to meet the nursing practice needs and career goals of nursing personnel.[46]

In the 1970s, a number of states enacted legislation requiring evidence of continuing education (CE) for relicensure of nurses (and of certain other professional and occupational groups). Under the stimulus of this legislative mandate, formalized programs have increased. They are given under the auspices of educational institutions, professional organizations, and commercial for-profit groups. Most now seek some sort of recognition or ac-

creditation so that their programs will be acknowledged by licensing boards as legitimate sources of continuing education. Most programs use the Continuing Education Unit (CEU), nationally accepted for unit measurement of all kinds of CE programs. (Ten contact hours equal one unit.)

Both the ANA and NLN and their constituent organizations have been engaged in planning and implementing a voluntary system of continuing education for nurses. The ICN has urged its members to take the lead in initiating, promoting, or further developing a national system of continuing nursing education. The ANA has set both standards and guidelines. The latter include such points as working with other organizations, employees, and educational systems to provide continuing education to nurses, but a major focus is development of Continuing Education Approval and Recognition Programs (CEARP) or Continuing Education Recognition Programs (CERP). Almost all state nurses' association (SNAs), except in those states where CE is mandatory, now have some form of CERP program. Generally, their purpose is to record and/or recognize nurses' voluntary participation in CE and approve CE offerings. Contact hours, or CEUs, or recognition points (one point is equal to one contact hour) are the time measurements used. A fee may be charged to the nurse if recording services are extensive. When the SNA also has an accreditation or approval program, the CE provider inevitably pays a fee.[47]

The ANA accreditation program, with its

regional accrediting committees, is a separate entity and provides the learner, employer, state board, or other interested consumer some assurance that the accredited program has met certain standards. To meet the criteria, the provider group usually must include information about its educational resources, qualifications of the teachers, objectives, outline, and evaluation techniques to be used for each program. CE programs of the schools accredited by the NLN are usually included in the total accreditation, but some also seek ANA CE accreditation.

More nurses seem to be attending formal programs. How much CE improves practice is still an arguable question, for measurement of direct results is seldom practical. However, it has been shown that the motivation of the learner and the opportunity to apply what is learned are key factors.

Although in-service programs are not always accepted for formal CE requirements, most employers make such programs available (or mandatory) for improvement of nursing practice. Because such programs can be quite costly, there is increased interest in providing educationally sound programs, directed toward meeting specific practice goals and building in an evaluation mechanism.[48,49] In some cases, evidence of CE is a job requirement or necessity for promotion. In other cases (fire prevention and infection control), formal CE is a requirement of the Joint Commission for the Accreditation of Hospitals (JCAH).

Opportunities and funds to attend programs are often part of some collective bargaining agreements. However, nurses, especially if they consider themselves professionals, should be prepared to pay for their own CE.

One of the greatest thrusts in CE in the last 15 years has been the nurse practitioner programs. When the first program was begun at the University of Colorado in 1965, it was as continuing education. Until recently, a majority of the programs either were or began in that mode. They ranged for some time from on-the-job training to organized programs of a year or more, culminating in a certificate. Those funded by HHS must be at least a year in length, according to governmental guidelines. The first semiformal approval mechanism was a joint statement of the ANA and the American Academy of Pediatrics, which issued guidelines in 1972. However, later there was some disagreement on the degree of physician control, and by 1974, the ANA had developed accreditation guidelines for CE that were specific to the various types of nurse practitioner programs. Although there is a definite trend toward master's degree education for NPs it is expected that the CE programs will not be completely phased out for some time.

Is CE readily available to most nurses? Despite some justifiable complaints that formal programs are not always available in certain geographic areas, there are many ways for nurses at all educational levels to continue their professional development. Examples of self-directed learning activities include self-guided, focused reading, independent learning projects, individual scientific research, informal investigation of a specific nursing problem, correspondence courses, self-contained learning packages using various media, directed reading, computer-assisted instruction, programmed instruction, study tours, and group work projects.* The first nursing journal to have developed self-learning programs that include evaluation, for a minimal fee, was the AJN, and others have followed. There have also been other innovative ways in which nurses are offered learning opportunities, such as through mobile vans, television, telephone systems, satellites, and other forms of telecommunication, as well as increased regional programs by nursing organizations.

The opportunities for CE in nursing are considerably greater than they were some years ago. What kind of CE a nurse chooses

---

*The ANA pamphlet, "Self-Directed Continuing Education," cited in the references, provides additional detail on how to manage self-learning.

will remain, to a large extent, an individual decision. However, the necessity to be currently competent is both a legal and ethical requirement for any professional. Equally important, nursing cannot advance unless all nurses accept the responsibility of lifelong learning.

REFERENCES

1. Division of Public Policy and Research, *Nursing Student Census with Policy Implications* (New York: National League for Nursing, 1984), p. 35

2. Jerome Lysaught, *An Abstract for Action* (New York: McGraw-Hill Book Company, 1970), p. 109.

3. Mildred Montag, *The Education of Nursing Technicians* (New York: G. P. Putnam's Sons, 1951), p. 70.

4. Ibid., pp. 94–100.

5. Mary Kohnke, "Do Nursing Educators Practice What is Preached?" *Am. J. Nurs.,* **73**:1572 (Sept. 1973).

6. Bonnie Bullough, "The Associate Degree: Beginning or End?" *Nurs. Outlook,* **27**:324–328 (May 1979).

7. American Nurses' Association, *Educational Preparation for Nurse Practitioners and Assistants to Nursing: A Position Paper* (New York: The Association, 1965), pp. 7–8.

8. Montag, op. cit., p. 73.

9. Lynne Beverly and Mary Junker, "The AD Nurse: Prepared To Be Prepared," *Nurs. Outlook,* **25**:514–518 (Aug. 1977).

10. Doris Wagner, "Nursing Administrators' Assessment of Nursing Education," Nurs. Outlook, **28**:557–561 (Sept. 1980).

11. Peggy Bensman, "Have We Lost Sight of the AD Philosophy?" *Nurs. Outlook,* **25**:511–513 (Aug. 1977).

12. Betty W. Martin and Dorothy Jean McAdory, "Are AD Clinical Experiences Adequate?" *Nurs. Outlook,* **25**:502–505 (Aug. 1977).

13. Virginia Allen and Connie Sutton, "Associate Degree Nursing Education: Past, Present and Future," *Nurs. and Health Care,* **2**:496–497 (Nov. 1981).

14. *The Graduate of Baccalaureate Degree Nursing Programs,* The Association (Boulder, Colo.: Western Interstate Commission for Higher Education, 1968).

15. *Nursing Student Census with Policy Implications,* op. cit. p. 43.

16. Fay Carol Reed, "Education or Exploitation?" *Am J. Nurs.,* **79**:1259–1261 (July 1979).

17. Ann Slavinsky et al., "College Graduates: The Hidden Nursing Population," *Nurs. and Health Care,* **4**:373–378 (Sept. 1983).

18. Ann T. Slavinsky and Donna Diers, "Nursing Education for College Graduates," *Nurs. Outlook,* **39**:292–297 (May 1982).

19. Rozella Schlotfeldt, "The Professional Doctorate: Rationale and Characteristics," *Nurs. Outlook,* **26**:309 (May 1978).

20. Mary Roberts, *American Nursing* (New York: Macmillan Publishing Company, Inc., 1954), pp. 533–534.

21. Ibid., pp. 535–536.

22. Department of Health, Education, and Welfare, *Toward Quality in Nursing. Report of the Surgeon General's Consultant Group on Nursing* (Washington, D.C.: The Department, 1963), p. 22.

23. *Facts About Nursing, '72-'73,* op. cit., pp. 10, 39.

24. *The Registered Nurse Population: An Overview* (Bethesda, Md.: U.S. Department of Health and Human Resources, Health Resources and Services Administration, 1982), p. 16.

25. American Nurses' Association, *Statement on Graduate Education in Nursing* (New York: The Association, 1969).

26. American Nurses' Association, *Statement on Graduate Education in Nursing* (Kansas City, Mo.: The Association, 1978), p. v.

27. Ibid., p. 4.

28. Ibid.

29. "Characteristics of Graduate Education in Nursing Leading to the Master's Degree," *Nurs. Outlook,* **27**:206 (Mar. 1979).

30. Ibid.

31. Report of the Committee to Formulate Guiding Principles for the Administration and Organization of Master's Programs in Nursing, in *Proceedings of the Meet-*

ings of Representatives of Graduate Programs in Nursing (May 1955) (mimeo).

32. Jean Campbell, "Post-master's Education in Nursing," *Nurs. Outlook,* **9**:554 (Sept. 1961).

33. Council of Baccalaureate and Higher Degree Programs, *Memo to Members* (New York: National League for Nursing, Feb. 1973), p. 2.

34. Martha Rogers, "Doctoral Education in Nursing," *Nurs. Forum,* **5**:69–74 (Spring 1966).

35. American Nurses' Association 1978, op. cit., p. 3.

36. Institute of Medicine, *Nursing and Nursing Education: Public Policies and Private Actions* (Washington: D.C.: National Academy Press, 1983), p. 141.

37. Jaunita Murphy, "Doctoral Education in, of, and for Nursing: An Historical Analysis," *Nurs. Outlook,* **29**:645–649 (Nov. 1981).

38. American Nurses' Association, 1978 op. cit., pp. 3 and 4.

39. U.S. Department of Health, Education and Welfare, *The Doctorally Prepared Nurse* (Bethesda, Md.: The Department, 1976), p. 5.

40. American Nurses' Association, *Nurses with Doctorates* (Kansas City, Mo.: The Association, 1981).

41. W. Carole Chenitz and Janice Swanson, "The Postdoctoral Research Fellow in Nursing: In Between the Cracks in the Academic Wall," *Nurs. Outlook,* **29**:417–420 (July 1981).

42. American Nurses' Association, *Facts About Nursing* (Kansas City, Mo.: The Association, 1983).

43. Helen Ference, "What LPNs Do," *Am. J. Nurs.,* **84**:799 (June 1984).

44. National Association for Practical Nurse Education and Service, *Statement of Practical/Vocational Nursing Entry Level Competence* (New York: The Association, 1981).

45. Kelly West, "Influences of the Scholar," *Bull. Med. Lib. Assn.,* **56**:43 (Jan. 1968).

46. American Nurses' Association, *Self-Directed Continuing Education in Nursing,* (Kansas City, Mo.: Association, 1978), p. v.

47. "The Status of Continuing Education: Voluntary and Mandatory," *Am. J. Nurs.,* **77**:410–416 (Mar. 1977).

48. Lynne Goodykoontz, "Evaluating a Continuing Education Program" *J. Cont. Ed.,* **11**:25–28 (July–Aug. 1980).

49. Dorothy del Bueno, "No More Wednesday Matinees," *Nurs. Outlook,* **24**:359–361 (June 1976).

Nursing Research: Status, Problems, Issues

HISTORICAL OVERVIEW

Like so many beginnings in nursing, research in nursing probably had its start with Florence Nightingale, who made detailed reports on observations of both medical and nursing matters during the Crimean War, documented the evidence, and pointed out significant data, which resulted in reform. After that, there was no other published research by nurses in the early periods of nursing. This was partly because it became an apprenticeship occupation in the United States and because, in the Victorian era, females were encouraged to leave intellectual initiative to males, and nurses often epitomized Victorian females. However, nurses gradually gained more education, moved into universities, and formed a professional organization.

Early studies that might be called a form of research were primarily for the improvement of nursing education and nursing service, because the early leaders were almost always responsible for both of those areas and there were obvious knowledge gaps. At a time when medicine was only semiscientific, it is natural that nurses, scientifically untrained, would

not attempt to establish a scientific base for nursing. But there was an attempt to gather data about nursing. One of the first, if not the first, study of American nursing education was Adelaide Nutting's survey of the field, published in 1906. Lillian Wald's school nursing project in New York was probably the first demonstration project reported in the *American Journal of Nursing* (by Dock in 1902). Wald herself wrote *House on Henry Street* in 1915, about that innovative experiment in public health nursing.* Other studies followed. In 1909 an ANA committee initiated a series of studies of public health. In 1912 Adelaide Nutting's survey of nursing education was published by the U.S. Bureau of Education, followed by the first major study of nursing, the 1923 Goldmark Report. These and succeeding studies by the Committee on the Grading of Nursing Schools, described in Chapter 5, greatly influenced the direction of nursing, and to some degree, nursing research. Although most of these studies focused on the nurse rather than nursing care, some of the nurse-teachers in universities did

_____
*See Chapters 3 and 4 for further details.

experiment with nursing techniques. In the late 1920s and 1930s, a few fellowships were granted to nurses in graduate programs who showed aptitude for research, and by 1930, nursing leadership had recognized the value of research and attempted to foster it. However, few were in positions to become involved in problems of patient care, and the nurses closest to the patient did not see themselves in a research role.[1]

Notter,[2] as well as Simmons and Henderson, cites a handful of nurses who did minor studies related to clinical nursing, most often of nursing procedures, in the 1920s and 1930s. But while medical research was plunging ahead and finding new answers to disease, research in nursing and about nursing was still related to the image, role, and functions of the nurse and was done as often as not by social scientists rather than nurses. Still, there was support by nurses of some of this research, such as the five-year ANA-initiated study of nursing functions, which yielded much useful data.[3,4] By 1970, ANA had also established a Commission on Nursing Research, and in 1972 a Council of Nurse Researchers was started.

The growth of the university schools of nursing had a definite effect on nursing research. As better-prepared faculty and students became involved in studies, sometimes a particular school concentrated on particular problems. Some universities also developed research centers, such as the Institute of Research and Service in Nursing Education at Teachers College in 1953, and Wayne State's Center for Health Research in 1969. This trend continued through the 1970s. In addition, the launching of *Nursing Research* in 1952* and the publication of several texts in nursing research at about the same time drew nursing closer to professionalism. The sponsorship of research by national health agencies and services, which emphasized the patient and patient care, may also have been a turning

*1977 was the twenty-fifth anniversary of *Nursing Research,* and that entire year's issues have articles on the historical development of research in nursing.

point toward clinical research. The American Nurses' Foundation was established by ANA specifically to further nursing research by conducting and supporting projects, as it still does today.

As might be expected, federal interest in nursing research was highly influential in its development. In 1955, a Research Grant and Fellowship Branch was set up in the Division of Nursing Resources of the U.S. Public Health Service, providing funds that enabled many nurses to complete their doctoral studies, as well as funds for other research, faculty development, workshops, and the nurse scientist programs.[5] A Department of Nursing was also established in the Walter Reed Institute (1957), and it was here that much of the early nursing research was done and where now prominent nurse researchers received their training.

In 1963 the surgeon general's report noted that research is one of the obligations of society and urged increased government funding because, with the rapidly changing patterns of medical care organization, the need for nursing research had outstripped resources available for studies of nursing care. "The potential contributions of nursing research to better patient care are so impressive that universities, hospitals, and other health agencies should receive all possible encouragement to conduct appropriate studies."[6] Even so, funds were not available in large amounts, and progress in the development of clinical nursing research was slow. Seven years later, the National Commission for the Study of Nursing and Nursing Education (NCSNNE) expressed dismay that so little research had been done on the actual effects of nursing intervention and care; the profession had few definitive guides for the improvement of practice. The kinds of clinical studies done by nurses were cited as major contributions to health, and it was urged that funds for nursing research be increased. Although funds were increased for a time, continued cutbacks in federal funds soon created a major problem in nursing research as well as in education. Still, nurses have been forging ahead in nursing research, particularly clinical research, seeking funds from foundations as well as the government.

WHAT IS NURSING RESEARCH?

Schlotfeldt's definition of the term *research* is classic: all systematic inquiry designed for the purpose of advancing knowledge.[7] Notter makes a useful comparison between problem solving related to patient care (sometimes also described as the *nursing process*) and scientific inquiries.[8] Both go through such steps as (1) identifying a problem, (2) analyzing its various aspects, (3) collecting facts or data, (4) determining action on the basis of analysis of the data, and (5) evaluating the result. In scientific inquiry, step 4 includes developing a hypothesis, as well as setting up a study design or method. After the analysis and evaluation of data in terms of the hypothesis, the findings of the research are reported. These steps may be relatively simple or very complex; they may involve laboratory equipment, human experimentation, or neither. Research may be designated as *basic,* the establishment of new knowledge or theory that is not immediately applicable, or *applied,* the attempt to solve a practical problem. Either way, the same steps are taken.

There are several types of research, and nurses may be involved in any of them, or more than one. *Historical* or *documentary* research provides more than a record of the past; because history tends to repeat itself, its study can prevent mistakes and help point new directions. Real historical research requires study of original records or documents (primary sources) to prevent distortion that comes with interpretation by succeeding historians. Historical research is having a new resurgence in nursing. Not only are the past and its human figures being studied on the basis of new hypotheses, but there is interest in preserving the ideas and attitudes of contemporary nursing leaders—while they are still alive. One good example of a technique being used is the

oral history, which involves audiotaped or videotaped interviews that may also be published, such as Gwendolyn Safier's *Contemporary American Leaders in Nursing, An Oral History* (New York: McGraw-Hill Book Company, 1977). (Also available for short-term loan are videocassettes in the Sigma Theta Tau Distinguished Leaders in Nursing Series.)*

Descriptive research describes what exists and analyzes the findings in terms of their significance. The purpose may be simply to get information, such as the periodic *National Sample Survey of Registered Nurses,* which reports on the nurse population and factors affecting their supply, or to gather facts that might be later used as a basis of a hypothesis of another type of study. Various techniques can be used: interviews, observations, case studies, or literature review. The studies can be both clinical and nonclinical.

In *experimental* research, the researcher manipulates the situation in some way to test a hypothesis. Preferably, one controlled setting or group in which certain factors or variables are held constant, and an experimental setting or group in which one or more variables are manipulated are used and the results compared. Such studies might be done in a laboratory, using animals, chemical or biological substances, or people. If the study involves human beings, whether in a standard laboratory, in a clinical setting, or in the field (the subject's home, school, workplace), the ethical principles and/or laws related to human experimentation must be observed. There are, of course, ethical principles that apply to all types of research. All of these kinds of research can also be nursing research, although there might be some argument about some of the examples given, depending on how nursing research is perceived.

The controversy about who should engage in what kind of research seems rather foolish in light of the need. There are proponents of

---

*Further information is available from Sigma Theta Tau (see Chapter 27).

"pure" or basic research, who feel that nursing needs a scientific base before practice can be studied. The separation is artificial. Basic research can be a foundation for applied clinical research but, given the unanswered questions in nursing care, there is no reason that there should not be research of both kinds, the abstract and the pragmatic. Equally pointless is the scientist/practitioner dichotomy. Probably all good nurses should have some configuration of practice, education, and research skills, because all are part of nursing's role. Clinicians who do not know, understand, or care about research are missing a source of knowledge that will enhance their practice; an investigator without sound clinical knowledge is not fully prepared.

One definition of nursing research is "research that arises from the practice of nursing for the purpose of solving patient care problems."[9] A noted nurse researcher describes nursing research as a "systematic inquiry into the problems encountered in nursing practice and into the modalities of patient care, such as support and comfort, prevention of trauma, promotion of recovery, health education, health appraisal, and coordination of health care."[10] She emphasizes as key words *patient* and *effect,* calling them the critical nucleus of nursing research. This type of research is also defined as clinical nursing research. However, it has been pointed out that *clinical* can have different meanings to different people: involving a place such a a hospital or clinic; pertaining to some form of disease or symptom; or the testing of an action considered a nursing action. Newman maintains that if the criterion "relevance to practice" is applied, then all nursing research is clinical research, but "the distinguishing factor between basic and clinical research is the purpose of the research: whether it is knowledge for the sake of knowledge or knowledge for a specific purpose."[11] Johnson and others see nursing research in a more abstract vein,* seeing new concepts developed by the nurse researcher from refor-

mulation of concepts from other sciences, leading to development of "theories of nursing intervention which will yield predictable responses in patients when implemented in nursing care."[12]

There are a number of other variations on the definition of nursing research and how it might be classified, and probably the arguments will persist. One of the most thoughtful nurse researchers (and one with a sense of humor) suggests that perhaps the best answer to "What is nursing research?" is "A good question."[13]

WHY NURSING RESEARCH?

Research of one kind or another has been responsible for the major advances in most fields, has resulted in modern technology, and has had a dramatic effect on medicine. The notion that much of the science of nursing is derived from medicine or the social sciences probably evolved because nursing did borrow many of its concepts and practice patterns from other disciplines. Some nurses began to recognize that many of these concepts had not been tested or tested recently and certainly had not been tested in relation to nursing practice. Others began to wonder what in nursing care made that critical difference in patient outcome. What was the impact of nursing care, how could it affect health care, and how could it affect health care of the future? The NCSNNE believed that the answer lay in nursing research.

This commission believes it is essential for the future of health care in this country to begin a systematic evaluation of the impact of nursing care. We advocate the development of objective criteria such as measurable improvement in patient conditions, evidence of early discharge or return to employment, reduced incidence of readmission to care facilities, and lowered rates of communicable disease. We do not suggest for a moment that nursing is wholly responsible for these or any other fac-

---

*Refer to the review of nursing theories in Chapter 9.

tors in the qualitative measurement of health care. We do believe, however, that nursing represents an important independent variable in our total health system. As such, we must learn how we can utilize nurses—more effectively, more efficiently, and more economically.[14]

More than a decade later, another National Commission* said much the same, adding, "Through research, nurses can test, refine, and advance the knowledge base on which improved education and practice must rest."[15]

Thus, it was once more affirmed that research is also necessary to determine just what nurses should be taught—the underlying theory or theories of nursing. Practice disciplines have always needed to develop their own bodies of verified knowledge and to evaluate that knowledge in practice, both for survival as a profession and for the well-being of their clients. This has been constantly reiterated by nursing leaders and scholars in the last few decades: that the primary tasks of nursing research are development and refinement of nursing theories that serve as guides to nursing practice and can be organized into a body of scientific nursing knowledge, and finding a valid means for measuring the extent to which nursing action attains its goals in terms of patient behavior.

As described in Chapters 9 and 12, these theories have gained an important place in nursing education, but not nearly as much in nursing practice. In fact, the question is raised, "Does nursing research affect practice?"

RESEARCH INTO PRACTICE

Over the years, a major issue has been the utilization of nursing research. After all, no matter how critical the findings of research studies may seem, if they are not tested in practice over a period of time, in a variety of settings, the results might still be questioned.

If they are not used at all, practice may change, but it will not change as a result of research. The first step is communication. Without communication, there can be no replication, application, utilization, or evaluation by others. In the last few years, means of reporting research and participating in peer review have increased considerably. As late as 1977, *Nursing Research* was the only journal in the United States devoted exclusively to reporting nursing research, but since that time several others have come on the scene. Because they are "refereed" journals, that is, the articles are reviewed and approved by a panel of experts before publication, the methodology, content, and analysis have been scrutinized by others in research and found appropriate. This may or may not be true of research articles in other nursing or non-nursing journals, but here, too, such articles are increasing in number, although they are not necessarily presented in as much detail.

Carnegie[16] lists other major avenues of reporting research: the federal government, state, regional, and national organizations, foundations, universities, and health agencies, all of which might be responsible for publication of newsletters, abstracts, reports, articles, monographs, books, and conferences, seminars, programs (with proceedings), as well as publishing houses that produce various indexes. *Dissertation Abstracts International* carries abstracts of all doctoral dissertations, complete photocopies of which can be purchased through the publisher, University Microfilms, Ann Arbor, Michigan. In addition, there are individual and university libraries, governmental and private networks of health science libraries, and professional association libraries which use computer-based retrieval service techniques to prepare bibliographies on requested topics.*

Does better communication guarantee utilization? Unfortunately, nursing has a history of ignoring the results or recommendations of research, or at least, delaying action. For in-

---

*See Chapter 5.

*See Chapter 29.

stance, early recommendations from studies of nursing education about educational preparation of nurses are only now coming to fruition, after about a seventy-five-year time lag. But here, at least, social and economic factors may have been contributors to such slow action. What about utilization of *clinical* findings?

Gortner and others have categorized practice-related research as studies: (1) building a science of practice (systematic identification of health problems and health needs of patients and relationships between nursing and patients), (2) refining the "artistry of practice" (laboratory and field studies on what nurses do), (3) concerned with descriptive, analytical, and experimental studies of physical and social environments in which nurses and their clients interact, (4) aiming to develop methodology or measurement tools, and (5) dealing directly with application of research findings to the field through replication on a small or large scale.[17] The extensive examples given show that there is useful practical application, but that often the results go no further than reporting at a research conference. For example, an author investigating the extent to which just one research finding was used by eighty-seven nurses, concluded, "A clear picture emerged: the practitioner either was totally unaware of the research literature relative to her practice, or if she was aware of it, was unable to relate to it or utilize it. There was an apparent isolation of research from practice."[18] This author also noted that most practicing nurses neither subscribe to nor understand nursing research journals, that because they are not researchers, they are not invited to (or interested in) research conferences, and that the researchers and practitioners tend to be in two different settings—universities and service agencies—with limited contact. These findings do not differ much from those of others exploring this dilemma. In a survey of 215 nurses, most of whom were involved in direct patient care, the obstacles most frequently cited related to use of re-

search findings were reading and understanding the report, relevance of findings for practical situations, inability to find research findings, suggestions too costly or time-consuming to implement, resistance to change in the workplace, and lack of worthwhile rewards for using nursing research.[19]

Probably in the majority of practice sites, this outlook is still prevalent. Most nurses in practice today, including nurse administrators, were not educated at a time when research was considered a part of nursing's responsibility and certainly were not trained to carry out any type of research. (In 1949, when a researcher sent the report of a study to a leading nursing journal, it was returned because "nurses do not do research, they are not interested in research, and . . . research has no place in nursing." Even in the 1960s, there was still debate as to whether it was appropriate for nurses to do research.)[20] Since most hospitals are not affiliated with university programs, where most of the research has been done, and since even in programs of higher education, most faculty do not do research, it is small wonder that research has not been a part of nursing practice.

However, some clear trends are emerging that may turn this situation around. First, some researchers are beginning to realize that they have a responsibility for *translating* the research into terms and concepts understandable to the clinician and disseminating their research results in places other than research conferences. They must make a distinct effort to reach out to nurses who are known as innovators and early adopters.[21]

Second, more practitioners are being oriented to nursing research in their educational programs. And, perhaps most important, nursing research is being done in clinical sites by nurse researchers and staff.[22,23] There are several models for clinical nursing research. The most common has been that of the university nurse researcher using a clinical site. The involvement of the clinician varies, and often little attention is paid to the potential usefulness of the research for practice. The agency-based model calls for either a researcher hired simply to help design and/or conduct a study (and then depart) or, more commonly now, a full-time employed researcher. In the latter case, clinical nurses are actively involved in defining and choosing the research and often participate in gathering the data. It is assumed that the staff would be motivated to use the findings, since the research reflects their concerns and questions. A problem is that the findings are often specific to that agency and are not generalized. One large research development project piloted another approach, the collaborative research development model, in which university-based researchers and agency-based clinicians functioned as equal contributors, each drawing on the other's expertise to achieve a mutual goal, a successful clinical research study.[24] The follow-up of this project was aimed at moving research and practice closer together by helping the nursing staff incorporate the new research-based knowledge in their practice.

The researchers describe research utilization as a "systematic series of activities that can culminate in the change of a specific nursing practice." The activities that comprise research utilization include (1) identification and synthesis of multiple research studies in a common conceptual area (research base); (2) transformation of the knowledge derived from that base into a solution (clinical protocol); (3) transformation of the clinical protocol into specific nursing actions (innovations) that are administered to patients and (4) a clinical evaluation of the practice to see whether it produced the predicted results.[25] The authors developed seven specific steps to produce "research-based" practice changes: systematically identifying patient care problems; identifying and assessing research-based knowledge to solve those problems; adopting and designing the nursing practice innovation; conducting a clinical trial and evaluation of the innovation; deciding whether to adopt, al-

ter, or reject the innovation; developing the means to extend (or diffuse) the new practice beyond the trial unit; and developing mechanisms to maintain the innovation over time.[26]

Oddly enough, another problem in nursing research is indiscriminate or unthinking application of nursing research findings. Nurses who become aware of research that seems to be pertinent to their field tend to use it without appropriate evaluation or validation. In some cases, this happens because most nurses currently practicing have not been taught to evaluate the quality of research, although guidelines are available in the literature. Moreover, there is a gap in providing guidelines for applying research to individuals' practice settings. To do so, the consumer (of research) must first make a critical validation of the study, that is, question each step of the author's assumptions, findings, and conclusions. If the conclusions are weak, tentative, or contradicted by others, convincing others to apply the research becomes a problem. If the settings or subjects are too different from the consumer's practice environment, the findings may not make a useful transition. If there are too many constraints in the practice environment, the attempt to implement the findings may require considerable groundwork. Nevertheless, assuming that the study is valid, each indirect application on the cognitive level has useful dimensions in expanding nurses' theory base and making them alert to other studies that might be more directly applicable.[27]

Undoubtedly, actually carrying out all these processes in a significant number of hospitals will take time, but the advances that have been made in less than ten years are impressive.

ISSUES AND PREDICTIONS

Besides the basic fact that there are not enough nurses prepared to do research, and that those who are do not always choose to do so, there are a number of other problems and issues related to nursing research.*

The quality of nursing research is sometimes raised as a problem or issue. Much, probably most, of the research in the past twenty years has been done as part of the requirements for a master's or doctoral degree. Although it may be of satisfactory quality, it is almost always limited in scope because of both monetary and time constraints. There are those who say that master's degree research particularly tends to be somewhat superficial, and even shoddy, lacking little more purpose than to complete the degree, with almost no follow-up or replication likely. This may be true, particularly in schools that have limited numbers of faculty prepared in research techniques. Those qualified may be overextended and others, whose own research experience is limited, may assume some of the responsibilities.

Because education and scholarship are frequently equated, why do so few nursing faculty engage in research, research in which their students might also participate? A number of reasons are given: most nursing faculty are not educationally qualified for university positions; their high number of student contact hours allows little time for individual research; they are not as clinically competent as they should be or do not have access to clinical facilities that permit clinical research; there is little research money available externally and lack of institutional support as well; most nurse faculty are women, and studies have shown that women prefer to teach rather than do scholarly research. A recent suggestion is that nurses have lacked mentors in research,[28] and suggestions are made about fulfilling such a role.[29] It has in fact been shown that nurses with mentors who encouraged them in scholarly activities did initiate research and publish more frequently than nonmentored nurses.[30]

Whatever the reason or combination of reasons, there is increased pressure for nursing

faculty to do research, particularly clinical research, in the area in which they teach. If teachers selected a particular problem to study over time, replication, now lacking, would be possible. If several teachers and/or other researchers studied clusters of problems, whether through consortia or cooperative groups of faculty and nursing service, nursing would have a more solid and extensive theory base. Then, too, peer evaluation and long-term experience would undoubtedly strengthen research skills.[31]

Another issue related to education is when and how to teach research. Many baccalaureate programs are including more or less research in their curricula, whether as a simple introduction or to involve the students in faculty research, but there is concern as to whether some approaches will actually discourage students' interest in research.[32]

Even more controversial are the rapidly multiplying doctoral programs, which are discussed in more detail in Chapter 13. Besides questions of quality (of faculty and resources particularly), there is considerable debate on what the curriculum should include in order to prepare a scholarly nurse researcher.[33]

An unexpected issue arose from what at first seemed very positive. In 1983, two major reports on nursing from the National Commission on Nursing and the Institute of Medicine* again reiterated the importance of nursing research. Both recommended that a high priority be given to nurse researchers and nursing research. The Institute group specifically commented on the "remarkable dearth of research in nursing practice" and noted that the lack of adequate funding for research and the resulting scarcity of talented nurse researchers have inhibited the development of nursing research. They also made the point that since the government grants were administered at the manpower unit in DHHS (the Division of Nursing), and not at a level of visibility and scientific prestige such as the Na-

---

*The important issues of ethics and patients' rights in research are presented in Chapters 10 and 22.

*See Chapter 5 for detailed information about these reports.

tional Institutes of Health (NIH), there was no encouragement for nurses to devote their careers to nursing research of patient problems. It was recommended, therefore, that the government "establish an organizational entity to place nursing research in the mainstream of scientific investigation."[34]

What is considered a probable follow-up on this recommendation was introduction of legislation in Congress in late 1983 to do just that—in this case, to create a National Institute of Nursing as part of NIH. While this might be seen as good news for nursing, it created a furor and a split opinion within nursing for a number of reasons.[35-38] For one thing, the nursing organization representatives who cooperated with the bill's sponsor failed to communicate adequately with the interested nursing community, and some of the concerns and political ramifications were not explained beforehand. For instance, the proposed institute was opposed by the head of NIH, and there was some concern that nursing research would be downgraded and underfunded in NIH. Some key nurses felt that it would be better to strengthen the Division of Nursing and have the research funding continue to come from there; in fact, there was concern that the Division would be irrevocably weakened if another nursing entity were established. Although the bill was passed by the House and Senate, it was killed by President Reagan's pocket veto at the end of the 1984 session. He called the creation of a nursing institute "unnecessary and expensive." Clearly, a reasonable consensus must be reached within nursing about this issue and a united legislative effort made to accomplish the underlying goal: adequate funding of, and opportunities for, nursing research.

One final problem should be mentioned. For various reasons, such as the fact that nursing's image does not include a scholarly component, many other disciplines and the public are not aware of what nursing research has done or even that there is such a thing. Not only does this situation tend to place nursing at a less than professional level, but it also limits the opportunities of nurses to promote nursing research as an endeavor worthy of support. Medicine has gained multi-million-dollar research grants, but nursing still must struggle for acceptance and funding. Thus, the need to make nursing research visible, to show the contribution it has made and can make to health care, is vital. One interesting suggestion is to learn the game rules of the health-industrial complex and use research to develop health care products and services.[39] Another is to involve client-advisory groups, who can provide crucial information and also act as advocates.[40]

The future of nursing research shows great promise. Despite concern that not enough faculty are involved in research, both faculty and administrators of educational programs have developed strategies for integrating research into the faculty work load.[41] A survey of schools given federal funds for research shows that a vital factor in success is the commitment of both faculty and institutions to research.[42]

Although there are still only a fraction of the doctoral nurses needed and very few pursue research activities after their dissertations are completed, the number is growing, the kind of research done has a rich diversity, and there seems to be collaborative research with other disciplines in which the nurse is an equal partner. According to one study of nursing research over the last three decades, the amount of research has risen considerably, the focus has shifted to clinical problems, and it has become more theoretically oriented and more sophisticated in its methods.[43] There is also reason for optimism about federal funding for nursing research, at least for some time after the Institute of Medicine report.

The ANA Commission on Nursing Research has published research priorities for the 1980s:[44]

Priority should be given to nursing research that would generate knowledge to guide practice in:

1. Promoting health, well-being and compe-

tency for personal care among all age groups;

2. Preventing health problems throughout the life span that have the potential to reduce productivity and satisfaction;
3. Decreasing the negative impact of health problems on coping abilities, productivity, and life satisfaction of individuals and families;
4. Ensuring that the care needs of particularly vulnerable groups are met through appropriate strategies;
5. Designing and developing health care systems that are cost-effective in meeting the nursing needs of the population; and
6. Promoting health, well-being, and competency for personal health in all age groups.

The members pointed out that while unanticipated problems will undoubtedly arise, new knowledge will bring about effective solutions. A preliminary statement also noted that "Accountability to the public for the humane use of knowledge in providing effective and high quality services is the hallmark of a profession. Thus, the preeminent goal of scientific inquiry by nurses is the ongoing development of knowledge for use in the practice of nursing . . . the complexity of nursing research and its holistic scope often require scientific underpinning from several desciplines. Hence, nursing research cuts across traditional academic/research lines and its research methods are drawn from several fields." That was a statement based on security, not apology. As one editor of a nursing research journal said, "research in nursing has finally come of age, and is entering a new era—one that will be marked by the acceptance of research as an essential commodity not only within the profession but outside of it as well."[45]

REFERENCES

1. Leo Simmons and Virginia Henderson, *Nursing Research—A Survey and Assessment* (New York: Appleton-Century-Crofts, 1964), pp. 7–24.
2. Lucille Notter, *Essentials of Nursing Research,* 2nd ed. (New York: Springer Publishing Company, Inc., 1978), pp. 9–10.
3. American Nurses' Association, *Nurses Invest in Patient Care* (New York: The Association, 1956).
4. Everett Hughes et al., *Twenty Thousand Nurses Tell Their Story* (Philadelphia: J. B. Lippincott Company, 1958).
5. Fay Abdellah, "Overview of Nursing Research 1955–1968," Part I *Nurs. Res.,* **19**:6–17 (Jan.–Feb. 1970); Part II, *Nurs. Res,* **19**:151–162 (Mar.–Apr. 1970); Part III, **19**:239–252 (May–June 1970).
6. Department of Health, Education, and Welfare *Toward Quality in Nursing,* Report of the Surgeon General's Consultant Group on Nursing (Washington, D.C.: The Department, 1963), pp. 51–53.
7. Rozella Schlotfeldt, "Research in Nursing and Research Training for Nurses: Retrospect and Prospect," *Nurs. Res.,* **24**:177 (May–June 1975).
8. Notter, op. cit., pp. 20–23.
9. Elaine Larson, "Nursing Research Outside Academia: A Panel Presentation," *Image,* **13**:75 (Oct. 1981).
10. Susan Gortner, "Research for a Practice Profession," *Nurs. Res.,* **24**:193–196 (May–June 1975).
11. Magaret Newman, "What Differentiates Clinical Research?" *Image,* **14**:88 (Oct. 1982).
12. Dorothy Johsnon, "Development of Theory: A Requisite for Nursing as a Primary Health Profession," *Nurs. Res.* **23**:373 (Sept.–Oct. 1974).
13. Florence Downs and Juanita Fleming, eds., *Issues in Nursing Research* (New York: Appleton-Century-Crofts, 1979), p. 75.
14. Jerome Lysaught, *An Abstract for Action* (New York: McGraw Hill Book Company, 1970), p. 85.
15. National Commission on Nursing, *Summary Report and Recommendations* (Chicago: The Commission, 1983), p. 11.
16. M. Elizabeth Carnegie, "Avenues for Reporting Research," editorial, *Nurs. Res.,* **26**:83 (Mar.–Apr. 1977).
17. Susan Gortner et al., "Contribution of Nursing Research to Nursing Practice," *J. Nurs. Admin.,* **6**:23–27 (Mar.–Apr. 1976).

18. Shake Ketefian, "Application of Selected Nursing Research Findings Into Nursing Practice: A Pilot Study," *Nurs. Res.*, **24**:89–92 (Mar.–Apr. 1975).

19. Jean Miller and Susan Messenger, "Obstacles to Applying Nursing Research Findings," *Am. J. Nurs.*, **78**:632–634 (Apr. 1978).

20. Jean Watson, "Nursing's Scientific Quest," *Nurs. Outlook.*, **29**:413 (July 1981).

21. Daniel King et al., "Disseminating the Results of Nursing Research," *Nurs. Outlook,* **29**:164–169 (Mar. 1981).

22. Larson, op. cit.

23. Helen Chance and Ada Sue Hinshaw, "Strategies for Initiating a Research Program," *J. Nurs. Admin.,* **10**:32–39 (Mar. 1980).

24. Maxine Loomis and Kathleen Krone, "Collaborative Research Development," *J. Nurs. Admin.,* **10**:32–35 (Dec. 1980).

25. Jo Anne Horsley et al., *Using Research to Improve Nursing Practice: A Guide* (New York: Grune & Stratton 1983), p. 2.

26. Ibid., pp. 7–10.

27. Cheryl Stetler and Gwen Marram, "Evaluating Research Findings for Applicability in Practice," *Nurs. Outlook,* **24**:559–563 (Sept. 1976).

28. Harriet Werley and Joan Newcomb, "The Research Mentor: A Missing Element in Nursing," in Norma Chaska, ed., *The Nursing Profession: A Time to Speak* (New York: McGraw-Hill Book Company, 1983), pp. 202–215.

29. Kathleen May et al., "Mentorship for Scholarliness: Opportunities and Dilemmas," *Nurs. Outlook,* **30**:22–28 (Jan. 1982).

30. Carol Spengler, "Mentor–Protege Relationships: A Study of Career Development Among Female Nurse Doctorates," Unpublished Ph.D. dissertation, University of Missouri, Columbia, 1982.

31. Nancy Bergstrom et al., "Collaborative Nursing Research: Anatomy of a Successful Consortium," *Nurs. Res.,* **33**:20–24 (Jan.–Feb. 1984).

32. Rona Levin, "Research for the Undergraduate: Too Much, Too Soon?" *Nurs. Outlook,* **31**:258–259 (Sept.–Oct. 1983).

33. Virginia Cleland, "Educational Issues Related to Research in Nursing," in Downs and Fleming, op. cit., pp. 25–38.

34. *Nursing and Nursing Education: Public Policies and Private Actions* (Washington, D.C.: National Academy Press, 1983), p. 217.

35. Rhetaugh Dumas and Geraldene Felton, "Should There Be a National Institute for Nursing?" *Nurs. Outlook,* **32**:16–22 (Jan.–Feb. 1984).

36. "Should There Be a National Institute for Nursing? Responses from Our Readers," *Nurs. Outlook,* **32**:74, 119–122 (Mar.–Apr. 1984).

37. "Letters: The NIN Debate," *Nurs. Outlook,* **32**:139 (May–June 1984).

38. Pamela Maraldo, "The National Institute of Nursing Bonus," *Nurs. and Health Care,* **5**:5 (Jan. 1984).

39. Joanne Stevenson, "Nursing Research and the Industrial Community," *Image,* **9**:3 (Feb. 1977).

40. Shirley Domrosch and Elizabeth Lenz, "The Use of Client-Advisory Groups in Research," *Nurs. Res.,* **33**:47–49 (Jan.–Feb. 1984).

41. Jacqueline Fawcett, "Integrating Research Into the Faculty Workload," *Nurs. Outlook,* **27**:259–262 (Apr. 1979).

42. Marjorie Batey, *Research Development in University Schools of Nursing* (Hyattsville, Md.: Department of Health, Education, and Welfare, 1978).

43. Julia Brown et al., "Nursing's Search for Scientific Knowledge," *Nurs. Res.,* **33**:26–32 (Jan.–Feb. 1984).

44. "Generating a Scientific Basis for Nursing Practice: Research Priorities for the 1980s," *Nurs. Res.,* **29**:219 (July–Aug. 1980).

45. Florence Downs, "What Does an Editor Think?" *Nurs. Res.,* **33**:3 (Jan.–Feb. 1984).

THE PRACTICE
OF
NURSING

15

Areas of Nursing Practice

One of the most exciting aspects of nursing is the variety of career opportunities available. Nurses, as generalists or specialists, work in almost every place where health care is given, and new types of positions or modes of practice seem to arise yearly. In part, this is in response to external social and scientific changes—for instance, shifts in the makeup of the population, new demands for health care, discovery of new treatments for disease conditions, recognition of health hazards, and health legislation. In part, these roles for nurses have emerged because nurses saw a gap in health care and stepped in (nurse practitioner, nurse epidemiologist) or simply formalized a role that they had always filled (nurse thanatologist).

Usually, further education is required to practice competently in specialized areas. Sometimes, this is part of on-the-job training, but frequently it requires formal or other continuing education. Practice in areas of clinical specialization will vary to some extent according to the site of practice and the level and degree of specialization. For instance, in a small community hospital, a nurse may work comfortably on a maternity unit, giving care to both mothers and babies; in a tertiary care setting, perinatal nurse specialists, psychiatric nurse specialists, and nurses specializing in the care of high-risk mothers may work together; in a neighborhood health center, the nurse-midwife may assume complete care of a normal mother and work with both the pediatric nurse practitioner and hospital nurses.

In addition, nurses hold many positions not directly related to patient care as consultants, administrators, teachers, editors, writers, patient care educators, executive directors of professional organizations or state boards, lobbyists, health planners, utilization review coordinators, nurse epidemiologists, sex educators, and even anatomic artists, airline attendants, and legislators.

Therefore, it is difficult to find any one way to present areas of practice. In this chapter, the approach used is first to describe positions and the responsibilities and conditions of employment for each.* Certain systems (armed forces, Public Health Service, Veterans Administration), which may have different requirements or opportunities, and international nursing are treated separately. An overview of the various health care settings is given in Chapter 7. Kinds of specialty nursing

---

*Guidance on job seeking is given additional attention in Chapter 30.

are considered briefly, although the NP role, because of its relative newness and its still somewhat controversial position in health care, is given more attention. Further information is available from the specialty nursing organizations, educational programs, and career articles published in various nursing journals.

In discussing conditions of employment, specific salaries are usually not given, because they are changing rapidly in the unstable economic climate and because they vary geographically (highest in the West, lowest in the North Central and Southern states, but rising in the Sunbelt) and according to whether they are urban, rural, or suburban. There is agreement that nursing salaries have been climbing, at least until the 1984 fiscal crisis in health care.[1] Other listings of current salaries are reported periodically in many nursing journals, in federal statistics, in the current ANA *Facts About Nursing,* and in ANA reports.

Patterns of employment have changed over the years. The largest single number of RNs is still employed in hospitals, but what was once a very popular field, private duty, has dropped considerably. Other changes are described in Chapter 11. One definite trend seems to be toward specialization.[2,3]

NURSING SUPPLY AND DEMAND

With all the career opportunities available for nurses, many of them barely emerging, it seems ludicrous to question whether there are too many nurses to fill these positions. However, because so much of nursing education is funded by the federal government, the issue of overproduction seems to arise with each new introduction of the Nurse Training Act (NTA). In the 1970s, particularly, attempts by various presidents to cut or virtually eliminate funding seemed to escalate. This is not unreasonable in some respects, because the original intent of the NTA (1964) was, in part, to increase the supply of nurses (Chapter 19). Since then, the number of nurses has in-

creased tremendously. Does that mean that the shortage has been overcome? By 1974 there were many dire warnings of overproduction of nurses, and it is true that in some geographic areas the job market was relatively tight. (At the same time, foreign nurses were being imported to work in hospitals, with accompanying legal problems.) The federal government engaged the NLN to conduct a study to determine whether new graduates were experiencing difficulty in acquiring positions and contracted with ANA to study the foreign nurse situation. Even before the results were available, there was some evidence that the need for nurses was still not met.

Rather, there was a tendency for some health agencies to "save money" by employing less prepared and, theoretically, less expensive nursing personnel (and fewer of any kind) regardless of need. There was, unquestionably, an unrelenting shortage of nurses prepared at the baccalaureate and higher-degree level, and, overall, a maldistribution of nurses. Poor use of nursing personnel is not new; it is also not resolved. One nurse, not underestimating the employer's problem, also saw a responsibility for nursing.

> Productive change in the system has to start with the values inculcated in nursing education. How do we capture the high motivation, human relatedness, and sense of justice that today's student brings, and channel it to postgraduation employment choices in areas other than affluent ones, for hours other than eight to four, for days other than Monday through Friday? How do we alter the elitism that governs nursing practice? Clearly, any solution to the health manpower problem which fails to explore ways and means of improving distribution and utilization in the broadest sense of these words is doomed to failure.[4]

When the NLN survey was completed, it showed no major changes in the job-seeking experiences of new graduates. The ANA foreign nurse study confirmed problems previously identified: that many foreign nurses recruited to this country had serious difficulties both in language and in practice, and because of these disadvantages were often grossly misused and underpaid. A number of state boards of nursing were already requiring that the state licensing examination be passed before permitting practice, and the failure rate was high. One effect of the ANA report was the formation of the Council of Graduates of Foreign Nursing Schools (CGFNS), which subsequently arranged for foreign nurses to take preliminary qualifying examinations before leaving their country. Regulations by the Immigration and Naturalization Service require that graduates of foreign schools of nursing (except those in Canada) pass this examination to be eligible for H-1 (occupational preference) visas. This was seen as a protection for both the public and nursing. (See Chapter 20.)

The factors that affect supply and demand in relation to all nursing manpower are currently in a state of flux, as they frequently are. On one side are the demands of the public—their perceived right to health care and their increased utilization of services. On the other are the overwhelming increase in health care costs and the demands of third-party payers to cut back. In hospitals, the cutbacks have taken a toll on nursing positions, but the shift in funding to HMOs, ambulatory care, and home health care has created a greater demand for nurses in these areas. (Sometimes NPs are also being employed instead of physicians, either because of a physician shortage or because of the high salaries of doctors.)

On the other hand, in the early 1980s, a state of hysteria seemed to sweep over the health care system in relation to nursing. First there was panic because of the nursing *shortage.* Hospitals seemed to be particularly affected, and recruitment for nurses was fiercely competitive, even to the point of offering bonuses to employees who could recruit a nurse. The reason for the shortage and what could be done was explained in every nursing hospital and related journal. The American Hospital Association itself did a national survey.[5] The

reports on nurse satisfaction/dissatisfaction described in Chapter 5 and even polls in magazines (Chapter 11) were read avidly. (Not that they revealed much more than a good administrator should have known anyway—nurses were unhappy about their salaries, working conditions, understaffing, lack of flexibility, lack of respect, poor administration, and inability to give good patient care.)

For a short while, it looked as though administration and medicine were going to reform, that strong, well-prepared nurse administrators would be appointed and placed in the top decision-making echelon, that doctors and administrators would treat nurses with courtesy and respect, and that nurses would be considered partners in patient care, with professional autonomy. Then suddenly a new day dawned: the federal government, with the enactment of Public Law 97-248,* initiated a new method of reimbursement for Medicare and cracked down on expenditures. Now the game was to cut back on nursing or, in some cases, to use less expensive nursing personnel, and miraculously the nursing shortage was over. By 1984, some nurses had difficulty finding jobs, and nursing journals began to note a precipitous drop in recruitment ads. By April 1983, it had already been reported that more than 40 percent of U.S. hospitals had no RN vacancies and 60 percent had no LPN vacancies.[6] There was no area of the country where rates did not decrease. The reasons for the decline were apparent. Because of the recession, more nurses went back to work and others who might have quit stayed. Combined with the cutback in budgeted positions, supply now overwhelmed demand, even in public health.

At the same time, there were predictions of an MD oversupply and warnings that NPs would have a worse time than ever in terms of physician opposition to practice.

The news was not all bad. In some cases, the information about the reasons for nurse

*See Chapter 19.

dissatisfaction had struck home; turnover is very expensive. New approaches in participatory management such as quality circles[7] were initiated, and ways to help new graduates, such as internships, were instituted.[8] Primary nursing was started in more hospitals, and clinical career ladders gave nurses opportunities for advancement without going into management.[9] All–RN staffs were beginning to be seen by the more progressive hospitals as a desirable staffing pattern resulting in better patient care.[10]

Nevertheless, new attention was also being given to what made a nurse marketable and what the best job opportunities were. One survey of 500 nurse executives[11] resulted in some predictions. Expected was particular growth in hospice, home care, ambulatory care, and short-stay units. (This is also reported in Chapter 7.) Need for specialization was definitely growing (except for psychiatric nursing), but certification,* preferably with advanced education, was going to be a must. And in general, there was a clear trend toward preference for nurses with a BSN. Others reported a favorable salary for BSN nurses.

As the career opportunities are presented in the succeeding sections, it might be helpful to keep these perspectives in mind.

HOSPITAL NURSING

Positions described in hospital nursing include all those in which the employing agency is a hospital, whether private or voluntary, general or special, hospitals of all sizes; and hospitals operated by a city, county, state, or the federal government, no matter how much they differ in policies and procedures. The one element all hospitals have in common is that they are in existence primarily to take care of patients. The greatest differences from an employment point of view are types of responsibility, advancement opportunities, and salaries.

*See Chapter 20.

NONGOVERNMENTAL HOSPITALS

Nursing service positions in hospitals follow a pattern that varies principally with the size and clinical services of the hospital.

General Duty or Staff Nurse

The first-level position for professional nurses is that of general duty or staff nurse and is open to graduates of diploma, associate degree, and baccalaureate programs in nursing education. Individual assignments within this category will depend upon the hospital's needs and policies and the nurse's preferences and ability.

Staff nursing includes planning, implementing, and evaluating nursing care through assessment of patient needs; organizing, directing, supervising, teaching, and evaluating other nursing personnel; and coordinating patient care activities, often in the role of team leader. It involves working closely with the health team to accomplish the major goal of nursing—to give the best possible care to all patients.

To help attain this goal, the ANA published, in 1973, standards of practice applicable to all nursing situations. Additional, more specific standards are also available for medical-surgical, maternal-child, geriatric, community health, psychiatric mental health nursing practice, and a number of subspecialties. The general standards of practice, which can also be guidelines for practice, are

1. The collection of data about the health status of the client/patient is systematic and continuous. The data are accessible, communicated, and recorded.
2. Nursing diagnoses are derived from health status data.
3. The plan of nursing care includes goals derived from the nursing diagnoses.
4. The plan of nursing care includes priorities and the prescribed nursing approaches or measures, to achieve the goals derived from the nursing diagnoses.

5. Nursing actions provide for client/patient participation in health promotion, maintenance, and restoration.

6. Nursing actions assist the client/patient to maximize his health capabilities.

7. The client's/patient's progress or lack of progress toward goal achievement is determined by the client/patient and the nurse.

8. The client's/patient's progress or lack of progress toward goal achievement directs reassessment, reordering of priorities, new goal setting, and revision of the plan of nursing care.[12]

Involved in meeting these standards are literally hundreds of specific nursing tasks, some of which can be carried out by less prepared workers; it is the degree of nursing judgment needed that determines who can best help any patient.

Because the goals of the various kinds of nursing education programs differ, theoretically the responsibilities of each type of nurse should also differ in the staff nurse position. Unfortunately, the tendency is to assign all to the same kinds of tasks and responsibilities, so that viable differences are not utilized. This is so common that there is even a tendency to praise as innovative those nursing services that do delineate nursing roles and responsibilities at the staff nurse level according to educational background.

Some hospitals categorize staff nurse positions as I, II, III, and so on, depending on education, experience, and clinical proficiency. Salary increases are given at each level, and this horizontal promotion allows the nurse competent in, and preferring, bedside care to be rewarded without being forced into an administrative role. This is often called a *clinical career ladder*. The increased utilization of clerical and nonnursing personnel to assume nonnursing tasks also frees the nurse for the patient contact for which nurses are prepared.

Three basic methods of assignment for patient care in the hospital are functional, team, and case.[13] In *functional nursing,* the emphasis is on the task; jobs are grouped for expediency and supposedly to save time. For instance, one nurse might give all medications, another all treatments; aides might give all the baths. Obviously, the care of the patient is fragmented, and the nurse soon loses any sense of "real" nursing; patients cannot be treated as individuals or given comprehensive care. Nevertheless, there is a tendency to use this approach in many hospitals, especially on shifts that are understaffed. The work gets done; there is generally little nurse or patient satisfaction.

Team nursing presumes a group of nursing personnel, usually RNs, PNs, and aides, working together to meet patient needs. It became popular after World War II, when the shortage of nurses was acute. For team leader, a baccalaureate degree had been suggested by the Surgeon General's Consultant Group on Nursing (1963),[14] but there are still not enough baccalaureate graduates to fill these positions, and it is usual to have either a diploma or AD graduate act as team leader. Other team members are under the direction of the team leader, who assigns them to certain duties or patients, according to their knowledge or skill. She or he has the major responsibility for planning care and coordinates all activities, acting as a resource person to the team. In addition, if there are few or no other RNs on the team, the team leader may perform nursing procedures requiring RN qualifications. Often, the team leader is the only nurse directly relating to the physician, but, too often, actual patient contact is infrequent or sporadic. The original concept of the team has been diluted. Planning and evaluation are seldom a team effort; conferences to discuss patient needs are irregular; and too frequently, the team leader does mostly functional nursing, doing treatments and giving medications in an endless cycle. Nevertheless, the professional nurse should expect to be part of a nursing team or, more likely, leader of this team, because most hospitals utilize some version of team nursing, at least to the extent that the registered nurse supervises and directs other nursing personnel in patient care.

Instituted in the 1970s and gaining in popularity is "primary" nursing, a somewhat confusing designation for the *case method,* in which total care of the patient is assigned to one nurse, which was the traditional caregiving pattern. A major difference between primary nursing and other methods of assignment is the accountability of the nurse. The patient has a primary nurse, just as she or he has a primary physician. A nurse is a *primary nurse* when responsible for the care of certain patients throughout their stay and an *associate nurse* when caring for the patients while the primary nurse is off duty. In most places, that nurse is responsible for a group of patients twenty-four hours a day, even though an associate nurse may assist or take over on other shifts. The primary nurse is in direct contact with the patient, family/significant others, and members of the health team, and plans cooperatively with them for total care and continuity. The head nurse then is chiefly in an administrative and teaching (personnel) role. Almost always the primary nurse is an RN, often with a baccalaureate. Sometimes the nursing team involved in primary nursing comprises all RNs, with the exception of aides who are generally limited to "hotel service," dietary tasks, and transportation. There is almost unanimous agreement that the primary nursing pattern is much more satisfying to patients, families, physicians, and nurses and that care is of a highly improved quality. Although there has been some concern over the increased cost of an all-RN staff and the more personalized care, data show that after the initial start-up time, costs are not greater and sometimes less than those of other staffing patterns.[15]

Almost half of all hospitals still have fewer than 100 beds, so there may be relatively little separation of specialties with the exception of obstetrics, pediatrics, and, more frequently now, psychiatric care. Even here, when there is a declining census, hospitals are beginning to cooperate by sharing such facilities. Therefore, the staff nurse is most often truly a generalist; even if he or she is assigned in a special area, rotating to other areas regularly (often

because of short staffing) may be necessary. A new graduate should, with appropriate orientation and individualized in-service education, be able to function at the staff nurse level in any of these areas. Positions in the emergency room and outpatient department (which are receiving an increasing number of patient visits), operating room, rehabilitation unit, or intensive care unit may require specialized training, but newly developed settings within the hospital, such as an outpatient surgery unit[16] or "overnight" unit[17] also present new challenges in nursing care without necessarily mandating more formalized education.

Hospitals with home care services usually require nurses to have had public health experience to function in this area. Nursing roles are changing in all of these clinical areas. In the operating room, for instance, many of the technical aspects are carried out by OR technicians, whereas the RN has overall responsibility for the safety of the patient, supervision and education of auxiliary nursing personnel, and sometimes support of the patient through pre- and postoperative visits. The increased utilization of nurse practitioners and clinical specialists, discussed later, adds another dimension to nursing care in these specialty areas. Although students usually do not have extensive experiences in the areas noted, even limited exposure may attract the nurse to certain kinds of practice. The emergency room and intensive care unit, where quick, life-determining decisions must be made, independent judgments are not unusual, and tension is often high, will probably not attract the same kind of individual as the geriatric unit or rehabilitation unit, where long-term planning, teaching, and a slower pace are the norm.

Qualifications and Conditions of Employment. The basic requirement for a staff position is graduation from an approved school of nursing and nursing licensure or eligibility for licensure. The nurse who has the latter qualifications may be designated as a graduate nurse (GN) and must take and pass the licensure examinations within a specific period of time.

Sometimes a lesser salary is offered until the RN is acquired, and the new graduate may be limited to a general nursing unit, that is, not the coronary care unit or another that requires an investment of intensive in-service education. Nevertheless, in the hospital, the variety of experiences is endless. Larger hospitals and those in medical centers may offer a greater variety of specialties, exotic surgery, and rare treatments, and the advantage of being in the center of hospital, medical, and nursing research. Smaller hospitals may be less impersonal, are often in the nurse's own community, and provide the opportunity to be a generalist on smaller patient units (which does not necessarily mean a smaller patient load). A nurse is usually hired for a particular specialty unit (except for very small hospitals), but it is not uncommon to be asked to "float"—replace a nurse on any unit. Floating should not extend to units that require special knowledge and skill unless the nurse is so trained. In some hospitals, there are "float pools"—highly skilled nurses who never have a regular unit.

In most cases, hospital nurses will be required to rotate shifts and work on holidays. For this reason, it is possible to work part time in most hospitals.[18] Usually there are salary differentials for working evenings and nights. In recent years, flexible hours and shifts have become popular.[19] Fringe benefits also vary greatly and may include health plans, retirement plans, arrangements for continuing education, holidays, sick time, and vacation time. The amount of autonomy varies considerably. Opportunities for promotion may be through clinical advancement or the managerial ladder. Most staff nurses are interviewed and hired by the hospital's personnel department and/or the nursing service department.

Another alternative is to be employed by a "Rent-a-Nurse" or temporary service company (TSC).[20] Those nurses most commonly using TSCs are nurses beyond a hospital mandatory retirement age, some new graduates, nurses enrolled in advanced educational programs, and nurses with small children who cannot work full time or all shifts. TSCs are businesses that employ nurses, and often other professional, technical, and clerical workers, paying them a salary for the hours worked, with the usual legal deductions, after billing the institution or patient/client using the worker's services. There are local and national services, and selecting a reputable one is extremely important. Job assignments may be made an hour or a week ahead, but the nurse is not obligated to take it; however, a no-show is usually dismissed. There is a great deal of flexibility and variety, but there are also disadvantages, even with a good TSC: no job security, no benefits, sometimes only the minimum rate paid by the area hospitals with no increases, and, of course, the constant reorientation to new nursing units and patients, even hospitals. Whether or not the TSCs will thrive in a tight economy is not clear. Some hospitals will use them for more flexibility, but others have started their own pools.

Clinical Nurse Specialist

The *clinical nurse specialist (CNS),* who may also be called a *nurse specialist, nurse clinician,* or *clinical specialist,* has become an increasingly important part of the nursing practice scene since the early 1960s. A clinical specialist is an expert practitioner within a specialized field of nursing or even a subspecialty. There are clinical specialists in all the major clinical areas, but also some concentrating on cancer, rehabilitation, and perinatal nursing, tuberculosis, care of patients with ostomies, neurological problems, respiratory conditions, epilepsy, and many other subspecialties.

The ANA Social Policy Statement describes nurse specialists in some depth. It lists the characteristic functions of a CNS, including:

- Identification of populations or communities at risk
- Direct care of selected patients or clients in any setting, including private practice
- Intraprofessional consultation with nurse specialists in different clinical areas and with nurses in general practice

- Interprofessional consultation and collaboration in planning total patient care for individuals and groups of patients, and in planning and evaluating health programs for population groups at risk related to the specialty or the public in general.[21]

In addition, the CNS frequently acts as a role model and teacher for the nursing staff and develops or is involved in nursing research.

To fulfill these responsibilities, the CNS must develop certain competencies:

Those competencies include ability to observe, conceptualize, diagnose, and analyze complex clinical or non-clinical problems related to health, ability to consider a wide range of theory relevant to understanding those problems, and ability to select and justify application of theory deemed to be most useful in understanding the problems and in determining the range of possible treatment options. Ability to foresee and discuss short- and long-range possible consequences is also to be demonstrated. While this is not an exhaustive list, the foregoing intellectual competencies are of the utmost importance in specialization.[22]

Originally, the intent was to give the CNS staff authority, that is, reporting directly to the chief nurse administrator and acting in an advisory capacity to the nursing staff and supervisors. However, a line position (superior-subordinate or direct vertical relations) gives administrative authority, and there have been some problems when a CNS as a staff member makes recommendations and the supervisor chooses not to accept them, especially in relation to personnel matters (such as disciplining an incompetent nurse), or when the CNS is seen as an outsider. There seems to be a trend now for the CNS to also assume a supervisory position focused on nursing care or to be given certain administrative authority. A clinical specialist in the traditional supervisor role of personnel manager is sometimes limited in the amount of time devoted to clinical nursing. The ANA has emphasized the importance of flexibility:

When nurse specialists are employed in health care settings, descriptions of their positions and functions ought not to be standardized. The work rules for the specialist must be jointly determined and negotiated by the applicant and the employing institution. The emphasis should be on developing negotiated positions and organizational arrangements that are most likely to result in freedom and responsibility for maximum use of the abilities of the particular specialist in the particular health care setting. In joint practices and partnerships, in which nurse specialists practice on a private basis with other nurses or other professionals, joint determination of working arrangements and shared responsibility also apply.[23]

Qualifications and Conditions of Employment. Generally, CNSs are expected to have a master's degree in nursing, with emphasis on the specialty area, although some are employed in the position because of experience, clinical expertise, and possibly continuing education without any degree. Certification by ANA or a specialty organization is often required. Salaries are expected to be on the level of supervisor or higher, but at times these salaries are individually negotiated, depending on education, experience, and the role expected by the employer. Basic fringe benefits may be the same as those of other nurse employees; sometimes more vacation is offered.

Frequently, there is a great deal of flexibility in the CNSs' time. They may work no specific shift but care for the patients selected according to the patients' needs, which may mean being available evenings or nights, or, by choice, even available on call if a problem arises. (Telephone consultations with patients who develop problems or need support at home are not uncommon.) There should be time available for library research and home visits. A CNS usually has office space, preferably near the clinical units.

Although there are not nearly enough clinical specialists to meet patient needs, not all hospitals employ this kind of nurse, or they employ only a limited number of them because they believe they cannot (or do not choose to) afford the increased salary. Clinical specialists are most commonly found in large hospitals, medical centers, or certain government hospitals such as those run by the Veterans Administration.[24]

NURSING SERVICE ADMINISTRATION

The administrative hierarchy in hospital nursing usually consists of a head nurse, supervisor, assistant or associate director of nursing, and director of nursing; the titles vary with the times and the philosophy of the hospital concerning nursing service administration.

Head Nurse

Head nurses are in charge of the clinical nursing units of a hospital, including the operating room, outpatient department, and emergency room. They may be called *charge nurses,* or more recently, *nursing coordinators.* In a hospital functioning as a line and staff organization (as most are), head nurses are responsible to the next higher person on the scale, usually the supervisor, or, in a smaller hospital, the assistant director of nursing or the director. The head nurse position is the first administrative position most nurses achieve (or perhaps that of assistant head nurse, who may share some of the head nurse functions and substitute for the head nurse in his or her absence).

It is the head nurse's function to manage the nursing care and assure its quality in a relatively small area of the hospital. How this is done again depends on the philosophy of nursing service and often on the individual's personality. If a democratic philosophy of administration prevails, the staff participates in decision making both on the unit and in the entire setting. The head nurse uses leadership skills in assisting the group to make decisions and coordinates the overall activities.

As the complexity of patient care increased, head nurses found themselves inundated with paper work, which limited their major role in managing nursing care. Hospital administrators began to realize that it was less expensive and more efficient to employ clerical personnel to answer phones and questions, to complete and route forms, to order and check supplies and drugs, and to perform the myriad other necessary clerical tasks that have kept the head nurse away from administration of patient care. *Ward clerks, ward managers, floor managers, unit managers, service assistants,* or whatever the local term is, have a wide variety of responsibilities, with some ward clerks even taught carefully to transcribe doctors' orders. Hospitals utilizing computers have been able not only to cut down on every nurse's paper work, but to add greater assurance of accurate, rapid communication interdepartmentally. Since there is now a trend toward decentralization of nursing authority, which means that nurses on individual units may make nursing care and other decisions without going through the nursing hierarchy, the head nurse is expected to give more attention to acting as a consultant and teacher for staff, to following the clinical progress of the patients, and to maintaining communication with physicians and other health personnel.

In 1978, ANA delineated responsibilities for three levels of nurse administrator. The first-line level is identifiable as the head nurse level. The responsibilities included for this role are:

1. Providing for direct nursing care services to clients.
2. Evaluating nursing care given and assuring appropriate documentation, guidance, and supervision of staff members.
3. Selecting nursing personnel for hire.
4. Evaluating staff, including disciplinary action and separation from service.
5. Providing for teaching and staff development.
6. Coordinating nursing care with other health services.

7. Participating in and involving staff in nursing research.
8. Providing clinical facilities and learning experiences for students.[25]

Where there is primary nursing, there is more emphasis on personnel management and teaching in the head nurse role. Regardless of the staffing pattern, staff evaluation is a major responsibility. Considered first-line managers, head nurses control the quality of care more than anyone else and often know best how to eliminate waste, improve utilization of personnel and dollars, keep communication systems open, and provide direct leadership.

Qualifications and Conditions of Employment. Qualifications for head nurses are usually evidence of successful nursing experience and preferably a baccalaureate degree. The need for a master's is predicted, and a few head nurses do have that degree; some have BSNs. Currently, most head nurses have no degree. The successful head nurse should have, besides nursing expertise, administrative ability. Unfortunately, in many hospitals, moving into administrative positions is still the only mode of advancement for RNs. Because a good clinician may not be interested or able in nursing administration, such promotions are not always successful. Employers may now offer managerial courses to aid the transition. To some extent, the assistant head nurse position offers this training opportunity, but additional training and education are considered vital for most nurses assuming this position.

Head nurses may earn between $500 and $2,000 more per year than staff nurses; other benefits may vary. Benefits acquired by staff through collective bargaining may or may not apply to the head nurse position. In most instances, the head nurse works only the day shift, but may alternate on weekends and holidays with the assistant head nurse.

Supervisor

It has been said that the role of the *nursing supervisor* is the most ill-defined in the hospital hierarchy. Because basic management principles for span of control usually specify that no more than six to eight people should report to an administrator, except in small hospitals, the supervisor usually is needed as the middle management person. Some hospitals have eliminated the supervisor, at least on the day tour of duty, putting responsibility directly on the head nurse. In general, however, the supervisor is responsible for several clinical units, delineated by either location or specialty. In a small hospital, the supervisor might be responsible for all the clinical units, and in any hospital, the evening and night supervisors usually have larger areas to supervise. In many hospitals, these supervisors are the only administrative personnel available for any department after 5 P.M. Therefore, they find themselves acting as temporary hospital administrators, devoting more time to overall hospital problems than to their main responsibility, nursing care. At times they dispense drugs because no pharmacist is present, thus violating the Pharmacy Practice Act in most states. Some of the larger and/or more progressive hospitals have now arranged for an assistant administrator to be available for general administration responsibilities, but this is still more the exception than the rule. Even when limited to nursing, the role of the supervisor often encompasses an enormous amount of responsibility and diversity: many aspects of personnel management, which may include hiring and firing; evaluation and improvement of patient care; and staffing and coordination of nursing systems (policies, procedures, resources). Stevens has suggested that for better management, these areas of responsibility be divided among different supervisors responsible for each. They would then deal with head nurses only in relation to those areas.[26] Responsibilities of this middle management role as delineated by the ANA Commission on Nursing Services are as follows:

1. Participating in nursing policy formulation and decision making.

2. Problem solving and supervising the delivery of nursing care.
3. Evaluating care provided.
4. Collaborating with other departments.
5. Coordinating staff activities.
6. Staffing and scheduling of personnel.
7. Arranging for equipment and supplies.
8. Recruiting and selecting personnel.
9. Evaluating staff for promotions and transfers, disciplinary action, and separation of service.
10. Providing orientation, training, and continuing education for staff.
11. Undertaking or facilitating research activities.
12. Providing and coordinating clinical learning experiences for students.[27]

Qualifications and Conditions of Employment. Generally, supervisors have been employed after showing evidence of ability in a head nurse or other administrative position. Clinical expertise may or may not have been a factor, but an advanced degree was probably a distinct advantage (even if not in administration). Increased emphasis is being put on the combination of clinical expertise, administrative skills, and at least baccalaureate degrees. In larger hospitals, master's degrees are stressed, preferably with experience and/or a nursing administration major in the educational program. Actually, the large majority of supervisors have no degree at all, although there is a trend toward enrollment in both degree programs and in continuing education programs that focus on middle management skills.

Salaries of supervisors tend to be from $2,000 to $3,000 more a year than those of head nurses, but salaries may vary according to education and experience. Some fringe benefits, such as vacation time, may be greater. Supervisors tend to remain on one work shift although they also work weekends and holidays. Even more than that of the head nurse, the supervisor position is considered administrative by employers. This has made it difficult for these individuals to be included in collective bargaining with other nurses. ANA has differentiated supervision of nursing care from managerial supervision in labor negotiations, and there have been NLRB rulings in that direction.

Assistant or Associate Director of Nursing

Assistant or *associate directors of nursing* work with the director of nursing in any or, occasionally, all aspects of the director's responsibility. Specific areas of responsibility may be assigned, particularly if the institution is large. If there is a diploma program of nursing, its head may also have the title of associate director of nursing. The assistant or associate is generally expected to have at least some of the qualifications of the director or to be in the process of acquiring them. As a rule, this individual is hired by the director and thus is expected to share a harmonious philosophical approach and be compatible in the work relationship with the director. Salary is often negotiable on the same basis as that of the director, although it is, of course, usually less. Probably a great majority of the nurses assuming assistant or associate positions do so for the experience and as a step toward becoming a top nurse administrator. They do get that experience, but in a large hospital, many of their day-to-day activities are more likely to be in a direct relationship with staff and somewhat less involved in top-level hospital planning. There are opportunities to represent nursing service on hospital committees and to chair key nursing committees. A good director will relate to the associates as peers who will participate in the determination of overall nursing service policies and strategies. It is a highly varied position, with no set routine, but extended hours.

Director of Nursing

The *director of nursing* position is the highest in the nursing service hierarchy. The title may also be *director of nursing service, chief nurse, nurse administrator,* or, if this individual is considered part of the top echelon of hospital administration, *assistant administra-*

tor for nursing, vice-president for nursing, or a variation of whatever title the administrator of the hospital carries. For years, nurses and others, including ANA and the American Hospital Association (AHA), have endorsed such a title with the concomitant responsibilities. Nursing service is generally the largest individual department in the hospital, often employing more than half the total number of employees. It affects and is affected by the functions of all other departments, and, as the AHA stated, "participation and cooperation of the administrator of the department of nursing service in formulating policies and procedures is an essential element in accomplishing the administration's objective of coordinating functions among the various departments of the institution."[28] Some directors are also formally responsible for other departments in the hospital.

It is generally agreed that those in the position of chief nurse administrator must be leaders, both of the nursing personnel and also in nursing generally, so that they can also represent nursing when relating to other health disciplines. ANA, in describing the role of the nurse administrator at the executive level, identifies that person as responsible for the nursing department and managing from the perspective of the organization as a whole, as well as responsible for the integration of nursing with other functional areas of the health care agency in the mutual achievement of organizational goals. "The nurse executive ensures that standards of nursing practice are established and implemented so that sound nursing care is provided to consumers.[29]

Unfortunately, a serious problem is that regardless of ANA and AHA recommendations, most directors are not yet part of the upper echelon of hospital administration; the National Commision on Nursing addressed this issue and strongly recommended a change.[30]

Actually, as a matter of two extremes, nurse administrators in very small hospitals or in large medical center hospitals have few similarities in areas of responsibilities. A director of a small hospital may be a jack-of-all-trades. Because small hospitals are also usually in rural areas or small towns, management takes on a personalized dimension.[31] On the other hand, in some medical centers, directors of nursing are also assistant or associate deans or deans of collegiate nursing programs and do little direct management.

The American Society of Nursing Service Administrators (ASNSA) provides the most current information about today's nursing service administrators, updating a 1977 survey.[32] A warning is in order, however. The sample of 500 (with 343 respondents) was drawn from ASNSA membership on the assumption that since society members are employed in hospitals representing over half of the total number of hospitals, the sample would be representative of that universe. The fallacy lies in the fact that probably only the best prepared, most motivated, and perhaps most affluent nurse administrators are likely to become members. Only thirty-three hospitals with fewer than 100 beds were represented and fifty-six in the 100–199-bed category, but these account for about half of all hospitals. They are inclined to have the least prepared, least powerful, and least paid directors of nursing. Even a comparison of the 1982 and 1977 samples is skewed, since the earlier survey had over 5,000 respondents.

Nurse administrators in hospitals, most still carrying the title of *director of nursing,* tend to be female, married (55.6 percent), and forty to forty-nine years of age. There were three under thirty and seventeen over fifty-nine. Most had reached the position through the traditional nursing management steps in the hospital, although the 1982 group had moved more rapidly, and the men most rapidly of all. Sixty-nine percent had been prepared in diploma schools and almost 23 percent in baccalaureate programs. All but one (an AD nurse) had higher education: 25 percent baccalaureate, 62 percent master's, and 2 percent doctorate. About half had had some training in administration. Since 1977, those with the master's had more than doubled. No hospital with over 500 beds had a director with less than a master's. With rare exceptions, the salary rose with the higher degree and the size of the hospital. Salaries ranged from $15,000 to over $65,000; a few directors are known to be in the $100,000 range. Both salaries and fringe benefits have increased since 1977. Only thirteen men were represented in this sample, but the major differences from the women were that all but one had a master's degree, they had moved to administration faster, with fewer interim positions, and most worked in hospitals ranging from 200 to 299 beds. Differences in other aspects, including salary, were not generally significant. Recognition that further education was necessary was demonstrated by the fact that almost half of the nurse administrators with the baccalaureate were taking academic courses for credit, compared to 17 percent of those with the master's. However, almost all had taken CE courses. A heartening note is that more than three-quarters participated in overall hospital budget planning and policy, although their degree of influence is not known.

Qualifications and Conditions of Employment. The ANA Commission on Nursing Services recommended the following qualifications for the administrator of nursing services in 1969 and they are still appropriate.

The competence of the administrator of nursing services involves an ability to facilitate and coordinate a diverse staff of nursing specialists who are making decisions about the nursing needs of individuals, families, and other social groups, and an ability to make decisions about the organization and delivery of nursing services. Two requisites for this leadership role are an understanding of the social, political, and economic influences affecting programs of health care and competence in dealing with any problems in the relationships of professional practitioners and within the complex social system in which nursing is practiced.

Abilities essential to the administrative leader of a program of comprehensive nursing care are the following:

1. The ability to think and act in terms of the total system of health care and to recognize the need for adapting that system to the needs of people.
2. The ability to think and act in terms of the distinctive and contributory role of the nursing profession.
3. The ability to use pertinent knowledge and methods of working with and through people who are concerned with, or affected by, health care.
4. The ability to use knowledge, methods, and techniques pertinent to directing, guiding, and assisting nursing staff members in fulfilling their responsibilities for nursing services.

Basic to these skills is the ability to coordinate, integrate, and reconcile the needs of nursing practitioners, and their goals for nursing service, with organizational requirements and objectives.

Minimum educational qualifications for administrators of nursing services should include completion of a baccalaureate program which has prepared them for professional nursing practice, and completion of a master's degree program with a dual focus on clinical nursing practice and on administration of organized nursing services. Professional experience should have contributed and enhanced the development of the competencies described above.[33]

The 1978 statement cites only educational qualifications: a baccalaureate in nursing and either a master's or a doctoral degree in nursing administration with prior competent administrative experience.[34] The AHA specifies no academic credentials, but rather "sound educational and professional qualifications in administration."[35]

There is some agreement that the nurse administrator must be clinically knowledgeable, if not proficient but that it is essential to have knowledge and skills in newer management techniques, including labor relations, personnel management, financial theories and skills, systems theory, and organizational theory, as well as knowledge of systems of health care delivery. Postprogram preceptorships are recommended by some.

Other nurse administrators have pinpointed some other essential skills and knowledge: quality assurance, planning; political sophistication; good communication; a sense of timing; knowledge about relationships within the health field; and awareness of community and consumer needs.

Salaries for directors of nursing are usually negotiated, but vary a great deal depending on location, size of hospital, responsibilities, and qualifications. This is a difficult, complex position with major responsibilities, frequently great pressure, and no routine forty-hour week, either in time or activities. The director is often expected to be active in community, professional, and other activities, which extend beyond working hours. In some cases, dismissal can be instant and with no reason given (particularly if there is no contract), if the director has not pleased the administration or the hospital board of directors. On the other hand, the leadership of a capable and farsighted director of nursing can create dramatic changes in the quality of nursing care and delivery of health care, and bring immense personal satisfaction and reward.

In-Service Education

A position that may be at the assistant-associate level and that is becoming an integral part of nursing service is that of *in-service education director,* also called *director of staff development* or *in-service coordinator.* At one time, the responsibility for orientation of all nursing staff, training of nonprofessional nursing staff, and in-service education was a fringe duty of an assistant or associate who had other major responsibilities. Rapid changes in health care, scientific and medical advancements, the great diversity in first-level staff nurse applicants, increases in ancillary nursing personnel, and concern about the continuing education (CE) of all nurses have brought the position of in-service education director and instructor into a new focus.

Although in-service education still has a major responsibility for orientation and development of new staff, it is no longer a matter of a few lectures by physicians or demonstration of new equipment. In some hospitals it is an organized, evaluated series of learning experiences based on nurses' needs, and sometimes done on the basis of self-learning.

Some of the current changes are planned programs of CE, based not just on the administration's concept of the learners' needs, but also on input from the learners; enlargement of in-service staff for around-the-clock teaching sessions; better-qualified teachers; the employment of knowledgeable outside speakers; the utilization of more sophisticated teaching media; planned teaching on the clinical unit; and self-learning packages.

The responsibilities of the in-service director include the organization, planning, evaluation, and often implementation of orientation, CE, and training programs for the nursing service department, and, increasingly, for other hospital departments. (For instance, all interested hospital personnel might be taught the fundamentals of emergency resuscitation and external cardiac massage.) This educator must be aware of other resources available for the teaching program, but is personally responsible for the overall development of courses and programs. If there is a large in-service department, one or more in-service instructors may share with the director responsibility for the teaching programs.

Despite the fact that most in-service divisions are still within nursing, a trend to be noted is the move toward hospital-wide training and education departments, which may include CE programs for all health professionals and support staff, and patient education. Nurses still tend to be directors of these departments (all but those involving medicine), but master's-prepared health educators with administrative experience are beginning to be recruited.

Qualifications and Conditions of Employment. Although some in-service directors and/or instructors have no degrees, it is desirable that they have at least a baccalaureate degree, with some knowledge of teaching principles and techniques (particularly in relation to the adult learner), clinical expertise, and preferably a master's degree (especially as in-service director). They should also be able to work through and with others, with enough self-confidence to assume a staff role with little inherent authority.

Because of the cost of in-service education, there is also a need to develop both strong evaluation tools and programs that meet the goals of the institutions as well as the learner.[36] Salary may depend on these qualifications and the kinds of responsibilities assumed; usually, salary and benefits are at the level of the supervisors for the in-service director, less for the instructor. Some sessions may be held in the evening or at night, but the majority of activities are usually scheduled during the day. This position is particularly attractive to nurses who are stimulated by teaching all levels of nursing personnel and who enjoy remaining in the hospital setting.

Other Positions for Nurses in Hospitals

There are a number of other employment opportunities for nurses in hospitals, although they may have only a tangential relationship to nursing and are often in a department other than nursing service. Nurses on the intravenous (IV) team are especially trained, and responsible, for all the intravenous infusions given to patients (outside of the operating room and delivery room). On the basis of a predetermined protocol, they may bring the appropriate intravenous solution to the bedside or obtain it on the unit, add ordered drugs, and start and/or restart the infusion. In some institutions they are also permitted to start a blood transfusion.

The nurse-epidemiologist or infection con-

trol nurse focuses on surveillance, education, and research.[37] The surveillance aspect is designed for the reporting of infections and the establishment, over a period of time, of expected levels of infections for various areas. Patients with infections are checked, and it is determined whether the infection was acquired after admission. Reports are used for epidemiologic research, and staff is educated in prevention of infection. Nurses have also been trained as epidemiologists in public health agencies, where they perform similar but broader duties that involve the total community.

The project director or manager in the hospital evolves from a new organizational framework in which the executive delegates individual responsibility for specific projects and activities. That person seeks information and ideas from others and develops a project approved by the executive. Usually, the project director has no staff, although when there is staff assigned temporarily, they continue to be accountable to their functional superior. Examples of projects are quality assurance, performance evaluation, or hospital construction.[38]

A challenging role is that of ombudsman, or patient advocate, in which a nurse acts as an intermediary between the patient and the hospital in an attempt to alleviate or prevent problems of the patient related to the hospital or hospitalization. Nurses are also being employed as utilization review agents.[39] This role originated with the Medicare regulation stating that if a Medicare patient's hospital stay was prolonged beyond a necessary length of time, the cost of the additional stay was not paid. A selected nurse or nurses check patients and their records at predetermined periods to gather data for the Utilization Review Committee. A more sophisticated and newer version of the role is that of nurse coordinator with a Professional Standards Organization. These nurses prepare a detailed patient profile assessing the patient's need in relation to appropriate level of care, length of stay, utilization of ancillary services, and discharge planning. Using their nursing judgment and experience, they decide whether medical care conforms to established criteria. These data are reviewed with the medical adviser, a practicing physician, who uses the information gathered and synthesized by the nurse in his review and evaluation of deviations from established norms and criteria.

Finally, new emphasis on health education in the hospital and community has resulted in the creation of a community health coordinator, who develops and/or coordinates the various aspects of patient teaching as well as the teaching of outpatients and other interested individuals in the community, on health matters. This nurse may not be a part of nursing service, and is more likely to direct the teaching program than to do the teaching personally.[40]

MUNICIPAL, COUNTY, AND STATE HOSPITALS

Municipal, county, and state hospitals are primarily intended to provide hospital accommodation for indigent citizens within prescribed political boundaries. In many instances, they operate on a much broader scale and accept patients who pay part or all of their hospital bills. The fact remains, however, that these hospitals are supported principally by city, county, and state funds which come from taxpayers. This means that decisions about the amounts allocated for operating them rest in the hands of a central board, which may also allocate funds for schools, prisons, and many other institutions, all of which invariably want and need more money than they receive. Furthermore, the hospitals are usually obligated to accept all patients who come to them for treatment, even though they may be overcrowded and understaffed. This often spreads money and personnel very thin. It is predicted that, because of the pressures of the health economy, an increasing number of people will be forced to seek care in governmental hospitals.

Many of these hospitals conduct outstanding educational programs for all categories of health personnel, and appointments to their staffs are considered highly desirable, particularly from the point of view of experience.

Nursing positions in these hospitals usually follow the same general pattern as in other hospitals. Staff nurses rarely need additional qualifications, except possibly for work in a hospital treating such specific diseases as tuberculosis or leprosy. However, in cities where a large part of the poor population comes from an ethnic group that speaks another language, nurses from that ethnic group or speaking that language are particularly welcome.

Staff nurses in a large city, county, or state hospital may find that a great deal of the nursing care is given by practical nurses and nurse's aides. The principal functions of RNs may be teaching, directing, and supervising other workers, in many instances doing very little bedside nursing themselves. They may find the patient load very heavy at times; however, there may also be more challenges and greater satisfaction here than in a comparable position in any other type of hospital, both because of the learning opportunities and the opportunity to be a change agent in providing quality care for the socially disadvantaged.

Because these hospitals are government-operated, nurses and all other staff members are eligible for the benefits given to any employee of the particular governmental entity concerned. These benefits, which are so important to one's economic security, vary throughout the country, but they often include an early retirement or pension system, not usually offered by nongovernmental institutions.

Nurses who work in a city, county, or state hospital are employees of the governing political body, not the hospital. Salary checks are issued from a central office. Salary increments are often given according to a scale based on length of employment. Nurses seeking employment in one of these hospitals may apply directly to the hospital they wish to work in or to the appropriate central agency, which is usually located in the municipal building, county courthouse, or state house. If there is no particular preference, the central office may give information about all available positions for which the nurse is qualified and help in the selection of the one best suited.

NURSING WITH THE FEDERAL GOVERNMENT

Professional nurses interested in a career with the federal government will find opportunities in both military and nonmilitary services. The military services include the Army, Navy, and Air Force. The Veterans Administration (VA) is not a military service, although it is closely allied. The other principal nonmilitary federal service employing nurses is the U.S. Public Health Service (PHS).

Many nursing positions in nonmilitary federal services are for specialists in education, administration, research, or clinical areas and therefore require education and experience beyond the basic program. There are many others, however, particularly with the PHS and the VA, for which newly graduated professional nurses may qualify to practice. Both the PHS and the VA employ new graduates temporarily, pending completion of the state board examinations.

The federal government owns and operates more than 400 hospitals in this country in which many government employees (and sometimes their dependents), veterans of the armed services, American Indians, and other special groups are eligible for care without charge, regardless of their ability to pay. In addition, the federal government also operates hospitals in other countries for members of the armed services stationed in these countries.

Among the various federal agencies operating hospitals—and sometimes other health services—are the VA, the PHS, the Air Force, the Army, the Navy, and the U.S. Department of Justice (Bureau of Prisons). All these hos-

pitals are supported financially by taxes. These hospitals usually have high standards of service, equipment, and facilities and are able to attract highly qualified personnel. Many of the country's outstanding physicians and nurses are members of their staffs. Research and teaching are integral parts of the work of many of the larger institutions. Although each branch of the armed services operates hospitals primarily to provide care for its own members, all branches will care for a member of any service in an emergency and until transfer is feasible. Sometimes, because of regional considerations, these patients are kept in the original hospital for the entire period of illness.

All those eligible for care in a government hospital—with the exception of prisoners and during wartime—may, if they prefer, go to a nongovernment hospital for care, but they have to pay their own bills unless authorized to make the change. In some instances it is more economical and practical for the government to pay civilian hospitals to care for members of the armed services and other federal employees than it is to operate federal hospitals in all localities or transport the patients long distances. Exceptions are also sometimes made for cases that would benefit from some special treatment facility not available in a government hospital.

Professional nurses who work in most hospitals operated by the federal government perform essentially the same functions as nurses in a civilian hospital in a comparable position. They give, teach, and direct nursing care. They coordinate the work of various health personnel and plan and implement patient care in cooperation with the health team.

Nurses who work in hospitals connected with federal prisons* have somewhat different duties, of course. But their primary concern and responsibility is to keep the prisoners well and give them skilled nursing care when they

---

*Nursing in state or municipal prisons is generally similar.

are ill. In addition, nurses sometimes teach prisoners to care for themselves.

The organization of nursing service within a federal hospital is similar to that of a civilian hospital, and the adaptable professional nurse would find little difficulty in adjusting to its few dissimilarities.

Qualifications and Conditions of Employment. Each branch of the federal government has set up basic qualifications for professional nurses who wish to join its ranks and has established criteria for advancement. The conditions of employment also follow a similar pattern in the several branches of the federal government nursing services.

U.S. PUBLIC HEALTH SERVICE (PHS)

Founded in 1798, the PHS is the federal agency specifically charged with promoting and assuring the highest level of health attainable for every individual and family. It is also responsible for collaborating with governments of other countries and with international organizations in world health activities. It is a vital force in advancing research in the health sciences, in developing public health programs, and in providing therapeutic and preventive services. The PHS offers opportunities for a variety of nursing assignments: the Clinical Center research hospital in Bethesda, Maryland; public health and clinical nursing in the Indian Health Program; and consultation in such fields as community health, environmental health, hospital services, clinical specialties, nursing education, and nursing research. Assignments depend on the nurse's education and experience, professional aptitudes, personal and career preferences, and needs of the service.

The graduate nurse may enter the PHS either by appointment to the Commissioned Corps or the Federal Civil Service. Minimum requirements are U.S. citizenship, at last eighteen years of age, graduation from an approved school of nursing, and physical eligi-

bility. Graduates from associate degree or diploma programs of less than thirty months are often appointed at a lower rank than other graduates; they are required to have an additional year of nursing experience to achieve the same rank as other graduates. The Commissioned Corps is a uniformed service comprised of professionals in medical and health-related fields. Pay, allowances, and other privileges are comparable to those of officers of the armed forces. Appointments may be made at the junior assistant grade, equivalent to ensign in the Navy or second lieutenant in the Army. The top rank is surgeon general, equivalent to rear admiral and major general. Currently, three nurse members of the corps have achieved the rank of assistant surgeon general. A candidate must have a bachelor's degree in nursing from an NLN-accredited college or university and, if without prior military service, must be under forty-four.

Opportunity for collegiate nursing students to become familiar with the careers in the PHS as well as to further their professional knowledge is offered through the Commissioned Officer Student Training and Extern Program (COSTEP). In the junior COSTEP, a limited number of carefully selected students are commissioned as reserve officers in the corps and called to active duty for training during "free periods" of the academic year. Assignments are made in the continental United States for 31 to 120 consecutive days in any twelve-month period, in the areas of medical and hospital services, research, or public health practice. Salary and privileges are at the junior assistant health service grade and include housing allowance, travel, and medical care. After satisfactory performance, a COSTEP officer may be retained in the Inactive Reserve Commissioned Corps of the PHS while continuing college education. Upon completing professional education, the officer may request active status and retain his or her commission. If active duty is not desired, the commission is terminated. To be eligible, students must have completed two years of a baccalaureate program, expect to return to college after each COSTEP assignment, and be otherwise eligible for appointment to the Commissioned Corps.

The civil service system is considered the basic mode of federal employment and comprises a range of professional and nonprofessional personnel. A civil service examination is not required for RNs before appointment. There is opportunity for advancement through a well-defined merit system. Nurses employed under civil service in PHS have Social Security benefits. They are eligible for retirement benefits, which they may receive upon resignation, depending on the length of employment.

One PHS hospital remains: the National Hansen's Disease Center located at Carville, Louisiana. it provides care and rehabilitation for patients with leprosy and for training and research in that disease.

The Indian Health Service is responsible for the health care of more than 925,000 American Indians, Eskimos, and Aleuts, operating approximately forty-eight hospitals and eighty health centers, most west of the Mississippi River. The clinical nurse in the Indian Service works in the clinics and hospitals. The community health nurse coordinates nursing services between the hospital, clinic, school, and home.

There are a number of other nursing positions in the PHS. The National Institute of Mental Health deals with basic research training activities for specialized manpower, and intensified programs on suicide, crime, and delinquency. The Center for Disease Control conducts national and international programs in research, prevention, and control of infectious diseases. The National Center for Health Services Research conducts and supports research and demonstrations related to the availability, organization, and financing of health services. The Maternal and Child Health Service employs nursing specialists in the field in its nationwide programs, providing comprehensive health services for mothers and children.

The Clinical Center under the aegis of the Department of Health and Human Services (DHHS) is a component part of the National Institutes of Health, the principal research arm of the Public Health Service. The National Institutes of Health are composed of a number of institutes—including National Eye Institute; National Cancer Institute; National Institute of Aging; National Institute of Neurological Diseases and Stroke; National Heart and Lung Institute; National Institute of Arthritis, Metabolic and Digestive Diseases; National Institute of Allergy and Infectious Diseases; National Institute of Dental Research; and National Institute of Child Health and Human Development. The hospital of the Clinical Center employs staff nurses to participate with the medical staff in planning for the total care of patients undergoing medical research. They may be assigned to any nursing service for an indefinite period of time or they may choose to rotate from one service to another when vacancies permit. Nurses at the Clinical Center are encouraged to be innovative in the development of new skills and to be active participants in determining their role.

The National Health Service Corps (NHSC) was create in 1970 "to improve the delivery of health services where health personnel and services are inadequate to meet the health needs." Under this broad mandate, the NHSC provided health care personnel to urban and rural communities that had critical health manpower shortages. That mandate continues today.

In 1972, an amendment to Title VII of the PHS Act authorized scholarships to be awarded to health professionals while still in school who agree to serve in the NHSC in a designated HMSA (underserved area) after completion of their training. The purpose of this program was to provide adequate supplies of trained physicians, dentists, nurses, and other health specialists for the corps. At the end of fiscal year 1983, there were over 2,700 scholarship recipients serving their obligations and over 5,000 still in training.

Evidence indicates that market forces have led to the diffusion of health personnel into less well served areas, and this trend will continue. The NHSC seeks to complement this process by placing personnel, mostly physicians and dentists, in designated shortage areas which have the most severe need and demand for health services and which can show that they have made unsuccessful efforts to attract and retain health manpower.

Although there are other major programs in the PHS, the others do not employ nurses. For information about job opportunities with the Department of Health and Human Services, contact the Federal Job Information Center in your area listed in the telephone directory under "U.S. Government."

VETERANS ADMINISTRATION NURSING SERVICE

The Veterans Administration (VA) was established in 1930 as a civilian agency of the federal government. Its purpose is to administer national programs that provide benefits for veterans of this country's armed forces. The VA operates the nation's largest organized health care system, comprised of 172 hospitals, over 200 outpatient clinics, more than 100 nursing home care units, and 16 domiciliaries. More than 1.3 million veterans receive hospital care through the VA system yearly. The VA's Department of Medicine and Surgery employs more than 30,000 professional nurses.

To accomplish its objective of providing high-quality health care, the VA has developed extensive programs in research and education. A majority of VA medical centers are affiliated with medical schools, schools of nursing, and other health-related schools in a network of health care facilities that cover the entire country. Individual hospitals range in size from approximately 110 to 1,400 beds most of which provide care for patients with medical, surgical, and psychiatric diagnoses. A few hospitals are predominantly for the care of patients with psychiatric diagnoses. Many VA health care facilities have outpa-

tient clinics and extended-care facilities, such as nursing home care units.

VA medical centers are administered through the Department of Medicine and Surgery, headed by a Chief Medical Director. The Nursing Service functions within this department under the leadership of a Deputy Assistant Chief Medical Director for Nursing Programs, who is the national Director of Nursing Service. The National Nursing Service office is located at the Veterans Administration Central Office, 810 Vermont Avenue NW, Washington, D.C. 20420.

To qualify for an appointment in the VA, a nurse must be a U.S. citizen, a graduate of a state-approved school of professional nursing, currently registered to practice, and meet required physical standards. Graduates from a professional school of nursing may be appointed pending passing of state board examinations.

There are several levels of salary grades for VA nurses, ranging from junior grade through associate, full, intermediate, senior, chief, assistant director, director, and the executive grade of director, the last reserved for the national leader of the VA Nursing Service.

Qualification standards relating to education, experience, and competencies are specified for appointment or promotion to each grade. The VA salary system recognizes excellence in clinical practice, administration, research, and education. Nurses, including those giving direct patient care, receive salaries commensurate with their qualifications and contributions. A Nurse Professional Standards Board reviews performance and recommends promotion or special salary advancement according to established criteria. A nurse appointed to one VA medical center may transfer to another with continuity of benefits and without loss of salary.

Personnel policies in the VA include a variety of health and life insurance options (partially paid for by the federal government), retirement plans, and liberal annual and sick leave benefits.

The VA Nursing Service emphasizes continued learning and advanced education. There is a Nursing Career Development Program to provide opportunities within the system. Nurse researchers are employed in some VA medical centers and in the national office. CNSs work in some VA health care settings. Also, NPs function in specific units, clinics, or satellite facilities. Applications and inquiries for full- or part-time employment should be directed to the Personnel Office at the VA Medical Center at the location of interest. A toll-free telephone number (800-368-5629) is available for information about nationwide employment opportunities.

THE ARMED SERVICES

Despite similarities, there are specific differences among the Army Nurse Corps, Navy Nurse Corps, and Air Force Nurse Corps. In recent years there have been a number of changes in qualifications and assignments to meet the changes in society and in the health field. All the armed services have a reserve corps of nurses established by acts of Congress to provide the additional nurses that are needed to care for members of the services and their families in time of war or other national emergency. Nurses may join the reserve without having joined the regular service; the requirements are similar. A certain amount of daily training (which is paid) is required, usually one weekend a month and two consecutive weeks a year, at local medical units related to that particular service. There are opportunities for promotion, continuing education, and fringe benefits such as low-cost insurance, retirement pay, and PX shopping. More information is available from the reserve recruiter of the particular service. In all the services, nurses have the economic, social, and health care benefits of all officers as well as the opportunity for personal travel. After discharge (or retirement, which is possible in twenty years), veterans' benefits are available.

The Army Nurse Corps

Because it is the oldest of the federal nurs-

ing services, the Army Nurse Corps has had considerable influence on the development of nursing and the status of nurses in all of the armed services. When the Army Nurse Corps was established as part of the Army Medical Department in 1901, nurses had a status comparable to that of enlisted men. Believing that they needed the authority of officers for disciplinary reasons related to giving nursing care, nurses, principally through the ANA, tried unsuccessfully for many years to persuade Congress to give them that recognition. During World War II, the federal government gave nurses serving in all branches of the armed services temporary commissions. But it was not until 1947 that women nurses achieved permanent commissioned status. Men in nursing had to wait until 1955 to be so recognized.

Qualifications for a commission in the Army Nurse Corps are that the person be:

1. A graduate of a baccalaureate program of nursing acceptable to the Department of the Army.
2. Between twenty-one and thirty-three years of age (unless with prior military service).
3. Currently licensed to practice nursing in the United States, the Commonwealth of Puerto Rico, or the District of Columbia, or a U.S. territory.
4. A citizen of or lawfully admitted to the United States for permanent residence.
5. Able to provide excellent professional, personal, moral, and scholastic references.
6. Able to conform to the physical standards prescribed for appointment in the U.S. Army.
7. Married or single; both women and men may have dependents of any age.
8. Engaged in practice as a registered nurse on a full-time basis for not less than six months within the one-year period preceding date of application.
9. Registered nurses from acceptable associate degree and diploma programs with at least twelve months of full-time experience as an RN may apply for appointment without concurrent call to active duty.

An RN just completing a baccalaureate program in nursing comes into the Army Nurse Corps as a second lieutenant. Additional professional experience and education may earn an initial appointment at a higher rank. Ordinarily, the agreed-upon length of service is three years. Generally, every newly commissioned officer is in the Army Reserve, in which the individual may continue indefinitely after release from active duty. In the Regular Army Nurse Corps, the nurse may now advance to the rank of brigadier general.

Army nurses may give direct patient care in any clinical specialty as staff nurses, head nurses, or nursing consultants. They may teach as directors or instructors for military courses in various hospitals and the Academy of Health Sciences, or be responsible for nursing education and training within a Department of Nursing. They may become involved in administration in various clinical services or at Army headquarters. They may also function as nursing methods analysts, nurse researchers, nurse counselors, consultants to the surgeon general, or advisor to military nurses of allied nations. Assignments may be in the United States or various parts of the world. There are numerous educational programs, such as the clinical nursing specialty courses. Army Nurse Corps officers may also be selected to attend a college or university for advanced degrees with all or part of the costs paid.

Further information may be obtained from the local Army recruiting station (ask for the Army Nurse Corps recruiter) or by writing to Army Nurse Opportunities, P.O. Box 7713, Clifton, N.J. 07015.

Navy Nurse Corps

Although the Navy Nurse Corps was officially established by Congress in the twentieth century, Navy nurses were recommended by the first chief of the Bureau of Medicine and Surgery in 1811, and sisters of the Order of the Holy Cross served on the Navy ship *Red Rover* as volunteers in 1862. They were the first female nurses to serve aboard the first U.S. Navy hospital ship. The first Navy nurses (called the *Sacred Twenty*) and a superintendent reported to Washington for duty in 1908. By 1910 nurses had expanded their activities to include the Far East, Hawaii, and the Caribbean. In World War I, women nurses were assigned to hospitals in England, Ireland, Scotland, and France. Throughout World War II, Navy nurses also brought nursing care to front-line casualties aboard twelve hospital ships and also to air evacuees. They served in foreign lands where American women had never been seen and some were prisoners of war. In 1944, the *USS Highbee* became the first combat ship to be named for a woman, the second superintendent of the Navy Nurse Corps.

Today, many Navy nurses not only care for patients, but also teach patients, corpsmen, and other nurses, and assume administrative positions. They are assigned to clinics, hospitals, and Hospital Corps schools in the United States and other parts of the world.

Appointments are made in grades of ensign to lieutenant (senior grade), depending upon age, education, and other professional qualifications, but the nurse may advance to the rank of commodore. Basic qualifications are that the person be

1. A graduate of an approved nursing school in the United States or Canada.
2. A registered nurse.
3. At least twenty and less than thirty-five years of age.
4. Single or married; applicants with dependents will be considered.
5. A citizen of the United States.
6. Physically qualified according to Navy standards.
7. Able to supply excellent professional, personal, moral, and scholastic references.

All Navy nurses are encouraged to continue their education through Navy in-service and CE courses, as well as courses leading to academic degrees. Qualified career officers may request assignment to full-time study for a baccalaureate or master's degree.

Further information is available from the local Navy recruiting station or from the Nursing Program, Navy Recruiting Command, Naval Department, Washington, D.C.

The Air Force Nurse Corps

In 1947, with the passage of the National Security Act, the United States Air Force was established as a separate service.

The United States Air Force Medical Service, including the nursing component, was established on July 1, 1949. Prior to that date, medical personnel in the Army Medical Service were assigned to duty with the United States Air Force.

The mission of the Medical Service is to provide the medical support necessary for maximum peacetime readiness and combat effectiveness of the Air Force. As an integral part of the mission, the Medical Service will provide, to the greatest extent possible, a peacetime health care system for all eligible beneficiaries. The Air Force Nurse Corps, as one of the five components responsible for medical support of the Air Force, has a vital role in this mission.

Since its establishment, the Nurse Corps has undergone many changes, including increased authorizations, increased rank, and new specialty codes. In 1955, male nurses were authorized to receive commissions, and now approximately one-quarter are men. Nurses can now be married and can have dependents of any age.

Air Force nurses provide quality nursing care in a variety of specialties and settings. They perform duties in one of twelve career fields, such as administration, mental health, operating room, anesthesia, clinical nursing, education, flight nursing, NP, midwifery, and environmental health. They are involved in clinical practice, patient teaching, supervision and teaching of paraprofessional personnel, administration, education, and research.

The majority of the nurses are assigned to medical centers, hospitals, and clinics in the United States and overseas. Most medical treatment facilities are small community hospitals, providing routine and emergency medical, surgical, pediatric, obstetric, and psychoneurological services for beneficiaries. One role unique to Air Force nursing is that of flight nurse. The Air Force has the Department of Defense responsibility for aeromedical evacuation in peacetime and during conflicts.

Nurses are assigned as flight nurses only after completing an intensive program at the School of Aerospace Medicine at Brooks Air Force Base, Texas. Since the first class graduated in February 1943, the course has been conducted continuously, with over 10,000 graduates. The course includes didactic and practical experiences in aerospace physiology, basic sciences, specialized techniques necessary for the safe and efficient transportation of patients by air, and survival and life support principles, procedures, and equipment. It provides students with the knowledge and skills required for management and nursing care of patients in flight.

Another unique role is that of environmental health nurse. The original environmental health nurses were called *aerospace nurses* and participated as members of the aerospace medical team in support of the Mercury series of manned space flights. Today they are leaders in preventive medicine, health promotion, and maintenance, and function in the occupational medicine, preventive medicine, and environmental health arenas. Environmental health nurses are prepared for this role during a two-year program that results in a master's degree in public health.

Air Force nurses are given every opportunity to grow—both academically and professionally. Nurses are encouraged to continue their formal education at civilian colleges and universities located near Air Force medical treatment facilities. Under a tuition assistance program, the Air Force may pay up to 75 percent of their tuition costs for off-duty courses. Many Air Force nurses compete regularly for undergraduate and graduate study opportunities. A certain number are selected each year to pursue full-time graduate studies in civilian universities. Air Force-sponsored students receive their normal pay during the school terms, plus educational assistance covering tuition and required expenses. Accepting this educational assistance requires an additional active duty obligation commensurate with the length of the educational program.

Tuition assistance is available for generic nursing students via the ROTC programs on most university campuses. Applications are accepted from BSN students who meet certain criteria during their senior year. This program offers an excellent opportunity for a wide variety of clinical experiences to new graduates. Applicants accepted for this program participate in a five-month nurse internship program before reporting to their first assignment. Nurses in the intern program have the opportunity to apply basic nursing knowledge and skills and acquire new, specialized skills. Rotations through several clinical areas help prepare nurses for a variety of nursing duties.

Air Force nurses have two professions—they are professional nurses, and they are professional officers. The ranks of Air Force nurses range from second lieutenant to brigadier general. All new accessions attend the military indoctrination for Medical Service officers. During this course, the Air Force nurse is introduced to life as an Air Force officer—a position of pride, leadership, and respect.

Most applicants receive their commissions as officers in the grade of second lieutenant. Nurses with additional professional experience and education may be appointed at a higher rank after review of records and in accordance with current policy.

To qualify for appointment, the applicant must

1. Be a graduate of a nursing school acceptable to the Surgeon General of the Air Force.
2. Have a current registration in any state, territory of the United States, or District of Columbia.
3. Meet physical and professional requirements.

4. Be at least eighteen years old.
5. Be a citizen of the United States.

Additional information may be obtained by contacting a local Air Force recruiter or by writing to headquarters, United States Air Force Recruiting Service/RSHN, Randolph Air Force Base, Texas 78150. In addition to a full-time career as an Air Force officer, commissions are also available via the Air Force Reserve and Air National Guard Programs. Information on Air Force Reserve Programs may be obtained by writing HQ Air Force Reserve/Sg. Robins Air Force Base, Georgia 31098 or HQ ARPC/Sg, Denver, Colorado 80280. Information on Air National Guard Programs may be obtained by writing National Guard Bureau/SG, Room 2E369, The Pentagon, Washington, D.C. 20310.

NURSING IN EXTENDED AND LONG-TERM CARE FACILITIES

Under Medicare and Medicaid, nursing homes that qualify for reimbursement are called *skilled nursing facilities.* The intermediate care facility provides for those who require care beyond room and board but less than that designated as skilled. These include institutions for victims of cerebral palsy or other neurological conditions and mental retardation. The older term *nursing home,* which might apply to either, is still used by most people. There are some 18,000 nursing homes in the country, about 75 percent under proprietary (for-profit) ownership.

Although the average bed capacity is around 75, the total number of beds is greater than hospital beds (about 1.3 to 1.5 million). There are more RNs working in nursing homes than there were even five years ago, although the majority of caregivers are practical nurses and aides.

Nurses may have positions in nursing homes similar to those in hospitals, with the additional role of facility administrator being assumed by some nurses. In this case, the nurse must be certified for the position, and although the individual's knowledge of nursing may be extremely helpful in understanding the need for quality care, being a nurse is not a requirement for certification.

The director of nursing, who has the same kinds of responsibilities as any other director of nursing, is sometimes expected to act as the administrator's assistant, whereas some administrators take over some of the director's prerogatives. In small nursing homes, the director might assume both roles. Because of the profit orientation, financial management is extremely important. The administrative nurse should be well prepared in managerial skills; unfortunately, that is rare.

A 1983 survey of 1,234 directors of nursing of long-term care facilities provides specific information. Typically the director is a white female about forty-five years old. Twenty-six percent have bachelors degrees, about 61 percent of which are in nursing. About 6 percent have a master's, about half in nursing. Almost seventy percent have no more than a diploma; about 16 percent report continuing their education formally. Supervision, management, gerontology, and professional issues are the subjects studied most often in continuing education. On the basis of an analysis of the director's perceived problem areas, educational needs could be grouped into areas of clinical nursing management, department management and supervision, administrative skills, and human resource management. About 11 percent of directors of nursing are licensed in nursing home administration. Sixty-five percent report that they belong to no nursing organizations; 13 percent belong to some health care group.

The average salary for these directors of nursing is $21,500, although 19 percent report earnings over $25,000.[41]

In most nursing homes the pace is slower and the pressure less. Nurses interested in nursing home care enjoy the opportunity to know the patient better in the relatively long-term stay and to help the patient maintain or attain the best possible health status. This is not the area of practice for someone impatient for quick results. Both rehabilitative and geriatric nursing require a large amount of patience and understanding. In rehabilitation, nurses work closely as a team with related health disciplines—occupational therapy, physical therapy, speech therapy, and others. In geriatric nursing, the nurse works to a great extent with nonprofesional nursing personnel and acts as team leader, teacher, and supervisor. It may well be that there is only one professional nurse in a nursing home per shift, with practical nurses as charge nurses and aides giving much of the day-to-day care.

Because the patients are relatively helpless and often have no family or friends who check on them, the nurse must, in a real sense, be a patient advocate. Physicians make infrequent visits and in some cases, where there are limited or no rehabilitative services, the nurse is the only professional with long-term patient contact.

For this reason, geriatric nurse practitioners (GNPs) are considered a tremendous asset in nursing homes. The GNP is responsible for assessing patients and evaluating their progress, sometimes performing certain diagnostic procedures. She or he usually manages medical problems within a general protocol, but a particularly important function is assessing personal and family relationships, patient and staff relationships, and life situations that may affect the patient's health status. In some nursing homes, the GNP is on twenty-four-hour emergency call and also performs the other usual NP functions.[42]

Qualifications and Conditions of Employment. Requirements for employment are similar to those in hospitals for like positions, although often the need for a degree is not emphasized. Conditions of employment and salaries have improved, but are not as good as those in hospitals. Because, under Medicare, orientation and subsequent in-service education are mandatory, the nurse has an excellent opportunity to learn about long-term nursing care and the concepts and techniques of geriatric nursing. Because the increase of older people is one of the trends in society, geriatric care is being given greater attention, and workshops, courses, and programs are available in the field. With an aging population, there are also likely to be good job opportunities for some time to come. It is unfortunate that so few are interested in care of the elderly.[43]

PUBLIC HEALTH (COMMUNITY HEALTH) NURSING

Although there is an increasing tendency to refer to *public health nursing (PHN)* and *community health nursing (CHN)* interchangeably, there are those who differentiate between the two terms. Two national organizations with large memberships of PHN/CHN nurses have slightly different definitions and orientations. The ANA says:

Community Health Nursing is a synthesis of nursing practice and public health practice applied to promoting and preserving the health of populations. The nature of this practice is general and comprehensive. It is not limited to a particular age or diagnostic group. It is continuing, not episodic. The dominant responsibility is to the population as a whole. Therefore, nursing directed to individuals, families or groups contributes to the health of the total population. Health promotion, health maintenance, health education, coordination and continuity of care are utilized in a holistic approach to the family, group and community. The nurse's actions acknowledge the need for comprehensive health planning, recognize the influences of social and ecological issues, give attention to populations at risk and utilize the dynamic forces which influence change.

In Community Health Nursing Practice the consumer is the client or patient. Consumers include individuals, groups and the community as a whole. For example, the consumer may be a single individual, family (interpreted in the broadest sense), a school population, an industrial population or selected at-risk segments of the population. Professional practitioners of nursing bear primary responsibility and accountability for the nursing care consumers receive.[44]

Translating this concept into specifics, the ANA Division on Community Health Nursing Practice stated:

The primary focus of community health nursing is on the prevention of illness and the promotion and maintenance of health. Therefore, community health nursing practice includes the provision of needed therapeutic services, counseling, education, direction, and advocacy activities. The community health nurse who is in constant contact with people in groups who seek and need health care has unique opportunities to identify discrete health problems, as well as potential health problems, and to evaluate current health status. The community health nurse is involved in the planning and coordination of community health programs and services.

The community health nurse, therefore, has responsibility in general and comprehensive areas of health practice for:

a. Determining health needs of the individual, the family, and the community;
b. Assessing health status;
c. Implementing health planning;
d. Evaluating health practices;
e. Providing primary health care.

The community health nurse needs to be aware of regulations which are developing, as well as new and existing regulations, policies, and laws that directly affect community health nursing practice.[45]

Shortly after this statement was published (1980), the Public Health Nursing Section of the American Public Health Association published its definition of PHN and delineated its scope of practice:

Public health nursing synthesizes the body of knowledge from the public health sciences and professional nursing theories. The implicit overriding goal is to improve the health of the community by identifying sub-groups (aggregates) within the community population which are at high risk of illness, disability, or premature death and directing resources toward these groups. This lies at the heart of primary prevention and health promotion. Public health nursing accomplishes its goal by working with groups, families, and individuals as well as by functioning in multi-disciplinary teams and programs. Success in the reduction of risks and in improving the health of the community is dependent upon a full range of consumer involvement, especially from those groups at risk as well as the community and its members, in health planning, in self help, and in individual responsibility for personal health habits which promote health and a safe environment.

Public health nursing practice is a systematic process by which:

1. the health and health care needs of a population are assessed in collaboration with other disciplines in order to identify sub-populations (aggregates), families, and individuals at increased risk of illness, disability, or premature death;
2. a plan for intervention is developed to meet these needs, which includes resources available and those activities that contribute to health and its recovery, the prevention of illness, disability and premature death;
3. a health care plan is implemented effectively, efficiently, and equitably; and
4. an evaluation is made to determine the extent to which these activities have an impact on the health status of the population.[46]

In fulfilling these responsibilities, PHN/CHN nurses practice in many settings. Most are employed by agencies that may carry the title of public health, community health, home health, or visiting nurse. They may be official—governmental and tax supported (such as a city or county health department); nonofficial or voluntary—agencies supported to a great extent by community funds (such as

a visiting nurse or home health service); or proprietary—for profit. These agencies range in size and services from small, employing only one or two PHNs, to very large, employing a sizable staff of professional nurses, other health professionals, practical nurses, and home health aides and homemakers. Some of the latter may be contracted for from an agency (see Chapter 8).

PHN employment opportunities are not limited, however, to these agencies. Nurses may also be employed by hospitals to conduct home-care programs or to serve as liaison between the hospital and community facilities, or by other institutions and agencies, private and governmental, in need of the kinds of services the PHN is prepared to provide in schools, outpatient clinics, community health centers, free walk-in clinics for drug addiction and venereal diseases, migrant labor camps, and rural poverty areas.

One type of practitioner prepared to assess community needs and assist the community in seeking appropriate help is the community nurse practitioner (CNP), a generally non-clinical nurse concerned with health care access, fragmentation, health promotion, and disease prevention.[47] CNPs, who usually have master's degrees, may be employed in both governmental and nonprofit agencies, but there are still too few to determine their impact.

PHNs may also work for various international agencies assisting less developed countries, because the need for PHN services in these countries is usually urgent. Because the PHN/CHN field is so broad, it offers almost unlimited employment opportunities for qualified professional nurses. As part of the traditional public health services, every state, every United States territory, and many counties, large towns, and cities have a public health department. (In some states, health and welfare units have been merged, but most still have separate health departments.) How effective it is in meeting the needs of the community it serves depends upon its finances, its physical facilities, its staff, and its leadership.

Originally, public health services were concerned with the control of such diseases as typhoid fever, cholera, smallpox, and yellow fever. Programs have expanded rapidly in the last few decades, on local, state, and national levels, to include diagnostic, therapeutic, and rehabilitative services as well as preventive health care and counseling. New areas of concern are mental illness, alcoholism, chronic illness, drug addiction, and the need for primary care. There is also active participation in civil defense.

Public health offers extraordinary opportunities for the imaginative, competent, and resourceful person to originate and develop ideas that may greatly affect the health of the community and, conceivably, of the entire world. Research and education are extremely important phases of public health and are carried on continuously, often under the auspices of, and supported financially by, the PHS.

Professional nurses make up the largest group of professional public health personnel, and their influence is considerable. Workers in the field of public health include physicians, social workers, sanitary engineers, nutritionists, dentists, physical therapists, speech therapists, and others. Members of these groups may work alone or in a team relationship. All public health workers, therefore, need an overview of the entire program to understand their place in the organization and the scope of their own work. An effective public health program requires excellent working relationships with other agencies, both health and nonhealth, because public health activities reach every segment of the community. Although situations differ, nurses in official agencies may make home visits, but their responsibilities are primarily in community health clinics focused on the needs of that agency's population. Traditionally, these have been family planning, maternal-child care, and communicable disease; in a number of communities these agency nurses are also the school nurses and, occasionally, are contracted to do some occupational health nursing. NPs are being employed to care for patients in the areas of their expertise, but all nurses observe and evaluate the patients' physical and emotional conditions and are involved in teaching, therapy, counseling and prevention; they make referrals as necessary and act in a liaison capacity with other agencies for needed services.

The visiting nurses, or home health nurses, regardless of their place of employment, also carry out these functions and may, in addition, give physical care and treatments.* If the nurse assessment indicates that such care does not require professional nurse services, home health aides/homemakers may be assigned to a patient/family, with nurse supervision and reassessment. Visiting nurses have also set up clinics that they visit periodically in senior citizen centers or apartments, as well as in the single-room occupancy (SRO) hotels commonly used for welfare clients in large cities. There are multiple liaison roles with hospitals, HMOs, clinics, geriatric units, and various residences for the long-term disabled and mentally ill or retarded, primarily to assist in admission and discharge planning, as well as coordinating continuing patient care.

Nurses in managerial positions in PHN/CHN agencies have responsibilities similar to those in hospitals in terms of general managerial skills. A major difference for the top nurse administrator is that that individual is frequently director of the entire agency, with direct responsibility to the agency board of directors (nonofficial agency) or the health officer (governmental agency).

As part of the administrative functions of management and administration of home health care services (planning, developing, and evaluating), certain specific responsibilities of the nurse administrator have been delineated:

- Uses statistical data to determine the quality and quantity of health services.

---

*With the advent of much earlier discharge from hospitals, patients are quite a bit sicker when they go home, and these nurses are required to know how to care for the acutely ill.

- Facilitates coordination of services within and outside the agency.
- Oversees responsibilities for management, education, and service functions.
- Oversees the fiscal affairs of the agency, with responsibility for budget preparation and control; secures financial resources for the agency.
- Initiates and participates in local, state, and national health and welfare programs.
- Promotes collaboration between the service setting and educational programs preparing service staffs.
- Employs, manages, and directs the human resources of the agency.
- Provides leadership and vision in developing the long-range plans for the agency in the context of community needs.
- Markets agency services.[48]

Some of the major changes that will affect public health nurses, as seen by some public health administrators are:

1. New health delivery systems—such as HMOs, comprehensive health centers, group practices, and satellite primary care centers—putting emphasis on preventive care as an incentive to economical operations.
2. New types of health and social manpower emerging in the community, placing a greater responsibility on the PHN to coordinate their activities.
3. Expanded responsibilities for service, resulting in PHNs providing primary care, particularly in areas of physician shortage.
4. Impact of management theory in the health field, requiring nurses to be knowledgeable about these concepts and still remain patient advocates.
5. Rising cost of home visits, necessitating great selectivity in choosing patients and developing new methods of health teaching.
6. Decentralization of health administration at state and federal levels, placing greater decision-making responsibilities at the local level.

7. Impact of profit-making agencies in competition with governmental and voluntary agencies.

Qualifications and Conditions of Employment. Schools of professional nursing have long recognized that nurses who plan to enter the field of public health need special preparation for it. Most diploma and AD schools give students theoretical instruction in public health nursing, conduct orientation visits to community health agencies, provide several hours of experience in prenatal and well-baby clinics, and integrate public health aspects of nursing wherever possible in all clinical areas. One of the problems in giving experience to students in these schools in the lack of clinical facilities (agencies) for practice. What experience is available is usually reserved for baccalaureate programs, because preparation for PHN is usually a major educational objective of these programs and students have taken a considerable number of courses in preparation. However, their experiences are also not limited to official and nonofficial agencies, as public health is seen in a broader perspective.

Besides state licensure, and for some agencies, prior nursing experience, one major qualification for PHN work is graduation from a baccalaureate nursing program. Many graduates of these schools go on to earn a master's degree and are thus prepared educationally for a lifetime career in this field. Because of the shortage of nurses with the prescribed PHN preparation at the present time, however, graduates of diploma and AD programs can and do find positions in this field, working at the beginning level and under supervision. In some areas they work only in clinics and do not make home visits. Some employers encourage nurses to work toward a baccalaureate degree by providing tuition or scholarship grants.

Pay and advancement at all levels are related to educational and other qualifications. On a national level, salaries are lower than for hospital nursing. Nurses may be promoted as they assume advanced or expanded role functions or administrative positions. Most agencies make available to all staff written personnel policies and conditions of employment. Many official agencies operate within a civil service system. In the states with strong labor laws permitting collective bargaining for nurses, nurses may organize either through a union or the SNA and bargain for better salaries and working conditions.

In the past, PHN/CHN nurses enjoyed standard daytime hours, with most working Monday through Friday. However, with the move toward more care in the community on a twenty-four-hour basis, rather than in institutions, PHN/CHN nurses will be expected to rotate shifts and work weekends, much the same as nurses employed in institutions.

There is another key point that relates to both the nurse as a practitioner and the conditions of employment. Because (PHNs) do not generally function in the protected controlling environment of an institution, where there is a degree of implied authority, but rather in the client's setting, where the client determines who will enter his home, and whether he will receive or follow the health teaching and counseling given, these nurses should have the personality characteristics to deal with such situations. Even if the setting is a clinic, there is no force that can make a client come to or return to a clinic, or, for that matter, follow any regimen given. There have been studies done indicating that the poor, especially blacks, may reject health services because they feel a prejudicial attitude among the providers of care, whereas at the same time average middle-class white nurses hold, or feel they hold, different values concerning health care. Even with the best of intentions, nurses (and other health workers in the community) may not be able to convince their clients that certain preventive measures are necessary. Not all nurses can deal with these frustrations or have the skills and personality characteristic that enable them to work and relate effectively with clients not of their own life-style.

Professional nurses who select PHN as a career need outstanding ability to adjust to many types of environments with a variety of living conditions, from the well-to-do in a high-rise apartment house to the most poverty-stricken in a ghetto or rural area, and to appreciate a wide range of interests, attitudes, educational backgrounds, and cultural differences. They must be able to accept these variations, to understand the differences, to communicate well so as to avoid misunderstandings and misinterpretations, and to be able to give equally good nursing care to all. PHNs in any position must use excellent judgment and are expected to use their own initiative. They have the opportunity to work with persons in other disciplines and other social agencies to help provide needed services to the clients, services that may include financial counseling, legal aid, housing problems, family planning, marital counseling, and school difficulties. In some instances, PHNs are not only case finders, but case coordinators—patient advocates in every sense.

OFFICE NURSING

Office nurses are employed by physicians or dentists to see that their patients receive the nursing they need, usually in the office. Office nurses may give all of this care or assign certain duties to other personnel who work under their direction and supervision. If working for several doctors or dentists in a group practice center, the nurse may need to supervise a staff of several employees.

Nurses may be employed in a one-doctor general practitioner's office, which requires a nurse with general skills, or they may be employed in a specialist's office, which requires special skills. For instance, a surgeon may employ a nurse who can also act as his scrub nurse in surgery done at the hospital or assist him in office surgery, providing adequate supplies and equipment and assuring adherence to aseptic principles. Becoming rapidly more popular is group practice, in which physicians of the same or different specialties provide comprehensive medical care for their patients.

Usually the several nurses employed are part of a team with other technical and professional personnel services. X-rays, laboratory tests, electrocardiograms, electroencephalograms, physical therapy, and splint and cast application may be done. On the other hand, in some of these offices, and even in certain one-doctor offices, nurses perform some diagnostic procedures.

Giving nursing care, often of a preventive or rehabilitative nature, is the primary function of office nurses, and if given the opportunity, they can contribute a great deal to the health and welfare of patients and their families. Unfortunately, in too many instances the employer expects the nurse to be hostess, secretary, bookkeeper, errand girl, housekeeper, purchasing agent, public relations expert, and laboratory technician as well, tasks that a medical assistant could do. However, although these extraneous nonnursing tasks do not appear to be the best utilization of a professional nurse's time and skills, it should be recognized that some nurses like the variety.

Office nurses responsible for nonnursing duties should learn to do them well. There is literature available on bookkeeping and secretarial procedures to which they can turn for help. Community colleges and adult education programs usually include secretarial and bookkeeping courses in their evening schedules. The nurse can soon master the information and procedures needed and will develop judgment as to which of these duties should have priority in a busy daily schedule.

What the office nurse does in terms of nursing will depend largely upon the employer's type of practice, philosophy of nurse utilization, and daily schedule of appointments. Tasks may be as routine as giving medications, chaperoning physical examinations, preparing equipment, and seeing that the patients' records are completed and filed at the end of the day. A more complete utilization of nursing skills would include observation, communication, teaching, and coordination with community health agencies. A few nurses

even make hospital patient rounds with or without the physician.

The office nurse should be free to do teaching and counseling of individual patients and even conduct formal classes for groups of patients at times. Therefore, the ability to teach effectively and evaluate the results is useful. There are pamphlets, charts, posters, and free samples that nurses can use as teaching aids, and, of course, the nurse, like the physician, is expected to keep current in the field, so that any teaching done is based on current data. A teaching program ideally is jointly planned by the doctor, nurse, and others involved in health care. The nurse explains to patients and families tests, treatments, and surgical procedures, how to prepare for hospitalization, and what to expect afterward, how to care for themselves at home and how to give self-medications and simple treatments safely and with a minimum of discomfort and pain. When indicated, they explain how families can take advantage of the health and welfare facilities in the community.

All of the community health agencies are of concern to office nurses. They must know the public health regulations for reporting communicable diseases, how to submit specimens for examination, and what to do with laboratory reports. When a patient is going abroad, they must be able to tell him what inoculations he will be required to have. They must be acquainted with the members of the visiting nurse staff and know how to work cooperatively with them in handling patient referrals and promoting community health measures. They must cooperate in all forms of communications with these agencies and others, such as the public schools.

Perhaps one of the most far-reaching effects on office nursing is the development of the NP, who is often part of the physician's private practice and assumes much responsibility for patient care. Some office nurses are now being taught by their employer to assume some of these tasks; more are taking CE or formal collegiate programs. Office nurses taught on the job are more likely to be (non-credentialed) physician's assistants, and frequently they identify themselves by this title.

Qualifications and Conditions of Practice. All office nurses must be licensed to practice and currently registered in the state in which they work. Although not usually required, education beyond the basic nursing program is desirable. In most cases, nurses have had previous nursing experience.

Salaries and working conditions in this field are, generally speaking, both flexible and variable, representing private arrangements between the individual office nurse and the employer. Office nurses sometimes say they are willing to make some sacrifices in salary because the hours or responsibilities of office nursing fit their tastes or general life situation. This type of nursing often gives the married nurse the morning free for household and family responsibilities, provides her with most, if not all, weekends off, and may not call for a full work week, depending on the doctor's office hours and his expectations of the nurse. There is, however, the possibility of evening hours or overtime if the doctor is delayed by an emergency.

Currently, the conditions of employment appear to be improving, with better salaries and a variety of fringe benefits (again depending on the employer). Some of the most common fringe benefits include paid vacation and holidays, paid sick leave, year-end bonus, and free medical care for the nurse and family. Less likely to be offered are medical-surgical or hospitalization insurance and pension or retirement plans. Nurses should carry their own malpractice insurance. Both salary and fringe benefits are likely to be lower than those for the hospital staff nurse. However, most office nurses seem to enjoy a friendly and congenial relationship with their employing physician or physicians and usually succeed in negotiating mutually satisfactory working conditions and remuneration. They

appear to stay in the job longer than most nurses, an average of nine years.

Those considering a career in office nursing will do well to discuss all aspects of their work and employment conditions in detail with their employer. It is important to make sure that they will be free to function primarily as nurses and that the employer understands what the nurse expects the role to be. A job description is highly desirable, and the office nurse who assumes a position without one would do well to formulate one while holding the position. A written contract setting forth the agreements between the nurse and her employer can also be mutually beneficial.

SCHOOL (STUDENT) HEALTH NURSING

School nursing began in 1900 as a function of disease control, to help cope with such epidemics as diphtheria, influenza, measles, and other communicable disease. State and federal legislation have a great impact on all aspects of the school nurse position, because funding for almost all schools is somewhat involved with public funding. For instance, Title 1, the Elementary and Secondary Education Act of 1965, provided money for school nurses in ghetto and rural poverty areas, and the number of school nurses doubled. On the other hand, some states have cut the number of school nurses, have hired less qualified nurses, or have turned over school nurse functions to PHNs when budget cuts were felt to be necessary. Nevertheless, the potential is great in terms of actual needs for preventive care, health teaching, and promotion of health.

Some school systems do not clearly delineate the responsibilities of a school nurse, or do not update the job description in line with modern concepts of health care. The nurse accepting such a position must be extremely self-directed; in many cases, health clerks and nursery assistants can do as much as school nurses within the legal context of the school setting.

One expert in school nursing states that there are three components of school nursing:

Health supervision involves such activities as health assessment, vision and hearing screening, emergency care, and health deficit identification.

Health counseling includes interpretation of health information, guidance and counseling regarding health behavior, and recommendations regarding individual and group health conditions.

Health education refers to planning, promoting, and implementing health instruction as well as providing consultation in health-related matters.[49]

However, in many job situations the school nurse is still primarily the giver of first aid in illness or emergency; helps in screening programs for diseases of the eyes, ears, and teeth; keeps records; and does limited health teaching and case finding. In a large school system, the nurse may be supervising practical nurses, aides, volunteers, clerical assistants, vision screening technicians, audiometric technicians, or other personnel, and may even become a supervisor of other nurses. In a small system, a nurse may assume all these responsibilities alone, even to the point of covering several schools in the same system. A physician may be on call or, more likely, may be available at stated times. The nurse–pupil ratio can vary from 1:800 to 1:11,000 or more.

School nurses become isolated from other nurse colleagues because, among other things, they are expected to become a part of the educational system, even sometimes to participate in PTA meetings, faculty meetings, and curriculum development (in areas related to health). Some choose to join the National Education Association (NEA) instead of ANA, and NEA becomes their economic security bargaining agent, as it may be for the teachers.

A fairly recent development is the school NP, who functions basically as other NPs

bringing much more comprehensive care to the pupils in those settings where nurses are permitted to function in this manner. A joint statement by ANA and the American School Health Association that defines the role of the school NP, and the necessary education, describes the added facets of the role. These include serving as a health advocate for the child, helping parents assume greater responsibility for health maintenance of the child; providing health instruction, counseling, and guidance; contributing to the health education of individuals and groups; applying methods designed to increase each person's motivation to take responsibility for his own health care; assessing and arranging management and referrals for children with health problems; securing and evaluating a thorough health and developmental history of the child and recording the findings; performing physical examinations; and the like.

The patterns of practice for school nurse practitioners vary according to the needs perceived and the limits set by the school boards. In one pattern, the nurse might assume responsibility for the total school health program, assisted by an aide to do clerical work and to triage simple conditions. In a second pattern, the nurse may visit a number of schools, assessing and evaluating children and leaving the follow-up to another nurse or an aide on location. In another, practice might be limited to doing physical exams, substituting for a physician, or evaluating children with learning difficulties.

Colleges and universities also provide a setting for the nurse interested in student health although obviously there is considerable adult health involved. Responsibilities vary according to the size of the institution and the types of services offered. College students often pay a health fee which entitles them to specific benefits. Services may include mental health counseling, family planning, and care for minor illnesses or accidents. NPs also function in these settings, although there are instances in which an affiliation with a teaching hospital or medical school makes student health a learning setting for residents.

Qualifications and Conditions of Employment. Obviously, nurses interested in school nursing must like children and adolescents and be able to relate well to them. Educationally, the nurse should have at least a baccalaureate degree, as recommended by the American School Health Association, ANA and the National Association of School Nurses, as well as specified courses related to the field of school nursing. Master's degrees are encouraged, as is CE. Individual states or school systems within states may vary from these requirements. Some require no degree; others ask for a few additional courses which may or may not relate to the field (in one state these are courses in the history of the state and audiovisual aids). A number of states require certification for employment as a school nurse. In some cases, school nurses are expected to have the same educational credentials as teachers. School NPs will often have had a CE or degree program as preparation for this role.

Theoretically, nurses apply to the local school board for a school nurse position, but actually, in smaller systems, the nurse may be able to obtain such a position on the basis of personal acquaintance or sheer availability. School nurse positions are often considered particularly desirable for women with families because the time schedule is the same as for teachers, with weekends and summers free. Salaries, particularly in the larger systems, may be equal to those of the teachers, (which are low) if the qualifications are equal; in smaller communities, the salary may be quite low.

Opportunities for advancement are found primarily in the larger systems, where the nurse may move to a supervisory position. However, there are many satisfactions to be gained, and there is the possibility of professional growth in those systems in which nurses are able to assume a full professional role.

NURSING EDUCATION

Teaching is so much a part of the professional nursing student's basic experience that it might seem reasonable to expect many young graduates to select teaching as a career. Fortunately, many do, but not nearly enough to fill the positions available to well-prepared teachers in all areas of nursing education. There are not enough nurses at present to meet the need in any field of nursing, but the shortage of qualified teachers is particularly acute. Without enough teachers, the problem of preparing an increased supply of nurses for present and future needs assumes serious proportions. At any given time the need is probably considerably greater than the figures indicate, partially because there are new programs in higher education opening yearly, and also because most nursing education programs, particularly in institutions of higher education, have had financial problems that prohibit budgeting of an adequate number of teaching positions. An even more vital factor is that most programs do not have fully qualified faculty. Master's degrees have been recommended as a minimum for teachers in all nursing programs, and doctorates for deans of collegiate programs and faculty of graduate programs. Because general university standards require a doctorate for teaching positions at almost any level, there is now more pressure for nurses to adhere to this standard also.

According to NLN, in 1982, almost 97 percent of bacalaureate and higher-degree nursing faculty had master's or doctoral degrees, as did almost 65 percent of associate degree faculty and abut 47 percent of diploma faculty. All rose from the 1978 figures. Very few practical nurse faculty have graduate education. Faculty with earned doctorates (about 13 percent) function primarily in programs offering baccalaureate or higher degrees. Both NLN criteria and many state board standards for accreditation suggest master's degrees and higher (preferably in nursing), and it is expected that faculty not holding the appropriate degree be enrolled in a nursing education program that leads to such a degree.

The philosophy, objectives, kinds of students, and conditions of employment vary in different kinds of nursing education programs.* Nurses planning to teach should give thought to the kind of program with which they can identify philosophically and in which they can function effectively. The number and types of positions within each program depend upon the size of the student body, the curriculum content, the faculty organization, and the school's philosophy, aims, and budget. There is a place in some schools for a nurse instructor of sciences, but in most schools, students take courses in physical and social sciences taught by nonnurse instructors at their own or another college or university.

Most nurse teachers are employed to teach nursing in the area of their clinical expertise, but trends toward nursing curriculum "models" may mean the adjustment of the teacher to differing approaches. In associate degree and practical nurse programs, the teacher may be expected to teach a variety of nursing subjects. Other specific differences in settings may also be noted.

There are certain aspects of a faculty position that are the same, regardless of the educational setting. Faculty have certain responsibilities to the total program, usually through committees. Some are development and updating of philosophy, objectives, and conceptual framework, and selecting appropriate courses to meet those objectives; selection, evaluation, and promotion of students; assisting in developing educational and faculty standards, policies, and procedures; participating in promotion and tenure of faculty; developing special projects; and planning for the future. In a collegiate setting, the teacher is expected to participate in college committees of the same nature. In relation to the student, a basic role is teaching in the classroom,

laboratory, and clinical setting, individually or in groups, using appropriate and effective techniques with current knowledge and practice in the area of expertise. Advisement and personal and career counseling of students are also important; some teachers are class or student committee advisors and consultants as well. In the college and university settings, research and publication are major expectations; generally the teacher must seek outside funding for research. Almost equally important is service to the profession and the community, as members or officers of organizations, as consultants, or as speakers.[50]

Differences in teaching in the various programs relate to both the setting and the level. In universities, particularly medical centers, there is a trend toward joint appointments, with the teacher carrying a patient case load and, occasionally, administrative responsibilities in the clinical setting.[51] In some cases, teachers are reimbursed additionally for this duty.[52] Some set up a group faculty practice in which they deliver direct care to patients.[53]

Graduate faculty are expected to be scholarly and research oriented, for, as well as teaching, they will be directing graduate students' research. They are likely to work closely with graduate faculty in other disciplines if courses are interdisciplinary. They may be expert teachers and practitioners in a particular clinical specialty and/or in nursing administration, nursing education, or other graduate-level studies. Working with graduate students on special projects and guiding or supervising their research may mean spending hours with the student in conference and in committee presentations for the master's thesis or doctoral dissertation, including certain administrative responsibilities. The paper work in most teaching is extensive.

There are students of superior academic and intellectual ability and high motivation in all programs, but certain baccalaureate and almost all graduate programs have a more homogeneous selection, because high admission standards generally screen out those of lesser ability. However, just about all students are

*See Chapters 12 and 13 for specific details on each program and issues in nursing education.

much more challenging and demanding than they were ten years ago; they want participation rights, they ask questions, and they don't accept pat answers.

Faculty in college- or university-based programs have the advantage of being in an academic setting with broad interdisciplinary contacts and campus activities. They may have joint appointments in other departments or schools and other responsibilities there. They also have the benefits and problems of being in such a setting; the policies and regulations are less directly controllable. Students in collegiate programs affiliate or rotate through a number of hospitals, agencies, or facilities. Unless the program is in a medical center, or unless the teacher holds a joint appointment, students and teachers maintain somewhat of a guest status and find it more difficult to affect care. If other students are also present, there is competition for good "teaching" patients.

On the other hand, in diploma programs, basic nursing education is controlled by a hospital. Nursing classes and often clinical practice are given in that particular school and hospital, although students may go to other clinical settings. Because of geographic proximity and the fact that hospitals often think of the diploma students as "their" students and future employees, there may be a closer relationship between nurses in the clinical area and the faculty. Often the director of nursing has overall responsibility for both nursing service and nursing administration, and there are opportunities for both service and education personnel to plan and work together on joint projects related to the hospital in general. Usually there is more national prestige in being affiliated with a university program, although this varies, and other schools with strong community ties are highly respected.

The teaching opportunities in practical nurse programs offer another type of challenge to the nurse educator. The method of teaching and the philosophy of vocational education differ somewhat from those of professional education. The course of study usually is limited to one year. The setting may be in hospitals, public schools, or community colleges, among which both philosophy and environment vary considerably. It is important that the professional nurse teaching in these programs understand and respect the role of practical nurses in giving patient care and be able to teach accordingly.

Qualifications and Conditions of Employment. Besides the educational requirements, teachers in all nursing programs are expected to have a knowledge of nursing in general and continuously updated knowledge and clinical expertise in the subject area in which they expect to teach. They also need knowledge and skill in curriculum development, the teaching-learning process, and teaching methods and techniques. It is equally important for any prospective teacher to establish rapport with students, and to be open-minded and secure enough to welcome differences in opinion. Evaluation of teacher effectiveness is an ongoing process in a progressive educational setting and includes self-evaluation and evaluation by students, peers, and administrative heads. The quality of teaching is considered in retention and promotion of faculty.

One classic study on qualities for effective teaching lists knowledge of the subject; sympathetic attitude toward, and interest in, students; interest in and enthusiasm for the subject; tolerance, broadmindedness, liberality; interesting presentation; personality to put the subject across; sense of humor, sense of proportion; ability to stimulate intellectual curiosity; organization; fairness; sincerity, honesty; and moral character. Other intangible factors of personality and appearance are also mentioned.[54] Studies in nursing seem to indicate that these qualities are still considered important, particularly in teacher–student relations.

It is also often expected that the teacher will be scholarly and make contributions to nursing through participation in professional activities and/or publications. A teacher in an institution of higher education may be appointed at any level from instructor to full professor, depending on his or her qualifications (and the need of that institution for that individual). Tenure and promotion depend on fulfilling stated requirements.[55,56]

Tenure in colleges and universities means basically that the individual has a secure place in that institution and cannot be dismissed except under unusual circumstances. Usually there is a span of time (seven years or so) during which the person must be tenured or leave, unless put in some special category outside the tenure track. The more prestigious the institution, the higher the standards for appointment, promotion, and tenure.[57,58] If college teaching is to be a nurse's career, plans for doctoral education are a must.

Salaries and fringe benefits vary, and in an institution of higher learning are supposed to be the same as for an individual in another discipline at the same rank.* A full professor at the last salary step may earn as much as or more than the administrator of that particular program. Salaries in 1984, according to the American Association of Colleges of Nursing (AACN), ranged from about $24,000 to almost $44,000, escalating according to rank (instructor to professor) and, usually, doctoral preparation. Salaries are rising at about 4 to 6 percent per year. Economic conditions may slow down this rate of growth.

Teaching positions in any educational program usually demand irregular working hours. Except for scheduled classes, the amount of time a teacher will spend at work is unpredictable because there are so many influencing factors, such as class and clinical preparation time, student conferences, student evaluation, participation in school committees and meetings, library study, and participation in student activities.

Teachers are also involved in professional activities, updating their own clinical practice, and advancing their education. Depending on where they teach, they may be able to set their own hours as far as presence in the school is concerned (except for scheduled classes) or

*See Chapter 22.

may be expected to put in a forty-hour or more week on a regular eight-hour daily basis. It is estimated that the average university nurse teacher spends about fifty-six hours a week on the job. However, faculty are usually freer than other nurses to attend educational and other meetings. Nurses selecting a career in this field will want to analyze the conditions of each employment opportunity to make sure that it offers them as much as possible of what they want most in both material and professional rewards, and an atmosphere in which they can do their best work. For a teacher, often the greatest reward is the intellectual and personal stimulation of an educational environment, including interaction with students and peers.

Administration in Nursing Education

At the head of each educational program in nursing is a professional nurse who is both administrator and teacher. Nursing education administrators need preparation in administration as well as teaching. Again, it is best, and sometimes required, that the director of the program take graduate courses in administration in a college or university.

Courses in nursing education administration are only rarely available in graduate nursing education programs, so those whose goal is educational administration often acquire experience as assistants to a top administrator or in minor administrative positions and apply principles from nonnursing management courses. Workshops on preparation for the decanal role have been a project of AACN. In some colleges and universities, department chairmen or deans are appointed administratively on recommendation of the faculty for limited terms, after which they return to nonadministrative faculty positions. This approach has advantages and disadvantages. It gives presumably competent faculty members an opportunity in the administrative role, but it may not be considered desirable by the individual whose primary interest is educational administration and who must then relocate to remain in a top administrative position.

Qualifications for nursing administration positions in education usually include experience in nursing and nursing education and frequently in administration of some kind. This nurse should be able to relate well to others in the nursing program, in the profession, in the particular setting of the school, and in the community. The need for leadership qualities is frequently cited. A minimum of a master's degree is usual, and the dean, director, or chairman of a collegiate or university program in nursing is expected to have a doctoral degree. It is also not uncommon to expect these candidates to have achieved national prominence in the nursing field, and to have published and done research. Frequently, when a top administrative position is open, a search committee, composed according to institutional criteria, looks for, screens, interviews, and recommends an individual after a national search.[59]

The top administrative post of any nursing education program usually requires both long hours of work on the job and active participation in professional activities. If in a college or university, the administrator is expected to be a leader in campus-wide committees and activities. There may be pressure from the faculty, students, administration, and community, all trying to achieve their own ends.[60] Often there are financial problems for the school. There is little time for nurse administrators to keep abreast of their own clinical field, for the demand to keep current on administrative, educational, and general nursing trends is immediate. This is not a position for someone who cannot learn and act quickly and who wilts under pressure. The rewards, however, can be great professionally, in the satisfaction of accomplishments of the nursing program, its faculty, and students, and in the opportunity to be in a leadership position in nursing and in health care.

Salaries, fringe benefits, and sometimes rank and tenure tend to be negotiable and usually depend on a number of factors related to the position, the community, and the qualifications of the nurse. According to AACN, salaries of deans ranged from under $30,000 to over $70,000 in 1984.

PRIVATE DUTY NURSING

For many years, private duty nursing was second only to hospital nursing in its attraction for professional nurses, but each year has seen a decrease in the total number of nurses in this field of practice, particularly younger nurses.

Private duty nurses are independent practitioners in almost complete control of where they will work, when they will work, the types of patients they will care for, and when they will take vacation or days off. They are limited in what they can charge for services only by the prevailing fee in their community, which is not legally binding.

Private duty nurses make their availability for service known through a nurses' registry, an employment agency, local hospitals, and personal contacts with other nurses, doctors, and members of the community. Individual nurses may build up a list of "clients" composed of families and doctors who always try to engage them whenever they need private duty nurses. Some work only as specialists.

A private duty nurse is usually employed (by the patient or family) to nurse one patient in the hospital or home. Wherever they are, the nurse is responsible for the patient's care while with him or her. When the nurse leaves for any length of time, arrangements must be made for care in the interim. This is also done if the nurse wishes a day or so off after being with a patient continuously for a number of weeks.

Most patients requesting private duty nurses are quite ill, or at least require a great deal of care physically and/or mentally. More than half the patients cared for have undergone surgery, and are relatively helpless afterward, especially if they have drainage tubes, IVs, catheters, and so on. Other patients who often prefer constant attendance are those with strokes, cancer, and burns. Moreover, there is always a percentage of patients who can afford three nurses around the clock and who simply wish to have someone constantly at hand. There are also patients who are not in critical condition but who require an enormous amount of individualized care. Free from the pressures of time and heavy patient care loads that often harass the general duty nurse, private duty nurses have the opportunity to give truly comprehensive professional care to their patients, with limited concern for hospital routines.

Qualifications and Conditions of Employment. For success in private duty nursing and greatest job satisfaction, the private duty nurse must have a genuine liking for people and must be able to adjust well to a wide variety of personalities, establishing and maintaining warm yet professional relationships with both patients and their families, no matter how long a case may last. This nurse must enjoy giving direct comprehensive nursing care to one patient. Naturally, it is necessary to be currently licensed in the state where the nurse practices, with the exception of times when patient and nurse may be traveling and residing temporarily in another state. It is also important to understand the legal implications of the position and use sound judgment to avoid inappropriate involvement or activities. Malpractice insurance is advisable.

As self-employed persons or independent contractors, private duty nurses are almost entirely on their own as far as retirement plans, Social Security payments, and payment of taxes are concerned. They have no sick leave benefits, or paid vacations. They are their own business managers in every sense of the word.

The responsibility to keep updated is likely to be the private duty nurse's individual responsibility. Hospital in-service programs are usually available, as are workshops, institutes, and other programs, but no one makes arrangements for the independently practicing nurse. Such CE may be even more important for these nurses than for institutionally employed nurses, because even though theoretically the hospital nursing service is responsible for the overall nursing care of all patients, private duty nurses generally function with little or no supervision. This is obviously more likely if the nursing care is given in the patient's home.

An eight-hour tour of duty is fairly standard throughout the country, but twelve-hour shifts are not uncommon. Fees vary considerably from place to place; they may or may not be higher than those of a staff nurse per diem. Although it is generally agreed that there is sufficient employment available for private duty nurses in most areas, those nurses who limit their practice to the day shift, certain kinds of patients, and limited length of employment may find that they do not have the opportunity to work as much as they would like. Moreover, LPNs are being employed for private duty, particularly in the home, but also in some hospitals. The increased number of well-prepared NPs who are setting up independent private practice may also bring about changes in the private duty picture.

OCCUPATIONAL HEALTH NURSING

Occupational health nursing (OHN) was initiated at the Vermont Marble Company in 1895, using the services of Ada Stewart and her sister, Harriet, or, some say, in 1888 in the mining town of Drifton, Pennsylvania.

Two department stores were the next to provide similar health services for their employees: John Wanamaker Company of New York in 1897, and the Frederick Loeser Department Store, Brooklyn, in 1899. Early in the 1900s, more and more industries on both the East and West coasts recognized the economic value of keeping employees healthy and established similar health services. Adding impetus to the trend was the enactment of workmen's compensation laws (beginning in 1911), which place emphasis on the importance of preventing accidents to employees on the job and giving immediate and expert attention to injuries received at work. This development brought industrial nurses into the plants. World Wars I and II were also strong influences in the growth of industrial nursing because they created a great need to conserve manpower.

For many years nurses employed in these positions called themselves *industrial nurses*. In 1958, however, the industrial nurses within ANA voted to call themselves *occupational health nurses* because *occupational* embraces banks, hotels, offices, department stores, and so on, whereas *industrial* connotes (in the minds of most persons) manufacturing industries. Other organizations also adopted the newer term, including the American Association of Occupational Health Nurses.

A key factor in the changes in OHN was the enactment in 1971 of the Occupational Safety and Health Act.* That act created the National Institute for Occupational Safety and Health (NIOSH) to research health problems and recommend safety standards and the Occupational Safety and Health Administration (OSHA) to guarantee a ''safe and healthful workplace.'' OSHA inspects the nation's workplaces for health and safety hazards, but its effectiveness has been blunted by lack of funds and the resistance of employers, who have sometimes sued and won to limit the access of OSHA's inspectors. Nevertheless, unions, environmentalists, and other interested citizens have pressed for more action.

Until recently, there has been almost no place that OHNs could receive formal, specialized education. Now new OHN graduate programs usually include NP skills and courses on environmental health and safety, although some also emphasize management skills.

The American Association of Occupational Health Nurses states in its philosophy that

> The occupational health nurse is a vital component of the health care system. Responsibilities are influenced by current patterns of

health service, legislation, social and economic factors.

> The occupational health nurse is a vital component of the health care system. Responsibilities are influenced by current patterns of health service, legislation, social and economic factors.

> The occupational health nurse is accountable to the medical director for all professional and administrative matters. When no medical director is employed the nurse will be directly responsible to a member of management for all administrative matters but will seek guidance on medical problems from the company's designated physician.

> The primary goal of the nurse working as a member of the occupational health team is promotion and maintenance of the general physical and emotional health of the worker, prevention of disease, and rehabilitation of the sick and injured. The occupational health nurse is concerned with environmental conditions of the work area as well as the physical and mental health requirements of particular jobs. Emphasis is on preventive approaches to health care in which health teaching, counseling and detection are implicit.[61]

The health department in which an OHN works may consist of a single room, or it may be a large department with several examining and treatment rooms, x-ray and laboratory facilities, and offices for nurses and physicians. Whatever its size, the administrative policies and scope of the program are decided by business management; the health services are under the medical direction of a physician who may work for the company full-time, part-time, or on an on-call basis. Many OHNs are employed in one-nurse health departments. In these instances, the nurse carries the department's work alone.

Whether this nurse functions in a sophisticated manner in the delivery of health care depends on his or her education and experience and policies of the employer. As a prepared NP or nurse clinician, the nurse may assess the worker's condition through health histories,

---

*Also discussed in Chapters 6 and 19.

observation, physical examination, and other selected diagnostic measures; review and interpret findings to differentiate the normal from the abnormal; select appropriate action and referral; counsel; and teach. The practitioner must also be concerned with the physical and psychosocial phenomena of the workers and their families, their working environment, community, and even recreation. If the nurse is working in a more conservative environment and/or without the appropriate background, the activities may be limited to first aid and some emergency treatment, keeping records, assisting with physical examinations, and carrying out certain diagnostic procedures. In many cases, most often when the nurse does not function in an expanded role, standing orders or directions, prepared and signed by the medical director, give the necessary authority to care for conditions that develop while the employee is on the job. The nurse refers employees with nonoccupational illnesses or injuries to their family doctors. However, a particularly interesting development that broadens the scope of the OHN's practice is a new emphasis of concern on worker health problems that may or may not be directly caused by the job but affect worker performance—alcoholism, emotional problems, stress, drug addiction, and family relations. In many cases, the nurse is involved in counseling and therapy.

In a large health department in an industry that employs one or more full-time physicians, the nurse may also function as a nursing care coordinator to develop, implement, supervise, and evaluate the delivery of health care to employees, working with professional and nonprofessional staff. In general, OHN in a health department of any size means much more than meeting the immediate needs of an ill or injured employee. The nurse uses interviewing, observing, and teaching skills, takes health histories, keeps health records, and is responsible for supplies and equipment. The ability to take and recognize abnormalities in electrocardiograms, to do eye screening, audiometer testing, and certain laboratory tests and x-rays is considered useful. In addition, the nurse must be vitally concerned with the safety of the employees and may tour the plant with management and the safety engineer to help them plan a practical safety program.

The nurse may also need to act as an interpreter of company health and safety policies and thus must know the company policy on personnel matters, sick leave, insurance benefits, pay rates, and the necessary information for myriad records. Health teaching to attain and maintain optimum health, usually done on an individual basis, is generally considered an important aspect of the job. On the other hand, the serious and not infrequent responsibility of giving immediate care to workers with serious injuries, often with no physician present, should not be overlooked. Such situations have major legal implications. OHNs should be familiar with the laws governing the practice of nursing and medicine in their state and discuss them with the physician and management to make sure that they all understand the legal scope of nursing functions.

Qualifications and Conditions of Employment. Graduation from a state-approved school of professional nursing and current state registration are basic requirements for the OHN. Comparatively few employers require a college degree, although many consider it desirable. Whether the evolving role of the NP, who has more education and can also assume more responsibilities, will change this attitude remains to be seen. Currently, only CE related to the job is considered necessary. However, a great percentage of OHNs are nearing retirement age and, as they are replaced with better-prepared nurses, their availability, interest, and the new educational programs will probably make at least baccalaureate education the norm.

A career OHN will be expected to seek certification by the American Board for Occupational Health Nurses, an independent nursing specialty board authorized to certify properly qualified OHNs.

Salaries and fringe benefits vary according to the size of the industry or business and its location. Both tend to be somewhat lower than those of other nurses. Some OHNs belong to a union, but this is discouraged by the AAOHN (and by employers). The usual company benefits include vacations, sick leave, pensions, and insurance. Working hours are those of the workers; thus, in an industry with work shifts around the clock, nurses are usually there also. As a professional person, the nurse may have some of the privileges of management, such as temporary absences to attend meetings. Although some industries carry professional liability insurance that supposedly covers the OHN, it may not apply in all cases of possible litigation. It is advisable, therefore, for these nurses to carry their own professional liability insurance.

NURSING IN THE EXPANDED OR EXTENDED ROLE—THE NURSE PRACTITIONER

In the emergence of any new role, there is considerable controversy in relation to terminology, function, and education. Not all of these problems have been resolved concerning the nurse practitioner (NP). There is still disagreement as to whether the role is expanded or extended, merely changing, or not new at all. Lillian Wald, pioneer in PHN, made house calls, prescribed and dispensed medications and treatments, and counseled her client families as needed. In more recent times, the Frontier Nursing Service of Wendover, Kentucky, which was noted for its "nursing on horseback" midwifery services, has been expanding its practice to overall family services.[62]

It is generally agreed, however, that the new wave of NPs began with two experiments: a clinic program at the University of Kansas Medical Center, which showed that nurse-run clinics were more effective with chronically ill women than were regular clinics,[63] and the Ford-Silver program at the University of Colorado that became the first PNP program.[64] The term *nurse practitioner,* although coming into common usage for anyone functioning in the expanded role, creates a semantic problem because technically anyone practicing nursing is a nurse practitioner.

Definitions of nurse practitioners also vary, but generally it is conceded that nurse practitioners have acquired additional knowledge and skills, some of which were previously considered medical, either in short-term or degree educational programs, and use fully all aspects of nursing skills, which enable them to provide more extensive health services to the patient/client, often in collaboration with a physician or physicians, but also independently, in consultation with a physician as needed.

Edith Lewis saw as the common denominator:

> First and probably foremost is that the nurse is oriented toward providing care for clients rather than services to institutions . . . she practices independently or interdependently, as the setting dictates; she makes her own decisions, assumes responsibility and accountability for them, and is subject to few if any hierarchal restraints.
>
> For the most part, she maintains a one-to-one relationship with her clients and sees them as part of the family-community constellation to which they belong. She may or may not possess, or feel the need for physical assessment skills; to the degree that she uses them, she does so to enrich the data base for her nursing judgments. For the nurse practitioner is not practicing medicine; she is practicing nursing.[65]

A useful description of the responsibilities of NPs in primary health care after completing a formal program is given in the *1977 Federal Rules and Regulations* that govern the educational programs for NPs funded by DHHS through the Nurse Training Act. It lists the ability to:

1. Assess the health status of individuals and

families through health and medical history taking, physical examination, and defining of health and developmental problems;

2. Institute and provide continuity of health care to clients (patients), work with the client to insure understanding of and compliance with the therapeutic regimen within established protocols, and recognize when to refer the client to a physician or other health care provider;

3. Provide instruction and counseling to individuals, families and groups in the areas of health promotion and maintenance, including involving such persons in planning for their health care; and

4. Work in collaboration with other health care providers and agencies to provide, and where appropriate, coordinate services to individuals and families.

Primary health care means care which may be initiated by the client or provider in a variety of settings and which consists of a broad range of personal health care services including:

1. Promotion and maintenance of health;
2. Prevention of illness and disability;
3. Basic care during acute and chronic phases of illness;
4. Guidance and counseling of individuals and families; and
5. Referral to other health care providers and community resources when appropriate.

The nurse practitioner practices in a variety of settings such as clinics, health centers, extended care and long-term care facilities, physicians' offices, industries, homes, schools, and acute care settings.[66] Probably the most comprehensive picture of current NPs, their education and practice, is presented in the longitudinal study done by DHHS, which funded most of the educational programs. The data present an almost complete census of the over 20,000 NPs because the response rate for the three studies (1973, 1977, 1980) averaged over 95 percent. Some additional 1982 data were also provided by DHHS. In addition, longitudinal studies have assessed the influence of various factors over time, and some comparisons were made in the latest reports.[67]

A major trend in the education of NPs during this time period was the shift from certificate programs to the master's degree. (Certificate programs may enroll nurses without degrees.) Although the total number of programs increased from over 130 in 1973 to about 200 in 1980, the graduate programs had increased two and a half times. Now both are holding steady. There was also a drop in the pediatric specialty, perhaps due to social trends, an oversupply of pediatricians, or early saturation of PNPs, and an increase in adult and family specialization. Two-thirds of the latter programs are now given at the master's level. Only maternity and midwifery are about equally split between certificate and master's programs. Most certificate programs are now about a year in length; the master's are one to two years long. However, the certificate programs actually give more class and clinical time to NP preparation, probably because master's degree programs are more broadly based and academic. However, more master's programs are now having preceptorships. Both types of programs are inclined to have NP directors, although some are co-directed by an MD. There has been a major increase in NP preceptors, in contrast to early programs in which MDs were almost always used as preceptors. Many programs use both NPs and MDs. Certificate programs are now more likely to exist in university settings, except for emergency, midwifery, and maternity programs, which are located in hospitals. All regions except the South have experienced growth in NP programs; the Midwest has the least number of programs. In 1981, over 2,000 NPs graduated from the various programs.

The demographic characteristics of the students changed somewhat between 1973 and 1980. Instead of being evenly divided among the four regions, as in 1973, by 1980, over one-third of the students attended school in the Northeast. The proportion of men, although small, more than doubled to 5.2 percent. Blacks decreased to 4.5 percent. Marital status remained constant, with slightly more than half being married. The class of 1980 was somewhat younger, with about 43 percent over thirty-five. In master's programs, the change in age was more dramatic—a drop to 22 percent in those over thirty-five. Membership in ANA, although higher for master's students, and higher than for the overall nurse population, also dropped to about one-third. As younger students entered NP programs, their work experience was also shorter, but most had come from hospital positions. Reasons for choosing to become an NP were almost the same as in 1973: greater influence in providing better patient care, additional learning opportunities, and more challenging work. In 1980, greater independence was also listed. Increased income, status, and working conditions were seldom mentioned as motivating factors.

Employment data extend to 1982. About two-thirds of the graduates in 1974 and 1982 were employed and were providing primary care. Fewer were employed as teachers and consultants, perhaps because those needs had leveled off. The unemployment rate rose slightly, from 9.7 to 13.1, although about half of those affected cited personal reasons; the other half mentioned lack of appropriate employment opportunities. Neither 1973 nor 1982 graduates usually returned to their previous employment setting; roughly 17 percent moved to another area of the country. Most certificate graduates were employed in ambulatory clinical practice, although there was a significant increase (to 24 percent) in those employed in private practice. They showed a decline in employment in hospital outpatient and college health departments.

In 1974, most NPs estimated that more than 50 percent of their clients were poor; 1982 figures were similar, with a slight shift in the upper-income patient population. Most NPs from both programs practiced in urban areas, but medium-sized and small cities were also well represented. Pediatric, midwifery, and maternity graduates were more likely to prac-

tice in urban areas; those from FNP and emergency programs were employed in significant numbers in rural areas.

Over 45 percent of all NPs reported salary ranges from $16,000 to over $20,000. Over 60 percent of the graduates of nurse-midwifery and adult certificate programs listed salaries over $20,000; maternity and PNP graduates were least likely to do so. There was less variation in master's graduates, but PNPs also had the lowest and midwives the highest salaries. Those in teaching and consulting positions had incomes over $24,000, compared to $21,000 for their service colleagues.

A positive change was that more NPs (76 percent) were functioning full time as NPs. In addition, only 26 percent reported the immediate presence of a physician. Both trends indicate better acceptance of the role. Employers almost unanimously indicated their satisfaction with NPs, citing improved quality of care and improved patient return rates. They also saw the NP as useful in teaching students and staff members—and as substitutes for MDs. NPs were also satisfied.

Probably because of the NPs' expansion into the gray areas between medicine and nursing, especially in the management of disease conditions and the use and interpretation of various diagnostic modes, there has been considerable evaluation of NP performance, acceptance, and cost effectiveness. Despite justifiable criticism of this research as being largely anecdotal, very specific to certain individuals, and frequently done by those involved in their training or employment, almost all the research* shows that NPs have performed at a level comparable to physicians, according to standards of that setting;[68] have provided continuity of care where it had been fragmented; are accepted by consumers; save physician time; and are profitable to some employers, particularly physicians (without receiving comparable financial re-

---

*The hundreds of studies reported cannot be listed, but many have been published in the nursing, medical, and hospital literature.

ward themselves). In some cases, NPs' thoroughness and extensive teaching did not enable them to see as many patients as did MDs, and cost effectiveness was questioned. A few studies have compared NPs with various educational backgrounds, but they have not been definitive. Unfortunately, almost none have evaluated the NP role according to recognized research protocols.

There are several serious problems that interfere with NP practice. The first is the resistance of many physicians who are unfamiliar with and distrustful of nurses in this role, and who feel threatened professionally and economically, particularly when patients other than the poor are involved. Such MDs usually prefer to utilize PAs, if anyone, because PAs are legally under the MDs' supervision and cannot practice independently. Retaliation comes in the form of medical licensing boards harassing NPs and their MD colleagues for, respectively, practicing medicine without a license and aiding and abetting such practice, which can result in loss of license. Although these accusations seldom stand up and are usually not carried through, they sometimes succeed in discouraging NP/MD teams. Some medical boards and associations also lobby against changes in the nurse practice act that would legalize NP practice. Prescriptive authority was another area that they resisted,[69] although in some states nurses do have such authority.[70] Thus, the nurse–physician colleague relationship that is inherent in team practice is not always present. More serious is the question of the NPs' right to practice, which will be considered in Chapter 20.

A major concern is general lack of reimbursement for services (unless the NP works directly under the supervision of the physician). Ironically, DHHS funds NP programs through one agency and withholds funding through another (Medicare), except in experimental programs and, to some extent, in approved rural clinics. A few states reimburse (through Medicaid), as do a few private third-party payers. Maryland was the first state to require third-party reimbursement for nurses

(1980), thanks in large part to a nurse legislator. In 1981, Congress authorized payment for the services of nurse-midwives. However, some physicians are making strong efforts to limit nurse-midwife practice.[71]

The issue involves nurse autonomy and power, which will be discussed in Chapter 16. However, it is useful to remember that physician resistance to NP practice may have a lot to do with the projected oversupply of physicians, some of which already exists, and the competition NPs might give MDs.[72,73]

In the following sections, the most common NP roles are discussed in more detail. These roles may vary according to the setting, with more or less independence and more or less broadening or narrowing of the role as needed. Sometimes there is a comprehensive role, such as the family NP in a health clinic, or the insurance physical examiner.[74] There are many articles and books describing the many NP roles, some of which are listed in the bibliography.

Family Nurse Practitioner (FNP)

Family nurse practitioners (FNPs) may function alone in clinics in isolated rural areas, with only long-distance contact with a physician, in mobile units, in doctors' offices, in urban community health centers, group medical practices, health departments, and hospital outpatient departments, as well as independently. They may be involved in:

1. Management of well children or treatment of their uncomplicated illnesses.
2. Management of uncomplicated maternity patients in the course of pregnancy and the postpartum period.
3. Family planning—counseling and examination.
4. Medical supervision of those patients in a relatively stable phase of their illness, recognizing complications and exacerbations that require physician referral or consultation.
5. Acute and emergency care as dictated by the situation.[75]

Pediatric Nurse Practitioner (PNP)

Pediatric nurse practitioners (PNPs) are most likely to function in clinics, doctors' offices, health departments, and group practices. Their activities include (1) management of well children, (2) management of selected common childhood conditions and illnesses, with appropriate referrals when necessary, (3) anticipatory guidance to parents about childrearing and to the child about his needs, (4) health teaching about illnesses, and (5) other counseling.

Adult Nurse Practitioner (ANP)

The adult nurse practitioner (ANP) role usually includes the care of long-term patients, but may be limited to geriatrics or another specialty. Settings are similar to those of the FNP, but are especially outpatient departments, community health centers, and some nursing homes. Responsibilities include:

1. Evaluating the history, physical findings, and laboratory data appropriate for the patient's illness, making adjustments in drugs, and other therapeutic measures.
2. Aiding the patient and family to cope with the illness.
3. Utilizing appropriate services to help the client solve health-related problems.
4. Taking initiative in providing social, physical, and emotional rehabilitation of the chronically ill when possible.[76]

Obstetric-Gynecologic (OB-Gyn) Nurse Practitioner

Obstetric-gynecologic (OB-Gyn) NPs may function in settings similar to those of other practitioners, but particularly in clinics. They may or may not limit their practice to gynecology (depending on the setting and, of course, their education). Among their functions are:

1. Eliciting a complete gynecological history and performing breast and pelvic examinations, recognizing abnormalities.
2. Teaching and counseling patients in areas

of family planning and general gynecologic health (some insert intrauterine devices).
3. Detecting venereal disease and counseling patients.
4. Performing cancer screening examinations and perhaps other diagnostic tests.

For obstetrics, their functions are:

1. Eliciting a complete obstetric history and performing obstetrically oriented examinations, recognizing deviations from normal.
2. Performing routine prenatal and postpartum examinations.
3. Counseling patients about normal pregnancy.
4. Checking newborns (in some cases).

In some states, the nurse in public health clinics develops and implements a management plan for prenatal care for all "normal" pregnant women, referring those with any abnormality to the physician.

Psychiatric-Mental Health Nurse Practitioner

Psychiatric-mental health NPs function particularly in community mental health centers, including crisis intervention centers, and in interdisciplinary groups, but they frequently carry a private case load in association with physicians, hospitals, or other health care institutions. It is not unusual for them to be called upon to give emergency psychiatric care, and they may specialize in specific areas such as child psychiatry.

The nurse may serve as a therapist in individual or group therapy, participate as a consultant in an interdisciplinary group, and do general mental health and preventive counseling. In many ways the role is similar to that of the clinical specialist in psychiatric nursing, although the latter may tend to function chiefly in subspecialty areas.

Qualifications and Conditions of Employment. (All NP's) Just what the appropriate educational credentials of an NP should be has not really been decided. Probably the eventual decision will be the master's degree, but, just now, NPs prepared in almost any type of structured program will be employed by someone. In some cases, when they are trained on the job, their mobility is limited without further education. The educational confusion of generic and RN programs teaching assessment skills, as well as certificate, and various degree programs, does nothing for the NP image. One commonality that is gaining acceptance is certification by ANA and/or a specialty organization. Certification for entrance into a specialty provides a certain baseline of qualifications, as do legal guidelines, regulations, or the nurse practice act if it is sufficiently specific. Neither is there a clear picture of the conditions of employment, because the situations vary so much. If an employee, the NP might expect the same fringe benefits as others on a similar employment level. Salary may or may not be higher than that of another nurse who does not have this additional preparation, as has been discovered by nurses who return to the same place of employment but function in an expanded role. Sometimes it is a matter of individual bargaining. Physicians' assistants who are mostly men (NPs are mostly women) appear to receive higher salaries. However, this is said to be because most physicians' assistants work for private MDs and work more than forty-hour weeks.

Nurse-Midwife

Although nurse-midwives are sometimes categorized as one of the NP roles, the nurse-midwife has been in existence for some time. The first school of nurse-midwifery was started in 1931 in New York City by the Maternity Center Association. According to the American College of Nurse-Midwives (ACNM):

> Nurse-midwifery practice is the independent management of care of essentially normal newborns and women, antepartally, intrapartally, postpartally and/or gynecologically, occuring within a health care system

which provides for medical consultation, collaborative management, or referral and is in accord with the *Functions, Standards, and Qualifications for Nurse-Midwifery Practice* as defined by the American College of Nurse-Midwives (ACNM).

> A certified nurse-midwife (CNM) is an individual educated in the two disciplines of nursing and midwifery, who possesses evidence of certification according to the requirements of the American College of Nurse-Midwives.

Nurse-midwives practice in a variety of settings, where maternity care is given—clinics, doctors' offices, hospitals, and the new birthing centers.[77] Their practice may be interdependent within a health care delivery system, for example, a hospital obstetric service largely staffed by nurse-midwives, where a physician might be a backup as needed. They might also have a formal written alliance with an obstetrician, or another physician, or a group of physicians who have a formal consultative arrangement with an obstetrician-gynecologist. The ACNM states that nurse-midwives practice within the framework of medically approved protocols. The fact that many mothers now seem to prefer a normal/natural birthing process, when there are no potential complications, has brought a resurgence of interest in nurse-midwifery. Ten years ago, few states permitted nurse-midwives to practice, but this new interest has brought about legal changes that permit the nurse-midwife to practice with only a nursing license and ACNM certification or under new nurse-midwifery licensure laws (that also usually require certification). In the states where nurse-midwives are controlled by the medical practice act, their practice can be arbitrarily limited at the pleasure of that board.

ACNM-approved (accredited) nurse-midwifery programs vary from eight months to two years in length and are usually given by an educational or clinical institution. There are post-RN certificate programs that do not require a baccalaureate degree, but the trend is toward a master's degree. All programs include theory and practice in prenatal care, management of a patient in labor, normal spontaneous deliveries in the hospital, immediate care of the newborn, care of the postpartum patient, and family planning. After completion of an ACNM-approved program, the nurse-midwife is eligible to take the certification examination.

PRIVATE PRACTICE AND INDEPENDENT PRACTICE

The terms *private practice* and *independent practice* are often used synonymously, but Keller maintains that this misinterprets the nature of the activities in private practice and confuses it with practice in the NP role. Private practice, she says, "indicates simply that nursing is conducted under the auspices of nurses in solo or group association *and* that the business of that practice belongs to that nurse or those nurses—not to the public, to another profession, or to the government. The responsibilities and delegations of authority are administered within the bounds of said ownership, much as any private duty nurse administers her own practice."[78]

This new model of practice is seen as having many advantages: there is one-to-one interaction and continuity of care, maximum participation by nurse and patient, the possibility for consumers to attach more value to nursing services as distinct from other health services and to recognize that nurses especially can do justice to certain kinds of health problems, the chance for the public to exercise more choice in selecting providers of care, and the built-in accountability to the client that is associated with fee-for-service.[79]

A private practice is a business, and setting it up and running it must be a business-like process or it will not survive.[80] There are basic decisions to be made: what kind of organization should be created (corporation, partnership, for-profit, nonprofit); by whom (nurses and other professionals); for whom; at what fees; what kind and how many employees will

be needed; how to get clients (marketing); types of advertising; how to relate to other health professions; where the services will be offered; at what hours; and policies about telephone counseling and/or home visits (house calls). Early expenses include lawyers' and accountants' fees, space, furniture, equipment, supplies, telephone, insurance, stationery, postage, flyers, and brochures. Repeated obstacles or problems to most are the normal business aspects: employee contracts, salaries, benefits, tax deductions, fee preparation and collection, and the multitude of forms and records that must be kept. When federal or other contracts are involved, still more records are necessary.

What kind of services would nurses offer in private practice? If nurses do not have NP training, the usual services offered are any combination of health teaching and health promotion, home health, professional education (CE programs), and consulting. For instance, one nonprofit group started with a free hypertension screening program from which they made no money, but which gave them enough visibility to win a contract to provide health counseling services at a senior citizen center. They also engaged in such diverse activities as acting as preceptors for students in a graduate nursing program and a school of pharmacy and teaching classes in university schools.[81]

NPs in private practice may have a backup physician, or they may have developed relationships with physicians from whom and to whom referrals are made. Some NPs are in full partnership in a group practice of physicians.[82] These NPs do all the things NPs are legally permitted to do in their state, which may or may not include writing prescriptions. Sometimes these practices are in an urban/suburban area, but frequently they are in rural areas with few physicians available, and the nurse is the only health care provider.

Assuming that the nurse does not have legal problems about the scope of practice, a major problem is getting enough patients and reimbursement to earn a living. Many nurses can afford to give only part of their time to the practice because of limited reimbursement, and perhaps hold university teaching positions or are subsidized by some organization. As noted earlier, third-party payment is still uncertain, and most patients cannot or do not choose to pay an independent practitioner if they can get clinic care which is covered.

Another problem has been individual practice privileges in health care organizations, especially hospitals and nursing homes.[83] What this means basically is the privilege of a nurse not employed by that institution to admit patients and/or write orders for their care or participate in any part of his or her patients' care. The ANA has delineated several levels of appointment privileges and guidelines for appointment. JCAH and AHA have also made statements. For nurses, it is particularly important that the nurse's credentials be reviewed by a *nursing* credentials committee, just as physician's credentials are reviewed by a medical staff committee. Because the JCAH has now indicated that hospitals "may" extend privileges to nonphysicians, changes may occur.

In rural areas where there is no source of health care, the NP may have the same physical, professional, and psychological problems as physicians—isolation, overwork, and some lack of stimulation. Nevertheless, independent practice provides a degree of professional autonomy that many nurses crave. As one of the first acknowledged independent practitioners stated, "in the twenty-fifth year of my nursing career, I have become professionally free and have removed the impediments to my practice of nursing."[84]

NURSE ANESTHETIST

A *certified registered nurse anesthetist* (CRNA) is a registered professional nurse who has graduated from an approved school of anesthesia for nurses and has passed the certification examination. Lists of approved schools

may be obtained from the American Association of Nurse Anesthetists (AANA). The postgraduate course in anesthesia takes about two years, and some programs give courses with credit, which will count toward an advanced college degree. There are now also a few master's degree programs for nurse anesthetists.

Anesthetists generally function under the direction of an anesthesiologist (MD), when available, in any setting where anesthesia is given—the operating room, the obstetric department, the inhalation therapy department, the emergency room or the dental office. Anesthetists provide the patient with preoperative psychological support in many situations, although patient contact in this respect varies according to the setting. In the operating room, oxygen and the appropriate anesthetics, other drugs, and IV solutions are administered while the patient's vital signs and blood loss are carefully monitored. The CRNA accompanies the patient to the recovery room.[85]

Although salaries equal or exceed other nursing salaries, anesthesia situations are usually considered stressful, the hours may be irregular, and because the service must be covered for twenty-four hours, the anesthetist may be on call in some employment situations. Malpractice (liability) insurance is necessary, sometimes difficult to get, and considerably more expensive than that of other nurses. Many men now find this field attractive; the AANA notes that more than 14 percent of the 18,000 plus nurses in this field are men.

NURSE RESEARCHER

For some time, nurses have been participating in medical research, often as gatherers of data rather than researchers. They still do, although some are gaining status as researchers in general health research. Since the 1930s, nurses have become more aware of the need for research in nursing, but few were academically prepared to carry it out. At first, most nursing research was directed by social scientists who were concerned with nurses, their attitudes, and their education. As nurses gained more advanced preparation in the social, physical, and biological sciences, they began to direct and carry out research themselves—first on nursing functions and nursing education, but gradually moving into patient-centered studies of nursing care. A need to develop a knowledge base for nursing and research into nursing practice has also been repeatedly emphasized.

Nurses in research may function in a variety of roles, depending on their educational preparation. If the nurse has not had doctoral preparation or research training, working on a research team as a research assistant or associate, collecting data, or doing some data analysis may be a start. Fully prepared nurse researchers are in great demand. They may find employment in universities and health institutions or may choose to freelance as consultants. The need is greater than either the supply of qualified nurses or the funds available for research. The majority of nurses with doctoral degrees have taken positions in universities and colleges, either as professors of nursing or as administrators, where they engage in both research and teaching. This is considered a compatible and necessary combination, because they not only increase knowledge of nursing, but train other nurses in research and guide their studies. The need to recruit nursing students early for graduate study and research is important for the development of nursing.

A particularly encouraging trend is the employment of nurse researchers in practice settings, such as medical centers and government. In these positions, nurse researchers may have responsibility for studying patients' nursing needs, defining and evaluating patient care effectiveness, setting up testing situations for development of new nursing techniques, equipment, or procedures, acting as advisors or consultants to nurses developing patient research projects, and planning with other disciplines for the improvement of patient care.[86] Nurse researchers may also become research project directors, directors of research institutes, or be full partners in an interdisciplinary research team.

Qualifications and Conditions of Employment. Nurses engaged in research as described here are expected to have research training and ability, and, preferably, a doctoral degree. Personally, they must have the ability to do both creative thinking and to carry through the orderly process of research, which with human beings is seldom static or orderly, and the writing skill to report their findings. Nurses holding university positions earn the same salaries and benefits as other nurse teachers in that setting. Although time may be allotted for research, the funding of this research is often the responsibility of the teacher-researchers, and they must become adept at grantsmanship. There are also nurses hired by universities to head or participate in specific research projects, without teaching responsibilities. These positions are often on a short-term basis and may have been initiated by someone else. Most researchers find that they devote considerable time to their studies, and working hours are often not in a regular forty-hour-a-week framework. This is particularly true if the researcher also has teaching and/or administrative responsibilities.

If employed in a clinical setting, the nurse researcher's salary is probably negotiable, depending on her background. Although such positions may be budgeted, there may be very limited budgeting for other personnel and equipment needed for specific research projects. Again, funds must be sought from other sources, such as foundations, individuals, or, most frequently, governmental agencies. The availability of these funds has fluctuated, which has been a detriment to nursing research (see Chapter 14).

For nurse researchers, however, the satisfactions are great, both in terms of the personal satisfactions of research and the knowledge that they have made meaningful contributions to the nursing field. With all the opportunities available to nurses with doctoral degrees, it is certain that those engaged

in research do so because it is their first preference.

NURSE CONSULTANT

There are professional nurse consultants
specializing in all areas of nursing—education, administration, and clinical practice,
particularly specialties—who provide assistance to individuals and groups. Because the
usual purpose of seeking consultation is to
bring about change of some kind, which may
be a tension-provoking situation for the clients, not just specific knowledge but also the
ability to understand and communicate in
complex human relations situations is especially important. Someone who cannot relate
to others in a way that is appropriate to the
situation will not be successful, regardless of
expertise. A good consultant must get a clear
and accurate picture of the total situation, attitudes, abilities, and commitment of the people involved, the problems, assets, resources,
and other factors that are not always overtly
presented or visible, and have the ability to
critique and assist. Because consulting is usually done in a limited time span, the clients
must be stimulated to think productively
about what they can and must do to continue
the task. There is a difference between giving
advice and being a consultant, for the professional role requires the ability to observe, assess, plan, and make accurate judgments and
to present them in a way that is workable for
the clients. Usually consultants are presented
with a problem or a request to help develop a
program or service. The consultant collects
data, does a preliminary review, and then an
analysis, based on information sent and frequently an on-site visit. The client may be
given resource materials and a final written report with an analysis of the situation and recommendations for action.

Although many well-prepared nurses in top
positions consult apart from their primary
jobs (and this kind of prestige is considered
desirable by some employers), professional
consultants are usually employed in local,
state, national, international, private, or governmental agencies and organizations. There
are, for instance, consultants with the National League for Nursing, DHHS, state
health departments, the World Health Organization, and private consulting firms, even
private businesses, by the nurse and/or a
group. In the last case, the same aspects of
business management apply as for nurses in
private practice.[87] Fees may be negotiated or
set according to specific criteria.

INTERNATIONAL NURSING

The nurse with a taste for adventure and a
desire to see the world may enjoy a position
with one of the agencies concerned with nursing in areas outside the United States. Such
positions are almost invariably challenging
and a little off the beaten track. At the same
time, the qualifications are usually high, including special preparation in the area in
which the nurse will be working.

World Health Organization

One agency to which nurses have turned for
international health employment is the World
Health Organization (WHO) and its regional
office, the Pan American Health Organization.* Their major concerns currently are in
primary care, but related activities in terms of
education may also have priority. Because of
changing emphasis and varying needs, it is
best to contact these agencies for information
on the type of positions available, the requirements, and the conditions of employment.
However, generally it is necessary to have advanced education, experience, and language
capability.

Peace Corps

Since the Peace Corps began in 1961, it has
employed both volunteer and staff nurses.
Staff nurses serve in many of the sixty Peace
Corps countries in the preventive and curative
program developed to care for the volunteer.

*See Chapter 28.

Here too, there are changing priorities and variable funding, depending to an extent on the politics of the moment. Whether one is interested in a paid or volunteer position, it is best to contact the Peace Corps, Washington, D.C. 20525 for available opportunities and requirements. As a rule, it has been necessary for the nurse to be an RN, a U.S. citizen, and to have appropriate language skills for the country assigned, good health, stamina, and, of course, the necessary nursing skills.

Project HOPE

The purpose of Project HOPE has traditionally been to bring the skills and techniques developed by the American health professions to other peoples of the world in their own environment, adapted specifically to their needs and their way of life. HOPE began in 1958, when a prominent Washington, D.C., heart specialist, Dr. William B. Walsh, submitted a plan for the world's first peacetime hospital ship. A reconverted 15,000-ton veteran of two wars consequently became the *S.S. Hope,* and Project HOPE was sponsored by the People-to-People Health Foundation, Inc. In 1960 the *S.S. Hope* left on her maiden mission to Indonesia and South Vietnam, followed by missions to other countries in various parts of the world; it was retired in 1973. Whereas nurses on the ship's medical staff were highly competent specialists or generalists who worked on a one-to-one basis with host country counterparts in a hospital, the emphasis shifted. Relatively long-term, land-based programs, always an essential component of Project HOPE, have replaced the ship as the milieu within which HOPE teams carry out their professional activities.

The focus has changed again in recent years, and HOPE is now engaged in a number of projects in the United States, as well as continuing some of its international activities. It is best to get updated information from Project HOPE, 2233 Wisconsin Avenue NW, Washington, D.C. 20007. However, as for the WHO positions, advanced education, experience, and language skills are required.

OTHER INTERNATIONAL NURSING OPPORTUNITIES

Almost every religious denomination supports some kind of missionary work in foreign countries. Nurses are usually welcomed in such activities because missionary work often includes some form of professional or semi-professional health care activities. Nurses who select missionary nursing as their life's work must have a strong desire to nurse the sick and underprivileged, often in primitive surroundings; ability to teach religious principles by example, and possibly in religious classes; and knowledge of the language of the people in the regions assigned. They will have many opportunities to teach citizens and health workers of other lands. Missionary nurses must expect to find their rewards principally in personal satisfaction because missionary nurses usually earn a low salary for long hours of hard work. Nurses can obtain specific information about missionary nursing from their own church. Some mission groups accept volunteers who are not of their own religious faith.

Another major possibility in international nursing is occupational nursing for major industries (the multinationals) with overseas branches. On occasion, the governments, universities, hospitals, or industries of foreign countries also seek American nurses with all types of educational preparation. In recent years, Mideastern countries, particularly, have employed recruiters to fill staff and other positions in their hospitals. It is especially important to clarify the job-role and functions, as well as personal living conditions, and to learn about the country, for some American women nurses have found it very difficult to adjust in Moslem countries. Limited opportunities are found with the federal government in countries where federal personnel are stationed, but these positions are first filled by transferring career personnel already in the agency.

In all cases, there are usually advertisements in newspapers or professional journals for these positions. If not, the nurse should make inquiries to the private company concerned or the appropriate federal agency.[88]

OTHER CAREER OPPORTUNITIES

It would probably be impossible, or at least extraordinarily lengthy, to give information about every career possibility available for nurses. A list of specific *positions,* directly related to nursing, not even including specialization or subspecialization, runs into the hundreds when the diverse settings in which nursing is practiced are considered. Overall, these are clinical nursing, administration, education, or research (or a combination of all), but the specific setting brings its own particular challenges. They may require knowledge of another culture and the physical psychosocial needs of these people, such as nursing in an Indian reservation,[89] or a new orientation to practice such as working in an HMO, or in juvenile court,[90] or the prison system,[91] or even camp nursing.[92]

In some cases, specialization or subspecialization, usually requiring additional education and training (because most generic education programs present only a brief exposure), becomes a new career path. There are any number of these, and as each becomes recognized as a distinct subspecialty, involved nurses tend to form a new organization or a subgroup within ANA or some related medical organization to develop standards of practice. There are also many articles in journals and papers given at meetings about nursing in these various areas, so that a practicing specialty nurse can keep abreast of current practice; other nurses may also develop interest in new fields.

Specialization and subspecialization are not really new; operating room nurses have been practicing since the beginning of American nursing[93] and coronary care nurses[94] or enterostomal therapists[95] are into their second decade. More recently, there is new emphasis and, consequently, a number of new educational programs in such areas as women's health care,[96] family planning,[97] thanatology,[98]

and sex education,[99] all of which have an interdisciplinary context that brings additional dimensions to the practice.

When nurses assume positions such as editors of nursing journals, or nursing editors in publishing companies, they draw not only on their nursing background, but must learn about the publishing field and acquire the necessary skills. Editing is not the same as writing, and the responsibility for putting out a journal or other publication has financial, administrative, legal, philosophical, and policy-making components. In the same vein, nurses employed as lobbyists, labor relations specialists, executive directors or staff of nursing associations, nurse consultants for drug or supply companies, and staff for legislators or governmental committees all use their nursing, but must learn from other disciplines not related to nursing and develop new role concepts.[100] If they choose to maintain a nursing role and orientation as well, nursing is enriched and strengthened; if they abandon all identity with the profession, it may lose valuable input.

As health care and nursing expand, some nurses will develop new positions themselves, for which the need and the qualifications cannot now be determined. It seems safe to say, however, that opportunities and challenges in nursing today are practically unlimited.

REFERENCES

1. Robert Gulack, "Nursing Pay: Climbing Faster Then Inflation," *RN,* **46**:27–33 (Nov. 1983).
2. Howard Lewis, "Specialism: The Best Career Path?" *RN,* **47**:40–47 (June 1984).
3. Robert Gulack, "The Main Chance," *RN,* **46**:35–41 (Mar. 1983).
4. Sister Bernadetta Armiger, "Nursing Shortage or Unemployment?" *Nurs. Outlook,* **21**:315 (May 1973).
5. Marjorie Beyers et al., "Results of the Nursing Personnel Survey, Parts 1, 2, 3," *J. Nurs. Admin.,* **13**:34–38 (Apr. 1983); 26–30 (May 1983); 16–20 (June 1983).

6. Ross Mullner et al., "Hospital Nursing Vacancies," *Am. J. Nurs.,* **83**:547 (Apr. 1983).

7. Julie Wine and John Baird, "Improving Nursing Management and Practice Through Quality Circles," *J. Nurs. Admin.,* **13**:5–10 (May 1983).

8. Shelagh Roell, "Nurse-Intern Programs: How They're Working," *J. Nurs. Admin.,* **11**:33–36 (Oct. 1981).

9. Florence Huey, "Looking at Clinical Ladders," *Am. J. Nurs.,* **82**:1520–1530 (Oct. 1982).

10. Ada Sue Hinshaw et al., "Staff, Patient, and Cost Outcomes of All-Registered Nurse Staffing," *J. Nurs. Admin.,* **11**:30–36 (Nov.–Dec. 1981).

11. Gulack, op. cit.

12. American Nurses' Association, *Standards of Nursing Practice* (Kansas City, Mo.: The Association, 1973).

13. Edythe Alexander, *Nursing Administration in the Hospital Health Care System* (St. Louis, Mo.: C. V. Mosby Company, 1978), pp. 230–235.

14. Department of Health, Education, and Welfare, *Toward Quality in Nursing: Report of the Surgeon General's Consultant Group in Nursing* (Washington, D.C. The Department, 1963), p. 19.

15. Gwen Marram et al., *Cost-effectiveness of Primary and Team Nursing* (Wakefield, Ma.: Contemporary Publications, 1976).

16. Ellen Davis and Gladess Crisp, "An Inside Look at Nursing in Outpatient Surgery," *RN,* **42**:38–43 (May 1979).

17. Kathryn Morrow, "Specialize in General Nursing—On An 'Overnight' Unit," *Nursing 79,* **9**:122, 124, 126 (May 1979).

18. Marjorie Godfrey, "Is Part-time Nursing the Answer for You?" *Nurs. 80,* **10**:66–72 (Oct. 1980).

19. "The Demise of the Traditional 5–40 Workweek?" *Am. J. Nurs.,* **81**:1138–1143 (June 1981).

20. Loy Wiley, "Should You Join Rent-a-Nurse for Temporary Service?" *Nursing 76,* **6**:81–88 (Sept. 1976).

21. American Nurses' Association, *Nursing: A Social Policy Statement* (Kansas City, Mo.: The Association, 1980), pp. 25–26.

22. Ibid., p. 23.

23. Ibid., pp. 26–27.

24. Mary Popka and Frances Fay, "Clinical Nurse Specialist—Alive and Well?" *Am. J. Nurs.,* **84**:661–664 (May 1984).

25. American Nurses' Association, *Roles, Responsibilities, and Qualifications for Nurse Administrators* (Kansans City, Mo.: The Association, 1978), p. 4.

26. Barbara Stevens, "The Problem in Nursing's Middle Management," *J. Nurs. Admin.,* **2**:35–38 (Sept.–Oct. 1972).

27. *Roles, Responsibilities and Qualifications for Nurse Administrators,* op. cit., p. 6.

28. American Hospital Association, *Statement on the Position of the Administration of the Department of Nursing Service in Hospitals* (Chicago: The Association, 1971), p. 3.

29. *Roles, Responsibilities and Qualifications for Nurse Administrators,* op. cit., p. 4.

30. National Commission on Nursing, *Summary Report and Recommendations* (Chicago: The Commission, 1983), p. 6.

31. Alice Behrens, "The Pleasures and Problems of the Director of Nursing in a Small Hospital," *J. Nurs. Admin.,* **5**:311–334 (Feb. 1975).

32. Myrtle Aydelotte, *Report of the 1982 Survey of Nursing Service Administrators* (Chicago: American Hospital Association, 1983).

33. American Nurses' Association, *The Position, Role and Qualifications of the Administrator of Nursing Service* (New York: The Association, 1969).

34. *Roles, Responsibilities and Qualifications for Nurse Administrators,* op. cit., p. 14.

35. AHA, op. cit.

36. Dorothy del Bueno, "No More Wednesday Matinees," *Nurs. Outlook,* **24**:359–361 (June 1976).

37. Mary Diane Nadolny, "What Does the Infection Control Nurse Do?" *Am. J. Nurs.,* **80**:430–434 (Mar. 1980).

38. Robyn Ravgiala, "A New Role for Nursing: Project Director," *J. Nurs. Admin.,* **9**:22–24 (May 1979).

39. Phyllis Schaeffer, "The Utilization Review Coordinator: A Different Kind of Nurse," *Nurs. 76,* **6**:95–98 (Feb. 1976).

40. American Nurses' Association, *The Professional Nurse and Health Education* (Kansas City, Mo.: The Association, 1975).

41. *Professional Practice for Nurse Administrators in Long-Term Care Facilities,* Annual report of a project by the American Nurses' Foundation and the Foundation of the American College of Health Administrators, 1984.

42. Ginette Pepper et al., "Geriatric Nurse Practitioner in Nursing Homes," *Am. J. Nurs.,* **76**:62–64 (Jan. 1976).

43. Eleanor Feldbaum and Merle Feldbaum, "Caring for the Elderly: Who Dislikes It Least?" *J. Health Politics, Policy and Law,* **5**:62–72 (Spring 1981).

44. American Nurses' Association, *Standards: Community Health Nursing Practice* (Kansas City, Mo.: The Association 1980).

45. Ibid.

46. American Public Health Association, *The Definition and Role of Public Health Nursing in the Delivery of Health Care* (Washington, D.C., The Association, 1981).

47. Clarence Skrovan et al., "Community Nurse, Practitioner—An Emerging Role," *Am. J. Pub. H.,* **64**:847–885 (Sept. 1974).

48. Council of Home Health Agencies and Community Health Services, *Characteristics of the Home Health Agency Administrator* (New York: National League for Nursing, 1977).

49. Dorothy Oda, "A Viewpoint on School Nursing," *Am J. Nurs.,* **81**:1677–1678 (Sept. 1981).

50. Hope Solomons et al., "How Faculty Members Spend Their Time," *Nurs. Outlook,* **28**:160–165 (Mar. 1980).

51. Ingeborg Mauksch, "Faculty Practice: A Professional Imperative," *Nurse Educator,* **5**:21–24 (May–June 1980).

52. Gloria Smith, "Compensating Faculty for Their Clinical Practice," *Nurs. Outlook,* **28**:673–676 (Nov. 1980).

53. Mary Ann Rosswurm, "Characteristics of 23 Faculty Group Nurse Practices,"
Nurs. Health Care, **2**:327–330 (June 1981).

54. John Riley et al., *The Student Looks at His Teacher* (New Brunswick, N.J.: Rutgers University Press, 1950).

55. Glendola Nash, "Faculty Evaluation," *Nurse Educator,* **2**:9–13 (Nov.-Dec. 1977).

56. Shake Ketefian, "A Paradigm for Faculty Evaluation," *Nurs. Outlook,* **25**:718–6120 (Nov. 1977).

57. Juanita Murphy, "Tenure: Achieved or Ascribed," *Nurs. Outlook,* **26**:176–179 (Mar. 1978).

58. Joyce Foster, "Tenure: Process and Procedures," *Nurs. Outlook,* **26**:179–181 (Mar. 1978).

59. Karen Nishio, "The Right and the Qualified," *Nurs. Outlook,* **25**:713–717 (Nov. 1977).

60. Gertrude Torres, "The Nursing Education Administrator: Accountable, Vulnerable, and Oppressed," *Adv. Nurs. Sci.,* **3**:16 (Apr. 1981).

61. American Association of Occupational Health Nurses, *Guide for Development of Functions and Responsibilities in Occupational Health Nursing* (New York: The Association, 1977), p. 4.

62. Helen Tirpak, "The Frontier Nursing Service—Fifty Years in the Mountains," *Nurs. Outlook,* **23**:308–310 (May 1975).

63. Charles Lewis and Barbara Resnik, "Nurse Clinics and Progressive Ambulatory Patient Care," *New Engl. J. Med.,* **277**:1236–1241 (Dec. 1967).

64. Loretta Ford and Henry Silver, "The Expanded Role of the Nurse in Child Care," *Nurs. Outlook,* **15**:43–45 (Sept. 1967).

65. "A Role By Any Name," *Nurs. Outlook,* **22**:89 (Feb. 1974).

66. Anne Warner, *Innovations in Community Health Nursing* (St. Louis: C. V. Mosby Company, 1978).

67. Harry Sultz et al., "Nurse Practitioners: A Decade of Change," *Nurs. Outlook,* Part 1. **31**:137–144, 188 (May–June 1983); Part 2, **31**:216–219 (July–Aug. 1983); Part 3, **31**:266–269 (Sept.–Oct. 1983); Part 4, **32**:162–164 (May–June 1984).

68. Janice Ramsay et al., "Physicians and

Nurse Practitioners: Do They Promote Equivalent Health Care?" *Am. J. Pub. Health,* **72**:55–57 (Jan. 1982).

69. Jeri Bigbee et al., "Prescriptive Authority for Nurse Practitioners: A Comparative Study of Professional Attitudes," *Am. J. Pub. Health,* **74**:162–163 (Feb. 1984).

70. Donna Munroe et al., "Prescribing Patterns of Nurse Practitioners," *Am. J. Nurs.,* **82**:1538–1541 (Oct. 1982).

71. Elisabeth Hyde, "Territorial Imperatives in Health Care," *Nurs. Outlook,* **32**:136–137 (May–June 1984).

72. Claire Fagin, "The Economic Value of Nursing Research," *Am. J. Nurs.,* **82**:1844–1849 (Dec. 1982).

73. Claire Fagin, "Concepts for the Future: Competition and Substitution," *J. Psych./Mental Health Serv.,* **21**:36–40 (Mar. 1983).

74. "RN Opens Office for Insurance Health Assessment," *Am. J. Nurs.,* **81**:1891, 1910 (Oct. 1981).

75. Mary Ann Draye and Betty Peszecker, "Teaching Activities of Family Nurse Practitioners," *Nurse Pract.* **7**:28–33 (Sept.–Oct. 1980).

76. Paul Repicky et al., "Professional Activities of Nurse Practitioners in Ambulatory Care Settings," *Nurse Pract.,* **7**:27–40 (Mar.–Apr. 1980).

77. Judith Rooks and Susan Fischman, "American Nurse-Midwifery Practice in 1976–1977: Reflections of 50 Years of Growth and Development," *Am. J. Pub. Health,* **70**:990–996 (Sept. 1980).

78. Nancy Keller, "The Why's and What's of Private Practice," *J. Nurs. Admin.,* **5**:15 (Mar.–Apr. 1975).

79. Ibid.

80. Rosanne Wille and Keville Frederickson, "Establishing a Group Private Practice in Nursing," *Nurs. Outlook,* **29**:522–524 (Sept. 1981).

81. Sarah Archer and Ruth Fleshman, "Doing Our Own Thing: Community Health Nurses in Independent Practice," *J. Nurs. Admin.,* **8**:44–51 (Nov. 1978).

82. Rosanne Wille, "Sharing Responsibilities and Rewards as a Nurse Associate in a Group Practice," *Nurs. 79,* **9**:120–124 (Apr. 1979).

83. Mary Manley, "Clinical Privileges for Nonhospital-Based Nurses," *Am J. Nurs.,* **81**:1822–1825 (Oct. 1981).

84. M. Lucille Kinlein, "Independent Nurse Practitioner," *Nurs. Outlook,* **20**:22–25 (Jan. 1972).

85. Betty Smith, "Should You Become a Nurse Anesthetist?" *Nurs. 77,* **7**:108–111 (Nov. 1977).

86. Susan Steckel, "If You Want to Make a Positive Difference in Nursing, Become a Nurse Researcher," *Nurs. 78,* **8**:78–80 (July 1978).

87. Catherine Norris, "A Few Notes on Consultation in Nursing," *Nurs. Outlook,* **25**:756–761 (Dec. 1977).

88. VeNeta Masson, *International Nursing* (New York: Springer Publishing Company, 1981).

89. Martha Primeaux, "Caring for the American Indian Patient," *Am. J. Nurs.,* **77**:91–94 (Jan. 1977).

90. Mary de Chesnay, "Do You Want to Help Troubled Teen-Agers? Be a Juvenile Court Nurse," *Nurs. 76,* **6**:80–83 (Oct. 1976).

91. Patricia Moritz, "Health Care in Correctional Facilities: A Nursing Challenge," *Nurs. Outlook,* **39**:253–259 (Apr. 1982).

92. Hollis Backman et al., "Camp Nursing: An Opportunity for Independent Practice in a Miniature Community," *MCN,* **1**:88–92 (Mar.–Apr. 1976).

93. Margaret Fay, "The Challenge of O.R. Nursing," *Nurs. 77,* **7**:98–100 (Oct. 1977).

94. Frances Storlie, "Do You Want to Specialize in CCU Nursing?" *Nurs. 78,* **8**:71–76 (Jan. 1978).

95. Jacqueline Lamanske, "Want to Specialize? Consider Becoming an Enterostomal Therapist," *Nurs. 77,* **7**:94–96 (Apr. 1977).

96. Jean Colls, "Want to Specialize? Consider Becoming a Women's Health-Care Nurse Practitioner," *Nurs. 77,* **7**:72–74 (Jan. 1977).

97. Miriam Manisoff et al., "The Family Planning Nurse Practitioner: Concepts and Results of Training," *Am. J. Pub. Health,* **66**:62–66 (Jan. 1976).

98. Joy Ufema, "Do You Have What It

Takes to be a Nurse Thanatologist?'' *Nurs. 77,* **7**:96–99 (May 1977).

99. Beverly Henshaw, ''Providing Patient Care as a Sex Educator,'' *Nurs. 79,* **9**:78–80 (June 1979).

100. Gale Robinson Smith, ''Alternative Careers in Nursing,'' *Imprint,* **30**:23–24 (Dec.–Jan. 1984).

16

Issues of Autonomy and Influence

Within the overall issues of autonomy and influence lie many other nursing issues and concerns: maintenance of ethical standards and accountability (Chapter 10); direction of nursing education (Chapter 12); growth of nursing research (Chapter 14); utilization of nurse manpower (Chapter 15); and participation in credentialing (Chapter 20). If other disciplines are able to control nursing practice, it will never be able to fulfill its potential. If the voices of other groups override that of nursing, the tremendous contribution the profession can make to improving the delivery of health care will be lost. There is some indication that nursing's perceived lack of autonomy has already been detrimental to its ability to influence public policy. It is therefore essential that nurses understand the meaning of nursing autonomy and their individual and group roles in enhancing what has lately been called *nurse power*.

NURSING AUTONOMY

Professional *autonomy* has been defined as the right of self-determination and governance without external control. Inherent is the understanding that the freedom and independence thus held also mandate responsibility and accountability. Sociologists have identified autonomy as the most strategic (and cherished) distinction between a profession and an occupation or semiprofession. Identified as components of autonomy are control of the profession's education, legal recognition (licensure), and a code of ethics that persuades the public to grant autonomy. A distinction has been made between "job content" autonomy, the freedom to determine the methods and procedures to be used to deal with a given problem, and "job context" autonomy, the freedom to name and define the boundaries of the problem and the price to be paid for dealing with it.[1] The keys to autonomy as applied to nursing are that no other profession or administrative force can control nursing practice, and that the nurse has latitude in making judgments in patient care within the scope of nursing practice defined by the profession.

There are a number of reasons why nursing does not have full autonomy. Early nursing in America did not assume an autonomous stance. In part, this was because most nurses were women, and female status was low at the time. Nurses, usually female, were constantly admonished to obey the physician, usually male, and to abide by his judgment about the patient's condition. Even though nurses were trained to observe, the next step was to report and wait for further direction. Acting on their own judgment of what to do for the patient lay within a very narrow area. Added to this was the nurse's position in the male-dominated hierarchy of the hospital (which, as it became larger, became a male-dominated bureaucracy).

As Ashley reported, nurses have been expected to be mother figures, giving freely (in the financial as well as the social sense) of their time and efforts to meet the needs of all members of the hospital family, from patients to physicians. She attributed nurses' lack of progress and accompanying low status to the fact that they are women and maintained that their work has been virtually ignored and trivialized in comparison to that of physicians. "Nursing's problems, rooted in the tradition of economic exploitation, inadequate education, and long-standing social discrimination, have plagued the profession for the greater part of its history."[2]

The fact that there were some early nurses who struggled free and were able to practice independently, primarily in public health settings, is evidence that there was from the beginning health care practice that was uniquely nursing. Today there are changes in nursing, initiated by nursing, that give greater opportunity for autonomy—primary nursing in the acute care unit and the NP role in primary care. Although the latter practitioners are still encountering the constraints and distractions of some physician opposition, they are establishing themselves firmly and achieving one of the goals they had in choosing NP programs— more autonomy.* The primary nurse, too, has found satisfaction, with almost unanimous support for that role. Brown, referring particularly to primary nurses, described the autonomous nurse as one who

- is responsible to patient and family for total, individualized care

---

*See Chapter 15.

- is capable of independent decision-making that need not be physician ratified
- has a thorough command of nursing practice
- provides direct care to patients and families, providing opportunities for their participation
- serves as consultant to patients and families, helping them to make informed decisions
- has professional parity with physicians and participates in providing patient care as a fully accountable member of the team
- provides the "complete professional model of service, education, consultation and research."[3]

Clearly, this model can apply equally to nurses in all settings.

Concepts of Power and Influence

All of the classic definitions of *power* include the concepts of influence, control, and strength—for instance: "the ability of a person, group, or system to use their concerted strategies, energy or strength to influence the behavior or actions of others."[4] Or, as others have said, it is the capacity to modify the conduct of others in the manner desired and prevent one's own conduct from being modified in a way one does not want. Power is usually seen as a social relationship, not necessarily the attribute of a person or group; it is given, maintained, or lost within those relationships. Some thirty years ago, in a model that attempted to measure the potential effects of the influence or power of one person or group (A) over another (B), certain crucial dimensions were identified:

a. *The base of power*—economic and other resources, prestige, popularity, numbers.
b. *The means of power*—the specific actions that might be used (promises, threats, providing what the other needs or wants).
c. *The scope of power*—the set of specific actions that A can get B to perform.
d. *The amount of power*—the increase in probability that B will actually take certain

specific actions because of A's use of power.

e. *The extension of power*—the set of individuals over whom A has power.[5]

Power and influence are sometimes equated, because both affect or change the behavior of others; however, when they are separated, it is on the theory that power is the potential that must be tapped and converted to the dynamic thrust of influence. Almost all authorities agree that a person or group must be valued in order to have power or influence. French and Raven have described six sources of such power: reward power and coercive power, which seem self-explanatory; legitimate power (power derived from certain cultural values that are held or from a legitimizing act such as an election); referent power (liking or identifying with another); expert power (based on the knowledge, abilities, and credibility of the person or group); and informational power (arising from the communication activity of the person/group exerting influence).[6]

Considering these concepts, it is clear that nursing has the potential for power with its overwhelming numbers, its special knowledge and skill, and its place in public trust, and is, in fact, already beginning to exercise that power legislatively, although not as much as it might.[7,8] It would be a pity if nurses wasted their efforts on the limiting power of the powerless, the petty tyranny of the captive nurse with the clock-in, clock-out mentality.[9]

Other concepts of power are also applicable to nursing. Jacobs sees it as "essentially coercive in nature," with one person able to punish or reward according to the other's compliance; one person is, in a sense, dependent on another to gratify or deny his needs.[10] This concept has made power seem bad or corrupt, in the mode of Lord Acton's famous remark, "Power tends to corrupt and absolute power corrupts absolutely." Many women and nurses shy away from being identified with such a concept. A contrasting view looks at power as a positive and reciprocal process in which people are motivated to invest their time and effort to achieve goals without coercion or threats.[11] While probably closer to the preferred nursing self-image, this type of power is much more complex and less easily achieved.

McClelland and Burham have identified two different types of power: personal and shared.[12] *Personal power* is accrued to achieve individual goals, a form of self aggrandizement. These power types fear that if someone else accomplishes anything to achieve a particular goal, their own power and influence are diminished. This notion that shared power is loss of power has been a deterrent in nurse administration–staff relationships, but shared power can actually enhance the power of the sharers. For example, one group of nurses worked with the support of their directors of nursing to resolve specific problems that prevented them from fully utilizing their nursing knowledge. Not only were the situations improved, but the nursing staff as a whole (not just the doers) and the director both found that their power was enhanced by this exercise of shared power. The latter concept is demonstrated in the socialized power concept. These power figures work to achieve the goals of a group or organization without using coercive/reward power and derive satisfaction from seeing others achieve. Power is shared, and both the organization's goals, and indirectly, the individual's goals are met.

A particularly interesting concept is *reputational power,* in which power is equated with a person's reputation for being influential. Thus, reputational power is equated with real power. This theory, too, has an opposite; it says that no one individual or group necessarily dominates, but that power is diffused in the community. Power may be tied to issues and shift accordingly.[13] Here we see what might be considered nursing power at a national level. Certain influential nurses are usually easily identified, often because of their positions, and may be courted or simply more likely to be heard because they are thought to have influence with nurses (and, of course, they may). On the other hand, there are times when power clearly resides in a group, as when, at the 1982 ANA convention, state nurses' association executives and officers were probably the key actors in moving ANA to adopt a federation model. When other issues arose, the power shifted to other groups.

Nursing and Feminism

When it is asked why nurses, with so much potential for influence, do not seem to be able to or want to use it, there is inevitable reference to the fact that nursing is still about 97 percent a woman's profession, and, even with changing legislation and attitudes, women as a whole are still subject to discrimination (see Chapters 6 and 17) and still often victims of female socialization.

For many years, most women nurses looked at nursing as a useful way to earn a living until they were married, a job to which they could return if circumstances required. Most nurses did marry and most married nurses did drop out to raise families, working only part-time, if at all. Unmarried nurses (like male nurses) were more inclined to stay in nursing but, unlike men, frequently did not plot an orderly path to positions of authority and influence. This is similar to the career patterns of other women. In business, most women have traditionally been in their thirties or forties before they realized that they either wanted to or would be forced to continue working, and by then they were often frozen in dead-end, low-prestige (but productive) jobs. When they decided to compete for power positions in management, they were up against an "old boy" network that prevented or deterred their progress. Moreover, they had to overcome their own reluctance to be aggressive and to reject traditional female social goals.[14]

Nurses have tended to move into the administrative hierarchy more through default than intent, perhaps gathering credentials on the way. But until the last few decades, relatively few had attained power *outside* nursing, either as recognized expert practitioners within a practice setting or as representatives of nurs-ing in health policy determination. Why? Do nurses lack a goal-oriented commitment to nursing? Bowman and Culpepper said:

> There must be a conscious decision to use power. It is this conscious decision to assume power which nurses, individually and collectively, have been unable or unwilling to make. Most nurses think they are powerless. Many nurses see themselves as objects of the power of others, and have internalized the attitudes of subordination projected by those in positions of authority and other health professions. This has contributed to the development of a negative self-image within the profession.[15]

Women nurses now entering the field are generally more comfortable with the tenets of feminism and see no need to take an inferior role in a profession they have chosen to make a career. Grissum states that this does not mean that nurses who do not hesitate to question the reasoning behind a doctor's order, or demand more money and better working conditions, who are not intimidated and want more control over their profession and input into overall decision making are necessarily trying to attain omnipotence and dominate men (although some, of course, do). Instead, they demand equality, for which they are still often castigated by women as well as by men.[16]

Nurses who opt for leadership have found that they frequently had an additional battle to fight—being women in a woman's profession. In a study of nursing "influentials" that is, leaders in the profession, sexual stereotyping, discrimination of various forms (income, status, education), self-image problems (subservience, low self-esteem and self-confidence, insecurity, passivity, lack of assertiveness), and isolation from the male perspective were listed as disadvantages to being in a woman's profession. Frequently, these leaders were seen by others as deviant from the cultural norms that expect women to seek approval, affection, conciliation, and to be "other directed" and conforming.[17] Other nurses have reported their nurse peers displaying prejudice against qualified married women with children who seek leadership positions, putting obstacles in the way of those breaking new ground, isolating those who have established joint practice modes who must now "prove" themselves not only to nonparticipant physicians but to their own nurse colleagues.

Le Roux also presents numerous examples of "female prejudice against females," not necessarily nurses. She views this in light of the "renegade theory" and quotes Waelder:

> The fact that someone is close enough to us so that we feel called upon to compare ourselves with him and is yet different, is conceived like a latent criticism of ourselves, an implied attack against the way we are, and an implicit invitation to mend our ways; and we resent it.[18]

Neither nursing nor women need that kind of attitude. There is enough discrimination against women. Take one quite overt example, evident in the words of the federal judge who heard the job discrimination case of a group of Denver nurses. Although he acknowledged that nurses working for the city and county of Denver were paid less than male workers with comparable levels of responsibility and education, this judge ruled against them because a favorable ruling would have the potential for "disrupting the entire economic system of the United States of America." He interrupted the testimony of a noted nurse to read from the Declaration of Independence and announced that it didn't say anything about *women* being created equal. The denigration of women by the judge and the defense attorney in that trial make incredible reading.[19]

Although nurses have not always been supportive of the women's rights movement, there is general agreement that the consciousness raising that helps women to see their worth, to love and value themselves, has not only affected individual nurses who were involved, but has made nurses in general more aware of and resistant to discrimination.

The Dilemma of Nurses in a Bureaucracy

It is generally agreed that one of the major constraints to nursing autonomy and professionalism is the status of most nurses as employees in bureaucratic organizations (especially hospitals) where nursing, unlike medicine, is a department in the institutional hierarchy. The director of nursing (whatever the title) reports to the hospital administrator. Most decision making occurs at the top hierarchical level, and the goals of the bureaucracy are those that receive first priority. If, in the care of patients, those goals conflict with the nurse's professional goals, the nurse is in a dilemma that has been called *reality shock* when applied to new graduates and is considered one of the reasons for nurses' restless nomadism, sometimes culminating in flight from the profession. The other alternative has been, too often, acceptance of goals not necessarily in the patient's best interest: getting the work done to suit the hospital's schedule, not nursing to meet the patient's needs—a metamorphosis of nurse professional to nurse bureaucrat. When a nurse is rewarded for this behavioral shift, there is inevitably a slow drift to a survival mentality that precludes creative risk taking. As Nightingale said, "A good nurse does not like to waste herself," and lack of adequate resources and apparent lack of respect by administrators and others for *professional* nursing practice not only creates great job dissatisfaction but may make the nurse's work "slovenly."[20]

Job satisfaction surveys of nurses almost inevitably reflect two major dissatisfactions: lack of professional autonomy and the perception that they are not respected, or at least not listened to as professionals.* This plaint may not be much different from that of any other employee: nonresponsiveness by management is the basis of many labor disputes. There is no question that some institutional/

---

*A number of these surveys, especially those published in *Nursing 78,* are discussed in Chapter 11. Professional studies and reports citing similar results are cited in Chapter 5.

agency administrators are extremely controlling and some nurse administrators are not strong, all of which has an extremely limiting effect on nurse autonomy. Such a combination of factors has in recent years brought about a number of job actions in which the right of nurses to be involved in patient care decisions was a key issue, and nurses have won.[21] A major breakthrough was probably the 1974 strike of a group of San Francisco nurses, in which a prime issue was their being rotated to intensive care units even if they did not have the expertise to care for those patients. After a bitter struggle, in a union contract negotiated by the state nurses' association, the nurses won a voice in how assignments were made to specialty units, how other staffing arrangements were made, an expansion of the professional performance committees for peer review, and greater opportunity to participate in professional decision making and CE.[22] This pattern of demands has been adopted by nurses in other settings.

It is obvious why hospital and other administrators resist such steps; they see it as weakening their management rights and power. That they do not seem to be as negative toward the distinct power held by physicians in the same setting has a lot to do with the community prestige and power of physicians. For instance, it has been noted that physicians are in the same social circles as most hospital trustees and therefore have informal access to them and more acceptance as equals than do hospital administrators, who are, in a sense, also employees. But a large part of physician clout is derived from the fact that they are the gatekeepers to the health care delivery system; they are virtually the only health providers who can admit to or discharge from health care facilities. Even in public health and other ambulatory care settings, there is often no reimbursement of services if a physician is not supervising care, at least on paper. Health care agencies depend on patients for income; in most cases, they need physicians to help provide that income, particularly if they are

independent, but, to an extent, also if they are employed by the institution or agency.

Part of the independent stance of physicians is in their collegially oriented organization within the hospital, as described in Chapter 7. Unfortunately, nurses have been slow in adopting either such an organizational pattern for professional decision making or any other that guarantees nurses not only equity in health care endeavors, but parity. Christman considers this an essential step in gaining autonomy and describes one model.[23] Stressing the accountability to both patients and governing boards that is concomitant to autonomy, he suggests:

To discharge this responsibility nurses must, in general, use a process similar to that employed by the medical staff. They must: 1) control access to staff and practice privileges; 2) confirm background education and certification; 3) review clinical work through appropriate committees; 4) see that shortfalls (less than adequate care) in practice are determined and remedied; 5) delimit practice privileges; 6) develop quality assurance mechanisms; 7) delineate requirements for continuing education; 8) participate in the educational preparation of nursing students; and 9) engage in research to improve care. Because specialization in nursing is increasing greatly, the departmental responsibility for peer review and quality of care is just as necessary as it is in the medical departments.

Through the committee structure and the directing body, usually an executive committee and an elected chief-of-staff, the autonomous staff will maintain consultative relations: 1) with the board of trustees over qualifications for nursing staff membership and appointments and for standards of care; 2) with administration over logistical, material, and management-related issues; and 3) with the medical staff and the departments of the other health professions, e.g., dietary, social work, physical therapy, occupational therapy, clinical psychology, and with whatever other departments may exist, in order to share power and accountability.[24]

Although nursing autonomy of the type described may need the agreement of the chief administrator in an employment setting, a good nurse administrator can negotiate such arrangements as a requirement for effective and productive nursing practice. This does not mean that a nurse administrator abrogates managerial responsibilities, for good management can enhance opportunities for nurse autonomy. One model of shared governance that has stood is that at Loeb Center in New York, where nurses have practiced autonomously for many years.[25]

That this kind of nurse-initiated action takes a great deal of commitment and struggle has been documented, for to change to autonomy requires both strong nursing leadership and nurses' willingness to take action and assume appropriate responsibility.[26,27]

A newer dimension of nurse autonomy is the process by which clinical privileges are granted to NPs. Currently, the usual pattern is total control by physicians, with or without preliminary screening by nursing administration.[28] If such decisions are to be jointly made, perhaps nursing also ought to have input in the determination of physicians' clinical privileges.[29] The fact that *physicians* can determine which *nurses* have privileges points out the differences in the recognition of autonomy.*

Physician–Nurse Relationships

Physician–nurse relationships are a large, if not major, factor in nurse autonomy. There is necessarily a fine line between overstating or understating the problems, or, as some would have it, between paranoia and servility. Physicians' recognition of nurses as co-professionals and colleagues has been present almost since the beginning of nursing, but a hard core of physicians who see and prefer a nurse-handmaiden role, although less common than

*See also articles in the bibliography of Chapter 21 for legal aspects of doctor-nurse relationships.

even a decade ago, still exists. Some individual physicians and, to some extent, a part of organized medicine seem to have limited, stereotypic images of nurses and resist nurse autonomy—either because they honestly doubt nurses' ability to cope with certain problems (bolstered, unfortunately, by the behavior of some nurses they work with) or because they are threatened by the expansion of nursing roles. One example that showed serious lack of understanding of changes in nursing roles was the report of a committee of a prestigious medical group that dealt with the "status-seeking behavior" of nurses and urged a return to the nurse role of yore.[30] More serious is the periodic action of certain medical societies and boards to restrict expanded nursing practice by lobbying against the newer expanded definitions of practice in nurse practice acts, by opposing reimbursement for nursing services unless there is physician supervision, or by using their power to limit nursing practice in a particular community or health care setting.

The reasons for problems in nurse–physician relationships have been examined repeatedly. One reason given is that physician education tends to impress on the medical student a captain-of-the-ship mentality and a need for both omniscience and omnipotence (Aesculapian authority), whereas nursing education often does not develop nurses as independent and fearless thinkers.[31] This is also seen as one cause of the doctor–nurse game in which the nurse must communicate information and advice to the physician without seeming to do so and the physician acts on it without acknowledging the source. This game Stein calls a *transactional neurosis*; it has an inhibitory effect on open dialogue both stifling and anti-intellectual.[32]

Other reasons include the different socioeconomic and educational status of doctors and nurses; the MDs' lack of accurate knowledge about nursing education and practice, and vice versa, which enables them to work side by side without really understanding each other or communicating adequately (prompting some authors to compare their behavior to the parallel play of toddlers); different orientations to practice, including physician disapproval of the nursing emphasis on psychosocial aspects of patient care; the difference in attitudes about their professions as a long-term career commitment; nurses' lack of control over their practice, particularly in hospitals; physician exploitation of nurses; and general male misogyny.[33-37]

With many nurses looking toward expanded practice, the fact that many physicians surveyed do not seem comfortable in having nurses carry out responsibilities that were traditionally medicine has caused considerable misunderstanding. This is particularly true when nurses feel that they must prove themselves to be accepted in new roles, and that there is a "role-challenge" thrown out by physicians.[38] Again, apparently interrelated is the male–female role, the dominance–deference pattern that has had such strong historical roots that as someone stated, the nurse/woman must "feel like a girl, act like a lady, think like a man and work like a dog."[39] That some nurses demonstrate this deference was illustrated clearly in a study in which various nurses were told over the phone by an unidentified "doctor" to give an overdose of a so-called research drug. Although all showed by voice and body language that they resisted the order, all but one carried it out.[40]

On the other hand, there is an increasing number of physicians who encourage and promote nurse–physician collegial relationships and see them as inevitable and necessary for good health care.[41] Joint practice and other collaboration, both at the unit level and in various manifestations of physician–NP practice, are evidence of this cooperation.[42-44]

Glib proposals for cooperation will not solve the problems of conflict, which are detrimental to both professions and to the public. However, practical suggestions at the grassroots level on how to deal courteously and effectively with each other may sometimes be useful for the nurse dealing with physicians on a day-to-day basis.[45] Resolving the overall issue is a part of the challenge that both medicine and nursing must face.

NURSES AS CHANGE AGENTS

It is recognized that nurses, the only health professionals in contact with every facet of the health care system, are in key positions to bring about change. However, planned change involves problem-solving and decision-making skills as well as the ability to work well with others. A change agent must be skilled in the theory and practice of planned change. Therefore, a brief introduction to change theory may be helpful.[46]

Lewin's theory of change is probably the basis for the adaptations of most other theorists. He identifies three basic stages: *unfreezing,* in which the motivation to create change occurs; *moving,* the actual changing, when new responses are developed, based on collected information; and *refreezing,* in which the new changes are integrated and stabilized. A further notion is that in all changes there are *driving forces* that facilitate action and *restraining forces* that impede it. Each must be identified—the first so that they can be capitalized on, and the second so that they can be avoided or modified.

Lippit's theory includes seven phases within Lewin's stages, a delineation that is useful in thinking through action:

Unfreezing:

1. Diagnosis of the problem.
2. Assessment of the motivation and capacity for change.
3. Assessment of the change agent's motivation and resources.

Moving:

4. Selecting progressive change objectives.
5. Choosing the appropriate role of the change agent.

Refreezing:

6. Maintenance of the change once it has been started.
7. Termination of a helping relationship.

Welch[47] applies the process of change to a situation a nurse might change, working through these steps in some detail, and Olson[48] uses Lewin's model to go through another situational change a nurse may encounter.

Of interest is the model developed by Reinkemeyer (a nurse), which was used by another nurse in dealing with an alcohol abuse problem in her community.[49] Also based on Lewin's model, its phases are summarized as follows:

1. Development of a felt need and desire for the change.
2. Development of a change relationship between the agent and the client system.
3. Clarification or diagnosis of the client system's problem, need, or objective.
4. Examination of alternative routes and tentative goals and intentions of actions.
5. Transformation of intentions into actual change behavior.
6. Stabilization.
7. Termination of the relationship between the change agent and the client system.[50]

Why do nurses (and others) resist change? There are a number of reasons—some quite understandable: satisfaction with the current situation; a lack of clarity about what the change is; a felt threat from the change agent; a feeling that the process and the result of the change have not been thought through; selective perception and retention (hearing and remembering only what one wishes); too much work involved; fear of failure or disorganization; lack of two-way communication; and the belief that the change seems to benefit the change agent, not necessarily the group. It is obvious that some of these objections could be quite valid and, if not solved, would weaken the proposed change. If recognized by the change agent, they can be overcome, if the project is worthwhile and the change agent is proficient in human relations. If not all participants are won over, the decision must be made to stop or go ahead, trying to anticipate the negative aspects of what may become covert resistance if the resister is outvoted.

Conflicts of some kind are probably inevitable. It is important that the change agent develop effective methods of dealing with conflict. Action, rather than reaction, is the better course, but it should be recognized that a compromise might quite realistically result. Key steps include keeping the issue in focus, clarifying the problems, encouraging two-way communication, creating dialogue that involves group members in full participation, and always remaining responsive.[51] Just how a nurse handles resistance may be a matter of individual style and the particular situation. Some nurse change agents function with a "soft" approach that can be effective. Smoyak advocates a confrontation model—a direct approach considered useful when there is a clear-cut issue and the situation and individuals concerned are "healthy" and not "sick."[52]

Being a change agent is part of the leadership role, but it is also a role that can be legitimately and effectively assumed by a nurse not yet at that stage of professional development. Whether working as an insider or an outsider, each of which has advantages and disadvantages, knowing the process of change, planning carefully and thoroughly, and acting strategically and with an appropriate sense of timing are essential. Because a change agent is a leader in that instance, the leadership role must be assumed and the individual usually must start out by selling herself or himself first before the idea for change is seen as acceptable for consideration.

THE ROLE OF NURSING LEADERSHIP

The cry for leadership seems to be universal, but what constitutes *effective leadership* is frequently debated. The term defies simple definition. Leadership has been defined as "a social phenomenon in which a group or aggregation of individuals accepts and acts upon the ideas of one person,"[53] but in its simplest context, it is the ability to influence others, to lead, guide, and direct.

There are a number of theories and studies about leadership:

- the "great man" theory: leaders are born, not made.
- the charismatic theory: there is a personal quality of leadership that arouses a special popular loyalty or enthusiasm and an emotional commitment.
- the situational theory: leadership depends on the situation, and a person can be a leader in one situation and a follower in another.
- the contingency theory: the effectiveness of leadership depends on leader–member relations, task structure, and position power.
- the path-goal (expectancy) theory: the leader facilitates accomplishment by minimizing obstacles and rewarding followers for completing their tasks.
- the trait theory: leadership is acquired because the individual inherits or acquires certain traits.

The trait theory has been particularly popular, although there is little agreement on just what the key leadership traits and characteristics are. Among those that a variety of research has seemed to identify are effective interpersonal relationships that include tactfulness; a high level of energy and drive; persistence; assertiveness; aggressiveness; enthusiasm; self-assurance; self-confidence; decisiveness; superior judgment; dependability; integrity; persuasiveness; verbal facility; humor; courage; and friendliness. Superior intelligence was seen as a possible detriment if it interferes with the individual's ability to communicate with followers; some authorities believe that people desire to be led by someone not too far detached from the group. Data on factors such as age, appearance, sex, and social status are inconsistent; although neither age, appearance, nor sex correlate with ability to lead, most people do not become leaders until mid-

dle age, not as many women as men achieve leadership positions, and high socioeconomic status may be an advantage.[54]

Probably the fact that there are, and have been, leaders with the opposite traits, and that few, if any, have all, weakens the trait theory considerably. Yet people do have definite feelings about what they want in leaders. The president of an executive recruiting firm once stated what he considered essential for an effective executive: drive, people sense, communication ability, and calm under pressure, which might be considered a short version of the composite picture developed by a major researcher on leadership:

> The leader is characterized by a strong desire for responsibility and task completion, vigor and persistence in the pursuit of goals, venturesomeness and originality in problem solving, drive to exercise initiative in social situations, self-confidence and sense of personal identity, willingness to accept consequences of decision and action, readiness to absorb interpersonal stress, willingness to tolerate frustration and delay, ability to influence other persons' behavior and capacity to structure social interaction systems to the purpose at hand.[55]

Much is written about the price of leadership: the loneliness at the top, for instance, and it has been said that a good leader must get over the need to be loved and must learn to function without the need for approval of others. No leader can please all of his or her constituents all the time. To lead inevitably requires commitment; at times the leader must sacrifice personal desires, interests, time. The rewards, of course, are to see goals that one believes in met and to know that this might not have happened without one's leadership.

When the issue of nursing leadership is raised, there is, as in other professions, a demand for more and better. One writer said cynically,

> Nursing has an overabundance of silly, odd, inadequate, insecure, sadistic, incompetent, weak "leaders"; now it is time to get our pro-

fessional house in order with some capable, courageous, intelligent, ethical and sophisticated professional leaders who will have the knowledge and the daring to lead us as a profession and to meet the challenge of the next century.[56]

Leininger, who is recognized as a leader, maintains that there is a critical shortage of capable, well-prepared nursing leaders. She identified a key factor influencing nursing leadership as conflict between past and present expectations of leadership. She noted that if nurses have been "socialized to the subcultural norms that it is not 'ladylike' to fight, to confront, to negotiate, or to be bold or aggressive, they will experience norm conflicts with present day confrontation-negotiation strategies."[57] Other factors cited were negative attitudes toward authority; image, status, and role of women; size and complexity of organizational structures in which nurses function; new expectations related to interdisciplinary service and education; the diversity of interests and education in nursing; and the positional turnover of nursing leaders.

Yura et al.,[58] in their long-term research on leadership, have formulated a process of leadership, which, they say, can be learned, just as the nursing process, research process, and teaching-learning process is learned (thus belying the "leaders are born, not made" myth). Noting that nursing is an interpersonal process and that a shortage of nursing leadership behavior exists, they flatly state, "Leaders in nursing can be deliberately prepared." The theoretical considerations underlying their work are based primarily on the work of Tannenbaum et al.,[59] who consider interpersonal influence as the essence of leadership, with the leader trying to affect the behavior of followers through communication. The goals may be organizational, group, or personal for both leader and follower. To meet organizational goals, which may have little or no motivational importance, the leader may use inducements relative to the needs of the followers. Group goals evolve through interaction of group members and reflect what the group decides. The follower's personal goals are met when the leader "uses his influence to establish an atmosphere of warmth, security and acceptance, and when, through interpersonal techniques, the leader helps another to reach ends that could not possibly be reached alone."[60] The leader's personal goals may be met primarily through his or her influence and may coexist with organizational or group goals. To function successfully, the leader particularly needs sensitivity, for influence is exerted through communication. Leadership, in this concept, is a "cyclical process in that events at any step may be fed back to the leader so that modification in behavior may be made and parts of the sequence can be altered,"[61] (if not successful).

As a basis for development of the nursing leadership process, Yura et al., define *nursing leadership* as a "process whereby a person who is a nurse effects the actions of others in goal determination and achievement."[62] The four components determined to be strategic in putting nursing leadership into operation, that is, achieving goals, were delineated as *deciding, relating, influencing,* and *facilitating,* in that order (see Figure 16-1). The "human actions" inherent in each were then identified;[63] communication and evaluation were seen as inextricably incorporated in these components. The authors then demonstrated how to use this concept in educational preparation for leadership and in implementation and evaluation of the nursing leadership process. They urged the development of further research on the concept.

Some studies on nursing leadership have, of course, been done, although many are simply first-level studies at the master's level. One topic that has particular potential is leadership styles. Commonly identified styles are autocratic, democratic, and bureaucratic, but new concepts have emerged: *multicratic* (moving flexibly back and forth along the continuum of leadership behaviors as the situation demands) and *professional* (basically a democratic style with much adaptability).[64]

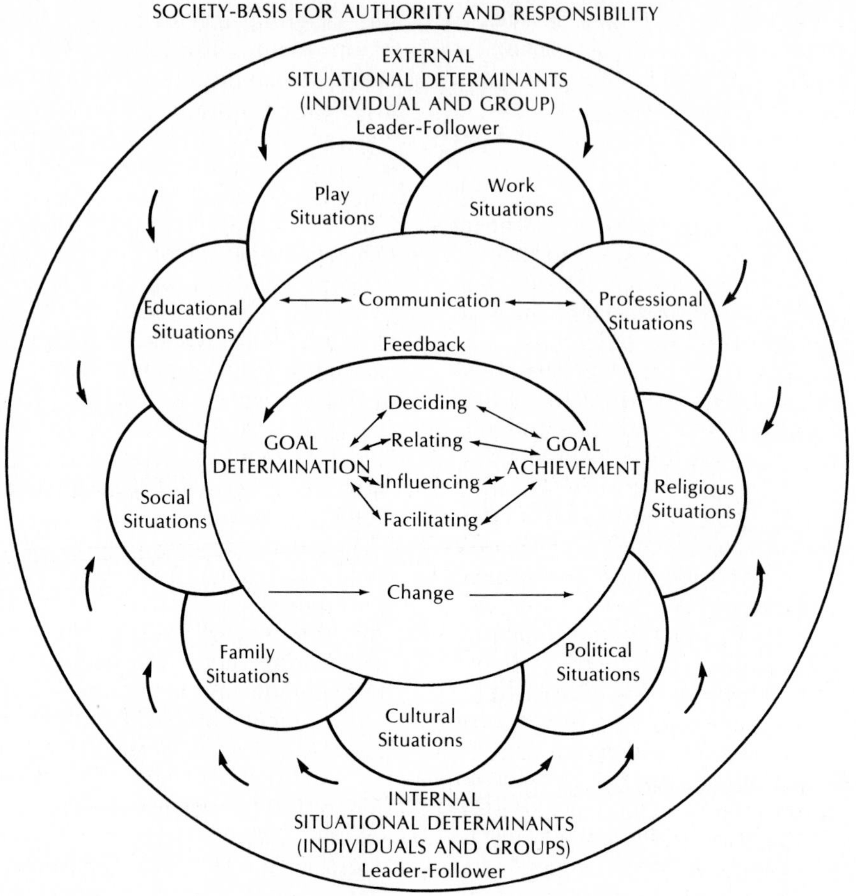

SOCIETY-BASIS FOR AUTHORITY AND RESPONSIBILITY

Figure 16-1. Models of nursing leadership process. (Reprinted with permission from Helen Yura et al: *Nursing Leadership Theory and Process*. 2nd ed. Norwalk, Conn.: Appleton-Century-Crofts, 1981, p. 98.)

Other nursing research on leadership has taken a people-oriented tack. In the last decade, there has been a new interest in learning about contemporary leaders. Safier's oral history gives an exciting insight into the lives and ideas of nurses who attained leadership during and after World War II, a crucial time of change for nursing.[65,66] Vance's doctoral study probably made available the first profile of contemporary nursing leaders, her so-called nursing influentials. Among other things, the composite profile of seventy women and one man (sixty-nine white and two black) showed an average age of fifty-five (range, thirty-eight to eighty); most coming from lower-middle-class (49 percent) and upper-middle class backgrounds (35 percent); 49 percent single and 35 percent married, with 33 percent parents of one to four children; 27 percent educational administrators; 22 percent educators; more than 11 percent administrators of nursing service, and 11.5 percent retired; 62 percent working in large cities, primarily in the northeastern and north-central United States;

and ninety-five having their master's or doctorate, most from eastern universities. Nurse influentials worked an average of forty-five to sixty-four hours a week (more than business executives surveyed), and most traveled from ten to sixty days a year. Almost all wrote (professional journals, books) and had appeared on radio or television, and all participated in some sort of political activity, primarily letter writing, testifying, and lobbying. An interesting comparison can be made between the leadership traits described earlier and what these nursing leaders identified as their source of influence. In order of importance, those traits and characteristics cited as highly important by at least half the respondents were communication skills, intellectual ability, willingness to take risks, interpersonal skills, creativity in thinking, ability to mobilize groups, recognized expertise in an area of the profession, charisma, and innovativeness. Having academic credentials, collegial support, and a professional work position of power/prestige were also considered important. Traits listed as most important for future leaders were scholarship, intelligence, courage, humanism, sense of self, vision, communication abilities, commitment, political abilities, competence, adaptability, drive, and integrity.[67]

About ten years later, Kinsey replicated the study.[68] Kinsey's subjects numbered forty-two, the top 25 percent of the ten nurse influentials identified by each positional nursing leader who was queried. Sixty-two percent (twenty-six) of these nurse influentials had also been included in Vance's study. (While the emergence of new influentials is inevitable, one wonders what, other than death or retirement, took the other forty-five off the new list. As it is, 9 percent of Kinsey's subjects reported retirement.)

There were many similarities between the two studies, with no real difference shown in the influentials' occupations, clinical specialty, geographic location, or sources of influence. The average age was a little younger, and one more man was added. In terms of

hours worked, the major difference was that fewer worked fifty-five to sixty-four hours, and more worked sixty-five and over. These nurses too were highly active and productive.

One interesting observation about these studies is that they show a phenomenon different from other professions, at least according to one educator. Houle notes that a profession's influentials, those who develop and apply new knowledge, are as likely to be drawn from the ranks of the practitioners as from the leadership elite. The latter he identified as *positional leaders,* with a slightly different connotation than that usually applied to this term. They are seen as facilitators—persons who maintain career identification but do not practice their profession directly. Instead, they "teach, do research, organize, administer, regulate, coordinate, and engage in other activities that advance the profession."[69] In nursing the influentials also tend to be the positional leaders.

What are a nursing leader's responsibilities? In the nursing literature, suggestions have been made over the years, many of them related to strengthening nursing, guiding nurses to greater autonomy, and speaking for nursing to other disciplines and to the public. But more than a decade ago, a respected nurse offered four major tasks to which nursing leaders must devote themselves, tasks not yet accomplished:

1. Advancing knowledge through research;

2. Making plans for and preparing personnel in sufficient numbers to meet the nursing needs of society;

3. Creating social systems in which exemplary nursing care, excellent nursing education, and significant scientific inquiry are demonstrated and can flourish; and

4. Identifying and developing nurse leaders who vitalize nursing itself and who utilize their very substantial talents toward identifying and promoting worthwhile and cher-

ished values of the larger society of which nursing is a vital part.[70]

STRATEGIES FOR ACTION

Yes, nursing does have influence. Yes, nursing does have power. This is evident in areas of politics and power. It is evident in the increased status of nursing and in the expansion of nursing practice to every conceivable setting. Hand wringing is not in order. It is probably a healthy sign that so many nurses are saying, "But compared to what we can do and should do, it's not enough." And they're right. The major problems within nursing are caused by the lack of cohesiveness, the lack of agreement on professional goals, the lack of planned leadership development, the heterogeneity of nurses in background, education, and position, the lack of internal support systems, and the divisiveness of nursing subcultures, all coping with a rapidly changing society. If nursing is to have the full autonomy of a profession, there must be unification of purpose and action on major issues. Leadership is vital, but it must be the kind of leadership described by Yura and her colleagues, focusing on shared power directed at accomplishing the profession's goals. Those goals must be agreed upon jointly. Although their selection may indeed be influenced by nurse leaders, the feedback from the grass roots must be a part of the final decision, or achievement of the goals will continue to be an uphill struggle. Therefore, the strategies that are suggested in the following sections are the responsibility not just of nursing leaders, but of all nurses.

Mentors, Networks, Collegiality: The Great Potential

The term *mentoring* is usually defined as a formal or informal relationship between an established older person and a younger one, wherein the older guides, counsels, and critiques the younger, teaching him or her (the protegé) survival and advancement in a particular field. The system has been described as the *patron system,* a continuum of advisory support relationships which facilitate access to positions of leadership, authority, or power.[71] Shapiro et al. selected this term, despite its negative connotations, because these helping individuals function literally as patrons—protectors, benefactors, sponsors, champions, advocates, supporters, and advisors.

At the far end of the continuum is the mentor, the most powerful, most influential individual, and the relationship with the protoegé is the most intense (and perhaps the most stressful). Next is the sponsor—a strong patron, but less powerful than a mentor in shaping or promoting the protegé's career. The guide is next, less able than either of the other two to serve as benefactor or champion, but capable of providing invaluable intelligence and explaining the system, the shortcuts and the pitfalls.

At the beginning of the continuum are the *peer pals,* peers who help each other to succeed and progress. The Shapiro group, which focused on ways to help women, saw this first step as highly important, more like the feminist concept of women helping women, more egalitarian, less intense and exclusionary, and therefore more democratic, by allowing access to a large number of young professionals. They admitted that it was the mentor relationship, restrictive though it might be, that could give the biggest career boost, whereas the peer pal relationship was often a bootstrap operation. However, mentorships are not democratic. Selection may be very idiosyncratic, as described later, and there are always strings attached—if nothing else, the demand to succeed.

Peer pals can create their own "new-order" networks.[72] There is a male corollary—the "good old boy" networks that, through an informal system of relationships, provide advice, information, guidance, contact, protection, and any other support that helps a member of the group, an insider, to achieve his goals, goals obviously not in conflict with

those of the group. The good old boys frequently share the same educational, cultural,
or geographic background, but whatever the
basis of their commonalities, mutual support
is the name of the game. It could be group
pressure; it could be a word to the right person
at the right time; it could be simply multifaceted information sources, but it exists. You can
count on it; you can take risks; you won't be
alone. (And you don't necessarily have to like
each other or agree on everything.) Could this
work for nurses? Why not?

Suppose a system of support could be developed in nursing. Not a good old girl network—no need to duplicate the nearsighted-
ness of the men in their narrow system that so
frequently excludes women—but a *good new
nurse network* that promotes the support *of*
nurses *for* nurses, men or women. A network
that provides backup for the risk takers until
all can become risk takers for a purpose. A
network that shows unified strength on issues
that can be generally agreed upon, so that the
profession as well as the individual practitioner can put into practice the principles of
care to which both voice commitment. A network that avoids destructive self-competition
and instead develops new leaders at all levels
through peer pals, mentors, and role models.
A network that encourages differences of
opinion but provides an atmosphere for reasonable compromise. In essence, a network
that develops and utilizes the essential abilities
of nurses to share, to trust, to depend on one
another.

Puetz describes how to start a network in a
formal sense, almost like a new organization.
It begins with a determination that it is needed
and wanted. Then a core of people can decide
who else to invite, "doers" and "stars" as
well as peer pals. Eventually a meeting is held,
goals are set, and the group is formalized. Actually, most networks start and function more
informally, although they always require that
core of interested people. The rest is almost an
analogy of the old chain letter concept, a
spreading out of contacts. Puetz also offers a
number of practical tips on networking and

notes other good advice about networking
given by Welch:

- learn how to ask questions
- try to give as much as you get
- follow up on contacts
- keep in touch with contacts
- report back to contacts
- be businesslike as you network
- don't be afraid to ask for what you need
- don't pass up any opportunities[73]

Because networking is "in" and is sometimes seen as what one writer called a "quick
fix for moving up," and because it is also new
to many women, it is being abused by some.
Besides the warnings noted above, networkers
are advised to observe both common and uncommon courtesies: don't make excessive requests; be appreciative; be sensitive to your
contacts' situation; and be helpful to others.[74]

There are already nurse networks in operation, often initiated by a nursing organization
or subgroup made up of nurses with common
interests, clinical or otherwise. The participants help each other make contacts[75] when
they relocate, or they supply needed information or suggest someone else who would
know. They alert each other to job opportunities and suggest their colleagues for appointments, presentations, or awards. They give
visibility to nurses, boost each other, and
praise each other, instead of being unnecessarily critical. But they also critique supportively
for professional growth.

Could this also be called collegiality? In a
sense. A *colleague* is usually defined as an associate, particularly in a profession. Yet, beyond this basic phrase, the term is rich in
meaning. In a thesaurus, we also find: ally,
aider, collaborator, helper, partner, peer,
friend, co-operator, co-worker, co-helper, fellow worker, teammate, or even right-hand
man and buddy. The implications are even
richer. Colleagues may be called upon confi-
dently for advice and assistance, and will give
it. Colleagues share knowledge with each
other, together rounding out the necessary information to enhance patient care. Colleagues

challenge each other to think in new ways and to try new ideas. Colleagues encourage risk taking when the situation requires daring. Colleagues provide a support system when the risk taker needs it. Colleagues are equal, yet different—that is, they may have varying educational preparation, experience, and positions, perhaps even belong to another profession, but when they work together for a particular purpose, that work is bettered by their cooperation. And to take it a step further, a collegium may be formed—a group in which each member has approximately equal power.[76]

Clearly, nurse colleagues are part of a nurse network. But developing that spirit of collegiality requires trust, and the trust must be mutually deserved. Then it can also extend beyond the borders of nursing to include other health professionals.

Now to return to the mentoring continuum. Neither the guide nor the sponsor has been given much attention in the literature, perhaps because of semantics. *Sponsor* is often used interchangeably with *mentor,* and both terms often refer to a relationship that is more at the guide level. (Pyles and Stern call this helping relationship the *gray gorilla syndrome.*)[77] For instance, in both nursing service[78] and education,[79] reference is made to neophytes being mentored, when actually those individuals are simply assigned to more experienced people for guidance. Mentors are never assigned; they choose. In the examples given, the level of participation is more at the guide level, perhaps progressing to sponsor if a suitable relationship is established. However, these senior persons are never mentors; they simply aren't powerful enough, and in the time given and considering the number of "protegés" involved, they probably haven't the interest or commitment to be mentors.

Mentorship is an intense relationship calling for a high degree of involvement between a novice in a discipline and a person knowledgeable and wise in that area. On a cognitive level, the mentor is involved with the novice as a whole person. The mentor-protegé relationship is a "serious, mutual, non-sexual, loving relationship," voluntary on the part of both. Levinson,[80] who studied mentor relationships extensively, said that the lack of a mentor is a developmental handicap. Mentoring is part of what Erickson calls *generativity,* in which the primary concern is establishing and guiding the next generation. A mentor acts as:

- teacher to enhance the young person's skills and intellectual development;
- sponsor to ease the neophyte's entry and advancement into the workaday world;
- host and guide to welcome the initiate into a new occupational and social world with its unique values, customs, resources, and cast of characters;
- exemplar to serve as a personal example of virtues, achievements, and ways of life;
- counselor to provide advice and moral support.

Sheehy[81] says that a mentor supports a younger adult's dreams and helps him or her to make them a reality, and is a protector and supporter who provides the extra confidence needed to take on new responsibilities, new tests of competence, and new positions. (Emphasis on competence is of paramount importance; the mentor teaches, supports, advises, and criticizes.) She also notes that the presence or absence of a mentor is enormously important in professional development. Sometimes the mentor is equated with a role model, preceptor, or the master in a master–apprentice situation. But it is more than that. Says Williams, "Achieving a mentor relationship with an older person is like falling in love—you can't force it to happen, and it only works if the chemistry is right. You can, however, make yourself receptive to such a relationship by displaying a teachable attitude and an eagerness to learn."[82] In other words, the apprentice has to show that she or he is someone worth investing in, someone who will show a measure of return by success in the field.

Mentors may be or have been role models

or preceptors, but role models and preceptors are not necessarily mentors. A role model can be merely that—someone to emulate and admire, even with minimal contact, and some perceptorships are carried out with almost total impersonality. Preceptors may overtly carry out their responsibilities to their students and yet withhold a vital element of development.

Because of the time and effort mentors put forth for their protegés (usually for one at a time), protegés are carefully selected. And they *are* selected. True, someone who wants another for a mentor can bring himself or herself to that person's attention, but the protegé must be seen as worthy. One group of executives cited certain qualities that they looked for in potential protegés: has depth, integrity, a curious mind, good interpersonal skills; wants to impress; has an extra dose of commitment; has a capacity to care; can communicate; understands ideas; can identify problems and help find solutions; ambitious; hard-working; willing to do things beyond the call of duty; someone looking for new avenues and new challenges; someone dedicated to a purpose; and always—someone who would be a good representative of the profession.[83]

There is no question that, although protegés get plenty of help, they are expected to produce, to be worth the mentor's time, to make him or her proud. The mentor's rewards are many—seeing someone's potential fulfilled, acquiring a following, and preparing other leaders for the profession. There are dangers to both. The mentor can be overwhelming and try to mold the protegé in his or her image, or the protegé can become too dependent. On the other hand, the protegé can take over the mentor's position; this is one reason that the relationship often ends on a bad note, usually in business, and happens most often when two men are involved. Protegés do outgrow mentors and may move on to another mentor or become mentors themselves. It also happens that a person may be mentor to one person and also give attention to another, although not as intensely.

There is now much literature on mentoring, particularly in business and education and in research studies. A selected list is found in the bibliography. Although almost everyone says that being mentored is a key to success, even quick success, others disagree.[84] After all, there are not enough true mentors for every ambitious person, and yet many succeed with no mentor at all. However, almost everyone had help from someone along the way, and everyone can find someone to be helped by and later someone to help, somewhere along the continuum of the patron system.

Nevertheless, interest in mentoring in nursing has risen in the last decade in terms of preparation for scholarliness,[85] research,[86] and leadership in general. In relation to this last item, it is particularly important to note several pieces of extensive research, all of which point to the importance of mentors in the development of today's nursing leaders.

In Vance's study,[87] 83 percent of the leaders reported having had mentors, and 93 percent were mentors to others. In Kinsey's replication,[88] the percentages were about the same. In both studies, the mentors were primarily women nurse educators (teachers) or teacher colleagues, advisors, and educational administrators. They, in turn, tended to mentor students and professional colleagues. All cited the importance of mentoring in their success. A more extensive nursing study of 500 women graduates of doctoral programs between 1974 and 1979 also showed the effect of mentoring.[89] Their average age was forty-four, and most had senior positions in nursing education. Fifty-seven percent had at least one mentor, who was usually a female nurse; of this group, many had other mentors later, often men. Those mentored attributed much of their development to their mentors, and those not mentored often cited the deprivation. Those mentored were slightly more productive and more satisfied with their work than the others. In answering the question "Would you choose nursing as a lifelong career again?" the mentored were more likely to say yes (56 percent) than the others (47 percent).

(Those who answered "no" said that their choices would have been medicine, law, or business.) Many other details on mentoring are given in this in-depth study. One interesting point is that with the exception of a very few, the mentors and protegés parted amicably and are now friends.

A final study to consider is one done on British women nursing leaders,[90] which likewise showed that most were and had mentors.

It is generally agreed that mentoring can help develop nurses to resolve the issues that face us. The commitment of nursing leaders to be those mentors is essential.

> There are influential nurses in many places. If they are willing to make the commitment of time and effort and caring that makes a true mentor, that influence will expand into more than a nurse's influence and become a nursing influence.[91]

Nurses as Risk Takers and Role Breakers

Grissum, like others, has identified the risk taker and role breaker as essential to changing the nursing image and to acquiring autonomy.[92,93] This involves personal and professional behavior on an individual level, being assertive, taking a stand on an issue, and laying claim to the part of health care that is nursing. It also means making a concerted effort to identify and change those aspects of the nursing image that are incorrect or negative, to help the public understand what nursing is and does.[94] One aspect of this new recognition is the effort made by ANA to get reimbursement for nurses.* Nursing services in institutions are frequently lumped in with the hotel services provided, and the distinct professional nursing services are not winnowed out. Thus, the public often has no idea what nursing care involves. Third-party reimbursement could provide nurses sufficient economic leverage to demand nurse-patient ratios appropriate for rendering of professional services, but nursing must also be able to jus-

tify expensive professional nurses in preference to less prepared personnel. And reimbursement of NPs would give the public greater choice in access to the health care system (and frequently much better care).[95,96]

Another aspect of role breaking is to reinforce the budding colleague relationship between nurses and other health professionals, especially physicians. This should be focused on all aspects of patient care in all places where professional nurses function. NPs and clinical specialists may, because of their specialized knowledge and skills, be quickly identified as colleagues. It has already been shown that primary nurses in hospitals and public health nurses who have full responsibility for nursing care of a group of patients are equally able to function effectively in collegial relationships. Joint practice committees on a state and local level should be nurtured. Too often they are token groups that are not effective and have little influence, particularly in changing medical attitudes.

Another responsibility is to change that in nursing which does not contribute to nursing as an autonomous profession. Some nurses look at nursing simply as a job, and perhaps they always will, unless there is enough peer pressure to stimulate them toward professionalism. Changes are already occurring. There is some indication that more married nurses are seeing nursing as a career and plan an ongoing commitment[97]: the same is true of many nurses just entering the profession.

Overcoming Sexism and Sexist Stereotyping

It is obvious that sexist attitudes have created problems for women nurses, but men nurses, too, complain of a reverse discrimination (Chapter 11). There is no more place for sexism, or male or female chauvinism, in nursing than in other aspects of society. Men and women need to support each other as professionals (and as human beings). Stereotypes are useless at best and destructive at worst. There are those who say that the answer is androgeny, the state in which both sexes feel free to choose from a full range of human behav-

---

*See also Chapter 15.

ior, without being restricted to the behavior ascribed by socialization.[98]

Nevertheless, given the pervasiveness of female sexual stereotyping, women nurses may have to make special efforts to attain overt power and influence.[99] Women and nurses must continue to polish their ability to be assertive, to express their own thoughts or feelings without anxiety and without imposing on the thoughts and feelings of others, and to do so better and more often, especially in the face of opposition. (Assertiveness has been contrasted to aggressiveness, which is not being concerned with others' thoughts and feelings.) Assertiveness helps an individual to resist manipulation, to feel more confident and self-assured. Withers says that for women, lack of assertiveness impairs personal and professional relationships and is one reason there is still widespread societal belief that women are incompetent. "Eventually the process becomes circular; women don't feel equal, so they don't act equal, so they aren't treated equally, so they don't feel equal . . . and so on."[100] Assertiveness training[101] has become popular, as have books on the topic,[102-104] but it is, first of all, important for unassertive persons to have confidence that their thoughts and feelings are worthwhile and to *want* to change. Actually, good assertiveness training builds on the effective ways in which an individual has always handled difficult situations, and many women already have the tact and sensitivity that is a useful base for assertiveness. A further step for women nurse leaders is to learn some of the techniques of gaining and holding power at top levels.

Political Action

Politics may be defined as the art or science of influencing policy. There is a legitimate tendency to think of politics in the context of government, but affecting policy and operations at the institutional level is often just as important in the work life of a nurse. The term *in-house law* has been used to describe the power nurses can have if they can determine policies and procedures that affect daily

practice. An example is policy stating that nurses may (or should or must) develop and implement teaching plans for patients or arrange for referrals to the visiting nurse, all of which have been blocked by physicians or administrators in some hospitals.

It is vital that nurses participate actively in the agencies or community groups where decisions are being made, such as local or state planning agencies.[105] The strategy used to gain input may vary. A basic principle is applicable: before, during, and after gaining entrée, nurses must show that they are knowledgeable, that they have something to offer, and that they can put it all together into an action package. There are many places to start, for most community groups are looking for members who work and are willing to hold office (for example, church groups, societies, and PTAs). These activities may be seen as (1) a way of getting experience on boards, using parliamentary procedure to advantage, politicking, gaining some sophistication in participating and guiding decisions, and (2) being visible to other groups and the public. Many community groups interlock, and, by being active in some, nurses come in contact with others. It also helps to gain support of women other than nurses. Organized women are becoming more successful in getting representation on policymaking groups. It pays for them to have someone who is ready and able to assume such responsibilities. But participating nurses must be capable; there is nothing worse than having an incompetent as the first nurse on a major board or committee. At this stage of nurses' reach for influence, it could do the profession more damage than having a non-nurse, for it appears that women (and nurses) still have to be better than those already in power to gain initial respect.

Another aspect to consider and use is the potential economic power of nurses. A director who controls a multi-million-dollar budget wields power in how that money is spent. On the other hand, those nurses who have major responsibility for patient care and have no budgeting control are at an immediate disadvantage. Budgetary control (and administrative control), which may include workers other than nurses, increases nurse administrators' circle of power, but they must act on it. The aura of status enables these nurses to move in power circles where they can cultivate individuals who influence public and private decision making. Community nurses are also particularly good resources, because most make strong community contacts. Today, the participation of the consumer in health care decisions is increasing. An activated consumer who supports nursing has impact on local decision making as well as on state and national legislation. A legislator is more inclined to hear the consumer who presumably is a neutral participant, as opposed to an obvious interest group. But nursing must sell that consumer the profession's point of view and balance consumer needs and nursing goals.

Although it is often through the influence of consumer groups and the community's traditional power figures that nurses get on decision-making committees, boards, and similar groups, after that, they're on their own and must be prepared, perceptive, articulate, and under control. In meetings, at coffee breaks, the politicking and the formation of coalitions may well determine which way a decision goes. Nurses who haven't learned to play that game had better take lessons: using role play, assertiveness training, group therapy, group process, speech lessons—whatever is necessary.

As Stevens advises power seekers:

• Pay the entry fee
• Have a voice
• Have something to say
• Look upward and outward (not just at nursing)
• Act like a powerful person[106]

This kind of political participation will be particularly important as the cost control mentality gains momentum.[107]

On the level of governmental politics, nurses can and have influenced not only such issues as Social Security, quality assurance, patient rights, and care of the long-term pa-

tient, but have a vital interest in such issues as reimbursement for nursing services, nurse licensure, and funds for nursing education. The specifics of the legislative process and guidelines for action are described in Chapter 18. However, there is no reason that nurses should not run for office. They are intelligent, frequently well educated, and know a lot about human relations. Although none have yet been elected to national office, those who have won state offices are not only effective, but often offer extraordinary insight into health issues. Some have been responsible for major legislative breakthroughs for nurses. For instance, in Maryland, not only was legislation passed providing reimbursement for the services of nurse-midwives and NPs, but effective July 1979, the General Assembly passed the first law requiring insurance companies to reimburse for any services "within the lawful scope of practice of a duly licensed health care provider"—all initiated or strongly supported by the nurse legislators. For those nurses who choose to run for office, it is important to learn all the tricks of the trade;[108] amateurs seldom win. The accepted route is to become involved first with local politics or to work in the campaign of an influential figure. For women, there are advantages and disadvantages. In a study of women officeholders in New Jersey, Tambarlane[109] found that some women were given opportunities or encouraged by their parties because they wanted to run one woman against another. However, an interesting finding was noted:

> When women's political work and/or success places strains on existing male dominant power relationships within the family or the party, men, perhaps fearing to lose their privileged positions—subtly or overtly—may withdraw their support.

This was certainly evidenced by some politicians' reactions to Geraldine Ferraro, first woman candidate for the U.S. vice-presidency, when her husband's financial affairs were criticized. It also has been found that women suffer discrimination by being excluded from certain all-male organizations such as the Jaycees, Kiwanis, Rotary, and Lions, where the groundwork for political and other appointments is often done. This may or may not change since the Supreme Court ruled against sexual discrimination; there are still back rooms, however.

One noteworthy item is the appointment of nurses to important state and national political offices, such as head of the U.S. Health Care Finance Administration.

Regardless of the setting, there are some basic guidelines for effective political action. First is to be a lifelong student of the social and technical aspect of professional practice; second, to know the current professional issues and the implications for various alternative actions; third, to be aware of emerging social and political issues and trends that will affect health care and nursing; fourth, to learn others' points of view (those of potential supporters or opponents) and come to terms with what policy changes are possible, as well as desirable; and fifth, to seek allies who can espouse or at least see the desirability of a particular course of action.[110]

Accountability and Professionalism

Without demonstrating accountability for practice, nursing will never be or be considered an autonomous profession. Standard setting, peer review, continued competence, and protection of patients' rights* all indicate that nursing is taking on the responsibilities to see that the public is protected. However, more nurses must also recognize that for nurses to be professional, the majority of practitioners must consider it a career and make the time, effort, and commitment necessary to participate in the key decision making.

Professional Unity, Professional Pride

It has long been a political precept that the most powerful groups are those that are

united. Almost always this means that an organization speaks for that group, and that is one of the purposes of a professional organization. Nursing has many organizations representing various interest groups (Chapters 24–28). At times they cooperate, but too often they are at odds or simply act separately. Fortunately, there is more concerted effort being made by most to form political coalitions in relation to important issues for nurses. Of serious concern, however, is what Lewis calls the *professionally uncommitted*. In an outstanding editorial even more appropriate today, she states:

It is scarcely newsworthy to observe that nursing is facing many problems today; that was equally true yesterday and will be tomorrow. But what troubles me today is the magnitude and import of our problems on the one hand, and the relatively small number of nurses taking part in the deliberations and decisions, on the other. Such issues as entry into practice, collective bargaining, and the credentialing recommendations must be resolved by the professional organization; yet the percentage of nurses in this country who are members of it is very small indeed. Sadder yet, some nurses seem almost unaware of the idea of nursing as a profession or of the issues that confront it. Why this alienation, deliberate or unwitting, from the profession of which all nurses are a part?

Nonmembership in the professional organization, I believe, is only one symptom of a deeper malaise: a pervasive lack of what I will call a professional identity. Many nurses are committed to nursing, as they perceive it within the boundaries of their particular job. Most of them, I'm sure, carry out their individual nursing functions to the best of their abilities, want to do whatever they're doing, better. But they are not committed to nursing as a self-determining, self-regulating profession and an important force in the health care field.[111]

Lewis maintains that it is essential to cultivate a professional identity early in nurses' educa-

---

*Patients' rights are discussed extensively in Chapters 10, 20, and 22; professionalism in Chapter 9; and accountability in Chapter 10.

tion and to make the profession and organization more relevant to their daily practice. The fact that nurses in influential positions, including faculty, also seem to lack professional identification deprives young nurses of professional role models. She concludes:

> But unless we take this problem seriously, there is a risk that nursing will cease to speak with a single, forceful voice, but will speak instead in the million and a half voices of individual nurses in this country, or in the fragmented voices of many specialty groups. Under those circumstances, who will listen and who will heed? Not the public, I'm afraid, nor the other health care professions, nor even nurses themselves.[111]

Others have agreed that the need for support of the professional organization, where unity and a resolution of internal problems must occur, is crucial if nursing is to be an autonomous, influential power group.[112,113]

Unity is hard to achieve, however, if you're not proud of yourself and your profession and what it stands for. If you're embarrassed by nursing's image or if, worse yet, you believe it. Because then, nurses are not a group with whom you want to be identified. Unity is not important because it doesn't seem worth the effort. The feeling of powerlessness is a comfort, in a sense, because it excuses you from taking action. That action can be taken is amply illustrated in the preceding pages. To look at the image of nursing is to see what you want to see. A nurse is not one kind of person, good or bad, handmaiden or entrepreneur. Nursing, like its components, has various images at various times. When you are that reflection, it should be what you want nursing to be. A small point—or, perhaps, a large one: the fashionable image might be woman as slob, but nurse as slob is distasteful. Twenty years ago, how to dress was taught in nursing schools to young working-class women. A sloppy uniform was cause for a reprimand. The same was true for the RN. Then that was no longer considered appropriate; modern women knew how to dress and behave in a so-

cially correct manner without receiving grammar school lessons. Are the results evident today? But perhaps we've come full circle. The business literature aimed at men and women is full of advice on "dressing for success," and now it might be nursing's turn. What is nursing's image when a patient is cared for by an unkempt nurse in nondescript clothes with long hair sweeping across the supine body? Yes, the public does notice. One individual being treated in a college health clinic reported, "I wondered who that person was in blue jeans and a top like men's underwear." A noted editor said at a meeting, "If you nurses are so worried about your image, you'd better clean up your nurses." Not you? Then perhaps a little peer pressure would help—a little direct or indirect action. Personal image and nonverbal behavior do convey a message—it could be a message of "no pride, no interest."[114]

Finally, it is time to look at what nursing has accomplished and is continuing to accomplish. It is a career of unlimited opportunities.[115] It has produced documented evidence that its practitioners make major contributions to health care.[116] It has exercised political power for the good of the public.[117] There's a lot to be legitimately proud of, even if there is unfinished business. Power and autonomy do not come to the spineless, the indifferent or downtrodden, or those who think they are.

Everyone has his or her own concerns, but individuals acting in isolation are vulnerable. Jordan notes that in this era of social revolution, more and more individuals are uniting to secure their legitimate rights and privileges.[118] Why would nursing want less? As Edith Draper, one of nursing's leaders, said in 1893, "To advance, we must unite."

REFERENCES

1. Christy Dachelet and Judith Sullivan, "Autonomy in Practice," *Nurse Practitioner,* 4:15 (Mar.–Apr. 1979).
2. Jo Ann Ashley, *Hospitals, Paternalism, and the Role of the Nurse* (New York: Teachers College Press, 1976), p. 93.

3. Barbara Brown, "The Autonomous Nurse and Primary Nursing," *Nurs. Admin. Q.,* **1**:33 (Fall 1976).

4. Merriam-Webster, *Webster's New Collegiate Dictionary* (Springfield, Ma.: G. & C. Merriam Company, 1975), p. 902.

5. John Harsanyi, "Measurement of Social Power, Opportunity Costs, and the Theory of Two-Person Bargaining Games," in Roderick Bell et al., eds., *Political Power* (New York: Free Press, 1969), p. 226.

6. John French and Bertram Raven, "The Base of Social Power," in Dorwin Cartwright, ed., *Studies in Social Power* (Ann Arbor: Institute of Social Research, University of Michigan, 1959), pp. 150–167.

7. Karen Dennis, "Nursing's Power in the Organization: What Research Has Shown," *Nurs. Admin.,* **98**:47–57 (Fall 1983).

8. Lucie Kelly, "Endpaper: Nursing Hegemony," *Nurs. Outlook,* **26**:224 (Mar. 1979).

9. Lucie Kelly, "Endpaper: The Power of Powerlessness," *Nurs. Outlook,* **25**:468 (July 1979).

10. T. Jacobs, *Leadership and Exchange in Formal Organizations* (Alexandria, Va.: Human Resources Research Organization, 1970), p. 4.

11. D. McClelland, *Power: The Inner Experience* (New York: Irvington Publications, 1975), p. 263.

12. D. McClelland and D. Burnham, "Power Is the Great Motivator," *Harv. Bus. Rev.,* **54**:100 (Mar.–Apr. 1976).

13. Cheryl Tatano, "The Conceptualization of Power," *Adv. Nurs. Sci.,* **4**:2–17 (Jan. 1982).

14. Margaret Hennig and Anne Jardim, *The Managerial Woman* (Garden City, N.Y.: Anchor Press/Doubleday, 1977), pp. 108–154.

15. Rosemary Bowman and Rebecca Culpepper, "Power: Rx for Change," *Am. J. Nurs.,* **74**:1054 (June 1974).

16. Marlene Grissum and Carol Spengler, *Womanpower and Health Care* (Boston: Little, Brown and Company, 1976), pp. 95–127, 193–213.

17. Connie Vance, "Women Leaders: Modern Day Heroines or Social Deviants?" *Image,* **11**:39–41 (June 1979).

18. Rose Le Roux, "Sex-Role Stereotyping and Leadership," *Nurs. Admin. Q.,* **1**:21–29 (Fall 1976).

19. Bonnie Bullough, "The Struggle for Women's Rights in Denver: A Personal Account," *Nurs. Outlook,* **26**:566–567 (Sept. 1978).

20. Lucie Kelly, "Endpaper: In Our Imperfect State," *Nurs. Outlook,* **27**:368 (May 1979).

21. Dorothy Brooten et al., *Leadership for Change: A Guide for the Frustrated Nurse* (Philadelphia: J. B. Lippincott Company, 1978), pp. 35–41.

22. Ruth Edelstein, "Management in American Nursing," *Int. Nurs. Rev.,* **26**(2):78 (1979).

23. Luther Christman, "The Autonomous Nursing Staff in Hospital," *Nurs. Admin. Q.,* **1**:37–44 (Fall 1976).

24. Luther Christman, "The Autonomous Nursing Staff in the Hospital," *Nurs. Digest,* **6**:72 (Summer 1978).

25. Genrose J. Alfano, "Healing or Care Taking—Which Will It Be?" *Nurs. Clinics of North America,* **6**:273–280 (June 1971).

26. Anonymous, "Change, Conflict, Continuing Education, Competency," *Sup. Nurse,* **10**:26–34 (Apr. 1979).

27. Juanita Murphy and Mary Schmetz, "The Clinical Nurse Specialist: Implementing the Role in a Hospital Setting," *J. Nurs. Admin.,* **9**:29–31 (Jan. 1979).

28. Paul Bergeson and Nancy Melvin, "Granting Hospital Privileges to Nurse Practitioners," *Hospitals,* **49**:99–101 (Aug. 16, 1975).

29. Nancy Melvin, "Developing Guidelines for Clinical Privileges for Nurse Practitioners," in *Power: Nursing's Challenge for the Future* (Kansas City, Mo.: American Nurses' Association, 1979), pp. 62–67.

30. Lucie Kelly, "Endpaper: The Eternal Fascination of Nursing Education," *Nurs. Outlook,* **26**:403 (June 1978).

31. Beatrice Kalisch, "Of Half-gods and Mortals: Aesculapian Authority," *Nurs. Outlook,* **23**:22–28 (Jan. 1975).

32. Leonard Stein, "The Doctor–Nurse Game," *Arch. Gen. Psychiat.,* **16**:699–703 (June 1967). Reprinted in *Am. J. Nurs.,* **68**:101–105 (Jan. 1968), and other publications.

33. Beatrice Kalisch and Philip Kalisch, "An Analysis of the Sources of Physician–Nurse Conflict," *J. Nurs. Admin.,* **7**:51–57 (Jan. 1977).

34. Joan Lynaugh and Barbara Bates, "The Two Languages of Nursing and Medicine," *Am. J. Nurs.,* **73**:66–69 (Jan. 1973).

35. Shirley Smoyak, "Problems in Interprofessional Relations," *Bull. N.Y. Acad. Med.,* **77**:51–59 (Jan.-Feb. 1977). Reprinted in N. Chaska, *The Nursing Profession: Views Through the Mist* (New York: McGraw-Hill Book Company, 1978).

36. Jo Ann Ashley, "Power in Structured Misogyny: Implications for the Politics of Care," *Adv. Nurs. Sci.,* **2**:3–22 (Apr. 1980).

37. Mariann Lovell, "The Politics of Medical Deception: Challenging the Trajectory of History," *Adv. Nurs. Sci.,* **2**:73–86 (Apr. 1980).

38. Jane Record and Merwyn Greenlick, "New Health Professionals and the Physician Role: An Hypothesis from the Kaiser Experience," *Nurs. Digest,* **4**:65–68 (Winter 1976).

39. H. Pratt, "The Doctor's View of the Changing Nurse–Physician Relationship," *J. Med. Educ.,* **40**:767–771 (Aug. 1965).

40. C. K. Hofling, et al., "Experimental Study in Nurse–Physician Relationships," *J. Nerv. Ment. Dis.,* **143**:171–180 (Aug. 1966).

41. Roseanne Krcek and Irving Krcek, "The Necessity for New Colleague Relationships Between Professionals," *Nurs. Digest,* **4**:83–85 (Summer 1976).

42. Pamela Devereux, "Essential Elements of Nurse–Physician Collaboration," *J. Nurs. Admin.,* **11**:19–23 (May 1981).

43. Anna Alt-White et al., "Personal, Organizational and Managerial Factors Related to Nurse–Physician Collaboration," *Nurs. Admin. Q.,* **8**:8–18 (Fall 1983).

44. Dianne Anderson and Mary Catherine Finn, "Collaborative Practice: Developing a Structure That Works," *Nurs. Admin. Q.,* **8**:19–25 (Fall 1983).

45. Patricia Trinasky, "Nurse–Doctor Dissension Still Thrives," *Sup. Nurse,* **10**:40–43 (Apr. 1979).

46. Lynne Welch, "Planned Change in Nursing: The Theory," *Nurs. Clin. North Am.,* **14**:307 (June 1979).

47. Ibid., 313–320.

48. Elizabeth Olson, "Strategies and Techniques for the Nurse Change Agent," *Nurs. Clin. North Am.,* **14**:323–329 (June 1979).

49. Agnes Reinkemeyer, "Nursing's Need: A Commitment to an Ideology of Change," *Nurs. Forum,* **9**:341–355 (1970).

50. Olson, op. cit., 329–330.

51. Ibid., 334–335.

52. Shirley Smoyak, "The Confrontation Process," *Am. J. Nurs.,* **74**:1632–1635 (Sept. 1974).

53. L. D. Haskew, "Dimensions of Professional Leadership," *J. Natl. Ed. Assn.,* **50**(2):30–32 (1961).

54. Helen Yura et al., *Nursing Leadership: Theory and Process* (New York: Appleton-Century-Crofts, 1976), pp. 17–23.

55. R. M. Stogdill, *Handbook of Leadership—A Survey of Theory and Research* (New York: Free Press, 1974), p. 81.

56. Margaret Colton, "Nursing's Leadership Vacuum," *Sup. Nurs.,* **7**:29 (Oct. 1976).

57. Madeleine Leininger, "The Leadership Crisis in Nursing: A Critical Problem and Challenge," *J. Nurs. Admin.,* **4**:30 (Mar.-Apr. 1974).

58. Helen Yura et al., *Nursing Leadership: Theory and Process,* 2nd ed. (New York: Appleton-Century-Crofts, 1981), pp. 84–127.

59. R. Tannenbaum et al., *Leadership and Organization,* (New York: McGraw-Hill Book Company, 1961).

60. Yura et al., *Nursing Leadership,* 2nd. ed., p. 88.

61. Ibid., p. 90.

62. Ibid., p. 94.

63. Ibid., p. 99–100.

64. Dorothy Brooten, *Managerial Leader-*

ship in Nursing (New York: J. B. Lip-pincott, Company, 1984), pp. 34–35.

65. Gwendolyn Safier, "Leaders Among Contemporary U.S. Nurses: An Oral History," in Chaska, op. cit.

66. Gwendolyn Safier, *Contemporary American Leaders in Nursing—An Oral History* (New York: McGraw-Hill Book Company, 1977).

67. Connie Vance, "A Group Profile of Contemporary Influentials in American Nursing," unpublished Ed.D. dissertation, Teachers College, Columbia University, 1977.

68. Dianne Kinsey, "An Updated Group Profile of Contemporary Influentials in American Nursing," unpublished Ed.D. dissertation, Lehigh University, 1985.

69. Andrea O'Connor, "Continuing Education for Nursings's Leaders," in Norma Chaska, ed., *The Nursing Profession: A Time to Speak* (New York: McGraw-Hill Book Company., 1983), pp. 156–165.

70. Rozella Schlotfeldt, "Knowledge, Leaders and Progress," *Image,* **2**:2–5 (Feb. 1968).

71. Eileen Shapiro et al., "Moving Up: Role Models, Mentors, and the Patron System," *Sloan Mgt. Rev.,* **19**:51 (Spring 1978).

72. Lucie Kelly, "Endpaper: The Good New Nurse Network," *Nurs. Outlook,* **26**:70 (Jan. 1978).

73. Belinda Puetz, *Networking for Nurses* (Rockville, Md.: Aspen Systems Corp., 1983), pp. 63–80.

74. Janice Handler, "Networking: The Rules of the Game," *Savvy,* **5**:90–91 (Apr. 1984).

75. Lucie Kelly, "Endpaper: Contacts," *Nurs. Outlook,* **28**:396 (June 1980).

76. Lucie Kelly, "Endpaper: This Is My Colleague," *Nurs. Outlook,* **29**:488 (Aug. 1981).

77. Sue Pyles and Phyllis Stern, "Discovery of Nursing Gestalt in Critical Care Nursing: The Importance of the Gray Gorilla Syndrome," *Image,* **15**:51–57 (Spring 1983).

78. M. Michael Fagan and Patricia Fagan, "Mentoring Among Nurses," *Nurs. and Health Care,* **3**:77–82 (Feb. 1983).

79. Stephanie Pardue, "The Who-What-

Why of Mentor Teacher/Graduate Student Relationship," *J. Nurs. Ed.,* **22**:32–37 (Jan. 1983).

80. Daniel Levinson, et al., *The Seasons of a Man's Life* (New York; Knopf, 1978).

81. Gail Sheehy, *Passages: Predictable Crises of Adult Life* (New York: E. P. Dutton & Co., Inc., 1976).

82. Marcelle Williams, *The New Executive Woman* (Radnor, Pa.: Chilton Book Company, 1977).

83. Sylvia Rivchun, "Be a Mentor and Leave a Lasting Legacy," *Ass'n. Mgt.,* **132**:71–74 (Aug. 1980).

84. Sharan Merriam, "Mentors and Protegés: A Critical Review of the Literature," *Adult Ed. Q.,* **33**:161–173 (Spring 1983).

85. Kathleen May et al., "Mentorship for Scholarliness: Opportunities and Dilemmas," *Nurs. Outlook,* **30**:22–28 (Jan. 1982).

86. Harriet Werley and B. Joan Newcomb, "The Research Mentor: A Missing Element in Nursing?" Chaska, ed., *The Nursing Profession,* pp. 202–215.

87. Vance, op. cit.

88. Kinsey, op. cit.

89. Carol Spengler, "Mentor–Protegé Relationships: A Study of Career Development Among Female Nurse Doctorates," unpublished Ph.D. dissertation, University of Missouri-Columbia, 1982.

90. Leslie Hardy, "The Emergence of Nursing Leaders—a Case of in Spite Of, Not Because Of," *Nurs. Times,* **79**:1–4 (Jan. 1983).

91. Lucie Kelly, "Endpaper: Power Guide—The Mentor Relationship," *Nurs. Outlook,* **26**:339 (May 1978).

92. Marlene Grissum, "How You Can Become a Risk Taker and a Role Breaker," *Nurs. 76,* **6**:89–98 (Nov. 1978).

93. Lucie Kelly, "Endpaper: How to Start a Counterculture," *Nurs. Outlook,* **27**:149 (Feb. 1979).

94. Denise Benton, "You Want to Be a *What*?" *Nurs. Outlook,* **27**:388–393 (June 1979).

95. Carole Jennings, "Nursing's Case for Third Party Reimbursement," *Am. J. Nurs.,* **79**:111–114 (Jan. 1979).

96. Donna Diers and Susan Molde, "Nurses

in Primary Care: The New Gatekeepers?" *Am. J. Nurs.,* **83**:742–745 (May 1983).

97. Lucie Kelly, "Endpaper: Goodbye, Appliance Nurse," *Nurs. Outlook,* **27**:432 (June 1979).

98. Patricia Dean, "Toward Androgeny," *Image,* **10**:10–14 (Feb. 1978).

99. Renee Lieb, "Power, Powerlessness and Potential—Nurses' Role Within the Health Care Delivery System," *Image,* **10**:75–82 (Oct. 1978).

100. Jean Withers, "Background: Why Women Are Unassertive," *Nurs. Digest,* **6**:70 (Fall 1978).

101. Holly Hutchings and Louise Colburn, "An Assertiveness Training Program for Nurses," *Nurs. Outlook,* **27**:394–397 (June 1979).

102. Manuel Smith, *When I Say No, I Feel Guilty* (New York: Dial Press, 1975).

103. *Woman, Assert Your Self: An Instructive Handbook* (New York: Harper & R w, Publishers, 1976).

104. S eehy, op. cit.

105. Melinda McLemore, "Nurses as Health Planners—Our New Legal Status," *Nurs. Digest,* **5**:59–60 (Spring 1977).

106. Barbara Stevens, "Power and Politics for the Nurse Executive," *Nurs. and Health Care,* **1**:208–212 (Nov. 1980).

107. Lucie Kelly, "On the Danger of Sawing Off Tree Limbs," *Nurs. Outlook,* **31**:155 (May–June 1983).

108. Thom, Mary, "Running for Office,"

MS. Magazine, **2**:61–68 (Apr. 1974).

109. "A Distaff 'Look' to Politics," *Weekend Dispatch* (New Jersey), Sept. 16, 1978, p. 2.

110. Mary Kelly Mullane, "Nursing Care and the Political Arena," *Nurs. Outlook,* **23**:697–701 (Nov. 1975).

111. Edith Lewis, "The Professionally Uncommitted," Editorial, *Nurs. Outlook,* **27**:323 (May 1979).

112. Beatrice Kalisch, "The Promise of Power," *Nurs. Outlook,* **26**:42–50 (Jan. 1978).

113. Sister Dorothy Sheahan, "Scanning the Seventies," *Nurs. Outlook,* **26**:33–37 (Jan. 1978).

114. Kathleen Stevens, "Personal Effectiveness of a Power Source," in Kathleen Stevens, ed., *Power and Influence: A Source Book for Nurses* (New York: John Wiley and Sons, Inc., 1983), pp. 217–246.

115. Lucie Kelly, "Endpaper: Debunking the Dead-end Dogma," *Nurs. Outlook,* **29**:200 (Mar. 1981).

116. Lucie Kelly, "Endpaper: A Celebration of Nursing," *Nurs. Outlook,* **30**:322 (May 1982).

117. Lucie Kelly, "Endpaper: Not Bad, Nursing," *Nurs. Outlook,* **25**:275 (Apr. 1978).

118. Clifford Jordan, "To Advance, We Must Unite," *Nurs. Outlook,* **29**:482–483 (Aug. 1981).

LEGAL RIGHTS
AND
RESPONSIBILITIES

17

An Introduction to Law

Law has been defined as "the sum total of rules and regulations by which society is governed. It is man-made and regulates social conduct in a formal and binding way. It reflects society's needs, attitudes, and mores."[1] The more complex the society is, the more complicated the legal system that governs it and also the more likely that the law will be in a state of change. Everyone dealing with law knows that there is no final or absolute answer—something that is quite frustrating for those who want to know exactly what they can or cannot do. Yet, there are certain principles that may serve as guidelines and as a basis of understanding American law.

ORIGINS OF MODERN LAW

The first "laws" were set up by the leaders of primitive peoples who found they could not live successfully in groups without rules or codes to govern them. Certain leaders, known as *lawgivers,* sometimes had prevailing customs and traditions set down as the basic law of the land. One of their early tasks was to distinguish between sensible laws and those that were merely taboos or superstitions.

The most illustrious lawgiver of ancient history was Hammurabi, king of Babylon (2067–2025 B.C.), who developed a detailed code of laws to be used by the courts throughout the empire. Known as the *Code of Hammurabi,* the text was inscribed on stone columns, the ruins of which are now in the Louvre in Paris.

The laws governing Greece remained unwritten until about 621 B.C., when Draco, an Athenian statesman and lawgiver, codified them. Although the code was a marked advance toward equal justice under the law for all people, it was so stern (demanding the death penalty for nearly all crimes) that the word *Draconian* is still used to describe an unduly cruel person or action. Draco's code was replaced by a milder one prepared under the direction of Solon (c. 638–558 B.C.) and was later revised by Plato (c. 428–c. 348 B.C.).

In Rome, Emperor Justinian 1 (A.D. 483–565) appointed a commission of legal experts to prepare a revision—actually a consolidation—of Rome's inefficient set of laws, which had developed over a period of approximately 1,000 years. This revision, the *Corpus Juris Civilis,* issued in four parts, served as a basis for civil law in most European countries and in England. Later it had considerable influence on the structure of laws in the United

States. The third part of the document, the *Digest* (A.D. 533), intended for use by judges and practitioners of the law, contained the law in concrete form and was by far the most important section, influencing jurists and scholars for many years, possibly even to this day.

Another famous code of laws, parts of which are still in effect in France, was prepared under the leadership of Emperor Napoleon of France (1769–1821). The legal system of the state of Louisiana, once a French colony, was originally based on the Napoleonic Code; all other colonies based their laws on the English system of common law.

In England, centuries ago, the king reigned supreme, but because of great distances and limited communication facilities, he found it necessary to enlist the help of lords and barons in settling disputes in their geographic areas. He, however, retained the privilege of overriding or vetoing their decisions if he deemed it to the crown's or the kingdom's advantage to do so.

The lords and barons, in turn, passed on authority for settling certain disputes to persons of lesser standing, retaining the power of veto over their decisions. To achieve a degree of order and uniformity, the same persons traveled from place to place in the manner of circuit judges to hear arguments pro and con and serve as mediators in settling controversies. It was quite natural for these "judges" to make similar decisions when cases presented similar sets of circumstances.

As so often happens, the administrative official (in this case, the king of England) became concerned lest some of his power be stripped from him, and he took steps to regain and centralize control over the dispensation of justice throughout his land. This he did by assuming responsibility for the appointment of judges to preside over hearings of disputes to be held in designated places called the *king's courts*. To help them in their duties and serve as guides for future deliberations, the judges often kept written records of their decisions for their personal use. Later, the keeping of such records became mandatory. These records and the principles found therein were the foundation of common law.

With the introduction of written decisions, one of the most important principles known in the law was born, the principal of *stare decisis,* which means to stand as decided or "let the decision stand."

> When a previous case involving similar facts has been decided in the jurisdiction, the court will be strongly inclined to follow the principles of law laid down in that prior adjudication. Unless precedents are carefully regarded and adhered to, uncertainty would be both perplexing and prejudicial to the public. However, when the precedent is out of date or inapplicable to the case before the court, the principle of *stare decisis* will not be followed and the court will announce a new rule.[2]

Courts of law presided over by competent lawyers quickly gained the confidence and respect of the English people. As a result, common law achieved extraordinary power, at times claimed to be even greater than that of the reigning monarch, whose arbitrary despotism remained almost unquestioned until the barons forced King John to sign the Magna Carta in 1215 at Runnymede. The following excerpts from the Magna Carta are applicable to some of the current issues in our society:

> No freeman shall be taken, or imprisoned, or outlawed, or exiled, or in any way harmed, nor will we go upon or send upon him, save by the lawful judgment of his peers or by the law of the land. [Article 39]
>
> To none will we sell, to none deny or delay, right or justice. [Article 40]

These clauses were the antecedents of due process of law and the guarantee of trial by jury. The charter also provided for a committee of twenty-five barons to enforce it. This was the beginning in England of a government that provided a system of checks and balances that would keep the monarchy strong but prevent its perversion by a tyrannic or inept king or queen. Though severely tested at times, government in England from then on meant more than the despotic rule of one person; custom and law stood even above the king.

The British Parliament, the supreme national legislative body, established in 1295 and actually an outgrowth of the Magna Carta, marked the beginning of self-government in England. It took its name from the French *parlement* (derived from *parler,* "to speak"), which in France was originally used to describe any meeting for discussion or debate. The English form *parliament* was first used to designate a debate, later a formal conference only. The laws enacted by this body were termed *statutory law,* as contrasted to *common law.* The rules and regulations developed to guide the deliberations of Parliament, and now widely used in other countries, are often called *parliamentary law.* They are not laws, however, and are more correctly termed *parliamentary procedure.*

THE UNITED STATES LEGAL SYSTEM

As the American colonies were founded one by one, the manner in which they would be governed was a vital and primary consideration. The edicts of the governments in the homelands of the settlers were a persuasive force, of course; in addition, the colonists were influenced greatly by their own previous experience and knowledge. From the beginning, self-government became their goal, a goal that seemed more attainable in the English colonies than in those originally settled by the Spanish and French.

One of the early problems was to establish methods of dealing with disputes over property and personal injuries. To handle such disputes, the Pilgrim Fathers adopted a system similar to that of the common law then in effect in England. Judges were appointed and courts established, but because the life and customs were so different here from those in England, it often proved impractical and unfair to apply decisions that had been made in the mother country. Furthermore, the problems within the colonies varied so widely that

a judge's decision regarding a dispute in one colony was not necessarily applied by another judge to a similar set of circumstances in another. Each colony, therefore, developed its own procedures and laws, both common and statutory, based on its own peculiar needs.

From this evolved the concept of *states' rights,* which has played such an important role in the history of the United States. For many years, any infringement of these rights either from the federal government or from other states was vigorously opposed, although in recent years there has been less resistance to the initiation of federal programs that assume or share responsibilities that for years were carried by the individual states alone.

It is not unusual, of course, for several states to adopt in their separate legislatures an identical law, such as that governing the age at which people may vote if they meet other qualifications. The fact remains, however, that a state that enacts its own laws can retain, revise, or repeal them without interference from other states or the federal government. Relinquishment of this right is a serious matter in a democracy, because doing so sets a precedent that may be difficult to overcome. On the other hand, variance in state laws also gives rise to a great deal of confusion, misunderstanding, and red tape. How much simpler it would be, for example, if the laws governing the licensure of nurses and the practice of nursing were uniform throughout the country—providing they were adequate laws, of course.

The founders of the United States did not depend on common law alone to govern the colonies; neither did they give unlimited power to the governors and councils appointed by the governments of their homelands. To establish and maintain a degree of control, each of the original thirteen colonies early in its history established legislative bodies elected by the voters. The first was the House of Burgesses, which met in Jamestown, Virginia, in 1619 and which was attended by two burgesses (citizens) from each of twenty-seven plantations.

Such localized government was considered adequate as well as advisable until 1774, when the colonies felt the need to unite to voice their collective grievances against England's colonial policies. In that year, the First Continental Congress, attended by representatives of all colonies except Georgia, met in Philadelphia from September 5 to October 26. The Congress did more than express grievances; it also created an association to impose extensive boycotts against British trade, thus firmly establishing the tradition of pooling strengths and resources in time of national stress and emergency.

By the next year, war had begun and the Second Continental Congress, meeting in session from May 10, 1775, until December 12, 1776, created a Continental Army under the direction of George Washington to oppose the British. With the Declaration of Independence, formalized on July 4, 1776, the colonies were launched on a course of liberty from which they—and the states that were later formed—never retreated, although discussions, disagreements, financial difficulties, jealousies, and friction hampered progress time after time.

The Continental Congress continued to meet annually for varying periods of time in several different cities. With limited funds and little experience in affairs of state, the representatives retained the will and courage to continue to advance toward full independence. In 1778, the Congress submitted the Articles of Confederation to the legislatures of the states for ratification; this was accomplished in 1781. The states considered themselves practically as separate countries, however, delegating to the central government only those powers which they could not handle individually, such as the authority to wage war, establish a uniform currency, and make treaties with other nations. They made no provision for an executive head of the central government.

The Articles of Confederation proved to be too weak to hold the colonies together, giving rise to fears that foreign powers might recon-quer part or all of the country. Under the leadership of farsighted patriots such as George Washington and Alexander Hamilton, a movement toward nationalization was given impetus. As a result, in 1787 a Constitutional Convention met in Philadelphia to draw up the Constitution of the United States, the idea for which had originated in English and earlier colonial history. Ratification of the Constitution by a majority of the thirteen colonies established the permanent structure of the Congress of the United States, which held its first meeting in New York, March 4, 1789. Its first meeting in our present capital, Washington, D.C., was held in 1800. The Constitution also designated that a president, elected by the people, should be at the head of the government.

Since then, the volume and complexity of problems facing the legislature have increased tremendously. Departments and councils by the score have been set up to assist in the work of making laws. But at the hub of the work, guiding the action, is always the Constitution of the United States—the law of the land—which, although amended twenty-six times (to 1985), could scarcely be improved upon were it rewritten from the start today. Its basic principles are as pertinent now as they were in 1789.

Constitutional Amendments

Shortly after the adoption of the Constitution, it became apparent that the government's police power needed to be limited by spelling out the rights of the states and the individual citizen. Congress, therefore, submitted to the states twelve amendments to the Constitution intended to clarify these rights, ten of which were ratified by the states in 1791, thus establishing the Bill of Rights, on which social and political developments in the last few decades have placed renewed emphasis. It may be well, therefore, to review these amendments here to help form a basis for later discussion of the legal rights and responsibilities of citizens including nurses.

The *First Amendment* guarantees United

States citizens freedom of religion, speech, press, and the right "peaceably to assemble and to petition the Government for a redress of grievances." This amendment is often the center of controversy in disputes related to the freedom guaranteed herein.

The *Second Amendment* gives the people the right to keep and bear arms, because a well-regulated militia is necessary to the security of a free state. The *Third* refers to the quartering of soldiers in a private home in time of peace or war.

The last seven amendments included in the Bill of Rights have direct or indirect bearing on crimes, trials, and other legal matters in which nurses might become involved. They, are therefore, reproduced here, in full.

Article IV [Fourth Amendment] Protection Against Search

Th right of the people to be secure in their persons, houses, papers, and effects, against unreasonable searches and seizures, shall not be violated, and no warrants shall issue, but upon probable cause, supported by oath or affirmation, and particularly describing the place to be searched, and the persons or things to be seized.

Article V [Fifth Amendment] Due Process of Law Assured

No person shall be held to answer for a capital, or otherwise infamous crime, unless on a presentment or indictment of a grand jury, except in cases arising in the land or naval forces, or in the militia, when in actual service in time of war or public danger; nor shall any person be subject for the same offense to be twice put in jeopardy of life or limb; nor shall be compelled in any criminal case to be witness against himself, nor be deprived of life, liberty, or property without due process of law; nor shall private property be taken for public use, without just compensation.

Article VI [Sixth Amendment] Rights of Accused in Criminal Cases

In all criminal prosecutions, the accused shall enjoy the rights to a speedy and public trial, by an impartial jury of the state and district wherein the crime shall have been committed, which district shall have been previously ascertained by law, and to be informed of the nature and cause of the accusation; to be confronted with the witnesses against him; to have compulsory process for obtaining witnesses in his favor, and to have the assistance of counsel for his defense.

Article VII [Seventh Amendment] Jury Trial in Civil Cases

In suits at common law, where the value in controversy shall exceed twenty dollars, the right of trial by jury shall be preserved, and no fact tried by jury shall be otherwise reexamined in any court of the United States, than according to the rules of the common law.

Article VIII [Eighth Amendment] Excessive Punishments Forbidden

Excessive bail shall not be required, nor excessive fines imposed, nor cruel and unusual punishments inflicted.

Article IX [Ninth Amendment] Unenumerated Rights of the People

The enumeration in the Constitution, of certain rights, shall not be construed to deny or disparage others retained by the people.

Article X [Tenth Amendment] The Rights of States

The powers not delegated to the United States by the Constitution, nor prohibited by it to the states, are reserved to the states respectively, or to the people.

Later Amendments. The *Eleventh Amendment* (1798) is concerned with judicial powers; the *Twelfth* (1804), with the method of electing a president and vice-president; the *Thirteenth* (1865) abolished slavery. The *Fourteenth Amendment,* added in 1868 during the reconstruction period following the Civil War, states, in part:

No state shall make or enforce any law which shall abridge the privileges or immunities of citizens of the United States; nor shall any state deprive any person of life, liberty, or property, without due process of law; nor deny to any person within its jurisdiction the equal protection of the laws.

The *Fifteenth Amendment,* ratified in 1870, reads:

1. The right of the citizens of the United States to vote shall not be denied or abridged by the United States or by any State on account of race, color, or previous condition of servitude.
2. The Congress shall have power to enforce this article by appropriate legislation.

The *Sixteenth Amendment* (1913) authorized Congress to "lay and collect taxes on income"; the *Seventeenth* (1913) refers to the election of United States senators; the *Eighteenth,* adopted in 1920 and repealed in 1933, prohibited the manufacture, sale, or transportation of intoxicating liquors for beverages within the United States and all territories subject to its jurisdiction.

The *Nineteenth Amendment,* known as the Women's Suffrage Amendment, went into effect August 26, 1920. It reads as follows:

1. The right of citizens of the United States to vote shall not be denied or abridged by the United States or by any state on account of sex.
2. Congress shall have power to enforce this article by appropriate legislation.

The *Twentieth Amendment* (1933) specifies the dates on which the terms of the president, vice-president, senators, and representatives shall assume office.

The *Twenty-first Amendment* (1933) repealed the *Eighteenth Amendment*; the *Twenty-second* (1951) limited the presidential terms of office to two; the *Twenty-third* (1961) gave citizens of the District of Columbia the right to vote for presidential and vice-presidential candidates.

The *Twenty-fourth Amendment* (1964) states:

The right of citizens of the United States to vote in any primary or other election for President or Vice President, for electors for President or Vice President, or for Senator or Representative in Congress shall not be denied or abridged by the United States or any State by reason of failure to pay any poll tax or other tax.

The *Twenty-fifth Amendment* (1965) deals with the disability of a president or a vacancy in the office of vice-president and stipulates how the offices shall be filled in event of an emergency.

The *Twenty-sixth Amendment* (1971) reduced the voting age to eighteen.

For a while, there was great hope that the Twenty-seventh Amendment would be passed, barring legal discrimination against women based on sex. The bill, passed by Congress (1971–1972) and sent to the states for ratification, read, "Equality of rights under the law shall not be denied or abridged by the United States or any State on account of sex." To be adopted, two-thirds of the states (thirty-eight) needed to ratify the amendment by a specific time. When it was apparent that this goal would not be reached by the legal deadline of March 22, 1979 (three votes were still needed by mid-1978), both the House and Senate voted to extend the deadline to June 30, 1982. At the same time, a proposal to allow states that had already ratified the amendment to rescind their decisions was defeated, but the final decision on whether rescinding is possible remained open. Most of the states in which the Equal Rights Amendment (ERA) was defeated were in the South (Florida, Georgia, Alabama, Mississippi, Louisiana, North Carolina, South Carolina, Virginia, Oklahoma, Arkansas), but the legislators of Nevada, Utah, Arizona, Missouri, and Illinois also voted not to ratify. The required number of states was never won, so the bill was defeated in 1982 by lack of ratification.

The Constitution and its amendments encompass some of the provisions made by the federal government to ensure the rights of individuals to protection under the law and to fair and just practices in the application of laws at any political level. Guards against usurpation of the privileges and authority of individuals, as well as state and local jurisdictions, are also provided. Beyond this, it is up to the states, counties, townships, and municipalities to develop laws and legal procedures to protect their citizens. It is the individual's responsibility to be well informed about the laws governing his or her geographic area and especially those that are applicable to his or her status and vocation. This will help avoid legal infractions and provide some protection against miscarriage of justice should an individual become involved in litigation.

LEGAL STRUCTURE OF THE UNITED STATES

Under the United States government, the law is carried out at a number of levels. The Constitution is the highest law of the land. Whatever the Constitution (federal law) does not spell out, the states retain for themselves (Tenth Amendment). Because they can create political subdivisions, units of local government—counties, cities, towns, townships, boroughs, and villages—all have certain legal powers within their geographic boundaries. On all levels, but most obviously on the federal and state levels, there is a separation of power: legislative, executive, and judicial. The first makes the laws, the second carries them out, and the third reviews them, a system which the founders of the United States believed would create a balance of power.

There are three basic sources of law: statutory law, executive or regulatory law, and judicial law.

Statutory law refers to statutes that are acts of legislative bodies declaring, commanding, or prohibiting something.* Statutes are always written, are firmly established, and can be altered only by amendment or repeal. The Nurse Training Act is one example of a federal law. A state law requiring professional

*The legislative process is described in Chapter 18.

nurses to be licensed before they can legally practice nursing is another example.

Executive or regulatory law refers to the rules, regulations, and decisions of administrative bodies. For example, the DHHS Division of Nursing develops the regulations that determine the requirements for the various programs in the Nurse Training Act; the State Board of Nursing spells out the requirements for a nursing school; a city Health Code may adopt a patients' bill of rights as a requirement for all hospitals in the city. All have the effect of law.

Judicial law, also called *decisional, case,* or *common law,* as distinguished from law created by the enactment of legislatures, comprises a body of legal principles and rules of action that derive their authority from usage and custom or from judgments and decrees of courts based on these usages and customs. Courts are agencies established by the government to decide disputes. (The term *court* is also sometimes used to refer to the person or persons hearing a case.) There is usually only one judge for a trial (with or without a jury) and two or more to hear the appeals (with no jury). The kind of court in which a case is brought depends upon the offense or complaint.

There are also various classifications of law.

Criminal or penal law deals with action harmful to the public and the individual and designates punishment for offenders. Three gradations of criminal acts are recognized by the law: (1) *offenses,* such as traffic violations or disorderly conduct; (2) *misdemeanors,* such as small thefts, perjury, conspiracies, and assaults without the use of weapons; and (3) *felonies,* which include major robberies, assault with a dangerous weapon, arson, rape, and murder.

Civil law states the rights of persons and stipulates methods of maintaining or regaining them. The word *civil* means "citizen"; civil laws, therefore, pertain to the individual citizen. The system of civil law is derived, in greatly modified form, from the law of Rome established by the Emperor Justinian. Many acts of negligence, libel and slander, and commercial disputes are examples of cases that are subject to the application of civil law. It is distinct from criminal law.

There are many subdivisions of civil law. One of particular interest to nurses is *contract law.* Laws of contract govern all legal actions related to the making, keeping, or breaking of legal contracts of any type—for example, employment contracts, marriage contracts, and contracts for the sale of property. Contract law also deals with fraudulent contracts. No fraudulent contract against an innocent person is binding unless he wants to make it so.

Laws are additionally classified by subject matter, such as labor laws, maritime laws, mercantile laws, tax laws, motor vehicle laws, and others. Two other major categories of law are martial and military law.

Martial law means the suspension of civil law in time of emergency and the enforcement of military law on the civilian population.

Military law is a branch of national (or state) law which governs the conduct of national (or state) military organizations in peace or war. The rules or laws are enacted by the legislative body and administered in court-martial—a court consisting of military officers where personnel are tried for breaches of military law or discipline. Nurses enrolled in the armed forces as commissioned officers are subject to military law, which applies to all branches of the military services.

Enforcement of Laws

Besides generally adhering to the principle of *stare decisis,* courts also abide by another basic legal principle—that the court must have jurisdiction over the person or thing involved, that is, that the proceeding commences in a court located where the defendant lives or is served a subpoena or where the property in dispute is located. An exception occurs when, because of extraordinary publicity or emotionalism about a situation, the defendant claims that she or he cannot get a fair trial in

that place and requests a change of venue—to be tried in some other jurisdiction.

The Constitution of the United States provides for the enforcement of federal laws by establishing a system of courts (sometimes called *constitutional courts* because they hear cases about matters mentioned in the Constitution), headed by the Supreme Court, the only one specifically mentioned in the Constitution. Other federal courts—courts of appeal, district courts, and others—have been established in all states and territories either on a permanent or a temporary basis. Staffed by judges, lawyers, and other personnel employed by the federal government, they try all cases arising under the Constitution and laws of the United States except those over which the Supreme Court has original jurisdiction. For example, cases involving violations of federal income tax laws and the passing of counterfeit money are tried in federal courts. These courts have no jurisdiction over state and local courts.

Most citizens are not involved in legal action handled by a federal court. Misdemeanors are usually dealt with on a local level, often by a justice-of-the-peace court, common in rural areas and small towns, or, in urban areas, a magistrates court, sometimes called a *municipal* or *police court.* A district court, often called a *county court,* may hear cases in one county or in several. Matters related to estates and wills often are handled at the county level in surrogate courts (sometimes called *probate courts*) under the direction of surrogate, or probate, judges.

At the state level, no two states have court systems that are identical. They may differ in the names of the courts, their methods of selecting and removing judges, the number of jurors needed to convict the defendant in criminal cases, and in other ways. They do not differ widely, however, on fundamental principles or in their conduct of judicial affairs.

State courts have jurisdiction over all cases arising under common law and statutory laws in their respective states, except in Louisiana, which still operates partially under the Code of Napoleon, which makes other provisions. All states have a high court for the trial of cases, usually called a *supreme court.*

To meet changing times in general and advances in the legal profession particularly, reform of the courts at all levels is almost constantly under consideration by the state legislatures. It is a slow process, however, because it involves a change in the law and possibly the enactment of a new one; in some states a constitutional amendment is necessary.

Juries

A **petit jury** is a group of persons, usually twelve, sworn to listen to the evidence of a trial and pronounce a verdict. The right to trial by jury is guaranteed by the Constitution of the United States and by the constitutions of the individual states.

A juror must have the qualifications specified by the statute that applies in a particular situation and be free from any bias because of personal relationships or interests. A person cannot serve as juror on a criminal case if she or he has formed an opinion beforehand on the guilt or innocence of the accused.

Jurors are selected impartially. Jury duty is one of the privileges of a citizen in a democratic society, and many persons find it challenging, educational, and enjoyable. It may also be boring. Some jurors never participate in a trial because they are not the type of person wanted by one or the other of the lawyers, who have a number of peremptory challenges, which require no explanation. Prospective jurors may spend their entire time of service in a jury room. There is a definite technique to jury selection, intended to be most favorable to a lawyer's client. In malpractice or accident cases, nurses are usually not selected to serve; they know too much and may be unsympathetic, say some lawyers.[3]

A woman is often excused from jury duty if she has home and family responsibilities that would suffer because of her absence, or if she is pregnant. In some states, however, nurses, or women in general, were not called or were quickly excused. Because this violates the woman's right to serve if she so chooses and is able, women's rights groups have fought those restrictive laws. In 1975 the Supreme Court ruled that it is constitutionally unacceptable for states to deny women equal opportunity to serve on juries. The decision was based on the Sixth Amendment guarantee of a jury trial from a cross-sectional representation of the community. Women comprise over 50 percent of the population; therefore, systematically excluding them would deny those rights.

A man must have a very good reason to be excused, although those with pressing duties, such as doctors, lawyers, members of a fire or police department and the armed forces, are usually exempt. Various reasons for requesting release from a call to jury duty are accepted in all states.

A juror receives a modest daily fee. Many employers keep an employee on full salary while he or she is on jury duty, usually for two weeks or a month, although he is expected to report for work when not actually in court.

A **grand jury** is a group of persons, usually numbering from twelve to twenty-three, whose principal function is to examine the accusations against someone charged with a crime and determine whether or not she or he should be indicted; that is, brought to trial before a petit jury. The grand jury system is based on the English system dating from the thirteenth century and is guaranteed to citizens by the Constitution.

Members of the grand jury are selected even more carefully than members of a petit jury; they are called for a month of duty at more or less regular intervals and are paid more for their services.

LEGAL STATUS OF YOUNG PEOPLE[4]

United States citizens of any age are endowed with the rights of freedom of religion, speech, press, petition, and others as set forth in the Bill of Rights. Furthermore most people agree that all are entitled morally (at least until they forfeit the privilege through their own actions) to respect, tolerance, and understanding from their fellow man. Children born into citizenship in the United States have certain civil rights and responsibilities, some of which are in effect all of their lives; others they relinquish when they become adults and take on new ones.

In the last few years that point of legal adulthood or majority has been in a state of flux, but even more so has been the question of the rights of young people in the nebulous state between minority and the age of majority. Legislation has begun to deal with the rights of children in relation to privacy, informed consent, and many health-related matters. Some of the major legal decisions concerning health care and youth are discussed in Chapter 22, but a few basic facts on the legal status of young people should provide useful background.

Infant, minor, child, and *juvenile* are terms, usually used interchangeably, for someone who has not yet attained majority. The *age of majority* is the age designated by state law at which a citizen of the United States becomes legally adult and is entitled, therefore, to assume full civil rights and responsibilities. This term, sometimes abbreviated to *majority,* is synonymous with *full* or *legal age.* Each state adopts its own law setting the age of majority. In most states, this had been twenty-one; however, since the passage of the Twenty-sixth Amendment, most states have changed to eighteen, the voting age. On attaining legal age, individuals are permitted by statutory state law to perform certain acts with or without the consent of parents or guardian. Nevertheless, even within a particular state, the law varies with respect to the activities or purposes involved. The state has the right to set the age of qualification for such activities as serving on a jury, marrying without parental consent, buying, possessing, and drinking alcoholic beverages, making a contract, drawing a will, inheriting money, working for wages, obtaining a license to drive a

motor vehicle, attending school, receiving juvenile court treatment for illegal or criminal conduct, using the court to sue another person or one's parents, and receiving medical care without parental consent.

In 1975, the United States Supreme Court forbade setting separate ages of majority for males and females, but some state laws have retained sexual differentiation in setting majority status. Moreover, young people under the age of majority are not only denied certain rights enjoyed by adults, but are denied others by their parents as well, although they also have certain protections.

Emancipation describes the condition whereby children are released from some or all of the disabilities of childhood and receive the rights and duties of adulthood before the age of majority. Emancipation may be partial or complete. Theoretically, only the court or a specific state law can determine emancipation except under certain classic circumstances such as the young person's marriage or membership in the armed services. Parents can petition the court for a declaration of emancipation, which releases them from their legal obligation to the child—the duty to support, maintain, protect, and educate. They give up the custody and control of their child and the right to receive services and earnings. When parents abandon their parental duties, it implies consent, even when formal action is not taken. On the other hand, when young people leave home, and/or earn an independent living, and are otherwise free from the authority and control of parents, this may be grounds for emancipation. Usually young people cannot petition for emancipation without parental consent, but the reality is that unless there is a serious problem, an individual in those circumstances is considered emancipated for all general purposes.

In cases involving consent for medical treatment, the term *mature minor* may be used, indicating that the child is sufficiently intelligent to understand the nature and consequences of treatment.

Right of Sustenance and Shelter

Besides the constitutional rights cited earlier, minors have additional legal rights. From the moment of birth until legal age, children are entitled by state law to such food, shelter, medical care, and clothing (legally termed necessities) as the parents can reasonably afford.*

Wherever minors may be—in school, recreation camp, hospital—they always have the right to food, clothing, and shelter as provided by their parents, either directly or through written or unwritten contract with the agency or individual under whose care any children have been placed temporarily. Failure to provide for a child in this way (including medical care) is termed *child neglect.*

In case of extreme parental neglect or abandonment, the state is obligated to intervene and either see that the parents resume their responsibility for the child's care or take the child from them, temporarily or permanently, and place the child in the custody of a guardian, foster family, or institution. The state also must assume financial responsibility for the child until or unless other means of support is available.

Although many young people are earning money—sometimes enough to live on—before they are eighteen or twenty-one, they theoretically are entitled by law to continue receiving sustenance and shelter as provided by their parents or a legally appointed guardian. Also theoretically, the parents are entitled to the minor's earnings. It is unlikely, however, that a court would require a parent to support a wage-earning child under circumstances of hardship without requiring the child to contribute at least part of his or her earnings. Neither is it likely to require the child to turn over a full paycheck to the parent.

When a person reaches legal age, parents no longer are liable for child support; neither are they permitted to confiscate the child's earnings. If the child is mentally or physically in-

---

*State laws are changing from the traditional focus on "father" to include the mother or the term *parent.*

capable of assuming the responsibilities of adulthood, however, the law will usually require the parents or legal guardian to continue to provide the necessities.

Right of Protection

The law requires parents to protect their children from danger and harmful exposures of all kinds. Failure to do so constitutes *negligence.* A parent who in a fit of rage or as a means of inflicting punishment seriously injures a child, is guilty of *assault,* which is unlawful beating or other physical violence inflicted upon a person without his consent.

Child abuse is reportable in every state. Hospitals, all health professionals (including nurses), and sometimes schoolteachers are required to report reasonable suspicion of child abuse. Failure to do so may expose the individual to civil and, perhaps, criminal charges. In most states, those reporting in good faith are rendered free from civil liability (lawsuits) for having made the report. This entire issue has become particularly sensitive since sexual abuse of children has become more visible. The question has been raised as to whether it is always in the best interest of the child and family to report the situation, if changes are being made.[5] On the other hand, health professionals, teachers, and social agencies have been sued for *not* reporting or following through on these cases.[6] The minor's right of protection extends to her or his school where, in most states, the law stipulates what punishment a teacher can employ to maintain discipline in a classroom or school. Private schools are not always subject to the same legal restrictions as public schools in this respect.

The law requires the administrative officers of schools, hospitals, places of amusement, all public buildings and vehicles, transportation systems, health and beauty salons, and others to observe specific rules of safety for the protection of all citizens, minors and adults alike. Such establishments must have and enforce regulations intended especially to protect the young child or else risk getting into legal difficulties of various degrees of seriousness. Furthermore, they must employ persons capable of providing the services they offer safely and competently.

Right to Give Consent

Under the law, *consent* means that a person gives permission in writing or orally for the performance of a certain act. In many cases, minors have not been able to consent to health care,* but many changes are occurring.

Female minors are protected against sex crimes to a certain extent by penal laws that state at what age a girl can legally consent to sexual intercourse. The age varies in different states—from ten to eighteen. A man who violates the law is guilty of rape and subject to the punishment prescribed by law. The law is frequently inadequate in its handling of sex offenses against both young boys and girls, but the issue is getting increased attention legally and socially.

Right to an Education

Children are legally entitled to an education until they complete elementary school, without cost, except indirectly in the form of taxes, transportation charges, and the like. This right makes it mandatory for parents or legal guardians to see that they attend school regularly. Children cannot legally be deprived of their rights, even if they are needed at home, without special permission from school authorities.

Rights of Marriage and Parenthood

Every state has its own statutory laws governing the right of a couple to marry with or without the consent of their parents, guardian, or a superior court, and with or without reputable witnesses. The majority of states permit a couple to marry without the consent of their parents or anyone else at age eighteen. The ages at which a couple can marry with the consent of their parents or other responsible

---

*Consent to medical treatment is discussed in Chapter 22.

person are also stipulated by state laws. They are usually lower than the ages required for marriage without consent. Although changing, many marriage laws are also very specific about other legal requirements such as mental ability, freedom from venereal disease, and family relationships. Minors who marry declare their independence by so doing and, therefore, assume the same legal responsibilities as adults who marry. The parents of the very young husband or wife often continue to help them financially, but the law does not make it obligatory. Neither are parents responsible for debts the minors incur for education or any other purpose after their marriage.

A number of states recognize common law marriages as legal. A couple is married under common law by declaring themselves man and wife and thereafter living together as such. An increasing number of court decisions concerning persons living together, whether homosexual or heterosexual, juvenile or adult, are expected to set new precedents in the legal status and rights of each. There are also new rulings emerging on the rights of single or unmarried parents. For instance, in 1979 the teenage father of a child born out of wedlock was able to prevent adoption of the child and was given custody himself. Minors in general have the right of custody over their children, but whether or not the mother can consent to adoption of her child without parental consent varies from state to state. Illegitimate children, those born when their parents are not married, have most of the legal rights of legitimate children, particularly within the last few years, as courts and legislation have overturned old statutes discriminating against these individuals.

Right to Make Contracts and Wills, Inherit Property, and Sue

Most states do not consider a contract binding if one of the parties is a minor. This does not mean that the contract cannot be carried out but that the child may disaffirm it. Therefore, many adults do not enter into contracts with minors unless there is a parental signature; the parent, as an adult, cannot repudiate legal contractual obligation. Contracts that cannot be voided by minors are those for "necessaries" (food, clothing, shelter, and medical care), marriage, enlistment in the armed forces, and, in some states, educational loans and automobile and motorcycle insurance.

A contractual agreement to work, written or unwritten, can be legal, subject to the laws of the state that delineate the kinds of jobs that children can hold, at what age, and under what circumstances (hours, hazards, and so on). Most states require work permits, which, in turn, require parental consent and proof of age. Acquisition of a social security card is also necessary. Generally, salaries and fringe benefits should be the same for adult and child, male and female. Exceptions may be in the areas of babysitting, housework, and agricultural work.

In most states, the law does not recognize a will made by a minor as a legal document. Exceptions are sometimes made, however, particularly if a minor is married. A minor may inherit money or property, but usually does not have control over it until a specific age or the age of majority, on the assumption that the minor cannot manage an estate. Therefore, the court or an adult designated in the will acts as a guardian of the minor. The guardian or trustee has the legal responsibility of safeguarding the estate. Sometimes the disbursement of money inherited by an infant is subject to the discretion of an orphans' court, which might release money to pay for the minor's education or medical expenses or for other purposes.

There appears to be no hard-and-fast rule that states at exactly what age a person may witness a will or other legal document or serve as a witness in legal action, or as a legal witness at marriages and other ceremonies. The courts have permitted testimony of children as young as seven years old. It is not so much a question of age as of intelligence and understanding. Some children have more ability and demonstrate better judgment than persons of considerably older age. A witness must be mentally capable of knowing what he or she is doing. This obviously excludes the mentally deficient witness and the child who is too young to realize the import of his or her acts.

A minor can sue or be sued to enforce any civil right or obligation. Before any action against the child can be taken, however, if there is no parent or legal guardian, a court of law must be asked to appoint a guardian to institute the action on behalf of the minor or to act for the minor. This person is generally referred to as a guardian *ad litem,* that is, the capacity as guardian ceases when the action or claim is settled.

If the child is suing, an adult—a lawyer, parent, guardian or "next friend"—must bring the suit for him or her. In a few states, a child may bring suit against parents or other family members for negligent or injurious harm; other states have an *intrafamily tort immunity* law. Even in the latter circumstances, a child can often sue for damage to personal property or *willful* personal injury.

Other legal action against juveniles in relation to arrest, detention, trial, and punishment has been in a constant state of change in recent years, both in terms of protecting the minor and protecting the public from the minor.

THE LEGAL RIGHTS OF WOMEN

There was a time when adult women were considerably restricted by the law, simply because they were females.* Married women were even more limited than single women, because husbands were entitled to the wife's worldly goods and usually represented them in the execution of all legal procedures. Even if the woman was not married, she was usually under the control of a male family member.

---

*See Chapters 3, 4, 6, and 16 for additional information on sexism.

The history of women's struggle for equal rights precedes the Constitution, at which time Abigail Adams warned her husband that if the new legal codes did not give attention to women, they would foment a rebellion; two hundred years later, women are still at a legal disadvantage.

The women's suffrage amendment drafted by Susan B. Anthony was introduced into the Senate in 1875, but ratification was not certified until 1920. Efforts toward an equal rights amendment have been under way for more than fifty years.

Between 1920 and 1963, little legislation useful in securing women equal rights was passed, but, probably because of the civil rights, black power, and women's rights movements that gained strength in the 1960s, new energies seemed to be released. Dumas cites and describes forty-three pieces of legislation related to women's rights or of special interest to women that were enacted into law between 1963 and 1978.[7] Among these were:

PL 88-38 (1963)—*Equal Pay Act*; PL 88-352—*Title VII of Civil Rights Act of 1964*; PL 92-157—*Comprehensive Health and Manpower Training Act of 1971*; PL 92-261—*Equal Employment Opportunity Act of 1972*; PL 92-318—*The Higher Education Amendments of 1972*; PL 92-496—*Civil Rights Commission Act of 1972*; PL 93-203 (1973)—*Comprehensive Manpower Act*; PL 93-259—*Fair Labor Standards Act Amendments of 1974*; PL 93-380—*The Education Amendments of 1974*; PL 94-106—*Department of Defense Appropriation Authorization Act of 1976*; PL 94-482—*Education Amendments of 1976*; PL 94-566—*Unemployment Compensation Amendments of 1976*; PL 95-79—*Department of Defense Appropriation Authorization*; PL 95-99—*National Science Foundation Authorization Act. 1978*; PL 95-207 (1977)—*Career Education Incentive Act*.

All of the laws cited by Dumas specifically prohibit sex discrimination in employment, military service, or education. However, with legal protection, women are not necessarily granted equal work opportunities and equal pay for equal work, even in state and federal agencies. Within the first five years of the Equal Pay Act, hundred of corporations were found in violation of the law and owed 46,000 women some $15 million in back pay. There were at the same time more than 7,800 complaints of sex discrimination filed under the 1964 Civil Rights Act.[8] Discrimination that is most difficult to combat is in the area of job promotion, appointment to key positions, or in gaining tenure in academia.[9]

Women have encountered discrimination, both subtle and blatant, in establishing their own credit, purchasing property, organizing a business, and receiving fair insurance or pension credits. Women have at least some recourse to the law through the enactment of the following laws:

PL 93-237 (1974)—*Small Business Act*; PL 93-383—*Housing and Community Development Act of 1974*; PL 93-495 (1974)—*Equal Credit Opportunity Act*; PL 94-63—*Public Health Service Act Amendments and Special Health Revenue Sharing Act of 1975*; PL 94-455—*Tax Reform Act of 1976*; PL 95-216—*Social Security Amendments of 1977*.

Many, if not most, insurance companies and retirement plans are reluctant to give women the same retirement benefits as men. They may also discriminate in the availability and amount of disability insurance on the grounds that women are more inclined to fake illness. The problem of sexual harassment of women by their employers or professors has also had some visibility, with limited positive legislation, but some judicial response.[10,11] For the time being, it seems as though there is likely to be more judiciary law than statuatory law on these issues. Legislation was introduced, but not passed, on the insurance/retirement questions. The argument was that women lived longer than men and therefore should not get as much as men. However, a series of Supreme Court rulings now ban employers from offering retirement plans with unequal male/female benefits.[12]

Comparable worth (equal pay for different jobs that require similar levels of training, education, and responsibility) has moved a giant step closer. The state of Washington was ordered, in 1984, to pay its female workers up to $1 billion in back wages because of pay inequity. This is expected to go the the U.S. Supreme Court.[13] Similar cases have been lost by women. It is also worth noting that a report by the distinguished National Research Council, completed in 1981, indicated that women were still concentrated in low-paying jobs and were "systematically underpaid." And today, women are still earning less than 60 percent of what men earn.

Supreme Court and state high court rulings have handed down mixed decisions concerning women's issues. Pregnant women have been both upheld and rejected on the question of time and/or pay for pregnancy leave (remedied in part by legislation). Courts have ruled for and against alimony for *either* husband or wife, and custody of children by either. Although the Supreme Court supported a woman's right to have an abortion, it also agreed that abortions need not be paid for by public funds, thus encouraging legislation that severely limited the ability of poor women to have legal abortions.

Women's rights issues that *have* resulted in legislation include rape prevention and control, and family planning such as: *Public Health Service Act Amendments and Special Health Revenue Sharing Act*—PL 94-63 (1975) and *Health Planning and Health Services Research and Statistics Extension Act*—PL 95-83 (1977); assistance in child care for working mothers: PL 94-401 (1976) *Child Day Care and Social Service Amendment* and PL 95-171 (1977) *Social Security Amendment*. A new concern is for "displaced homemakers," widowed or divorced spouses who have lost their source of income. A bill was first introduced in 1977 that would provide counseling, training, and referral centers, but no action was taken.

Women have become more militant about seeking legal relief from discrimination on the job or elsewhere. Cross suggests some ways to proceed:

1. File charges with the federal agency that has jurisdiction, following the specific protocol for action. For instance, in filing with the Equal Employment Opportunity Commission (EEOC), there are certain steps that have to be followed and time periods elapsed. If the EEOC (as an example) cannot get the company to end the discriminatory behavior, it gives the woman "notice of right to sue" and she must then get a lawyer and sue. The EEOC itself also sues in some instances. (Unfortunately, with the backlog of cases for many of these agencies, a two- to three-year time span may elapse before any action is taken.)

2. File a class action suit, getting help from your own lawyer or the American Civil Liberties Union. The process and validity of class action suits is now in question, so this too might be lengthy.[14]

Cross also provides information about action to be taken in specific cases and how to attain legal assistance.

The fact that action on women's rights has been so fragmented, frequently contradictory, and not always implemented is a major reason that the ERA is considered so important. The misunderstanding about what it will or won't do has been widespread, particularly in relation to support and protection of women. (It is important to remember that the ERA prohibits discrimination against either sex.) Some of the projections of what ratification of ERA would mean in relation to some controversial issues are:

1. Decisions about the support obligation of each spouse and about alimony after divorce would be based on individual circumstances and resources, instead of on sex. It is unclear what would happen in the distribution and control of marital property.

2. Women would be permitted to volunteer for military service, or be drafted, if neces-

sary, with appropriate exemption. They would be assigned to duty compatible with their physical and other qualifications and service needs.

3. In school, enrollment in certain kinds of courses could not be limited to a particular sex; only legitimate, activity-related physical qualifications could be used to set restrictions.

4. Labor laws that provide real protection for women would probably remain and be extended to men also, but those barring women from certain occupations would be invalidated.

5. The constitutional right to privacy is expected to permit continued segregation of public toilets and sleeping quarters in dormitories, prisons, and so on.

6. Homosexual marriages would not automatically be permitted or prevented; this is generally a state decision.

7. Private or business relationships between men and women would not be affected in any legal sense.

Because some of these changes are already occurring as a result of the action of individual states, courts, or a lack of objection, there are attorneys and others who say that ratification of the ERA is not necessary and that the trend toward equality between women and men is so strong that lack of a constitutional amendment will not stop it. Nevertheless, because trends do not take care of the problems of here-and-now and equal rights decisions, and because laws are so inconsistent, grossly unjust treatments for thousands have resulted. The fight for passage of the ERA will undoubtedly continue.

REFERENCES

1. Mary Hemelt and Mary Ellen Mackert, *Dynamics of Law in Nursing and Health Care* (Reston, Va: Reston Publishing Co., 1978), p. 3.

2. Helen Creighton, *Law Every Nurse Should Know,* 3rd ed. (Philadelphia: W. B. Saunders Company, 1975), p. 7.

3. Robert Cartwright, "Jury Selection," *Trial,* **13**:26–31 (Dec. 1977).

4. Much of the material in this section has been taken from Alan Sussman, *The Rights of Young People: An American Civil Liberties Union Handbook* (New York: Discus Books, 1977), pp. 15–18.

5. Ferdinand Schoeman and Frederick Reamer, "Should Child Abuse Always Be Reported?" *Hastings Center Report,* **13**:19–20 (Aug. 1983).

6. Donald Brass, "Professional and Agency Liability for Negligence in Child Protection," *Law, Med. and Health Care,* **11**:71–75 (Apr. 1983).

7. Rhetaugh Dumas, "Women and Power: Historical Perspective," in *Nursing's Influence in Health Policy for the Eighties* (Kansas City, Mo.: American Academy of Nursing, 1979), pp. 68–73.

8. "The Women—They Want Action," *Dun's,* (June 1970).

9. Terry Selby, "Nurse Educators Charge Sex Inequities at Universities," *Am. Nurse,* **14**:10 (July–Aug. 1982).

10. Suzanne Perry, "Sexual Harassment on the Campuses: Deciding Where to Draw the Line," *Chron. Higher Ed.,* **27**:21–22 (Mar. 1983).

11. Karen Lindsey, "Sexual Harassment on the Job and How to Stop It," *Ms.,* **5**:47–51, 74–79 (Nov. 1977).

12. Cheryl Fields, "Court Declares Women Must Get Equal Benefits in Pension Plans, Sends Back 2 T1AA Cases," *Chron. Higher Ed.,* **26**:1, 13–18 (July 1983).

13. "A Worthy But Knotty Question," *Time,* **123**:30 (Feb. 6, 1984).

14. Susan Cross, *The Rights of Women: An ACLU Handbook* (New York: Discus Books, 1973).

The Legislative Process

IMPORTANCE OF ACTION

The successful functioning of a democracy depends on the willingness of its citizens to participate in their government. Perhaps the most important activity involved in a successful democracy is exercising the right to vote, with understanding of the issues concerned and the potential impact of election of the candidates. Further involvement might include participating actively in campaigns or in organizations that promote or oppose certain legislative issues; contacting legislators about issues; giving testimony at hearings; and even helping to originate and encourage the passage of specific legislation.

Nurses, particularly, need to take on these responsibilities of citizenship, not only on general principles, but because so much of their professional lives are, and will continue to be, affected by legislation. The nursing practice act of each state controls nursing education and practice and can be eliminated, amended, or totally rewritten in the legislative process. Any law involving health care, general education, or almost any other social issue might well have an impact on nursing. For example, at the end of one session of a state

legislature, there were 149 bills of interest to nurses in some way. Included were bills for changes in the practice act of professional nurses, vocational nurses, physicians, physical therapists, podiatrists; pharmacists, dentists, and chiropractors; licensing of certain paramedical workers; practice of other paramedical workers; treatment of drug addiction; use of certain drugs; funds for nursing education; funds for scholarships; funds for health facilities; abortion; birth control; health profession planning grants; malpractice; venereal disease; and matters related to consumer protection. On the national level, existing or pending legislation such as Medicare, Social Security, health projects, health care planning, Nurse Training Act, development of health maintenance organizations, national health insurance, health research, mental health grants, public health services, and labor relations all have an impact on nursing practice.

Although there has been a tendency for nurses to underestimate their strength in influencing legislation, there has also been an increasing recognition that they must become involved or suddenly find that someone else is making the legislative decisions on health care in which nurses should have a major part. An interesting development is that a number of nurses have successfully run for office. In fact, over half of the states report nurses holding political office, usually on a local level.

Many students, with political know-how and recognizing the power of the new youth vote, are taking a part in legislation at all levels. (However, studies to determine the effect of the eighteen-year-old vote have shown that powerful though the youth vote can be and has been in certain geographic areas, many of the young are as lax in voting as their elders.) Nursing students, in their heterogeneous groups of the young and the not so young, with their variety of backgrounds, have become increasingly active, and their impact has been felt. In one state they were a powerful influence in the enactment of child-abuse legislation. They have been effective in giving testimony on federal funding for nursing education. As a group, nurses have become more sophisticated in the legislative process, but they have not yet achieved their full influence as individuals, as members of a profession that numbers over 1.7 million, and as members of other power groups. In part this results from a lack of knowledge of the process itself, the ways in which they can make their power felt, and the *best time* to take action. To help remedy this situation, this chapter presents a pragmatic view of the legislative process.

BECOMING KNOWLEDGEABLE IN THE LEGISLATIVE PROCESS

There are a number of ways in which nurses can become more knowledgeable in the legislative arena. To begin with, ANA and its state and local constituent groups take an active part in legislation. Because ANA represents a profession, it may take part in developing a bill, testifying, and lobbying in behalf of its members, and has the responsibility to do so. (For example, ANA is responsible for nurses coming under the Social Security law; state organizations initiated the nursing practice acts.) The major legislative activities of the

nursing organizations are discussed in the chapters on these organizations. Pertinent at this point is the means by which members are kept informed about legislation. All major nursing journals, particularly the *American Journal of Nursing*, report key legislative movements on the national level, and, if particularly significant, those on the state level. *Capital Commentary,* written by the ANA Washington staff, who are also the ANA lobbyists, is included in *American Nurse,* and special legislative reports are sent to state and district offices, legislative committee members, directors of nursing service, heads of nursing education programs, and selected others. States or districts are permitted to reproduce this information, which is particularly important if membership action is required. They may also publish legislative newsletters or have legislative sections that describe legislation on national, state, or local levels in their journals or other means of communicating with members. Directors of nursing or heads of nursing education programs often post these legislative newsletters so that all nursing personnel have access to them. (And if not, they can certainly be requested to do so.) Some institutions have special legislative groups who keep abreast of pertinent legislation and see that the other nurses are informed. Students may be involved in these groups or their own. The National Student Nurses' Association, with its various communications, is also a means of gaining current information about legislation important to nursing. NLN's newsletters and legislative reports in its journal are excellent.

The kind of legislative information available in the newspapers depends on their editorial policies. Feature articles, news stories, and editorials on particular legislation are usually found, but these may not include legislation necessarily of special interest to nurses. Some newspapers list the major bills in the state legislature and/or in the Congress, report action taken, and current status. They may also report the vote of the legislators of that particular region on major bills. This enables readers not only to follow the action of a particular bill, but also to see how their own legislators vote in general. The League of Women Voters and various political action groups often publish some sort of legislative roundup for varying subscription prices. Legislators may also send newsletters to voters.

There are several ways for individuals to find out the names of their legislators. Calling the local municipal building or the county clerk's office will usually elicit this information, as well as the numbers of the legislative districts in which one lives. (It is politically expedient for local legislators to know those on a state or national level, because, at the least, local areas may benefit or suffer from such legislation.) However, some patience may be required because experience has shown that a prompt and complete answer is seldom forthcoming at the first extension to which one is connected.

A local or state League of Women Voters branch will usually give this information, and for a minimum fee will often send pamphlets or more detailed and useful information, such as the committees on which the legislators serve. Similar detailed information should be available from the district and state nurses' association. It is quite possible that other organizations to which a nurse belongs may also have such information, because other groups are also oriented to legislative action. It is always possible to call the local newspaper, asking for the political editor or reporter, but the request for information may be greeted with more or less enthusiasm, depending on the newspaper. Another possible source is local political clubs. It might even be educational to see whether family, friends, or neighbors know the names of their legislators. Although most pertinent health legislation is usually at a state or national level, it is also useful to become acquainted with local legislators, because of their potential contacts and influence.

Because a voter is more influential than a nonvoter, registration and voting are important. Local registration boards can give all

necessary information, including the place and time of registration and the polling places.

THE LEGISLATIVE SETTING

It is not possible to influence legislation unless there is a clear understanding of how a bill becomes a law and the setting in which this happens. Presumably, legislators, whether state or national, are elected on platforms of their own and/or their party's which set their goals, and on certain promises for action that they make to their constituents. Fulfillment of these goals and promises, of course, means successful passage of appropriate legislation, but also voting on other, perhaps unforeseen, legislation to the general satisfaction of the "folks back home." *It is important to remember that most legislators want to be reelected at the same or a higher level, and many of their actions reflect this desire.* It is equally important to know that it is not unusual to have hundreds or even thousands of bills introduced in a state assembly (or house) and senate. On the national level, over 25,000 bills may be introduced in the two-year course of a congressional session. Although not all of these are voted on finally, and not all are of interest to nurses, a legislator must have pertinent information on at least those that are likely to be of importance to his* areas of interest and his constituents. For this, legislators have staffs of varying size, depending on seniority and other factors. The staff total for both houses is well over 13,000 and rising. Some perform secretarial and other similar duties, but others act as aides, assistants, and/or researchers. These are individuals who gather, sort out, and sum up background material on key bills and brief the legislator on specific issues and on his constituents' feedback. The legislator generally uses this infor-

---

*In order to avoid constant reiteration of the phrase "his or her," the masculine pronoun is used in this chapter when referring to legislators; most legislators in the Congress are men.

mation to decide how he will vote. The men and women who are administrative assistants share the power of the legislators, if not the glory. Committee staff do the preparatory work that comes before committees and sub-committees, drafting bills, writing amendments to bills, arranging and preparing for public hearings, consulting with people in the areas about which the committee is concerned, providing information, and frequently writing speeches for the chairman.

Because these assistants get information from numerous sources, representatives of organizations, individuals, and lobbyists find it wise to become acquainted with them, maintain good relations, and provide accurate, pertinent information about the issues with which that particular legislator must deal. When representatives of nursing have not done so, they have found that the information about nursing that a legislator gets may be inaccurate, incomplete, out of date, or simply skewed in the direction another informant favors. A reported instance of the danger of maintaining poor relations with legislative staff was the difficulty that a certain presidentially appointed agency had in getting the appropriations it wanted from the Congress. It was clearly pointed out that the agency staff's indifference to the congressional staff and their negligence in keeping them informed of the agency's plans and activities caused a negative reaction in the appropriations committees.

A measure of the influence a legislator has is his placement on committees, where most of the preliminary action on bills occurs. Appointments are influenced or made by party leaders in the House or Senate. It is customary that the chairmanships of committees, extremely powerful positions, are awarded to members of the majority party, usually senior members of the House or Senate. Some committee assignments are more prestigious than others and are eagerly sought. Although there are cases in which the chairmen of some of these committees, particularly on the national level, have remained for years, the makeup of a committee may change with each new ses-

sion. The legislator's performance on his assigned committees may be a means of gaining attention and prestige with his colleagues and his constituents, particularly if major issues arise and there is attendant news media coverage. It is, however, not unknown for him to lose a favorable position because of clashes with his party heads. It is vital to know on which committee one's legislators sit, because the action of committees affects the future of a bill.

Another useful person to know is the party "whip," both at the state and national levels. They are selected by their party/delegation and have the job of "whipping in" the vote, seeing that all party members are present for a particular vote, and/or persuading the recalcitrant to vote a certain way. In times of stress, the whips can offer all kinds of political favors. If they fail, the party leaders take over. The function of the whip goes back to 1769, when the British parliamentarian Edmund Burke, in a historic debate in the House of Commons, used the term to describe the ministers who had sent for their friends as "whipping them in"—derived from the term *whipper-in,* the man who keeps the hounds from leaving the pack.

Influencing the Legislative Process

There are many elements to be considered before a legislative body or even individual legislators make a final decision on how to vote on a piece of legislation. Some are undoubtedly personal—how the legislator feels about an issue. Some are internally political—support of the party leadership or a favor owed to a colleague. But likely to be most influential is the voice of the legislator's constituency—"the folks back home."

> Congressmen are in a political situation in which significant rewards accrue to those who perceive their constituency's attitude correctly and vote on that basis. The deprivations are so severe that little room can be allowed for the Congressmen's own attitudes to distort this perception. In fact, representatives are moti-

vated to bring their own attitudes (or, at least, their public attitudes) into line with their perception of constituency attitude.[1]

In other words, if the constituents do not see that legislator, whether national or local, voting as they wish, the intractable or insensitive legislator is replaced. Of course, what may be important to them is not the great national or international issues, but those that affect their own lives and livelihood. But just who are these powerful constituents—the ordinary householder or a power conglomerate? Actually, both, as interested individuals or interest groups.

Kalisch and Kalisch define an *interest group* as "an association of people concerned with protecting and promoting shared values through the use of the political process."[2] Their purpose is basically to represent and promote the policy preferences of their constituents and use the power of the group to influence public decisions that affect them. Interest groups have been categorized as economically motivated, such as business and labor; professionally motivated, with emphasis on service rather than economic gain, such as ANA and AMA; and public interest groups that claim to speak for the public (even if they do not always seem to express popular views), such as Common Cause and Congress Watch. The reality is that such categorization does not hold in the rough-and-tumble of politics and in today's environment of overlapping interests. The professional groups often lobby for economic gains to their constituents, such as ANA's involvement with labor legislation and AMA's attempt to exempt medicine from the Federal Trade Commission's authority. Moreover, because success in influencing legislation is most often a matter of power and members, the increasing tendency of a variety of interest groups to form coalitions to support or oppose an issue, sometimes on a very short-time basis, not only demonstrates this overlapping, but confirms an old saw: "politics makes strange bedfellows."

One method used to influence legislation is support of a legislator, either for election or for reelection. For many decades, making political contributions has been illegal for certain incorporated groups such as ANA, and more recently, tighter constraints have been placed on contributions and spending. Because the law requires that campaign contributions be kept as a separate fund and that no organization money may be used for this purpose, many groups have created separate organizations for political activity. These are known as *political action committees,* or *PACs.* They may be located in the same office as an organization, such as ANA's Washington office, but funding activities are carefully separated, if not unrelated. PACs are powerful determinants of legislative action since the first priority of any legislator is to get elected, and campaigning is becoming extraordinarily expensive. While limits are set by law on the amounts that can be given to candidates, there are ways of manipulating the system. For instance, AMA, often identified as the largest contributor in congressional races, has in some years contributed close to $2 million to a campaign. A legislator important to the group's interests can receive maximum contributions from AMA's AMPAC at the national and state levels for each election, including primaries and run-offs, on top of any number of maximum individual gifts—all quite legal. Does this "buy" the legislator? "While substantial contributions may not actually 'buy' votes," stated Common Cause, "they do ensure easy access to public officials and create an unhealthy atmosphere of familiarity."[3]

Common Cause, which seeks to limit this kind of influence, reports that apart from campaign contributions, $1 billion is spent in congressional lobbying efforts, only a small part of which is disclosed. In fact, other ways of assisting candidates have been identified, such as using union dues (or company funds) and resources to provide computers, telephone banks, printing, mailing, sound equipment, and the salaries of union or company people assigned to specific campaigns. The legality of these practices is being questioned, but variations continue.

The ultimate effect of such support can be documented. Periodically a consumer group will publish a legislator's voting record, matching it to the source of his campaign contributions—and they do match more often than not. Moreover, when a particular interest group such as the Moral Majority targets a legislator for defeat and pours money and people into that effort, that candidate is often defeated. That is not to say that there is anything illegal or necessarily unethical about these activities. However, there *are* unethical aspects, as when distortion, false information, scandal, and a variety of other "dirty tricks," some quite serious, are used to destroy a candidate's reputation. Many examples of this can be found in some of the issues in which nurses have been involved, such as ERA and family planning.

On the other hand, a commissioner of the Federal Elections Commission, although admittedly a previous AMPAC executive, avers that the assumption of quid pro quo in PAC giving is faulty. "I have never known of a candidate changing a vote on the basis of who gave him a contribution. Money does not affect a legislative change; it supports a political philosophy."[4] Others are in agreement, since electing a candidate who is in general agreement with your point of view might be quite a bit easier than changing someone else's mind, once elected. Porter also maintains that people who spend their money through a PAC spend it more wisely than those who simply support a candidate whose name is in the papers.

Another important, if unofficial, component of lawmaking is lobbying. *Lobbying* is generally defined as an attempt to influence a decision of a legislature or other governmental body. Since it is a type of petition for redress of grievances, lobbying is constitutionally guaranteed. Lobbying exists at several levels, from a single individual who contacts a legislator about a particular issue of personal im-

portance to the interest groups that carefully (and often expensively) organize systems for monitoring legislation, initiating action, or blocking action on matters that concern them.

Professional lobbyists must be registered, and there are regulations concerning the types of organizations that may employ lobbyists. They spend all or part of their time representing the interests of a particular group or groups. Sometimes they are former legislators, aides, or employees of the executive branch and are able to get information and access.

A good lobbyist makes it his or her business to "know everyone" and to cultivate such friendships. There are numerous ways in which lobbyists attempt to influence legislators; much lobbying is done on a personal level, sometimes in the semisocial setting of a lunch, dinner, cocktail party, golf date, or other such activity. Lobbyists provide information to legislators and their staff (not necessarily objectively) and introduce resource people to them. Lobbyists are knowledgeable in the ways of legislation and are often familiar with legislators' personalities and idiosyncracies. They are invaluable in keeping their interest group informed about any pertinent legislation and the problems involved, and in aiding the group in taking effective action. It has been said that the skill with which a lobbyist monitors, analyzes, and participates in the political process is a major influence on success, but the interest group's ability to use a "unique mix of resources to influence political allies, neutral figures and opponents"[5] may be of even greater importance.

A skilled lobbyist can have great influence on lawmakers, and many times this is all to the good. When it is done properly and is controlled, lobbying is a desirable and accepted way of bringing important information and sound arguments to the attention of legislators, frequently by giving testimony before them. In this sense, lobbyists act as ombudsmen. Unfortunately, some lobbyists present biased information in order to influence opinions and decisions in a group's favor. Lobbying may lead to bribery, which has already created state and national scandals and caused great public concern. Legal measures have been taken to curb dishonest lobbying, rarely with complete success. The Congressional Reform Act of 1946 requires lobbyists to register and file statements of expenses incurred to influence legislation.

This organized approach to lobbying, effective though it is, should not overshadow the efforts of the individual who, in effect, lobbies when she or he contacts the appropriate legislator about an issue. Groups such as nurses, who do not necessarily have millions of dollars to spend, have proven to be very effective in lobbying by coordinating the efforts of individuals for unified action on an issue important to nursing. Therefore, how well and how much the individual citizen lobbies can be crucial in political action.

One influential lobbyist noted that ultimate power lies with the constituent. "The guy is hired by the voters. Getting a letter from a constituent is like getting a note from your boss."[6] This type of grass-roots lobbying activity is sometimes referred to as *outside lobbying* and includes telephone, telegram, and letter-writing campaigns, as well as letters to the editor, press conferences, and various other media activities. It is often most effective if it includes not only the group most involved, but also other influential people. The aim is to educate and/or mobilize at the local level to influence a policy decision.

Inside lobbying attempts to influence in a more direct manner through submission of testimony, drafting of legislation, amendments, or regulations, and face-to-face visits with legislators and their staff. A good lobbyist can "count heads" to determine which legislation should be targeted, especially the uncommitted swing vote, and can coordinate inside and outside lobbying efforts to the best advantage.

To influence the legislative process requires, first of all, information and, second, lobbying strategies. Later in the chapter, some sources

of information are listed, as well as effective techniques for grass-roots lobbying.

HOW A BILL BECOMES A LAW*

Anyone can initiate a bill. Legislation is basically a citizen's demand for action because of discontentment with an existing situation or because of an emerging need. It may well be that a bill is not a result of the voice of the majority of people, but it may be what the legislators or governmental officials think is wanted by the majority with whom they are concerned. A vocal group is more likely to get action than one that is silent. A citizen who takes his or her complaints to a legislator is more likely to get a response than one who just complains. And the larger and more politically active the complainer group, the better the chance of being heard. There have been instances of legislation based on the concerns of one individual, but most commonly ideas for a bill are suggested by groups, which may or may not be organized. Some common originators of bills are organizations representing various interest groups, a governmental administrator, agency, or department, a delegation of citizens in a legislator's district, a legislative committee, or the legislator himself. A prolific source of legislation is the executive communication—a letter from the President, a member of his Cabinet, or the head of an independent agency transmitting a draft of a proposed bill to the Speaker of the House and the President of the Senate. This communication is then referred to the standing committee that has jurisdiction over that particular subject matter. The chairman of that committee usually introduces the bill promptly, either in the form received or with changes he considers necessary or desirable.

In general, the enactment of a law follows the same procedure in all states and the federal government. The differences are slight and do not have an effect on the citizen's par-

---

*See Figure 18-1.

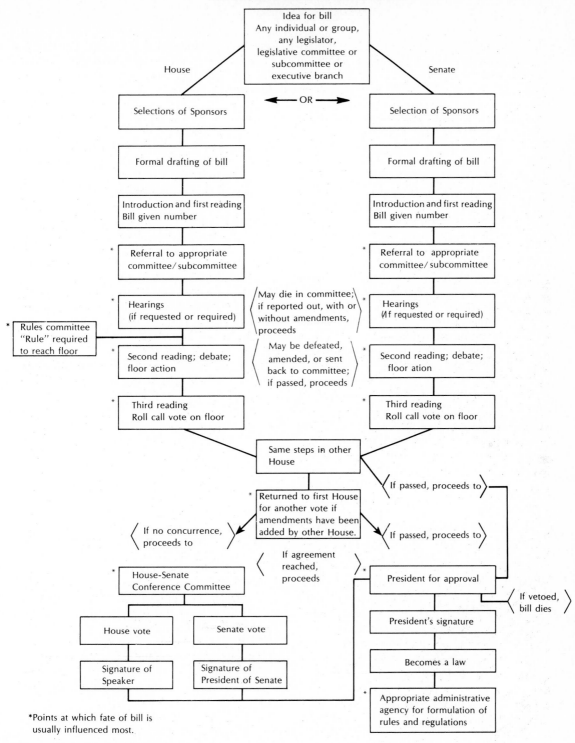

THE LEGISLATIVE PROCESS
How a bill becomes a law at the Federal level

Idea for bill
Any individual or group,
any legislator,
legislative committee or
subcommittee or
executive branch

House

Senate

←— OR —→

Selections of Sponsors

Selection of Sponsors

Formal drafting of bill

Formal drafting of bill

Introduction and first reading
Bill given number

Introduction and first reading
Bill given number

* Referral to appropriate
committee/subcommittee

* Referral to appropriate
committee/subcommittee

* Hearings
(if requested or required)

May die in committee;
if reported out, with or
without amendments,
proceeds

* Hearings
(If requested or required)

* Rules committee
"Rule" required
to reach floor

* Second reading; debate;
floor action

May be defeated,
amended, or sent
back to committee;
if passed, proceeds

* Second reading; debate;
floor ation

* Third reading
Roll call vote on floor

* Third reading
Roll call vote on floor

Same steps in other
House

If passed, proceeds to

* Returned to first House
for another vote if
amendments have been
added by other House.

If passed, proceeds to

If no concurrence,
proceeds to

If agreement
reached,
proceeds

President for approval

If vetoed,
bill dies

* House-Senate
Conference Committee

House vote

Senate vote

President's signature

Signature of
Speaker

Signature of
President of Senate

Becomes a law

* Appropriate administrative
agency for formulation of
rules and regulations

*Points at which fate of bill is
usually influenced most.

Figure 18–1. The legislative process.

ticipation in the legislative process. To keep the matter as simple as possible, introduction of a bill in the House of Representatives will be used as an illustration. Only the major steps are given, but the details, which can be quite complex, are both useful and interesting.[7]

A bill may be sponsored or introduced by one or more legislators. The legislator whose name appears first on the bill is often known as the *author* and has the responsibility for the procedural handling of the bill. Although a legislator may be requested to sponsor a bill simply because he is from an interested citizen's district, sophisticates in legislation choose more carefully. The more senior, more prestigious a legislator is, the better the chance for a bill's enactment. Bipartisan sponsorship is desirable, but on occasion a key member of the majority party alone can be just as effective. To have one or more sponsors who are members of the committees to which the bill will be sent is also a highly positive factor. Junior members of Congress often seek senior co-sponsors to enhance the opportunity for their bills to succeed.

Before a bill can be introduced, it must be couched in legal language. Although an organization may have its own knowledgeable attorney to do this, the bill is always put in its final form by a government legislative counsel; drafting of statutes is an art requiring considerable skill and experience.

After introduction in the House (which is commonly called *putting the bill in the hopper*), the bill is assigned a number by the Speaker.* Numbers are given consecutively as bills are introduced in each session; if the bill is reintroduced in the next session, it is unlikely to have the same number. The number is preceded by an HR in the House (an A or AB for Assembly in some states), or an S in the Senate. When the bill is "read" in the House by its number only, that is known as

the *first reading.* (In a Senate the sponsor introduces the bill more fully.) The Speaker then refers the bill to an appropriate committee or subcommittee (health, education, judiciary, and so on), and the bill is released for printing. Usually the printed bill includes the branch of Congress, the legislative session, bill number, by whom introduced, date, reference committee, and amendment to particular law (if pertinent). Consecutive numbers precede each line of the bill for easy reference. Definitions of key words may be given. Amendments to an existing law may be shown by have deleted words or phrases crossed out or put in parentheses and having new words or phrases put in italics or underlined.

Bills may be obtained from the sponsor or from one's own senator or representative. However, it is preferable to obtain them personally or by mail from House Documents Room, U.S. Capitol H226, Washington, D.C. 20515. (For Senate bills: Senate Documents Room S325, U.S. Capital, Washington, D.C. 20510. States also have document or bill rooms.) The bill title and number should be given, if possible, or at least the subject of the bill and approximate date of introduction. Free copies are limited to one of each bill requested, and a self-addressed mailing label should be included.

A great deal of a legislator's time is spent in committee. Some committees may go on simultaneously with the House session, and when the bell rings to indicate a roll call, members quickly go to vote, presumably having made their decisions previously. The committee to which the bill is referred is the first place where its fate can be influenced. If the bill is never put on the committee agenda or is not approved, it will generally proceed no further. The chairman has the power to keep the bill off the agenda or, conversely, to introduce it early or at a favorable time.

Open or public hearings may be held, at which any interested person may present testimony. The date and time of public hearings are published. The committee then considers the bill—sometimes in executive (closed) ses-

*The Speaker of the House is a member selected by the House membership to preside. He is usually of the majority party.

sion, if it is so agreed by open roll-call vote—and either kills it or approves it (reports it out) with or without amendments, or drafts a new bill. This activity is called *mark-up*.

Committee action is determined by a voice vote or roll call, but no record is kept of individual votes. (For this reason, there is some pressure toward having open committee meetings and voting.) For favorable action, the majority of the total committee must vote affirmatively. To get the desired vote, interested persons begin their legislative action at the committee level. Letters, phone calls, telegrams, and personal contact are used in reaching the chairman and other committee members. This is usually most effective if done by the legislator's own constituents, by whom he is understandably more influenced. Here, also, written testimony and/or oral statements can be given. The techniques for such action, which are highly important, will be given at a later point.

In Congress, the Director of the Congressional Budget Office submits a financial estimate of the cost of the measure enacted. This is included in the Committee Report written by a member of the committee. If the bill is recommended for passage, it is listed on the calendar and is sent to the Rules Committee (House only). In the House, the Rules Committee, with more majority than minority members, is most powerful; it can block the bill or clear it for debate. Presumably, the purpose is to provide some degree of selectivity in the consideration of measures by the House. The Rules Committee may also limit debate on the bill at the second reading. If a bill is blocked (no rule obtained), the discharge petition signed by a certain percentage of the House members can clear it, but this seldom succeeds.

A bill that survives all committee action is then scheduled for action "on the floor," meaning the total membership of the House. When the bill and number are read, that becomes the second reading. Amendments may be proposed at this stage and are approved or rejected by the majority. Lobbyists and inter-

ested citizens may view the proceedings from the gallery but cannot express their views. (These views should have been expressed through contact with their legislators by now.) The sponsor usually "manages" the bill (sees it through).

Debate is cut off by moving the previous question. If it is carried, the Speaker asks, "Shall the bill be engrossed and read a third time?" If approved, first the amendments and then the bill are voted on; but if the required number of objections exist, action may be postponed. If a group whose bill of interest seems to be in danger of defeat (or the reverse, if the aim is defeat) can influence at least the minimum number of congressmen to object, they can buy time to try some other approach to achieve their goals. Delay may also be desired if the amendments appended in committee or in the House are undesirable to concerned individuals. Locking on amendments to a bill that seems sure to pass is a technique for putting through some action that might not succeed on its own and that may be only remotely or not at all connected to the content of the original bill. (For instance, in one year in which the administration wanted to authorize only $12.2 million for the Nurse Training Act, the congressionally approved appropriation of $52.5 million was tagged on to another appropriations bill that the President could not veto for political reasons.) On the other hand, amendments that are totally unacceptable to the bill's sponsors may be added as a mechanism to force withdrawal or defeat of the bill. In general, amendments are introduced to strengthen, broaden, or curtail the intent of the original bill or law. If passed, they may change its character considerably. When debate is closed, the vote is taken by roll call and recorded. Passage requires a majority vote of the total House or a two-thirds vote for certain types of legislation. (Some legislators who, for some reasons, do not wish to commit themselves to a vote find it convenient to be absent at the roll call.) If a House member expects to be unavoidably absent, he may arrange to have his vote recorded by being "paired" with another absent member who would be voting on the opposite side of the question.

If the bill is passed, it goes to the Senate for a complete repetition of the process it went through in the House, and with the same opportunities to influence its passage. A bill introduced in the Senate follows the same general route with certain procedural differences. Also, the President of the Senate is the Vice-President of the United States.

A major difference is that bills that are not objected to are taken up in their order and debated. Filibustering is also a unique senatorial process—a motion to consider a bill that has been objected to is debatable, and senators opposed to it may speak to it as long as they please, thus preventing or defeating action by long delays. It takes a three-fifths vote to invoke cloture (closing debate and taking an immediate vote). This is quite difficult to achieve for political reasons of senatorial courtesy. At times, the same or a similar bill is introduced in both houses on certain important issues. The introduction of bills for nursing funding is an example. If these bills are not the same when passed by each house, or if another single bill has been amended by the second house after passing the first and the first does not concur on the amendments, the bill is sent to a conference committee consisting of an equal number of members of each house. The conference committee tries to work out a compromise that will be accepted by both houses. Sometimes the two houses are not able to arrive at a compromise and the bill dies, but usually an agreement is reached.

After passing both houses and being signed by each presider, the bill goes to the President, who may obtain opinions from federal agencies, the Cabinet, and other sources. If he signs it or fails to take action within ten days, the bill becomes law. The President may choose the latter route if he does not approve of the bill but for political reasons, such as a big margin of votes, cannot afford to veto it. He may also veto the bill and return it to the house of origin with his objections. A two-thirds affirmative vote in both houses for re-passage is necessary to override the veto. Because voting on a veto is often along party lines, overriding a veto in both houses is difficult. If the Congress adjourns before the ten days in which the President should sign the bill, it does not become law. This is known as a *pocket veto*.

Another type of legislation is a resolution. Joint resolutions originating in either house are, for all practical purposes, treated as a bill, but have the whereas-resolved format. They are identified as *HJ Res.* or *SJ Res.* with a number. Concurrent resolutions usually relate to matters affecting both houses. They are not legislative but are used to express facts, principles, opinions, and purposes of the two houses. They do not require the President's signature if passed. These are identified as *H. Con. Res.* or *S. Con. Res.* with a number. Simple resolutions concern the operation of one house alone and are considered only by the body in which they are introduced. They are designated as *H. Res.* or *S. Res.* with a number. State legislatures use similar procedures.

All bills that become law are assigned numbers, not the same as their original number, are printed, and attached to the proper volume of statutes.

One of the criticisms of the legislative process is that action is slow at the beginning of a session and relatively few bills are introduced, debated, and voted on. Often, many bills are introduced near the end of a session and receive inadequate attention. A tremendous number of bills are frequently acted on in the last weeks of a session (often passed), with some question as to whether they have been studied carefully. A technique used by some state legislatures is "stopping the clock"; the clock is figuratively stopped before midnight of the last day of the session (which has been predetermined), and all-night legislative action goes on until the necessary bills, often budgetary in nature, are acted on.

With so many checks and balances provided by "due process of law" in this democratic government, often accompanied by extreme political pressure from within the government and the influence of lobbyists, one can readily understand why it is so difficult and time-con suming to translate an idea for legislation into statutory law, urgent though the need may seem to those who originated and promoted it. A particularly good illustration of this time-consuming process is found in Figures 18-2 and 18-3, which follow the budget pro cess of what could be the Nurse Training Act from its inception in the Division of Nursing in the executive branch to final resolution.

Moreover, action on a law does not end with its enactment. Laws are usually general, for too much specificity makes them obsolete too rapidly and requires another trip through the legislative process to add amendments. Therefore, rules and regulations are devel oped by the governmental agency or depart ment within whose purview the law falls. For instance, amendments to the Nursing Practice Act are the responsibility of the department under which the state board of nurse exam iners falls, and this group will develop the reg ulations. On the national level, health legisla-

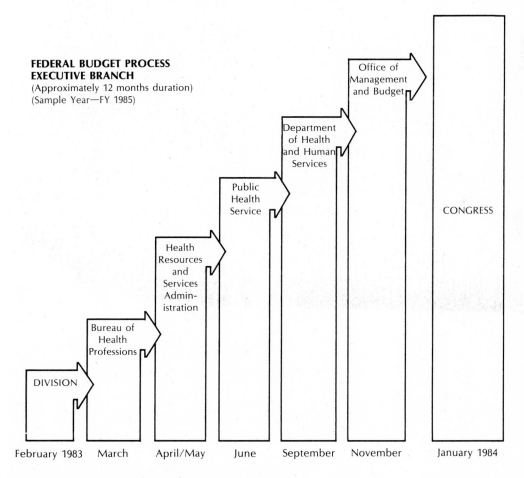

FEDERAL BUDGET PROCESS EXECUTIVE BRANCH
(Approximately 12 months duration)
(Sample Year—FY 1985)

Office of Management and Budget

Department of Health and Human Services

Public Health Service

CONGRESS

Health Resources and Services Admin- istration

Bureau of Health Professions

DIVISION

February 1983   March   April/May   June   September   November   January 1984

Figure 18-2. (Source: DHHS, FMB, BHPr, January, 1984.)

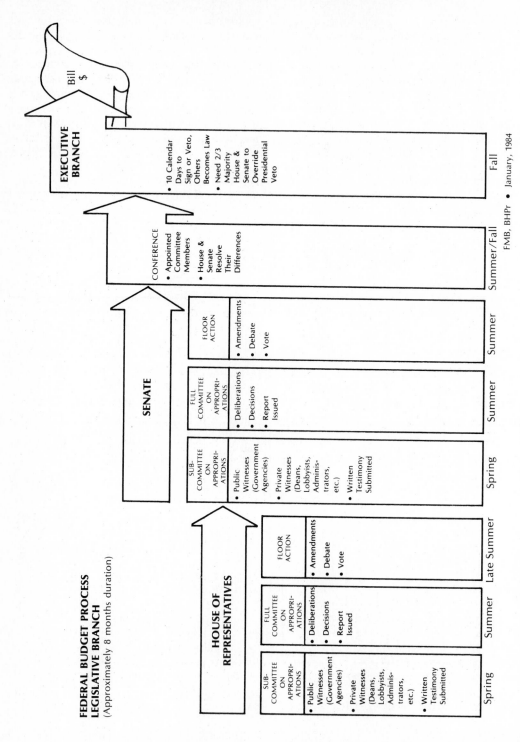

Figure 18-3. (Source: DHHS, FMB, BHPr, January, 1984.)

tion is sent to DHHS. Advisory committees of citizens are usually appointed, as spelled out by the law or the department. There is public notice of hearings for the proposed rules so that interested individuals may respond. These are published in the *Federal Register*. (States have counterparts.) Regulations are as important as the law itself, because they have the force of law and spell out the specifics of how it is to be carried out. It is also possible to influence legislation at this point and to strengthen or weaken the intent of the law. For example, rules and regulations that delineate the curriculum for a nursing education program may be flexible, rigid, or extremely loose, and a nursing school must adhere to them to become and remain approved. The opportunity to contribute to the development of regulations is available to interested organizations, which may make recommendations for individual appointments on advisory committees or offer informal participation and cooperation. They may also testify at the hearings on regulations. Regulations have been changed after hearings because of major protests by interested groups or the presentation of well-thought-out alternative regulations.

NURSES AND POLITICAL ACTION

As noted in Chapter 16, nurses as individuals and as a group are becoming more active for a variety of reasons. On the political scene, momentum has been building for a number of years, and organizations such as the ANA, NLN, and American Association of Colleges of Nursing (AACN) have taken leadership roles in mobilizing nurses in grass-roots lobbying. Among the approaches are educational programs and political consciousness-raising sessions both to teach nurses techniques and strategies and to make them aware of issues. ANA and other nursing organizations have set up networks, where the lobbyist or a monitoring group in the state or national capital alerts the organization about the status of a bill at a crucial time and an action plan

begins. Usually not all members are mobilized, only certain volunteer activists. The network is activated through a state legislative committee and a "telephone tree" that passes on the "act now" directive, or simply by mail-gram or first-class mail. If, as is often true, mass action is not needed, the difficult part is to select the nurses who have the right contacts with the right legislators. One organization sends mailings to all of its members to identify those who know legislators personally and are willing to contact them. Members are then categorized as to whether they have close, casual, or more formal relationships; an attempt is made to have at least four or five solid contacts for each legislator. Another type of categorization is by expertise. Using but not overusing the network is essential to success, as is follow-through to determine its success. While various techniques are used for lobbying, selection of one or a combination is part of the strategy. For instance, if the legislator is particularly sensitive to a constituency such as the elderly, or an influential citizen, or a particular part of his district, the members fitting that category are called on to act.

Such strategies and an active PAC (N-CAP is described in Chapter 25) have made nursing increasingly influential, particularly in Washington. A study which examined health policy influence in the 1970s placed ANA among the top fifty organizations, the top fifteen if government groups were discounted.[8] *The Congressional Quarterly* of January 1984 gives nurse lobbyists as good a rating, calling nursing "a sleeping giant" in the health lobbying community. ANA was seen as not generating the same kind of "heavy-handed lobbying campaign as AMA" but as representing far more people.

This simply points out once more the importance of skilled participation in the political process. Nurses and students of nursing have a large stake in legislation. Acting as individuals or part of a group, they can make an impact on public policy. However, learning how to communicate effectively with legislators is essential. Legislators want to hear from their constituents, but because they are extremely busy, carefully planned and organized contacts are most effective.

Personal Contact

It is sensible for nurses to become acquainted with their legislators before a legislative crisis occurs. This gives them the advantage of having made personal contact and shown general interest, and gives the legislator or staff member the advantage of a reference point. In small communities, legislators often know many of their constituents on a first-name basis through frequent contacts. This personal relationship may be more difficult to achieve in large areas, but the effort to meet and talk with legislators is never wasted.

Having identified and located the legislator, the nurse may call for an appointment or check when the legislator is available in his local office (or in his capital office if this is convenient for both). Before the visit, it is helpful to know

1. The geography of his legislative district and district number.
2. His present or past leadership in civic, cultural, or other community affairs.
3. How he voted on major controversial issues recently under consideration.
4. How he has voted in the past on major bills of concern to nurses.
5. The subject areas of his special interest such as health, consumer affairs, and so on.
6. His political party affiliation.
7. His previous occupation or profession with which he may still have some involvement.
8. What bills of major importance he has authored or coauthored.

This information may be available from the state nurses' association, political action groups (of which a partial list is included in this chapter), or literature about him from his own office.

No one can say how such a visit should be conducted—it is obviously a matter of personal style—but generally it is wise to be dressed appropriately, to be friendly, to keep the visit short, to identify oneself as a nurse and, depending on the nurse's own level of expertise, to offer to be a resource. It is always thoughtful to comment on any of his bills or votes of which the nurse approves. If the first visit coincides with pending health legislation, it is suitable to ask whether he has taken a stand and perhaps add a few pertinent comments. Not more than three major issues should probably be discussed, and it is useful to recommend specific solutions to problems if at all possible. A *brief* written account of the key points and/or documentation of facts can be left, along with an offer to provide additional information if he wants it. Legislators respond best if what is discussed is within the context of what his other constituents might want. In other words, is it good for the public and not just for nursing?

It is important to be prompt for the visit, but the constituent must be ready to accept the fact that the legislator may be late or not able to keep the appointment. The administrative assistant who substitutes will probably be knowledgeable and attentive, and the time will not be wasted. If distance and time make visiting difficult, a telephone call is a good approach. The same general guidelines can be followed, and here also, speaking to the legislator's administrative assistant serves almost as good a purpose as speaking to the legislator.

Although personal visits and calls are considered useful in trying to influence a legislator, especially if an initial introductory visit has already been made, letter writing is also effective and is the most frequent way to communicate. Legislators are particularly sensitive to communications from their constituents. They give far less attention to correspondence from outside their state or district and are often annoyed by it. If a local address is not known, addressing the letter to the state or federal house or senate is satisfactory. However, addresses should be on hand before the need arises, and some say that mail received in the local office is apt to get more attention, since the letters don't compete with other mail at the capital.

Accepted ways of addressing public officials are found in Table 18-1.

After the proper salutation, the writer should identify herself as a nurse and a constituent and state the reason for the letter. A good letter persuades not by emotionalism, vague opinion, threats, or hostility, but by reason, good sense, and facts. The letter should be brief, to the point, specific, and without trivia. In developing arguments to support a position, it is best, when possible, to cite specific local situations that will be affected by the legislation of concern. It is vital that the information about the bill be complete and accurate and the reasons for a particular stand honest and reasonable. A simple objection without reason may have some influence on the legislator, if he tends to count letters, but has little value in educating him on the issues. The writer should include in the letter the bill number, author or authors, or at

least its popular title, its status, the general purpose or interest of the bill, the specific recommendation to the legislator regarding the bill, how this stand is justified in terms of public interest, not just the profession, and what other organizations or groups have a parallel stand. If the legislator is the bill's sponsor or is on the committee considering it, the content of the letter is altered to take this into consideration.

Berating or threatening the congressman, pretending to wield vast political influence, making promises, or demanding a commitment are all counterproductive. Writing too often or too lengthily on nothing much is just as bad. For professional nurses, incorrect grammar or spelling reinforce a negative image and are inexcusable.

A letter requesting support on an issue is obviously more effective if letters are also written by other nurses and especially by non-nurses in the community. Nurses who can persuade family, friends, neighbors, or groups to

TABLE 18-1
How to Address Public Officials

Official	Address	Official	Address
President	The President of the United States The White House Washington, D.C. 20500 Dear Mr. President:	Assemblyman	The Hon. Mary Doe *The State House Trenton, N.J. 08625 Dear Ms. Doe:
Governor	The Hon. John Doe Executive Chamber Albany, N.Y. 12224 Dear Governor Doe:	Mayor	The Hon. John Doe City Hall New York, N.Y. 10007 Dear Mayor Doe:
U.S. Senator	Senator John Doe *Senate Office Building Washington, D.C. 20510 Dear Senator Doe:	City Councilman	The Hon. John Doe City Council New York, N.Y. 10007 Dear Mr. Doe:
Congressman	The Hon. John Doe *House Office Building Washington, D.C. 20515 Dear Mr. Doe: or Dear Congressman:	Judge	The Hon. Mary Doe (Address of Court) Dear Judge Doe:
State Senator	The Hon. John Doe *Senate Chambers Albany, N.Y. 12224 Dear Senator:	Other officials	(not included above) The Hon. John Doe Dear Mr. Doe:

*The local office, or if none, the home address may be used. *Note:* Addresses at state capitals vary.

support their viewpoints may supply guidelines for writing, if desired, but a form letter should *never* be written. Mimeographed letters and petitions could end up in the legislator's wastebasket.

The amount of mail reaching the capital on a sensitive issue has been known to bog down the congressional mail system for days, and it was reported that with the periodic flood of mass-produced mail, congressmen and senators were never sure how much seriousness to attach to a campaign. What does catch the eye is an example or an anecdote about how a particular bill would affect people. Some politicians have framed whole speeches around constituent anecdotes.

Some information can best be communicated to a legislator by telephone or telegram, particularly if speed is important, as when a vote is pending. Night letters are generous in the number of words allowed and inexpensive, and a fifteen-word public interest telegram can be sent to any congressman, President, or Vice-President for about a dollar.

Nurses using these methods should find that they have an increasing amount of influence with their legislators. Over a period of time, the legislators will come to recognize these nurses as persons of integrity and reliability who are accurate and confident about their facts and who are interested in the legislators' positions, attitudes, and problems. Nurses who generally agree with their legislator's approach will find that is is also politically astute to contribute to his reelection campaign and/or offer their services in the campaign. These might include house-to-house canvassing to check voter registration or to register voters, supplying transportation to the polls, making telephone calls to stimulate registration and voting, acting as registration clerk and watcher, poll clerk and watcher, block leader, or precinct captain, raising funds, preparing mailing pieces, planning publicity, writing and distributing news releases, making speeches, answering telephones and staffing information booths, planning campaign events, or having "coffees" to meet the candidate. Groups or organizations can become more extensively involved if they are able to do so legally and financially. Most nurses who have participated in political action have found it stimulating and educational.

Testifying at Hearings

Committee hearings are intended to get the opinions of citizens on particular bills or issues. Student nurses and nurses can be effective speakers for health care, but, if poorly prepared, can cause just as negative an impact. Criticisms made by legislators about nurse testimony include unfamiliarity with the bill and its revisions; a tendency to "talk down" to legislators and use professional jargon; losing equanimity when questioning becomes abrupt or abrasive; and an appearance of having more concern for their own well-being than that of the patient or public.

Attending public hearings of the committee to which health issues are referred is both an educational experience and a good preliminary before testifying oneself. It gives the opportunity to become more familiar with the atmosphere and setting of hearings, as well as the attitudes and personalities of the committee members, and to become acquainted with them individually. Although hearing rooms vary in appearance, and small states often have much simpler arrangements, generally the committee members are seated behind a raised table on which are microphones, nameplates, and copies of pertinent materials. Committee staff members and perhaps a stenotypist are seated below and to one side. A table with microphones is placed directly below for those testifying. It may be disconcerting for someone testifying to find only the chairman present at a hearing or, on the other hand, to find a full committee and hundreds in the audience. A nurse or organization may or may not be specifically invited to give testimony. Either way, it is a courtesy (and may be mandatory) to notify the committee in writing of the intent to appear or to request placement on the agenda and to provide a copy of the testimony if possible. Prior presentation of testimony does not exclude the possibility of adding appropriate remarks verbally or in answer to committee questions.

It can have a negative effect to request the opportunity to present testimony on bills of marginal interest or if a written statement inserted in the record would serve as well. Testimony should be prepared well in advance, or as much so as possible, because hearings may be called on short notice and sloppy testimony is worse than none. The ground rules applicable to the hearing (time limitations, length of testimony, number of copies to be submitted, deadline for submitting advance copies) should be requested from the committee staff and be followed.

Legislators, lobbyists, and others interested in legislative action have suggested some guidelines for giving testimony before legislative bodies:

1. Be prepared to adjust your schedule so that you can participate as the committee schedule permits. Hearings may start late, be cut short, run late into the night, be recessed and reconvened later, or otherwise changed.

2. Learn about your audience in advance, with accurate names and titles. Pronounce names correctly.

3. Although you have the right to disagree with your professional organization, totally independent action confuses the issues for legislators. It is better to work within the organization, ironing out differences. A collective voice usually carries more weight than isolated testimony.

4. Pay attention to protocol; be sure to thank the committee for the opportunity to address it.

5. Introduce yourself with a very brief biographical sketch; state the issue on which you are testifying, and note whether you represent a group or only yourself.

6. If the testimony is in writing and has been given to the committee, they may prefer that the information be briefly recapitulated rather than read completely. Be prepared with both a long and a short text.

7. Be brief and concise (about ten to fifteen minutes); discuss only the specific bill or issue concerned, refrain from irrelevant comments, and speak plainly and without professional jargon. Relate your arguments to people, not abstractions.

8. Be secure in your knowledge of the facts, totally honest, and comfortable in speaking to a group. Have additional data available to help in answering questions accurately. It is disastrous to present false information or a dishonest interpretation. If possible, know the data on which your testimony is based and do not simply read a statement prepared by someone else.

9. When being questioned, it helps to be able to think under pressure, remain cool, not become angry, and have a sense of humor. (Some legislators use committee hearings as stages; some may not be friendly to the nurse's cause; others have predetermined ideas and prefer to keep them.) Never try to bluff; if you do not know the answer, it is best to say so and perhaps volunteer to provide the answer to the committee before the vote or have it placed in the record.

10. As in any other situation, appearance is important. Be appropriately dressed; a uniform is not appropriate except in unusual circumstances.

11. Be aware that appearing at a hearing is often all that is necessary. Testifying may not be the best action for various reasons and should not be forced. The appearance of a large number of nurses and students at a hearing indicates that it is of major concern to them. Behavior should be courteous. This is also no time for intraprofessional quarreling.

12. Be aware that everyone appearing before a committee represents a special interest

group; legislators weigh conflicting views to make their own decision.

13. Don't be shocked or disillusioned if the vote goes against you at the hearing. Votes may have been promised to colleagues at this initial stage, even before the hearing, but may be reversed on the floor. If the bill is filed, a new version may be introduced, with changes made to minimize the opposition.

Politics is often a matter of compromise. Adherents of a bill must be prepared to yield on some issues as necessary, meanwhile holding firm on the most vital issues and allowing opponents to compromise on these points. Most of all, it is essential that nurses continue to be involved in political action, becoming ever more knowledgeable, sophisticated, and effective.

Other Means of Influencing Legislation

There are times when individual nurses are selected to participate in legislative and governmental advisory committees on the local, state, and national levels. Most often such a nurse comes to the attention of the appointing individual through professional achievements, political or professional activities, or recommendation by organizations. Organizations such as the ANA and NLN keep alert for the inception of pertinent committees and exert pressure to have nurses included. More and more nurses and students are being appointed to such multidisciplinary and advisory groups. The contributions of thoughtful and informed nurses to committee deliberations, actions, and recommendations can change the course of health care. Nurses have shown that they can be a positive force in legislation, and have found, in addition, personal and professional satisfaction in participation in what Woodrow Wilson called the dance of legislation: "Once begin the dance of legislation, and you must struggle through its mazes as best you can to the breathless end—if any end there be."

REFERENCE SOURCES FOR POLITICAL ACTION AND/OR LEGISLATION

Primary sources of information in Washington, D.C. are:

1. Government agency staff experts.
2. Congressional committee and subcommittee staff members.
3. Staff members of senators and congressmen.
4. The Library of Congress.
5. Private research organizations.
6. Professional, trade, and labor organizations.
7. Directories.
8. Publications.

Many government publications and directories are available from the Government Printing Office, Washington, D.C. 20402. If information is needed but you are not sure which federal agency to contact, the Federal Information Center (General Services Administration, 7th & D Streets, S.W., Washington, D.C. 20407; [202] 755-8660) can refer you to the proper agency.

For vacation, adjournments and recess, or scheduling of bills for a floor debate or vote, phone the Senate or House majority whips' offices or the Senate or House Democratic or Republican Cloakroom (recorded message). For committee hearings and schedule, see the *Congressional Record* for the next day (the last issue of the week lists the following week's schedule); United Press International or Associated Press Datebook; *Washington Star;* or *Washington Post,* "Today's Activities in the Senate and House." To check if the President has signed a particular bill passed by the Congress, contact the White House Records Office (give bill number) or Archives. To determine the status of a bill in the House or Senate, call or write to the House or Senate Status Office.

Organizations

American Association of University Women

2401 Virginia Avenue, N.W.
Washington, D.C.

Americans for Democratic Action
1411 K Street
Washington, D.C. 20005

American Nurses' Association and
N-CAP (Nurses' Coalition for Action
   in Politics).
Government Relations Department
American Nurses' Association
1101 14th Street, N.W.
Suite 200
Washington, D.C. 20005

Common Cause
2030 M Street, N.W.
Washington, D.C. 20036

League of Women Voters
1730 M Street, N.W.
Washington, D.C. 20036

National Health Council, Inc.
Government Relations
1740 Broadway
New York, NY 10019

National League for Nursing
Public Information Division
10 Columbus Circle
New York, NY 10019

Women's Political Caucus

1302 18th Street, N.W.
Room 603
Washington, D.C. 20036

REFERENCES

1. Charles Cnudde and Donald McCrone, "The Linkage Between Constituency Attitudes and Congressional Voting Behavior: A Causal Model," in Roderick Bell et al. eds., *Political Power* (New York: Free Press, 1969), p. 206.
2. Beatrice Kalisch and Philip Kalisch, *Politics of Nursing* (Philadelphia: J. B. Lippincott Company, 1982), p. 391.
3. "Common Cause: Money Talks on Health Issues," *The Nation's Health,* **8**:5 (Dec. 1978).
4. Margo Porter, "Put the Myths About PACs to Rest," *Assn. Mgt.,* **34**:35 (July 1982).
5. Kalisch and Kalisch, op. cit., p. 421.
6. Jonathan Walters, "Multiply Your Clout with A Grassroots Lobbying Network," *Assn. Mgt.,* **35**:61 (Apr. 1983).
7. The legislative process is given in full detail in Charles Zinn, *How Our Laws Are Made* (Washington, D.C.: U.S. Government Printing Office, 1978).
8. "Study Ranks APHA Relatively High in Health Policy Influence," *The Nation's Health,* **13**:16 (May 1983).

19

Federal Legislation Affecting Nursing

Both federal and state laws have a major impact on nursing practice and education. At the state level, nurses need to know about their own nursing practice acts and should be acquainted with the licensure laws of other health practitioners. These are discussed in Chapter 20. Other state legislation affecting the health and welfare of nurses may be equally important, and nurses should keep abreast of both proposed and enacted legislation.

In this chapter, the focus will be on federal legislation that affects the practice of nursing and the rights of nurses; occasionally, state laws that are almost universal or closely related to federal laws will be included. Obviously, all health legislation fits into that category, but those laws that seem to have particular significance will be highlighted here.

SOCIAL INSURANCE

Social insurance differs from personal, or private, insurance in that it is compulsory and, for the most part, operated under governmental auspices. The local, state, or federal government raises funds by taxation to pay the benefits of social insurance. This type of insurance is common in many European countries, but because of the traditional American belief that the individual should be as self-sufficient as possible, the United States was slow to establish a system of social insurance.

Workmen's Compensation

The first such insurance to be held constitutional was the *Workmen's Compensation Act*, enacted by the state of Washington in 1911. Today all states require employers in industry to carry workmen's compensation, but in some states, nonprofit organizations, including hospitals, are exempt. However, most nurses are covered by one or another of this type of insurance. Federally, employees are usually covered by the *Federal Employees' Compensation Act*, enacted in 1952.

Workmen's compensation insurance, the cost of which is carried entirely by the employer, pays to employees who are injured on the job a proportion of their regular salaries for the time they are unable to work because of their injuries. If they are permanently disabled, they are entitled to additional compensation.

Workmen's compensation insurance laws do away with the requirement of proof that the employee was negligent or that the employee was free from contributory negligence. They also prevent court action for injuries and provide instead an administrative procedure for securing awards of compensation.[1]

Many states have extended the coverage provided by workmen's compensation laws to include occupational diseases; other states have enacted separate occupational disease acts, some of which cover all types of occupational disease; others specify which ones are covered. The major breakthrough on the federal level was the enactment of the *Occupational Safety and Health Act of 1970* (also discussed in Chapters 6 and 15), which established administrative machinery for the development and enforcement of standards of occupational health and safety.[2] There are still no standards for the health care industry, which means, according to the law, that state safety rules remain in effect. These vary from state to state and even among specific communities. Of course, in case of negligence, the employer is liable to employee suits. This is important to the nurse who may acquire a communicable disease, a staphylococcal infection, or another illness on the job, for which she or he might be entitled to benefits under the state law.*

State laws governing workmen's compensation are not all alike, but most cover the majority of employees. They do not cover those employees who were intoxicated at the time of their accidents or those who willfully injured themselves. Every employee and every employer should know the terms of the workmen's compensation law in a given state. However, some changes may be coming.

In 1972, the National Commission on State Workmen's Compensation laws reported to the President and Congress that the protection furnished by workmen's compensation was, in general, "inadequate and inequitable." Between 1972 and 1977, hundreds of state laws were enacted in response to the Commission's

recommendations. However, a 1979 survey found that only about twelve of the nineteen recommendations were being implemented, particularly in relation to rehabilitation and prevention. In addition, research studies show that some 10 million workers, usually in low-paying jobs, are not covered at all. The fact that the cost of compensation insurance is rising so quickly is a further problem.

These laws are likely to remain on a state level; there is resistance to enacting a national law. One expert in the field recommended that each state have an advisory commission to study its act and make recommendations, and that the federal government encourage the states with technical and financial assistance.[3]

Social Security

Beginning in the early 1930s, the tradition in this country that every person was almost entirely responsible for his or her own health and welfare began to be challenged by many forces, particularly the federal government. As time went on, social welfare legislation to help the masses and sometimes specialized groups was enacted more and more often with less and less resistance by the legislators and their constituents.

As the social movement grew, the federal government became aware of people's needs that they either had not noticed or had not considered their business in the past. Many believed that the individual states should shoulder this responsibility and objected to the usurping of states' rights by the federal government. As the composition of the Congress changed with each new election, attitudes toward government involvement in social welfare also changed, to the extent that under President Dwight D. Eisenhower a Department of Health, Education, and Welfare (DHEW) was created by act of Congress in April 1953.* The then existing United States

---

*See Chapter 6 references for information about specific occupational hazards for nurses.

*Through the Department of Education Organization Act (PL96-99), enacted in 1979, an independent Department of Education (DOE) was created, and the remaining functions of DHEW were reorganized under the new Department of Health and Human Services (DHHS).

Public Health Service (PHS) became part of the new department. From that time on, health care facilities and personnel received increasing attention in the White House and on Capitol Hill.

The *Social Security Act*, passed in 1935 and amended many times since, is administered by the Department of Health and Human Services (DHHS), of which the Social Security Administration is a part. The lawmakers who produced the original act based it on the conviction that a program of economic security must "have as its primary aim the assurance of an adequate income to each human being in childhood, youth, middle age, or old age—in sickness or in health" and that it must "provide safeguards against all of the hazards leading to destitution and dependency."

The attainment of that goal requires, above all else, the broad economic objective of productive employment for those who are able and want to work. Second, and in proper perspective, is the goal to prevent dependency, which requires, on an ever-broadening scale, highly organized and efficient administrative procedures, and adequate financing.

The Social Security Act and its later amendments provide many benefits: federal Old-Age, Survivors', and Disability Insurance; unemployment compensation; federal grants-in-aid to states to promote special health and welfare services for children; matching funds to help finance state-administered relief programs for dependent children and needy persons who are aged, blind, or permanently disabled. Since 1965, the Medicare program (Title XVIII) has financed a large share of the hospital, nursing home, and home health care costs (and, on an optional basis contingent on the payment of a small monthly premium, the medical care costs) of persons over sixty-five who are eligible for Social Security benefits. Title XIX, Medicaid, passed at the same time, was a hasty compromise on the part of the Congress and can probably be best described as a cooperative federal-state medical assistance program for the poor.

By 1965, the Social Security Act provided four welfare programs administered by the state: Aid to the Totally Disabled (ATD) and the Blind (AB), Old Age Security (OAS), Aid to Families with Dependent Children (AFDC), and Medicaid; as well as the Social Security program for the retired and disabled wage earner and Medicare. The Social Security Amendment of 1972 federalized ATD, AB, and OAS, and these programs became known as the Supplemental Security Income program (SSI). The level of these federal payments to recipients is uniform throughout the states and higher than that paid by some states previously. Total assistance received by the SSI recipient must be no lower than before SSI; states may also add to the benefits voluntarily.

To a great extent, Social Security was originally and still is slanted toward the male wage earner, with the assumption made that most couples would remain married, that the husband would be the main breadwinner, and that the wife would stay at home.

Because of the aging population, the expenses of Social Security are becoming greater. Therefore, there is periodic legislation to try to keep the fund stable, such as the Social Security Amendments of 1983. Major changes are discussed in the following sections.

Old-Age and Survivors' Insurance. The average citizen who talks about Social Security benefits is usually referring to the federal Old-Age and Survivors' Insurance program. It provides a monthly payment from the government after retirement age; an income for the widow or widower (if over sixty-two years of age) and for dependent children (if they are under eighteen) if he or she dies; and a small lump-sum payment to help cover funeral expenses.

The amount of these benefits is based on the individual's average earnings and length of employment during his or her working life. Retirement age is officially sixty-two for both men and women. If she or he prefers, however, an individual may wait until sixty-five to start drawing benefits; if so, monthly checks will be larger than if begun at sixty-two. If a person continues to work for a salary after retirement age, the amount of annual earnings affects the Social Security benefits. Beginning in the next century, the retirement age will gradually be increased until it reaches sixty-six in 2009 and sixty-seven in 2027. Meanwhile, delayed retirements (beyond sixty-five) will gain higher benefits (after 1989). Social Security benefits became taxable in 1984.

If both a husband and wife work, each is eligible for retirement benefits in his or her own right. The working wife, on retirement, is entitled to her own retirement benefit and also to a wife's benefit, based on her husband's earnings, on a prorated basis. She would not receive the *full amount* of both her own retirement benefit and her wife's benefit, but if the husband dies, the wife receives the larger of the two benefits, or her own plus part of her husband's to make the highest possible benefit.

Because of the male-female differentiations and inequities in the Social Security Act, these benefits are changed periodically through amendments or by Supreme Court decisions. For instance, child care benefits were once denied to the widower of a deceased female wage earner, and widowers now have the same survivor's pension rights as widows (see above).

Major areas of inequity that still exist include no pension for divorced women if they have not been married for a certain number of years or if the husband is not retired at the time of divorce; no individual pension for women who work at home only; and less coverage for a two-earner family than for a one-earner (the wife usually gets no extra benefits for working). Of further concern is the limited amount a person can earn without losing Social Security insurance benefits between the ages of sixty-two and seventy, a serious problem in inflationary times.

The report of the Social Security Advisory Council, a group of prominent private citizens established by the law, has periodically made several suggestions (with no guarantee of acceptance), among them that all Social Security credits and benefits be shared equally by husbands and wives and that every retired person have minimal Social Security benefits at age sixty-five plus whatever benefits may be earned as workers.

Some employers not participating in Social Security, notably the federal government, had plans of their own and therefore felt that they were giving their employees adequate protection without Social Security coverage. However, beginning in 1984, all federal employees and those in nonprofit organizations must be covered by Social Security.

Disability Insurance. An insured worker of any age, male or female, who becomes totally disabled can begin receiving benefits after a six-month waiting period. To be eligible for these benefits, the worker must (1) have been covered by social security for a specified number of years (five to ten); (2) have a physical or mental disability of indefinite duration; and (3) be so badly disabled that she or he cannot work at gainful employment.

Again, women are at a disadvantage because benefits are not given to anyone who has dropped out of the work force for five years unless she or he has worked five years after that. This does not take into consideration that many women drop out of full-time work for child care.

Unemployment Insurance. Another major provision of the Social Security Act of 1935 is a system of unemployment insurance to protect workers who are unemployed through no fault of their own. Although it seems unlikely that many professional nurses will need this kind of financial assistance because jobs are generally available for qualified nurses, it is possible that a nurse may, for various reasons, need this protection. Situations involving discharge of a nurse are not always clear-cut. For example, one nurse, discharged from her position in one hospital because of her legitimate activities in behalf of her state nurses' association's economic security program, found other hospitals reluctant to employ her. Having demonstrated to her local employment service office that she was unemployed through no fault of her own (her association activities were entirely ethical), she claimed and received unemployment insurance until she found a more openminded employer.

Unemployment insurance is administered by the state governments. Federal law specifies a maximum and minimum benefit, and the states must remain within these limits. Each state has its own law governing the amount of weekly benefits allowed the unemployed person and the number of weeks for which it will be continued. This is because the cost of living and employment conditions vary so widely in different sections of the country.

To collect unemployment insurance, a person must have been out of work for at least a week; be able to work and willing to take a job in his or her line of work at the prevailing rate; must not have left the previous job without good cause or have been asked to resign because of misconduct. In some states, marriage, pregnancy, and further education do not qualify one to claim unemployment insurance, and a mother cannot collect unemployment benefits for a certain period after childbirth.

Some states do not qualify certain classes of workers for unemployment insurance. These may include farm and domestic workers, members of the employer's family, workers in nonprofit organizations, students, medical interns, and others.

Employers of fewer than four employees were not included until 1972, when states were also required to extend to each of their subdivisions the option of participating. In 1969, only 12 percent of management and 19 percent of government nurses had unemployment insurance coverage, but federal legislation required that by January 1972, this coverage be extended to all nurses except those employed by local government.

Medicare-Medicaid

Medicare-Medicaid is a form of national health insurance proposed in one way or another since 1915. Health insurance provisions were deleted from the 1935 Social Security Act by President Roosevelt because he believed this would be necessary to ensure passage of the bill. When enacted into law in 1965, the Medicare title provided hospitalization for Social Security recipients, as well as allowing purchase of insurance for physicians' services at a nominal monthly fee. The Medicaid title expanded the Kerr-Mills law, which provided payments to states for health care of the "medically needy" aged, to include persons in programs for aid to dependent children, the blind, and the permanently disabled. This law was extremely controversial, with some citizens and legislators not completely committed to the idea and the AMA rigorously and uncompromisingly opposed to it. ANA, however, supported it. Passed in 1965, Medicare went into effect on July 1, 1966.

Benefits and Coverage. There are two parts to Medicare, and in both the benefits are limited to those who are sixty-five years of age or older and some under sixty-five who are disabled. Upon its initiation, Medicare benefits were available to any citizen of the United States within this age group who had lived in this country more than five years and regardless of whether or not he or she was covered by Social Security. However, at that time it was stated that after 1968, individuals would have to have Social Security coverage to qualify for Medicare.

Part 1 of Medicare (HI) is designed to pay the major share of the costs for the individual over sixty-five who needs care in a hospital, HMO, extended care facility (a nursing home, for instance), or care at home. The coverage is not total: the patient pays a small deductible (which has been increasing) for hospital care, and the government pays the rest for a given period. Hospital stays longer than that period are financed partly by the patient and partly by the government. There are also limitations on the circumstances under which costs of care in an extended care facility will be paid for, and on the number of days covered. Outpatient hospital diagnostic services are paid for, again after a deductible, and with certain other stipulations. Payment is also made for visits by staff of a home health agency—such as a visiting nurse association—to care for a patient at home, if "skilled" nursing services are required. Part 1 is financed by Social Security taxes.

Part 2 of Medicare is an optional supplemental medical insurance program (SMI), available to the person over sixty-five upon payment of a small monthly premium matched by the government. This plan pays 80 percent of the individual's costs for physician's services (in the hospital, home, or office), diagnostic tests and x-rays, therapeutic equipment such as braces and artificial limbs, and additional home health visits over and above those provided by Part 1 of Medicare. The patient must pay the first x number of dollars of these expenses in each calendar year; after that, the 80 percent coverage goes into effect. Individuals have the same right to choose their own physicians that they always had.

SMI is financed through premiums paid by those enrolled or by someone (the state) paying in their behalf, plus general revenues.

Care covered in all cases must be "necessary and reasonable." Custodial care that could be provided by people without training is not included. Also not covered are certain services the elderly often need: drugs, routine eye and dental care, preventive care, or long-term care.

The Medicare program is the responsibility of the Social Security Administration, which enters into contracts with Blue Cross–Blue Shield, commercial carriers, and group prac-

tice prepayment plans to serve as administrative agents.* This arrangement is considered by some as not only adding another layer of bureaucracy, but also increasing costs.

In 1966, Medicare covered all "aged" persons (over sixty-five). Beginning in 1968, at least three calendar quarters in covered (Social Security) employment were needed; by 1975, the individual had to have the required number of quarters to be eligible for retired worker benefits. This automatically excluded from HI those not covered by social security, although the 1972 amendments allowed the noneligible to enroll in the program by voluntarily paying a monthly premium that was rather high. Any aged person can enroll in SMI. At the end of the first ten years of Medicare, of all the aged enrolled in HI, about 98 percent were also enrolled in SMI.[4]

The Medicaid program had two major objectives: ensuring that covered persons received adequate medical care, and reducing the financial burden of medical expenditures for those with severely limited financial resources. Before Medicaid, most poor people had little or no health insurance and often went without needed care or had to depend on charity. Medicaid was intended to cover all people eligible for welfare (ATD, AB, OAS, and AFDC) plus, at the option of the state, other poor people not eligible for welfare, such as the aged, blind, disabled, or dependent children whose incomes were slightly more than the welfare level. As the program became more and more expensive, legislative amendments altered and cut back eligibility requirements. The categories are complex and, unfortunately, many who need Medicaid's health care fall into the cracks. The law does not define the amount and duration of the service for which it requires the state to

---

*The term *intermediaries* is used for those handling claims from hospitals, home health agencies, and skilled nursing facilities; *carriers* is used for those handling claims from doctors and other suppliers of services covered.

pay, and, as the program has become more burdensome, many states have cut drastically the amount of services.[5] An instance of this might be the denial of payment for abortion except under limited circumstances, although in this case there are also other related emotional factors. The Hyde Amendment (attached as a rider to the appropriation bill since 1977), which outlawed most federal fundings for abortions, and its counterparts in some thirty-nine states that prevented the use of state funds, cut payment for abortion by public monies by 99 percent, as estimated by the Alan Guttmacher Institute in 1979. Some 34,000 women annually were probably denied legal abortions. However a ruling by a federal judge early in 1980 declaring that abortion aid limits for the poor were unlawful had the potential for change. The potential evaporated when, some months later, the Supreme Court upheld the constitutionality of the congressional ban on federal financing for abortions.*

Nevertheless, the long history of lower utilization of health services by the poor changed with Medicaid. By 1974, there was evidence that the poor saw physicians 13 percent more than did persons with high incomes; and children of poor families increased their use of physician services, whereas those of high-income families reduced theirs. Considered improved was the care of pregnant women. However, whether the quality of care in general is the same is moot.[6] It is predicted that it will get worse. Moreover, there is some question of whether services really reach those who need them. This is especially true of some of the special programs related to Medicaid, such as the Early and Periodic Screening, Diagnosis, and Treatment Program (EPSDT), which served only about 2 million of an eligible 12 million children.

Financing of Social Security

All federal benefits under the Social Security Act are financed by special taxes paid by employees, employers, and self-employed per-

sons. (Certain groups are excluded.) The tax is calculated on a percentage of the worker's income on which the employee pays one-half and the employer the other half. The self-employed person earning more than a minimal, set amount pays the entire tax, but at a lower percentage of income rate than the employed person whose employer pays half the tax. Deductions on a paycheck stub appear under *FICA*.

In recent years, there has been some concern about the fiscal stability of Social Security. FICA payments by the working person are increasing dramatically to support the older and disabled, as people live longer and receive increased (and necessary) benefits. Eliminating inequities will increase the cost even more. Whether or not Social Security can continue to be funded in the same way is being questioned.

Major Social Security Amendments Affecting Health Care

In the years following enactment, much criticism was directed toward Medicare-Medicaid because of the cost of the program. Increased costs were caused in part by the compromises forced by opposition to the bill, which established private insurance companies as fiscal intermediaries and allowed physicians and health care providers to set their own fees. Cost abuses received considerable publicity, and the frequent subsequent amendments were aimed at reducing the costs. A number of amendments since 1966 have been geared, to a great extent, to controlling the soaring costs of the program. There are now rigid regulations about the length of institutional stay that will be reimbursed, the level of care requirements for skilled nursing home services, payment for specific services, and coverage of particular groups. The second major concern, quality of care, also resulted in legislative amendments, for despite the fact that any institutions participating in Medicare must be certified by DHHS and those participating in Medicaid must abide by standards

---

*See Chapter 6.

ing over control of the money to the states. With block grants, there is little accounting to the federal government as to how the funds are spent, and state politics have an immediate effect. The final outcome was a compromise, the creation of four block grants: preventive health, combining eight programs; health services, combining mental health, alcohol abuse, and drug abuse programs; a primary care block, composed only of the community health center program; and maternal and child health care, combining seven programs. The categorical programs that survived were family planning, childhood immunization, venereal disease research and treatment, migrant health centers, tuberculosis grants, and primary care research and demonstrations. Newly approved was a new adolescent family life (AFL) program. Some of these funds were to be used to continue to provide services to pregnant teenagers, and new funds were to be used to provide counseling to teenagers to "encourage self-discipline." (AFL had a rather nonproductive three-year tenure, but strong conservative groups supported it for refunding.) All of these grants ran out in 1984. Continued cuts in PHS grants were expected by public health experts during the second four years of the Reagan administration, but at the beginning, the PHS lived under HR 6028, the 1985 *Appropriations Bill* for DHHS, signed by the President. Of the block grants cited above, all survived as new bills were signed into law at the end of the 98th Congress, except the primary care block and the migrant health centers. As is usual, these were then funded on continuing resolutions until the new Congress could write new bills. Also passed was *PH 98–551 Prevention Centers*, which established an Office of Disease Prevention and Health Promotion in the Office of the Assistant Secretary for Health and created 13 new research centers for disease prevention techniques, to be located in schools of public health.

Even more dramatic were the provisions of the *Tax Equity* and *Fiscal Responsibility Act of 1982* (TEFRA) (PL 97-248). The major

provisions affected Medicare and PSROs. Briefly, TEFRA extended Medicare to federal employees and required employers to offer employees aged sixty-five to sixty-nine and their dependents the same health benefits offered to younger employees; it permitted states to cover, under Medicaid, certain disabled children who reside at home; it discontinued the nursing salary cost differential (which had been allowed for inpatient services to older patients on the assumption that they need more intensive nursing care); it allowed hospitals to opt out of the Social Security system (although this was seen as a technicality); and it allowed reimbursement to hospitals for certain anti-union organizing activities. Most far-reaching of all, it required the Secretary of DHHS and certain congressional committees to develop Medicare prospective reimbursement legislative proposals for hospitals, SNFs, and, to the extent feasible, other providers. Other cost-cutting mechanisms affecting health care facilities and providers were also included.

The work on the prospective payment mechanisms resulted in enactment of PL 98-21, variously called the *Social Security Amendments of 1983*, the *Social Security Rescue Plan*, or simply the *DRG law*. This legislation established a "prospective payment system based on 467 Diagnostic Related Groups (DRGs) categories that allow pretreatment diagnosis billing categories for almost all United States hospitals reimbursed by Medicare."[10] Separate payment rates apply to urban and rural areas; psychiatric, long-term care, and children's and rehabilitation hospitals will continue to be reimbursed under the cost-based system. (Most experts expected them to be included later, as well as home care.) The system was to be phased in over three years, and some states that had already initiated their own plan were temporarily excluded (but with a check on their results). Capital-related costs were excluded, and direct and indirect teaching costs would continue to be paid. (Again, this was expected to change.) The Secretary of DHHS was required to collect data and report to Congress on the advisability and feasibility of including physician payments. What DRGs mean to a hospital is that if a patient is kept more than the number of days designated by the patient's DRG category, the extra costs must be absorbed. If the patient goes home early, the amount designated for the scheduled days is the hospital's clear profit. Some predicted that hospitals would encourage doctors to admit more patients who were not potential "problems" or those who were self-paying or insured.

Needless to say, the DRG system had a direct impact on nursing.* In some cases, hospitals, desperate to cut costs, chose to retain lower-paid nursing personnel, rather than RNs. Others chose to turn to all-RN staffs that could actually save money by teaching patients or by anticipating potential complications, so that the patient would be discharged before the DRG designated days. As noted in Chapter 15, the job market for nurses also became tighter. However, some nurses felt that this was also a good time to identify nursing services, so that they could be separated from general daily charges. Others identified ways of determining the acuity of nursing care so that these could be considered in the DRG system.[11,12] The next several years will probably see considerable additional legislation aimed at cost control.

Health Planning Legislation

One of the early health services laws that provided funds (on a matching grant basis) for constructing and expanding health care facilities was the *Hospital Survey and Construction Act of 1946*, popularly known as the *Hill-Burton Act*. It was highly successful, providing funds for more than 30 percent of the hospital beds in this country in its first twenty years, and funding was renewed several times.

Part of the original intent of Hill-Burton was planning. States received money for developing a planning program, supposedly

based on need. As might be expected, however, politics was a more important factor than any rational basis for planning. This resulted in a substantial oversupply of hospital beds and contributed to inflation of health care costs as it became imperative to keep those beds filled.

Another *carrot-and-stick approach* to planning, as Wing calls it,[13] was the Regional Medical Program (RMP), originally labeled the Heart Disease, Cancer, and Stroke Amendments of 1965, although never limited to those diseases. RMP did not involve direct financial aid to health facilities, but was intended to finance the coordination of research efforts and to finance the distribution of information from research institutions to the whole health care system. More than $1 billion was spent in the first ten years of the program to both local RMPs and the projects they sponsored. Projects included research, training, data exchange, direct patient care on a demonstration basis, or the construction of equipment and facilities related to these activities. (Nurses were involved in RMPs on a secondary level but benefited from the many educational programs.) RMP was federal funding for "needed" change in health care delivery; it was planning money for private providers to change the system. Partly because of medical politics, it failed to serve its purpose; there is little evidence that the money was well spent.

The first real federal attempt to institute a national system of health planning was through the *Comprehensive Health Planning and Public Health Services Amendments of 1966*, known as *Partnership for Health*. This legislation set up five new programs related to health planning. Two are most pertinent. One provided funds to state governments to maintain a state health planning agency and a consumer-dominated advisory council and to establish a state plan for health planning activities (CHP "A" agency.) The second provided funds to locally based, nonprofit private or publicly owned agencies designated by the state CHP agency as the approved areawide planning agency (CHP "B"

---

*See the bibliography for specific articles on how nurses may, should, and do work within the DRG system.

agency). Although a nationwide network of planning agencies was established under CHP, both money and authority were limited. The only comprehensive authority was to "review and comment" on requests for federal funding. "Most CHP agencies (were) so ineffective, understaffed, and administratively inept that this review and comment process was little more than added paperwork for the funding applicants,"[14] especially since the federal agencies paid little attention to the comments. CHP also failed.

The most comprehensive of these planning laws was the *National Health Planning and Resources Development Act of 1974*, designed to set up a new system of state and local health planning agencies and to integrate into those agencies a program for the support of certain kinds of health facility construction. It has been described by some as a mere reorganization and revitalization of the CHP, RMP, and Hill-Burton programs after their statutory authorization drew to a close. The objectives of the act included (1) increasing access to health services; (2) maintaining continuity of care; (3) restoring increases in health care costs; (4) preventing unnecessary duplication of services; and (5) assuring effective utilization of manpower resources. Each state was required to establish a state health planning and development agency (SHPDA) and a state health coordinating council (SHCC) that serves as advisor to the agency. SPHDA prepared state health plans for budget review. (A national council developed guidelines for state councils). The SHPDA was delegated to conduct state health planning and functions related to both the state and health systems agencies (HSAs). The HSAs in various geographic areas of the states had the responsibility to collect and analyze data concerning the health care status of the residents in their designated health service area, the state of the area's health care delivery system, and its utilization, among other things. Each HSA was required to develop a health systems plan (HSP) and an overall implementation plan (AIP). Most were private, nonprofit organizations with govern-

ing boards of ten to thirty persons, the majority consumers.[15] Nurses served on a number of these boards. Their power lay in their ability to review and approve or disapprove use of certain federal funds in their areas. PL 93-641 was an immensely complex, multifaceted law. HSAs were always accused of "playing politics." Communication and coordination among HSAs, state, and national agencies have not been adequate, and there have been multiple objections to the health planning guidelines that were four years in the process and did not go into effect until 1978.

In 1979, the Health Planning and Resources Development Amendments of 1979 were signed into law, with some weakening of the planning agencies' authority to rein in spending and unneeded facility building. Agreement on the amendments had been delayed for three years because of the various conflicts about the effectiveness of the law. Too much provider influence was one accusation. Another was related to the "certificate of need" power of the HSAs, without which existing health facilities cannot buy certain expensive equipment, and none can be developed in the first place without a certificate. Health planning squeaked through in OBRA 81, but, its long-term future is uncertain. A number of states have already dismantled the state planning group, but in others, they are strong.

Health Services Legislation

Various other laws providing health care programs and services of interest to nurses include the following:

The Community Mental Health Center Act of 1963 was a three-year program authorizing $150 million for the construction of community mental health centers. The act also provided for increased federal aid to state and local communities in conducting research to lessen the incidence of mental retardation through improved maternal and child health programs at the state and local levels. In 1965, an amendment to the act provided funds for staffing the centers as well as for providing physical facilities. Refundings have been inadequate, and mental health is now in a block grant.

The Maternal and Child Health Law (1963) gave matching grants to help the states provide better care, particularly for mothers and children in low-income families. Most maternal-child services were put in the block grant cited earlier. However, in late 1984, the Child Health Assurance Program (CHAP) was passed as part of the huge Deficit Reduction Act of 1984. It mandated health coverage for certain types of women and children not eligible for AFDC or Medicaid.

The *Older Americans Act of 1965*, amended again in 1975 to substantially increase appropriations for senior citizens' social, health, and nutrition services and funded through 1978, was the first major law besides Social Security to concentrate on the needs of the elderly. This law was last reauthorized in 1984.

The Health Maintenance Organization Act of 1973 authorized the spending of $375 million during the next five years to help set up and evaluate HMOs in communities throughout the country. The concept is an arrangement in which subscribers pay a predetermined flat fee monthly or yearly that entitles them to basic health care services as needed, (Chapter 7). Emphasis is on preventive care and health teaching. This was extended and amended in 1976, relieving some of the rigid requirements imposed in 1973. All funding was to end by September 1980, but in 1979 the federal government announced a ten-year plan to encourage the growth of HMOs. Discrimination for or against HMOs concerning certificates of need was an issue in the amendments to PL 93-641; the final result was exemption of HMOs from certificates of need. Because the Reagan Administration believes HMOs should be competitive in the private sector, funding for HMOs is indefinite. Start-up grants were eliminated in 1981, and elimination of the other funds was sought in 1984. However, funding was reauthorized.

The Indian Health Care Improvement Act (PL 94-437) of 1976, designed to improve federal health programs for Indians, includes provisions to recruit and prepare more Indians for the health professions and to authorize continuing education allowances to encourage health professionals to join or continue in the Indian Health Service. It too was up for reauthorization in 1984 and vetoed, but put on a continuing resolution.

The Alcoholic Abuse and Alcoholism Prevention Treatment and Rehabilitation Act of 1970 provided and increased service in this area of health care. A block grant was created in 1981, and reauthorization was given in 1984. Extended in 1976, the *National Health Service Corps Program* (PL 91-623) of 1971 provided for health services by physicians and nurses, in underserved areas. (The story of its enactment is told in Eric Redman's *Dance of Legislation*.) The Corps, through the requirement to repay NHSC scholarships and through volunteers, has provided needed services,* but the Reagan Administration wished to reduce authorization levels significantly in 1984 and, as part of the vetoed PHS Act further funding was eliminated. That program too, was put on a continuing resolution.

The Emergency Medical Services Act of 1973 authorized $185 million over three years to states, counties, and other nonprofit agencies to plan, expand, and modernize emergency medical services. After its expiration, the law was extended.†

The Disease Control and Health Promotion Act (PL 94-316), 1976, to provide authority for health information, education, and promotion programs and to extend disease prevention control programs, was a long-awaited health education law, but the health education aspects were meagerly funded. This too was changed to a block grant in 1981, combined with other programs. Some of the latter were to be split off in FY 1985.

It is sometimes confusing to follow the changes in these and other programs, or even their continuation. Some are amended or continued in a straightforward way as amend-

---

*See Chapter 15.
†See Chapter 8.

ments to a given law. If extension of funding is defeated or vetoed, a program may be carried by a continuing resolution until a new bill can be introduced. Sometimes a substitute bill providing a variation of the same services is passed. Other times, funding is picked up in an omnibus bill such as the amendments to the Public Health Service Act or one of the omnibus budget acts.

If a particular program is extended by one of these omnibus bills, it retains its name. This type of political maneuvering is one reason that legislative information provided by the professional nursing and other health organizations is so useful, although it must be read with the understanding that each organization or group presents such information colored by its own interests.

EDUCATION IN THE HEALTH FIELD

It was not until the *Health Amendments Act* of 1956 was passed after fourteen years of effort by devoted and dedicated citizens that *people* in the health professions received substantial financial assistance. This act, now a section of the Public Health Service Law, provided funds (called *traineeships*) to prepare nurses for administration, teaching, and supervision, and nurses and physicians for public health work. The traineeship program was successful—more than 67,000 nurses took advantage of funds for long-term, full-time study and/or short-term courses from 1956 to 1971—and the fact that it came up for periodic renewal before Congress helped to emphasize the importance of advanced preparation within the nursing profession.

As the population of the country and the world increased rapidly, and as the federal government urged the enactment of legislation to provide care for the aged under Social Security, health facilities and personnel became matters of urgency to Washington. More and more funds were channeled into health and education projects. At the same time, nurses were becoming more vocal, their organiza-

tions stronger, more self-assured, and more convincing when their representatives met with legislators and appeared before legislative committees. As a result of these and other factors, several new laws were enacted in the early 1960s that supported nursing and the individual nurse.

Most significant among these was the *Nurse Training Act* of 1964 (Title VIII of the Public Health Service Act). The purpose of this law, based on the report of the Surgeon General's Consultant Group on Nursing (Chapter 5), was to increase the number of nurses through financial assistance to diploma, associate degree, and baccalaureate degree nursing schools, students, and graduates taking advanced courses, and thus to help assure more and better schools of nursing, more carefully selected students, a high standard of teaching, and better health care for the people. Signed into law by President Lyndon B. Johnson on September 4, 1964, the law, which provided $287.6 million for a five-year program, was supported by both ANA and NLN. In passing through the legislative process, the bill was altered considerably, but it still emerged as a strong law, acceptable to most nursing leaders and nursing organizations. Subsequently, aid to students and schools of nursing was continued for two years under Title II (Nurse Training) of the Health Manpower Act of 1968.

The enactment of the *Nurse Training Act of 1971* expanded and extended federal aid to nursing education until June 30, 1974: the maximum federal share of costs for nursing school construction was increased; funds could be used to construct interim education facilities, and authority was granted for guarantees and interest subsidies on nonfederal loans for the building of nonprofit private nursing schools. In addition, funds were allotted for financial-distress grants; to help schools of nursing achieve quality nursing education or meet accreditation standards; and start-up grants to plan, develop, and establish nursing schools. New capitation provision grants were made to encourage nursing schools to expand their enrollment. (At the same time, this law added to the standing prohibition against race discrimination a prohibition against sex discrimination.) Variable amounts were granted to schools according to the number of full-time students they enrolled and graduated (called *capitation grants*). Additional support was given for schools preparing nurse practitioners (NPs) such as family nurse practitioners (FNPs), nurse-midwives, and pediatric nurse practitioners.[16] However, to receive the capitation grants, the schools were required to develop and/or maintain three special projects related to recruitment and retention of minorities, interdisciplinary education, preparation of NPs, innovations in curriculum and other specified areas. It was possible to include projects that were already supported by a special project grant from the division, also available under the Nurse Training Act, but continued commitment was required even if these funds were cut or eliminated. Although far short of the 1972 authorizations, the allocation still increased federal support for nurse training significantly. Then in 1973, the Nixon Administration refused to release a large amount of the appropriated funds, withholding completely those allotted for capitation. Although a suit against DHEW by NLN resulted in a favorable judgment for release of the capitation funds by the end of the year, limitations on traineeship funds prevented large numbers of students from beginning or continuing in baccalaureate and graduate programs.

Overall, it was estimated that DHEW withheld (impounded) a total of $1.1 billion in health funds in FY 1973. Other health groups also initiated suits for release of these funds, with usually favorable action. The struggle for adequate health funding in 1974 resulted in repeated vetoes by the President and a failure of the Congress to override the vetoes. In a final bill of 1973, approved congressional appropriations for nurse training were still approximately three times more than requested by the President, and a veto was expected. In his budgetary plan, the President had eliminated *any* funding for capitation, financial distress,

traineeships, construction grants, and educational grants and contracts; and alloted considerably less than had the Congress in all other areas. After months of prodding by the Congress and national organizations, the president signed the 1974 DHEW appropriations bill, in part because it contained an agreement that the administration could withhold up to $400 million of the total appropriation where the Congress had voted larger amounts for specific programs than the presidential budget.

This negative administrative attitude was particularly unfortunate because the funds granted as of 1964 had been well utilized. Some of the accomplishments included the starting of forty new nursing education programs, salvaging and/or increasing 26,000 places for first-year students; providing remedial services for disadvantaged students in twenty-four programs; supporting a number of innovative open-curriculum programs; providing nurses with training for primary care responsibilities; aiding recruitment of minorities, including men; and providing traineeship for 67,000 nurses in teaching, supervision, administration, and clinical specialities.[17] In addition, federal nursing funds over the years have supported nursing research and preparation of nurses in research, a great need in the development of the profession.[18] An elimination or cut in federal funds also endangered growth in this area.

The Nurse Training Act and three other health training acts were to expire June 30, 1974, but for various reasons, including consideration of a study on health manpower education costs, no legislation was introduced by mid-year. By that time, the funding had run out and the Nurse Training Act and the other education acts were supported by a continuing resolution. As a matter of interest, the *Congressional Budget and Improvement Act*, which would allow the Congress more control over the budgetary process and force it into long-term planning, had just been signed into law. This law also prevented the President from impounding unremitted funds, although rescission, cutting back on allotted program funds, was legal. Rescission had to be approved by the Congress within a specified time period. In the last minutes of the 93rd Congress, the Nurse Training Act of 1974 was passed. It was vetoed by President Ford on January 3, a pocket veto because the Congress had adjourned.

In the 1975 session, a new bill was introduced, passed, and again vetoed, but the veto was overriden by large margins of both houses—the first successful over-ride of that session. Grass-roots support by nurses was given much of the credit by key senators. In all, $106.5 million were appropriated for the Nurse Training Act for FY 1976, including capitation, traineeships, and special projects. Again, the President vetoed and again there was an override.[19] The Nurse Training Act of 1975 became Title IX, PL 94-63.

In 1978, the Congress, ignoring President Carter's claim that there was no longer a shortage of nurses, passed a two-year extension of nurse training programs. Without such authority, the program would have run out at the end of 1978. President Carter pocket-vetoed the NTA, claiming that the measure was inflationary. He later attempted massive rescission of Nurse Training Act funds, but through the extensive lobbying of nurses and their supporters, the Congress refused to go along with Carter and nursing did better than any other health profession. Meanwhile, when the Congress reconvened in January 1979, a new Nurse Training Act was introduced, later passed, and finally signed by President Carter. Funding was at $103 million, almost $3 million over 1979 spending levels. Included was funding for capitation, NP, nurse anesthetist, and advanced nurse training programs, traineeships, student loans, special projects and construction. A special stipulation was that DHEW contract out a two-year study of the supply, demand, and education of nurses. In 1980, it was time for introduction of a new Nurse Training Act.

Data were presented to Congress concerning the need to extend the Nurse Training Act and describing what it had accomplished. Unfortunately, Congress adjourned before final action could be taken on the Health Manpower Act, of which the nurse training funds were a part. Once more, the existing programs were extended through a continuing resolution. And once more, in the next session of Congress, another administration attempted to eliminate a large part of the funding in the proposed Nurse Training Act.[20] Eventually, however, the programs dealt with under the Nurse Training Act became a part of OBRA 81.

OBRA 81 continued institutional support for nursing education by extending and amending the special projects, advanced nurse training, and NP programs. The former authority for grants to assist schools of nursing in serious financial distress was reinstated. Authorization for capitation grants, nursing school construction grants, loan guarantees for construction projects (never used), and interest subsidies (never used) were not extended. Continuation of student support was authorized through nursing student loans and scholarships, professional nurse traineeships, and NP traineeships. Along with the other programs in that law, the nursing education provisions were up for reauthorization in 1984, and although some cuts in funding were anticipated, it was expected that most of the programs would continue, particularly the areas of research grants and graduate education because of the Institute of Medicine (IOM) report.* However, the NTA was part of S2574, the PHS Act Amendments of 1984 vetoed by President Reagan and current funding was extended under a continuing resolution.

Support for other health professions education (medicine, osteopathy, dentistry, veterinary medicine, optometry, podiatry, and pharmacy), known by the acronym, MODVOPP, had been supported by such early laws as the *Health Professions Education Assistance Act of 1963*, which provided matching grants over a three-year period for

---

*See Chapter 5.

the construction of new teaching facilities for health personnel (including collegiate schools of nursing). Later, PL 94-484, the *Health Professions Educational Assistance Act of 1976*, made the first important changes in federal support for medical education since 1971, when Congress had instituted basic federal aid to medical schools because of the growing physician shortage. PL 94-484 authorized a total of $2.3 billion for FY 1978-1980 for basic federal aid to health profession schools, student assistance and scholarships, and other health manpower training projects. Although designed to assist medical, osteopathic, and dental schools, the act contained provisions for other health professionals, including nursing (as noted earlier). It too was reauthorized in 1981, with cuts, and endangered in 1984 by the same veto cited above and was also put under a continuing resolution. Other workers in health care are federally funded, and such funding tends to increase their numbers tremendously. Among these are practical nurses, aides, emergency medical technicians, and physicians' assistants.

The *Manpower Development and Training Act* of 1962 was designed to prepare unskilled and poorly educated workers for jobs that require some degree of technological skill and to reduce unemployment by training quickly at government expense large numbers of these unskilled persons to fill available jobs. The act covered such health workers as practical nurses, orderlies, nurses' aides, psychiatric aides, and surgical technicians. Many hospitals, educational programs, and other groups took advantage of this law, and large numbers of these ancillary workers were trained. Because of the variety of programs and a tendency to produce subspecialty categories of workers, this not only tended to increase fragmentation of care, but also resulted in many dead-end jobs.

In 1963, the *Vocational Education Act* provided funds to help provide training facilities for practical nurses, and in 1965 this was broadened to include enrollees in associate degree programs (for practical nurse training).

Continued federal funding of practical nurse programs has been responsible, to a large degree, for the major increase of both programs and students enrolled. A leveling-off began in the 1970s, however.

The *Health Manpower Act* of 1972 provided the stimulus for substantial development of PA programs.* The *Emergency Medical Services Act* of 1973, mentioned earlier, also funded training programs for emergency medical technicians.*

CIVIL RIGHTS, EMPLOYMENT, AND LABOR RELATIONS

Beginning in the 1960s, a number of laws were passed to prohibit discrimination based on sex as well as race, color, religion, and national origin. Many of these are particularly meaningful to women and are cited in Chapter 17. Some of the most important are the following:

The *Equal Pay Act* of 1963 was intended primarily to end wage inequities based on sex and thus to assure women the same financial return as men receive for the same work. This did not apply to hospital employees, because it applied only to workers in industries covered by the Fair Labor Standards Act, and hospitals were not among these industries.

The *Civil Rights Act* of 1964, called by some the most far-reaching social legislation since Reconstruction, intended to create a rule of law under which the Untied States could deal with its race problems peaceably through an orderly, legal process in federal courts. Title VII of the Civil Rights Act (the Equal Employment Opportunity Law) has affected the job status of nurses because it includes a section forbidding discrimination against women in job hiring and job promotion among private employers of more than twenty-five persons. Executive Order No. 11246 as amended extended the law to include federal contractors and subcontractors. Hospitals and col-

---

*See Chapter 8.

leges are subject to this order because of their acceptance of federal grants of various kinds.

One year later, the *1965 Voting Rights Act*, with direct bearing on the Civil Rights Act, was passed, requiring that the procedure for registering persons to vote within a given county must be the same for everyone. Intended to ensure the right to vote promised in the Fifteenth Amendment, this law attempted to eliminate the practice of disqualifying potential voters on the basis of discriminatory literacy tests. This legislation represented an alteration in federal-state power, for the states had had the authority for nearly two centuries to set, for the most part, the standards for voting eligibility within their own borders.

The *Educational Amendments* of 1972 had three provisions of economic importance to women: (1) equal treatment of men and women in federally funded educational programs (especially admissions to programs); (2) minimum wage and overtime pay benefits to employees of nursery schools, private kindergartens, and other preschool enterprises; (3) extension of the federal Equal Pay Act of 1963 to executives, administrators, and professional employees. The same pay was guaranteed to men and women doing substantially equal work, requiring substantially equal skill, effort, and responsibility under similar working conditions in the same establishment.*

The *Employee Retirement Income Security Act*, 1974 (ERISA), established minimum federal standards for private pension plans to protect workers already covered by pension plans. The rigidity of the enacted programs and the confusion and overlap caused by dual enforcement by both the Department of Labor and Department of the Treasury caused many problems, and a delineation of functions was offered in later legislation.

The *Age in Employment Discrimination Act Amendments* of 1975 was intended to eliminate "unreasonable discrimination on the basis of age." Among other things, it banned certain kinds of mandatory retirement. The *Fair Labor Standards Act Amendments* of 1974 (originally 1938) increased the minimum wage and extended coverage to 7 million workers, including state, county, and municipal employees.

Among other civil rights that have been given new protection are the rights of patients, children, the mentally ill, prisoners, and elderly, and the handicapped.* Actions to protect these rights have come through a variety of legal means at state and national levels. Protection has increasingly been specified through regulations of various laws such as the amendments and subsequent regulations of the Social Security Act. Another is the *Rehabilitation Act* of 1973. Section 504 reads, "no otherwise qualified handicapped individual in the United States shall, solely by reason of his handicap, be excluded from the participation in, be denied the benefit of, or be subjected to discrimination under any program or activity receiving federal financial assistance." The definition of *handicapped* includes drug addicts and alcoholics, as well as those having overt physical impairment such as blindness, deafness, or paralysis of some kind. (A 1984 expansion of the definition relates to deformed newborns, as discussed in Chapter 22). Because most health facilities and health professional educational programs have some federal support, this law applies both to admission to a nursing school, for instance, and to employment in a hospital. Some cases have already reached the Supreme Court. In 1979, a PN with serious impairment of hearing sought admission to an AD nursing program. The Court upheld denial of admission because "nothing in the language or history [of the law] reflects an intention to limit the freedom of an educational institution to require reasonable physical qualifications for admission to a clinical training program."[21]

The right to privacy also affects nurses. One of the most important federal laws in this area

---

*Comparable worth issues will be discussed in Chapter 22, and are also mentioned in Chapter 6.

*These rights are discussed in Chapter 22.

is the *Freedom of Information Act* (FOIA) of 1966 and the *Privacy Act* of 1974. The purpose of the FOIA is to give the public access to files maintained by the executive branch of government. Recognizing that there were valid reasons for withholding certain records, the law exempted broad categories of records from compulsory public inspection, including medical records. To further clarify the situation, the FOI Act of 1974 was passed to amend the 1966 law. It had been necessary to set some time and expense limits for federal agencies because, in their frequent reluctance to give up information, they tended to use bureaucratic red tape to delay transmission of the requested records and imposed high fees to photocopy them. The next question that arose was whether a person shouldn't have the right to see all information about himself or herself in government files. The result was enactment of the Privacy Act. Its purpose was to provide certain safeguards for an individual against invasion of personal privacy by requesting the federal government, with some exceptions, to:

1. Permit an individual to determine what records pertaining to him are collected, maintained, used, or disseminated by such agencies.
2. Permit an individual to prevent records pertaining to him and obtained by such agencies for a particular purpose from being used or made available for another purpose without his consent.
3. Permit an individual to gain access to information pertaining to him in federal agency records, to have a copy made of all or any portion thereof, and to correct or amend such records.
4. Collect, maintain, use, or disseminate any record of identifiable personal information in a manner that assures that such action is for a necessary and lawful purpose, that the information is current and accurate for its intended use, and that adequate safeguards are provided to prevent misuse of such information.

5. Permit exemptions from the requirements with respect to records provided in this act only in cases in which there is an important public policy need for such exemption as has been determined by specific statutory authority.
6. Be subject to civil suit for any damages which occur as a result of willful or intentional action which violates any individual's rights under the act.

Such access includes the hospital record of patients in federal hospitals and, possibly, under Medicare-Medicaid. Another part of the law was aimed at protecting the confidentiality of patients' records.* Ten years later, many business, professional and civil libertarian groups agreed that the protections of the Privacy Act had been made out of date by computer technology and urged Congress to enact appropriate legislation. Of special concern was lack of adequate legal assurances of privacy and inaccurate information.

Another step in providing access to one's own records was enactment of the *Family Educational Rights and Privacy Act* of 1974, also known as the *Buckley Amendment*. The basic intent of this law was to provide students, their parents, and guardians with easier access to and control over the information contained in academic records. Educational records are defined broadly and include files, documents, and other materials containing information about the student and maintained by a school. Students must be allowed to inspect these records within forty-five days of their request. They need not be allowed access to confidential letters of reference preceding January 1975, records about students made by teachers and administrators for their own use and not shown to others, certain campus police records, certain parental financial records, and certain psychiatric treatment records (if not available to anyone else). Students may chal-

---

*Some states have also enacted FOI acts relating not only to records, but to meetings which must be open to the public (sometimes called *sunshine laws*).

lenge the content, secure the correction of inaccurate information, and insert a written explanation regarding the content of their records. The law also specifies who has access to the records (teachers, educational administrators, organizations such as testing services, state and other officials to whom certain information must be reported according to the law). Otherwise, the records cannot be released without the student's consent. The law applies to nursing education programs as well as others.

The rights of research subjects have also been incorporated in diverse federal laws, especially in the last decade. PL 93-348, the *National Research Act* of 1974, not only provided some funds for nursing research, but also set controls on research, including the establishment of a committee to identify requirements for informed consent for children, prisoners, the mentally disabled, and those not covered by the DHEW regulations, and required an institutional committee to review a research project to protect the patient's rights. The 1974 Privacy Act required a clear, informed consent for those participating in research. The 1971 *Food and Drug Act* also gave some protection in regulating the use of experimental drugs, including notification to the patient that a drug is experimental. The *Drug Regulation Reform Act* of 1978 took further steps to protect the patient receiving research drugs. Other drug and narcotics laws* also affect nursing.

In recent years, drug manufacturers have been developing many highly potent drugs in their attempt to supply an increasingly aware public with medicine to prevent and cure their ailments. Many of these drugs produce side effects ranging from a slight rash or a mild gastrointestinal upset to much more serious consequences, sometimes even death. When one drug—thalidomide—was proved in 1962 to cause major deformities in babies born of mothers who took the drug, Congress was

motivated to enact legislation to control more rigidly the production and distribution of new pharmaceuticals and thus protect the public against dangerous drugs.

The main provision of the law passed by Congress in 1962, called the *Drug Amendments of 1962* (to the Food, Drug, and Cosmetic Act of 1938), provides that manufacturers of drugs who seek Food and Drug Administration (FDA) approval must prove through extensive preliminary clinical testing, often a long, slow process, that the drug is safe to use and that it will have the intended therapeutic effect; misleading or false labeling and advertising by drug manufacturers are forbidden; and drug manufacturers, processors, and packagers must register with the FDA each year, be inspected by the FDA at least once every two years and be open to inspection at any time.

The *Comprehensive Drug Abuse Prevention and Control Act* of 1970 (Controlled Substance Act) replaced virtually all other federal laws dealing with narcotics, depressants, stimulants, and hallucinogens. It controls the handling of drugs by providers, including hospitals. The *Drug Regulation Reform Act* of 1978 took further steps in protecting the patient; at the same time, the FDA set requirements about sharing product information on drugs with consumers.

Also within the broad categories of rights are those laws related to labor relations. The first was the *National Labor Relations Act* (*NLRA*), one of several laws enacted to pull the country out of the Great Depression. The thesis, according to Werther,[22] was that labor unions could prevent employers from lowering wages, resulting in higher incomes and more spending. To achieve the growth of unions, employers had to be limited; for instance, they could no longer legally fire employees who tried to unionize. The National Labor Relations Board (NLRB), created by law, was empowered to investigate and initiate administrative proceedings against those employers who violated the law. (If these admin-

*These are discussed in Chapter 21.

istrative actions did not curtail the illegal acts, court action followed. Only employer violations were listed.)

In 1947, the NLRA was substantially amended, and the amended law, entitled the *Labor Management Relations Act* (or *Taft-Hartley Act*), listed prohibitions for unions. Section 14(b), for instance, contained the so-called right-to-work clause, which authorizes states to enact more stringent union security provisions than those contained in the federal laws. More than twenty states have enacted such laws. Usually they prohibit union security clauses in contracts that make membership or nonmembership in a labor union a requirement for obtaining or retaining employment. Such laws prohibit the closed shop, union shop, and sometimes the agency shop in which employees who do not join a union must pay a fixed sum monthly as a condition of employment to help defray expenses.

In 1959, a third major modification was made. One of the purposes of the law, the *Labor-Management Reporting and Disclosure Act* or *Landrum-Griffin Act*, was to curb documented abuses such as corrupt financial and election procedures. For this reason, it is sometimes called the union members' Bill of Rights. The result is a series of rights and responsibilities of members of a union or a professional organization, such as ANA, that engages in collective bargaining. Required are reporting and disclosure of certain financial transactions and administrative practices and the use of democratic election procedures. That is, every member in good standing must be able to nominate candidates and run for election and must be allowed to vote and support candidates; there must be secret ballot elections; union funds must not be used to assist the candidacy of an individual seeking union office; candidates must have access to the membership list; records of the election must be preserved for one year; and elections must be conducted according to by-laws procedures.[23]

Highly significant for nurses is the 1974 law that again amended the Taft-Hartley Act, PL 93-360, the *Nonprofit Health Care Amendments*. This law made nonprofit health care facilities that had, through considerable lobbying, been excluded in the 1947 law, subject to national labor laws. These employees were now free to join or not join a union without employer retribution, a right previously denied to them unless they worked in a state that had its own law allowing them to unionize. It also created special notification procedures that must precede any strike action. Included in the definition of *health care facility* were hospitals, HMOs, health clinics, nursing homes, ECFs, or "other institutions devoted to the care of sick, infirm, or aged persons." Whether doctor's offices could be included was left to be settled by the NLRB.[24] Employers of all kinds, however, must abide by the various civil rights and other protective laws noted earlier. The *Civil Service Reform Act* of 1978 also had an influence in the labor relations activities of nursing because its definition of *supervisor* allowed nurse supervisors to be included in collective bargaining units. It also wrote into law collective bargaining, previously sanctioned only by executive order.

Another right that should be reported is the revision of the *Copyright Law*, amended in 1976 to supersede the 1909 law. The categories of work covered include writings, works of art, music, and pantomimes. The owner is given exclusive right to reproduce the copyrighted work. The new law has some significance in this time of photocopying from journals and books; there are certain limits and need for permission to copy anything beyond certain minimums. Libraries can provide the appropriate information. Some books and journals specify their copying permission requirements.

NATIONAL HEALTH INSURANCE(NHI)

National Health insurance (NHI) has been debated in Congress for more than a decade. The plans offered were diverse and were always changing. As expected, a crucial question is that of cost.[25] Opposing viewpoints focus on comprehensive versus catastrophic plans, with some inclination to a phasing in of any plan by first concentrating on certain groups (infants and children, mothers, or the elderly). NHI tends to be a political football because of the public's "right to health" stance and the problem of funding (total governmental funding or private insurance plans).[26,27]

These differences can be seen in the varying opinions of physicians[28] and those who look toward a national health service (NHS). A differentiation must be made between national health *service* and national health *insurance*. NHS would make all health workers government employees, and all care would be provided in government hospitals and health centers (as in many European countries). Financing is mainly by general revenues, but some insurance funds are used. In NHI plans such as Canada's,[29] the crucial feature is that all health providers, including institutions, are independent entrepreneurs who contract with the government to provide services.[30] Both ANA[31] and NLN[32] favor a comprehensive NHI plan that includes inpatient and outpatient care, twenty-four-hour emergency care, home care, clinic services, rehabilitative care, and preventive and supportive care. However, no form of national health insurance is expected in the immediate future.

AGENCIES AND REGULATIONS

Follow-up of federal legislation requires close attention. It is not just the law itself that affects the public, but the proliferating federal regulations. Legislators have charged that regulations have been used specifically to circumvent the intent of the law; at the least, regulations often shape the legislation they are intended to carry out. Among President Carter's goals was clarification of the language of regulation (plain English, please) and allowance of sufficient time for comment by consumers. Otherwise, the process can become

the exclusive prerogative of the federal agencies. In the following chapters, examples will be given of how regulations can influence health care.

Of equal importance are the agencies created by the various laws, such as the FDA and Federal Trade Commission (FTC). The FTC, for instance, goes back to 1914, when the Federal Trade Commission Act was passed. It has extensive power; it can represent itself in court, enforce its own orders, and conduct its own litigation in civil courts, and it seems to have relative freedom from the executive branch of government. Its forays into the health field, with rulings on professional advertising,* licensure, and other aspects of health care delivery never thought of in 1914, may indicate a direction for other administrative agencies.[33] On the other hand, the subjects of the FTC rulings have banded together to lobby for limitation of FTC powers. This occurred, for instance, in 1982, when attached to the FTC reauthorization bill was an amendment exempting state-licensed professionals from its jurisdiction. A major supporter was AMA; an opponent, ANA. The underlying issue was whether, for instance, if professionals were exempted from fair trade practices, physicians could legally restrain the practice of competitors, such as nurse-midwives.[34] That time the FTC won, but the problem will not be immediately resolved.

REFERENCES

1. Helen Creighton, *Law Every Nurse Should Know* (Philadelphia: W. B. Saunders Company, 1975), pp. 60–61.
2. William Curran, "Major Reform in the Oldest of Health Insurance Programs: Workmen's Compensation and Industrial Health and Safety," *N. Eng. J. Med.*, **288**: 35–36 (Jan. 1973).
3. Irvin Stander, "The Future of Worker's Compensation," *Medicalegal News*, **8**:7–9 (Apr. 1980).
4. Marian Gornick, "Ten Years of Medicare: Impact on the Covered Popula-

*See Chapter 10.

tion," DHEW Publication No. 55A. **76**: 1170 (1976).

5. Kenneth Wing, *The Law and the Public Health* (St. Louis: C. V. Mosby Company, 1976), pp. 70–90.

6. Karen Davis, "Achievements and Problems of Medicaid," *Public Health Rep.* **97**:309–316 (July–Aug. 1976).

7. Kenneth Wing, "Recent Amendments to the Medicaid Program: Political Implications," *Am. J. Pub. Health*, **74**:83–84 (Jan. 1984).

8. "Federal Legislative and Executive Action," *Am. J. Law and Med.*, **7**:221–222 (Summer 1981).

9. Richard Sorian, "Reconciliation: Most Programs Cut: Some Retain Identity," *Nation's Health*, **11**:1, 16 (Sept. 1981).

10. Franklin Shaffer, "DRGs: History and Overview," *Nurs. Health Care*, **4**:388 (Sept. 1983).

11. Jane Hamilton, "Nursing and DRGs: Proactive Responses to Prospective Reimbursement," *Nurs. Health Care*, **5**: 155–159 (Mar. 1984).

12. Lucille Joel, "DRGs and RIMs: Implications for Nursing," *Nurs. Outlook*, **32**: 42–49 (Jan.–Feb. 1984).

13. Wing, op. cit., pp 132–134.

14. Ibid., p. 135.

15. Edyth Alexander, *Nursing Administration in the Hospital Health Care System* (St. Louis: C. V. Mosby Company, 1978), pp. 49–51.

16. Jessie M. Scott, "Federal Support for Nursing Education 1964–1972," *Am. J. Nurs.*, **72**:1855–1861 (Oct. 1972).

17. Ibid.

18. Susan Gortner, "Research in Nursing; the Federal Interest and Grant Program," *Am. J. Nurs.*, **73**:1052–1055 (June 1973).

19. Lucie Kelly, "The Nurse Training Act— How Legislation Is Formulated, Adopted, and Implemented," in *People, Power, Politics for Health Care* (New York: National League for Nursing, 1976), pp. 37–48. (This article includes considerable detail on how the 1975 Nurse Training Act became law.)

20. M. Gaie Rubenfeld et al., "The Nurse Training Act: Yesterday, Today, and . . .," *Am. J. Nurs.*, **81**:1202–1204 (June 1981.)

21. "Supreme Court Rules Against Handicapped," *Am. Nurs.*, **11**:6 (June 1979).

22. William Werther and Carol Ann Lockhart, *Labor Relations in the Health Professions* (Boston: Little, Brown and Company, 1976), pp. 6–8.

23. Ibid., pp. 22–27.

24. Yvonne Bryant, "Labor Relations in Health Care Institutions: An Analysis of Public Law 93-360," *J. Nurs. Admin.*, **8**:28–39 (Mar. 1978).

25. Victor Fuchs, *Who Shall Live?* (New York: Basic Books, Inc., 1974), pp. 127–146.

26. Theodore Marmor, "NHI in Crisis: Politics, Predictions, Proposals," *Hosp. Prog.*, **59**:68–72 (Jan. 1978).

27. Jeffrey Prussin, "National Health Insurance: A Political Issue at the Crossroads," *Nurse Educator*, **3**:23–27 (Nov.–Dec. 1978).

28. John Colombotos et al., "Physicians View National Health Insurance: A National Survey," *Medical Care*, **13**:369–396 (May 1975).

29. Gordon Hatcher, "Canadian Approaches to Health Policy Decisions," *Am. J. Pub. Health*, **68**:881–889 (Sept. 1978).

30. Milton Terris et al., "The Case for a National Health Service," *Am. J. Pub. Health*, **67**:1183–1185 (Dec. 1977).

31. American Nurses' Association, *Position Statement on National Health Insurance* (Kansas City, Mo.: The Association, 1979).

32. National League for Nursing, *Position Statement on National Health Insurance* (New York: The League, 1979).

33. Joseph Avellone and Francis Moore, "The Federal Trade Commission Enters a New Arena: Health Services," *N. Eng. J. Med.*, **291**:478–483 (Aug. 1978).

34. Lucie Kelly, "FTC: Dragon or Dragon-Slayer," *Nurs. Outlook*, **30**:490–492 (Nov–Dec. 1982).

20

Licensure and Health Manpower Credentialing

Despite a variety of patchwork reforms, the health care system remains the target of serious criticism. A major focus has been the undeniable fragmentation of services, accelerating costs, and poor utilization and maldistribution of health manpower. Therefore, credentialing of health manpower, as one of the factors that probably contributes to these problems, has been given special attention by legislative, governmental, and consumer groups. This pointed scrutiny has subsequently aroused new, or at least renewed, interest on the part of the health occupations and professions.

Licensing of individuals is probably one of the most authoritative mechanisms of credentialing, because it is a function of the police power of the state. Its primary purpose is to protect the public; therefore, the state, through its licensure laws, sets standards and qualifications for the licensed practitioner and holds the power to punish those who violate the law. At the same time, licensure, as it stands currently, has definite advantages for the licensee: status, protection of title (RN, LPN, MD), and certain economic gains. Other methods of credentialing for individuals or institutions have also evolved. Whether official, quasiofficial, or voluntary,

most purport to provide a certain assurance of quality or safety to the public as well as benefits for the credentialed. And therein lies the dilemma. As one expert in the credentialing field noted:

> It is true that any professional society or group, no matter how socially oriented, will tend to develop barriers to protect itself. . . . Among the contemporary protective mechanisms for the health professions are accreditation, certification, licensure, and registration. All four of these mechanisms medicine has employed with excellent results, if not always for the benefit of society, at least for the benefit of most members of the profession. And now many of the numerous other health professions wish to adopt, if they have not already done so, the same steps which medicine had fashioned to meet the needs of society *and its own protection* (emphasis mine)[1]

This phenomenon has not escaped the notice of the consumer or the government. Because the health professions, as a whole, did not seem to show rapid progress in remedying the more questionable aspects of credentialing, particularly licensure, a series of blue-ribbon panels, high-level committees, and prestigious task forces at state and national levels were formed. For instance, since 1968, federal government committees have produced at least six major publications on credentialing of health manpower personnel.[2-7] Furthermore, in 1970–1971, the Carnegie Commission on Higher Education looked at both higher education and some aspects of health professional education.[8,9] In 1972, the Commonwealth Fund supported an extensive study of accreditation (Study of Accreditation of Selected Health Education Programs, or SASHEP).[10] All of these groups presented firm recommendations for strengthening, changing, or eliminating various forms of credentialing, but it was the 1971 DHEW* (PHS) report that stirred the health professions to action.

This report made it clear not only that health manpower credentialing was no longer immune from public criticism and that it must be fused with the public interest, but also that the federal government had every intention of seeing that action was taken by using its authority in very specific ways. Preceding the recommendations was an invitation—and a warning:

> This Department has a definite role in the process of credentialing progress—a role for catalytic action and support. While the Federal Government cannot solve these problems by itself, it is also apparent that meaningful solutions may not be forthcoming, on a timely basis, without a greater Federal interest. The needs in this field offer real opportunity for significant public-private cooperation.[11]

There is clear evidence that the recommendations made in this and the final report (1977) were a strong impetus to changes in the various forms of health manpower credentialing.

The 1971 PHS report also gave definitions for the major credentialing process[12] that

have, since then, been used almost universally:

Accreditation*:   The process by which an agency or organization evaluates and recognizes an institution or program of study as meeting certain predetermined criteria or standards.

Licensure: The process by which an agency of government grants permission to persons to engage in a given profession or occupation by certifying that those licensed have attained the minimal degree of competency necessary to ensure that the public health, safety, and welfare will be reasonably well protected.

Certification or registration: The process by which a nongovernmental agency or association grants recognition to an individual who has met certain predetermined qualifications specified by that agency or association. Such qualifications may include (1) graduation from an accredited or approved program; (2) acceptable performance on a qualifying examination or series of examinations; and/or (3) completion of a given amount of work experience.

Another acceptable definition of *registration* given in the working papers of the nurse credentialing study† is: the process by which individuals are assessed and given status on a registry attesting to the individual's ability and current competency. Its purpose is to keep a continuous record of the past and current achievements of an individual.

INDIVIDUAL LICENSURE: PROBLEMS AND RECOMMENDATIONS

As noted earlier, licensure is a police power of the state; that is, the state legislative process determines what group is licensed, and

---

*The Department of Health, Education and Welfare (DHEW) preceded the current Department of Health and Human Services (DHHS) and the separate Department of Education. The Public Health Service is still part of DHHS.

---

*Nursing accreditation is discussed in Chapters 12 and 26.

†The nurse credentialing study is referred to later, but is also discussed in depth in Chapter 5.

with what limits. It is the responsibility of a specific part of the state government to see that that law is carried out, including punishment for its violation. Although licensure laws differ somewhat in format from state to state, the elements contained in each are similar. For instance, in the health professions laws, there are sections on definition of the profession that delineates the scope of practice; requirements for licensure, such as education; exemptions from licensure; grounds for revocation of a license; creation of a licensing board, including member qualifications and responsibilities; and penalties for practicing without a license.

Licensure laws are either mandatory (compulsory) or permissive (voluntary). If mandatory, the law forbids anyone to practice that profession or occupation without a license on pain of fine or imprisonment. If permissive, the law allows anyone to practice as long as she or he does not claim to hold the title of the practitioner (such as registered nurse).

Licensing of the health occupations was advocated in the early nineteenth century, but it was not until the early 1900s that a significant number of such licensing laws were enacted. They were generally initiated by the associations of practitioners that were interested in raising standards and establishing codes for ethical behavior. Because voluntary compliance was not always forthcoming, the associations sought enactment of regulatory legislation. To some critics, this movement is also seen as a means of giving members of an occupation or profession as much status, control, and compensation as the community is willing to give. It is true that as the health occupations proliferate, each group begins to organize and seek licensure. Because many of these occupations are subgroups of the major health professions, or are highly specialized, licensure creates problems in further fragmentation and increased cost in health care—according to the critics.

In all of the proposals for changes in health manpower credentialing, criticism of individual licensure is implicit or explicit. Particu-

larly in the last ten years, the evils were cited, but there was little recognition of actions taken to remedy the faults. Evolving changes (often slow in evolving) were dismissed as too little and too late. Edward Forgotson, a physician-lawyer who directed a study of licensure for the National Advisory Commission on Health Manpower, enumerated some of the key criticisms of individual licensing.

1. Most licensure laws for the health professions do not mandate continuing education or other requirements to prevent educational obsolescence. Therefore, the minimal standards of safety, theoretically guaranteed by granting the initial license, may no longer be met by some (perhaps many) practitioners.

2. Educational innovations in the health professions may be stifled by the rigidity of statutorily specified courses and curricular requirements. Changing these requirements to make them responsive to the rapid informational and technological explosion is a difficult and time-consuming process, and the result is the possibility that existing minimal standards may lag behind the practice realities.

3. Definitions of the area of practice are generally not specific, so that allocation of tasks is often determined by legal decisions or interpretations by lay people. On the other hand, some limitations of practice— ones that are not congruent with changing health care needs—are delineated.

4. Most licensing boards are composed of members of that particular profession (or, in some cases, the professional superior of that group), without representation by competent lay members or allied health professions. This is seen as allowing these professionals to control the kind and number of individuals who may enter their field, with the possibility of shutting out other health workers climbing the occupational ladder, and also limiting the number of practitioners for economic reasons. Moreover, the members of a one-profes-

sion board may lack overall knowledge of total expertise in the health care field, so that the scope of functions which could be delegated to other workers is not clearly determined. This creates the possibility that others capable of performing a particular activity may be prevented from doing so by another profession's licensing law.[13]

Not all health occupations are licensed. A recent unpublished government report listed forty-four health occupations* licensed in at least one state, about ten more than existed just five years ago. Of these, thirteen are licensed in every state: chiropractors, dental hygienists, dentists, nursing home administrators, optometrists, pharmacists, physical therapists, physicians (MD and DO), podiatrists, professional and practical nurses, and veterinarians.† The 1971 DHEW report pointed out the lack of geographic mobility for some of these health professionals, who may be licensed in one state but barred from another unless a new license is obtained.[14] Only nursing, with its state board examinations, now called the National Council Licensure Examination (NCLEX), that are used in every state, allows for licensure by endorsement. That is, assuming that other criteria for licensure are met, a nurse need not take another examination when relocating to another state. Even then, nursing does not completely escape the mobility criticism, because, in the last few years, various state boards of nursing have adopted rather idiosyncratic criteria.

Nevertheless, it seems that almost all of the established or fledgling health occupations, more than 250 at last count, consider licensing as a primary means of credentialing. The licensure problems of one health occupation obviously are not necessarily the same as those of all the others. Yet, because the majority of all kinds of health workers function in institutional settings, the various weaknesses of all health occupations' licensing laws, the incon-

sistencies and varying standards of those seeking licensure, and the sheer numbers involved appear to be the bases for whatever enthusiasm exists for alternatives to licensure, such as institutional licensure.

Given the many criticisms of licensure, it was not surprising that the 1971 DHEW report made major recommendations related to this form of credentialing. These included support of a moratorium on licensure of new health personnel; expansion of current acts to extend broader delegational authority; the use of national examinations and the development of meaningful equivalency and proficiency examinations; and strengthening of licensing boards to help maintain quality health services, such as assurance of the practitioner's continued competence. However, the most immediately controversial was probably the last:

The concept of extending institutional licensure—to include the regulation of health personnel beyond the traditional facility licensure—has important potential as a supplement or alternative to existing forms of individual licensure. Demonstration projects should be initiated as soon as possible.[15]

Institutional Licensure

Institutional licensure is a process by which a state government regulates health institutions; it has existed for more than thirty years. Usually, requirements for establishing and operating a health facility have been concerned primarily with such matters as administration, accounting requirements, equipment specifications, structural integrity, sanitation, and fire safety. In some cases, there are also minimal standards of square footage per bed and minimal nursing staff requirements. The issue in the "new" institutional licensure dispute is whether personnel credentialing or licensing should be part of the institution's responsibility under the general aegis of the state licensing authority.[16]

There are various interpretations of just what institutional licensing means and how it

*Health occupations seem to be designated differently in various publications, even within DHHS.

†Some of these are not licensed in the territories.

could or should be implemented. Lawrence Miike, a physician-lawyer, suggested that it was "instructive to view institutional licensure not as a developed concept, but, more appropriately, as a convenient descriptive term applied to the concept of a unified health delivery system."[17] He added that the *Hershey model* had become synonymous with institutional licensure to many people, which led to some confusion.

Nathan Hershey, then professor of health law at the University of Pittsburgh, had criticized individual licensure for years. In a number of papers, he advocated that institutionally based health workers be regulated by the employing institution within bounds established by state institutional licensing bodies:

> Because the provision of services is becoming more and more institution-based, individual licensing of practitioners might be legitimately replaced by investing health services institutions and agencies with the responsibility for regulating the provision of services, within bounds established by the state institutional licensing bodies.
>
> The state licensing agency could establish, with the advice of experts in the health care field, job descriptions for various hospital positions, and establish qualifications in terms of education and experience for individuals who would hold these posts. Administrators certainly recognize the fact that although a professional nurse is licensed, her license does not automatically indicate which positions within the hospital she is qualified to fill. Individuals, because of their personal attainments, are selected to fill specific posts. Educational qualifications, based on both formal and inservice programs, along with prior job experience, determine if and how personnel should be employed.[18]

Hershey further suggested the development of a job description classification similar to that used in civil service. Personnel categories could be stated in terms of levels and grades, along with descriptive job titles. Under such a system, the individual's education and work experience would be taken into consideration by the employing institution for the individual's placement in a grade; basic qualifications for the position, expressed in terms of education and experience, would be set by the state's hospital licensing agency.

Thus, a professional nurse returning to work after ten or fifteen years, Hershey indicated, might be placed in a nurse aide or practical nurse (PN) position, moving on to a higher grade when she "regained her skills and became familiar with professional and technological advances through inservice programs."[19] Hershey was, then and later, rather evasive as to the place of the physician in this new credentialing picture, implying that the current practice of hospital staff review was really a pioneer effort along the same lines and might as well continue to function. However, he did list as sites all institutions and agencies providing health services, such as hospitals, nursing homes, physicians' offices, clinics, and the all-inclusive "et cetera."

In the three years after the publication of Hershey's article (and prior to the DHEW report), institutional licensure as an alternative, or, in some cases, an adjunct to individual licensure, was a point of some discussion by assorted groups, especially the American Hospital Association and its affiliates. This interest is not immediately visible in the nursing literature, however. A survey of papers, articles, and position statements issued in that period, some of which are cited in the 1971 credentialing study,[20] described a number of variations of the concept.[21]

One advantage cited for institutional licensure is that job descriptions and classifications, combined with inservice training or other experiences and education, would allow health practitioners to move from one classification to another—not a new idea. This plan had already been adopted by some of the more progressive hospitals of that time. More to the point, then and now, is to determine whether all agencies would be willing to initiate the expensive and extensive educational, evaluative, and supervisory programs necessary to fulfill the basic tenets of institutional licensure. Hospital administrators, particularly, have been complaining about the expense of orientation and inservice education programs, cutting back on them as much as possible. Now, with even greater pressure to control costs, extensive staff education programs are even less likely. This raises the specter of a return to the corrupted apprentice system of early hospital nursing in the United States. Probably a hospital's own personnel would be used as teacher-preceptors. Who then would do their job? How would they be compensated? How long would "students" be expected to function in their current positions with the current salary while they "practice" the new role? And with what kind of supervision? What kind of testing program for each level? Testing by whom? With what kinds of standards? Such sliding positions might well cut manpower costs, but might they not also indenture workers instead of freeing them with new mobility?

Problems of criteria for standards are obvious. If fifty states cannot now agree on criteria for individual licensure, why would institutional licensure be any different? Considering the almost 7,000 profit and nonprofit hospitals with bed capacities ranging from the tens to the thousands, in rural and urban areas, with administrators and other key personnel prepared in widely varied ways, and the even larger number of extended care facilities, clinics, and home care agencies that are equally dissimilar, a state of confusion, diversity, and parochialism becomes an over-whelming probability. Instead of facilitating interstate mobility, institutional licensure would more likely limit even interinstitutional mobility. A worker could qualify for position X in institution A, with absolutely no guarantee that this would be acceptable to institution B. Moreover, the disadvantages to those health professions that have fought to attain, maintain, and raise standards might be disastrous to patient welfare. Nurses, who are just beginning to fulfill their roles in the delivery of total health care, accountable to the patient and not

to an administrative hierarchy or a physician for their professional acts, may find themselves relegated to increasingly technical tasks, substituting for a more expensive physician and being substituted for by the less prepared. (Not an NP, but a PA; not giving primary nursing, but resurrecting nursing by direction.) Will this save the patient money, or cost him optimum health?

Whether or not it is argued that many of these practices exist today—de facto institutional licensure, as one proponent asserted—it hardly seems progressive to legalize what is already considered an unsatisfactory situation. And let there be no mistake: under this proposed system, an institution would have the power to determine the specific tasks and functions of each job and indicate the skill and proficiency levels required, regardless of the employee's licensure, certification, or education. Control would be almost complete, because guidelines to be developed by the state institutional licensing agency are intended to be general.

But then, would not the state guidelines protect the consumer, if not the employee? Presumably, the state licensing agency would be empowered to review the institution's utilization and supervision of health personnel to determine whether employees are performing functions for which they are qualified. How feasible would such an evaluation be? No one believes that an army of experts knowledgeable in all the subcategories of health care could be recruited, employed, and dispersed to check the hundreds of thousands employed in the multiple subcategories of workers in the thousands of caregiving facilities in any state. Therefore, one more paper tiger would be created—inspection by paper work. To determine the effectiveness of such surveillance, it is only necessary to look at the nursing home scandals and the admitted deficiencies of various municipal, state, and proprietary hospitals, to name a few. In all of these situations, the institution reviewed was given an official blessing; in truth, the conditions varied from unsafe to life-threatening. Generally, approval was given on the basis of the written self-report, with or without a visit by harassed, overworked surveyors. (What's more, when surveyors did recommend closings of the institutions, they were frequently overruled or ignored, if it was politically expedient.) Would institutional licensure suddenly, miraculously avoid these pitfalls?

Nurses are periodically assured that institutional licensure would not include or affect them or their practice, because the focus would be on ancillary personnel. In the first place, serious discussions soon reveal that nurses *would* be a part of the overall scheme. Even if they were not, it is difficult to see how institutional licensure would *not* affect them when, at the least, others would decide upon the duties of nursing personnel whom nurses would supervise. It is also unrealistic for nurses to expect to be exempted when many of the tasks once considered part of professional nursing have now been assigned to those with less preparation, when expedient. Alternatively, tasks that have been part of another group's responsibility suddenly become nursing's, when it serves the purposes of the institution.

A final question remains, concerning those health professionals who provide care outside the walls of a health institution. Is the possibility of independent practice eliminated? Or will multiple systems of credentialing add to the confusion?

Given the inconsistencies of institutional licensure, the economic advantages to certain employers, and the perceived threat to established professions, a polarity of reactions was to be expected. Continuing to voice general approval were the hospital and hospital administrator groups, but organized nursing arose to rally an opposing constituency. The first major action was a strong resolution approved by the ANA House of Delegates, followed by a statement by NLN asserting unalterable opposition to the institutional licensure concept. Soon, most of the major RN and PN organizations, as well as AMA, stated like opposition.

Meanwhile, the federal government funded two institutional licensure projects, one in Pennsylvania and one in Illinois. The first never seemed to get off the ground; the Illinois project was completed, but the recommendations of the final report concluded that although technically the concept could probably be carried out, "Implementation of the institutional licensure concept should not be undertaken at this time unless a significant commitment to this concept, far greater than exists now, occurs. This commitment would have to be on the part of those in the health industry, at every level, as well as those in government health agencies."[22]

The strong protests plus the report seemed to cool DHEW's enthusiasm for this particular means of solving the credentialing problems. In 1977's *Credentialing Health Manpower* the only reference to institutional licensure was that on the basis of "studies of the feasibility of a national certification system and institutional licensure as alternatives to the traditional model of occupational licensure in health . . . the Public Health Service (PHS) has concluded that the certification alternative should be further developed, whereas the institutional licensure approach—because of the intense controversy that it generated—should not receive further consideration at this time."[23]

Does this eliminate the threat of institutional licensure? Not really, for it seems now that the concept is reappearing, if it ever disappeared, without its label.[24] In some states, overt attempts to legislate institutional licensure (which had been kept in committee or killed primarily through the efforts of organized nursing) keep emerging. One expert in the field predicts that with the trend toward multi-institutional ownership, especially by for-profit groups, and the concomitant trend for physicians to become employees, "corporate-wide credentialing" would be sought by the corporate giants.[25] He speculated on whether the professional groups would have the political clout to prevent it.

EXHIBIT 20–1

CREDENTIALING HEALTH MANPOWER
DHEW 1977 Recommendations

RECOMMENDATION I: A NATIONAL VOLUNTARY SYSTEM FOR ALLIED HEALTH CERTIFICATION

A broadly representative national (non-Federal) certification commission should be established to perform the following functions for allied health occupations:

1. Develop and continually evaluate criteria and policies for the purpose of recognizing certification organizations and monitoring their adherence to these criteria.
2. Participate in the development of national standards as proposed in Recommendation II.
3. Provide consultation and technical assistance to certification organizations.

RECOMMENDATION II: NATIONAL STANDARDS

National standards for the credentialing of selected health occupations should be developed and continually evaluated. Professional organizations, other elements in the private sector, and State governments should play a significant role in this process. The standards thus developed should be utilized for the various purposes for which standards are required, including professional certification, licensure, private sector and civil service employment, and third party reimbursement.

RECOMMENDATION III: CRITERIA FOR FUTURE STATE LICENSURE DECISIONS

States should entertain proposals to license additional categories of health personnel with caution and deliberation. Before enacting any legislation that would license additional categories of health manpower, States should consider the following factors:

1. In what way will the unregulated practice clearly endanger the health, safety and welfare of the public, and is the potential for harm easily recognizable and not remote or dependent on tenuous argument?
2. How will the public benefit by an assurance of initial and continuing professional competence?
3. Can the public be effectively protected by means other than licensure?
4. Why is licensure the most appropriate form of regulation?
5. How will the newly licensed category impact upon the statutory and administrative authority and scopes of practice of previously licensed categories in the State?

RECOMMENDATION IV: IMPROVED LICENSURE PROCEDURES

States should take new steps to strengthen the accountability and effectiveness of licensure boards that will allow them to play an active role in assuring high-quality health services. These include:

1. Allocate increased funding, staffing, legal assistance and other resources.
2. Assign high priority to disciplinary procedures and responsibilities.
3. Adopt relevant national examinations and standards.
4. Expand membership on boards to include effective representation of consumers and other functionally-related professionals.
5. Establish appropriate linkages with the various health licensing boards and between such boards and other governmental health agencies responsible for the planning, development and monitoring of health manpower and services.
6. Develop a data capacity that is relevant to the formulation of health manpower policy.

RECOMMENDATION V: COMPETENCY MEASUREMENT

Certification organizations, licensure boards, and professional associations should take steps to recognize and promote the widespread adoption of effective competency measures to determine the qualifications of health personnel. Special attention should be given to the further development of proficiency and equivalency measures for appropriate categories of health manpower.

RECOMMENDATION VI: CONTINUED COMPETENCE

Certification organizations, licensure boards and professional associations should adopt requirements and procedures that will assure the continued competence of health personnel. Additional studies of the best mechanisms to assure continued competence should be supported on a high-priority basis by professional organizations, the proposed national certification commission, State agencies, and the Federal Government.

Other Developments

When the 1971 credentialing rep. † suggested that there be a two-year moratorium on
licensing new categories of health personnel,
with "statutorily defined scopes of functions," there seemed to be a reasonable response. AMA, AHA, ANA, and other groups
had already suggested such action, and many
state legislatures were becoming concerned as
each emerging health occupation sought recognition through licensure. Still, the recommendation for an additional two years' moratorium in the 1973 report was only a stopgap
that did not persist. What are the alternatives?
The final 1977 DHEW recommendations
pointed the direction for future action (see Exhibit 20-1). The ultimate weapon is the government's power to give or withhold funding.
For instance, if requirements that health personnel must be certified or licensed under national standards and must give evidence of
continued competence were written into regulations for Medicare-Medicaid reimbursement, few employees or practitioners could
afford to ignore the matter. Because concern
for the public is shared by state governments,
some of the recommendations on licensure
were quickly adopted. Others, like national
standards, are much slower in being implemented.

Certification

As a follow-up to the 1971 credentialing report, a project to determine the feasibility of a
national certification system, aimed particularly at allied health personnel, was explored—with federal funding. The results
seemed to be positive, and DHEW concluded
that this concept, a voluntary national certification system, should be developed further.

By 1978, a Certification Council, later
called the National Commission for Health
Certifying Agencies (NCHCA), had been organized. Its general purpose was to certify the
certifiers—an overall group that would include the organizations that certified allied
health professionals but also set certain uniform standards and guidelines. At the same
time, certification of nurses* was also undergoing reorganization and expansion, as was
certification for PAs.† Nurse-midwives and
nurse anesthetists had been certified for some
time, but in the period following the credentialing reports, their system also underwent

---

*See Chapter 25.
†See Chapter 8.

Source: U.S. Department of Health, Education, and Welfare, *Credentialing Health Manpower* (DHEW Publ. No.
(OS)77–50057), 1977, pp. 7–17.

change. In general, certification was and is attracting considerable attention as a substitute for, or an adjunct to, licensure; in the latter case, it is a means of identifying specialists within a field. For instance, many of the health occupations described in Chapter 8 are only certified, but physicians with all-encompassing licensure increasingly use certification to differentiate specialists. It is anticipated that board-certified physicians will grow from 70 percent in 1980 to almost 100 percent in 2010.[26]

Still, certification is not a clearly understood credentialing mechanism. Two points are essential for comprehension: (1) certification is voluntary on the part of the individual, and (2) the organization or agency that certifies is nongovernmental, and is usually comprised of experts or peers in that particular field. This "private credentialing" differs fundamentally from "public credentialing" (licensure) in that the latter can legally prohibit unlicensed practice. Those who lack private credentials "still possess a legal right to practice, although they may be disadvantaged in the marketplace because independent decision-makers such as consumers, hospitals, and public or private financing plans value their services less highly."[27] Havighurst and King describe private credentialing* as serving solely informational purposes, a sort of "seal of approval" from the professional association or nongovernmental board that grants it.[28] It gives the consumer an opportunity to make more informed decisions, in that certification indicates that the certified person has voluntarily met certain standards that similar caregivers have not. Because the public needs to know that the certifying group and its standards have some legitimacy, there is a second-tier credentialing organization, like the NCHCA noted above, that can be either voluntary or governmental.

---

*Accreditation of educational programs, as done by NLN, or of health care facilities, as done by the Joint Commission on Accreditation of Hospitals (JCAH), are other examples of private credentialing.

Criticisms of certification are remarkably like those of licensure. One is that individuals as well qualified as those who are certified are denied certification and are thus disadvantaged in the marketplace. The denial may be due to the lack of a certain educational background or failure to pass an examination. The latter is a common certification mechanism. This was indeed challenged in a legal suit, and the certifying board settled out of court. The issue is often the validity of the examination and whether it discriminates against minorities, for instance—a matter that has also arisen in licensure. Examinations for both types of credentialing are now undergoing close scrutiny, with continual involvement of test experts. Nevertheless, some persons question whether *any* examination can really identify the competent practitioner.

Secondly, there is the question of grandfathering, also a licensure problem. Usually those who practiced a speciality before certification existed are "grandfathered in," that is, permitted to hold certification without fulfilling the usual requirements. Thus, the information given the public—that these persons fulfill certain criteria—is not accurate. Here the answer may lie in requirements to demonstrate ongoing competency for recertification—providing that that measure is valid. More certifying groups now have a recertification mechanism.

Finally, there is the concern that certification is done by the professional organization that also accredits the educational program from which the candidate must graduate in order to qualify for certification. Clearly, that mechanism provides complete control by the occupation and can also shut out potential candidates. This problem was resolved, to a large extent, by the FTC rulings that such arrangements were illegal restraint of trade.[29] Professions then gradually separated these functions into independent entities. Two examples are the nurse-midwives and nurse anesthetists, whose organizations are described in Chapter 27.

Despite these criticisms, certification is generally advocated as a way to assist the consumer in making choices. As will be described later, certification rather than specialized licensure is the route preferred by ANA to identify nurse specialists/practitioners. The ANA Social Policy Statement says:

> Certification of specialists in nursing practice is a judgment made by the profession, upon review of an array of evidence examined by a selected panel of nurses who are themselves specialists and who represent the area of specialization . . . the public needs clear evidence that a nurse who claims to be a specialist does indeed have expertise of a particular kind. The profession of nursing has a social obligation to the public to satisfy that need, which it does by means of certification of specialists and by accreditation of the graduate programs that educate specialists in nursing practice.[30]

Unfortunately, one major problem in certification of nursing specialists is that both ANA and certain speciality organizations each certify, so that both nurse and consumer must decide which, if either, is most reliable.

Sunset Laws and Other Public Actions

Besides considering alternatives, improving the licensure process has become a national mandate. Although the speed of the action taken has varied from state to state, steps taken almost universally at one level or another include adding consumers and sometimes other functionally related health professionals to each board, giving more attention to disciplinary procedures, and gradually developing proficiency and equivalency examinations. In a number of states, boards have been consolidated, sometimes under committees of lay people (or at least a majority of consumers), who make the decisions about licensing, with the individual boards acting in an advisory capacity. Although one reason given is improved efficiency, some nurses fear that this is an indirect approach to institutional licensure because these reorganizations tend to attenuate nursing's control over its practice.

For some professions, improving the licensure laws to protect the public was a new experience. A motivating factor was the enactment of "sunset laws" which "require the periodic reexamination of licensing agencies to determine whether particular boards or activities should be established."[31] By 1984, two-thirds of the states had enacted such laws. These laws were a result of a lobbying compaign by Common Cause, a consumer group, to bring about legislative and executive branch oversight of regulating boards and agencies of all kinds. Common Cause identified ten principles to be followed, including a time schedule. An important component was that an evaluation was to allow for public input, as well as that of the boards and occupations involved. Consolidation and "responsible pruning" were encouraged. Although the review would be done by appropriate legislative and executive committees, safeguards were to be built in to prevent arbitrary termination of boards and agencies.[32] These principles are generally adhered to, but states do vary in their management of sunset reviews. If a sunset law is in effect, the data and justification for existence are a joint staff–board responsibility, although the professional organizations are also usually helpful.

In 1976 the first sunset law was enacted in Colorado, requiring periodic, automatic termination of regulatory boards unless they were specifically re-created by statute.[33] When the nursing board was reviewed in Colorado, and later in New Hampshire, both were sunsetted. This meant that there would be no licensure law, no nurse could be licensed or relicensed, and no schools approved. In each case, the board, the association, and nurses in general had not prepared adequately. They had underestimated the importance of educating the public and legislators on what nurses do. The New Hampshire commission stated that "unregulated nursing would not frequently result in major irreparable harm to [public] health or safety because state regulation was not the most effective means of providing adequate recourse in cases of improper practice."[34] In both states, nurses later managed to get a new law enacted, but they also became much more aware of how important it was to plan for the sunset review and for nurses to work cooperatively for reauthorization of their licensure law.* They also learned many political lessons.

By 1985, most nursing boards had undergone sunset reviews, and the new or amended laws usually reflected changes in practice and society. These changes, and some instituted earlier, also reflected the impact of the DHEW reports. Most practice acts have broadened the scope of practice, added consumers to their boards, and sometimes required evidence of current competence through various means, including continuing education. State boards have given increased attention to removing and/or rehabilitating incompetent nurses. Meanwhile, educators are working seriously on equivalency and proficiency examinations and other methods of providing flexibility and upward mobility for nursing candidates. ANA and NLN have taken positive action on the issues of open curriculum, continuing competence, and certification. Nurses in the field have continued to improve techniques of peer evaluation, implement standards of practice, and encourage voluntary CE.

Finally, a major study of credentialing sponsored by ANA[35] made some daring proposals in 1979, suggesting the establishment of a national nursing credentialing center, run by a federation of organizations with "legitimate interests" in nursing and credentialing, "as the means of achieving a unified, coordinated, comprehensive credentialing system for nursing."† While this recommendation was not accepted by nursing, except "in principle," it did increase the nurses' understanding of credentialing issues, especially in nursing.

LICENSURE: THE LEGAL BASIS OF NURSING PRACTICE

Enactment of nurse licensure laws was one of the primary purposes of ANA at its inception. The first permissive nursing practice law in this country was enacted in North Carolina on March 3, 1903. Weak though it was compared with present-day laws, it represented a great achievement for nursing leaders, who had been working toward this goal for a decade. Within a month, New Jersey had passed a state nursing practice act, followed closely by New York and Virginia. In 1904, Maryland was the only state to pass such an act, but in each succeeding year from 1905 until 1917, legislation was enacted to govern the practice of nursing, although it was not always just what nurses desired. By 1917, forty-five states and the District of Columbia had nursing practice acts; by 1923 the last of the forty-eight states in existence adopted such an act. In 1952 all states and territories had such laws. Hawaii's first nursing practice act was passed in 1917 and Alaska's in 1941.

In every instance, the original state law was permissive. The first mandatory nursing practice act was enacted in New York in 1938, but it was not put into effect until 1947. One of the real dangers of permissive licensing is that correspondence and other schools with poor curricula and inadequate clinical experience produce workers who can legally "nurse," although they are potentially dangerous practitioners. Such programs also tend to defraud unsuspecting students who do not know that they will not be eligible for licensure, because a school must maintain minimum standards set by the state board before graduates may sit for licensing examinations. Theoretically, any person with or without schooling can practice as a nurse if someone is willing to hire him or her. The kind of nurse most likely to be hired is one who has graduated from a legitimate program but has not been able to pass the licensing exam.

As of 1985, there were no states with permissive licensure laws for professional nurses;

---

*Both Grobe and Thomas suggest specific strategies.

†See also Chapter 5.

a few states had permissive licensure for practical nurses (PNs). A review and report of the state boards indicated that only the District of Columbia lacked a mandatory RN law, although others were loose in their interpretation of mandatory. States that have such global exemption clauses in licensure laws stating that almost anyone can be a "nurse," providing that there is some kind of "supervision," are sometimes seen as permissive states regardless of a mandatory clause.

Objections to making licensure laws mandatory come from many sources. Some feel that mandatory laws are used to keep out individuals who might be capable but lack the formal education and other requirements for licensure. It is true that some laws are rigid in these requirements, but more and more states are beginning to consider the use of equivalency and proficiency examinations and other means of demonstrating knowledge and skills.

Another concern is that those already practicing in the field will be abruptly removed and deprived of their livelihood. This is, however, untrue because mandatory laws are forced, for political and constitutional reasons, to include a grandfather clause. A grandfather or waiver clause is a standard feature when a licensure law is enacted or a current law is repealed and a new law enacted. The grandfather clause allows persons to continue to practice the profession/occupation when new qualifications are enacted into law. Although the concept goes back to post-Civil War days, it is also related to the Fifth and Fourteenth amendments of the Constitution. The U.S. Supreme Court has repeatedly ruled that the license to practice a profession/occupation is a property right and that the Fourteenth Amendment extends the due process requirement to state laws. Many nurses currently licensed were protected by the grandfather clause when a new law was passed or new requirements were made, although most probably never realized it. For instance, when the Missouri Nursing Practice Act was repealed in 1976, the new law had a grandfather clause, and all nurses holding a valid license continued to be licensed. When the various states began to require psychiatric nursing as a condition of licensure, those who had not had those courses in their educational programs did not forfeit licensure. When the grandfather clause is enacted in relation to mandatory licensure, those who can produce evidence, that they practiced as, say, a PN, if applying for LPN status, must be granted a license. However, grandfathering does not guarantee employment. Thus, some employers chose not to employ "waivered" PNs, just as they had not employed them as unlicensed practitioners. Because of these problems, and often because of their need and desire to be safe, competent practitioners, many took courses to fill the gaps in their knowledge and chose to take the state board examinations later.

CONTENT OF NURSING PRACTICE ACTS

Unfortunately, many nurses know no more about the law that regulates their practice than that it requires them to take state board examinations in order to become licensed. More details about the procedure for obtaining a license will be given later; however, it is vital that nurses understand the components of their licensure law and how these affect their practice.

Because each state law differs to a degree in its content, it is important to have available a copy of the law of the state in which you practice and the regulations that spell out how the law is carried out. These may be obtained from the state board or agency in the state government that has copies of laws for distribution. The language in all laws often seems stilted because they are written in legal terms. However, a little effort or discussion with someone familiar with the law will soon enable you to become almost as familiar with legal jargon as with nursing jargon. This is particularly important, for the majority of states anticipate some change in their nursing practice act in the near future or have recently passed amendments often in relation to sunset review. Changes made or contemplated are generally in relation to the definition and scope of nursing practice, the makeup of the nursing board, and actions to ensure competency.

Most nursing practice acts have basically the same major components, although not necessarily in the same order: definition of nursing, requirements for licensure, exemption from licensure, grounds for revocation of the license, provision for reciprocity for persons licensed in other states, creation of a board of nurse examiners, responsibilities of the board, and penalties for practicing without a license. All states do not, unfortunately, have the same requirements in these categories. Some follow the 1980 ANA guidelines,[36] some the model act of the National Council of State Boards of Nursing (NCSBN);[37] others enact what is politically feasible or necessary in their particular state. Only the RN (not LPN) licensure law or component of the nursing practice act will be discussed in the following sections.* However, ANA recommends that, because nursing is one occupational field, it should be controlled by one law and one state board. (Definitions and requirements would, of course, still be separate.) LPN definitions are presented with RN definitions to show their interrelationships.

Definition and Scope of Practice

The definition of *nursing* in the licensure law determines both legal responsibilities and the scope of practice of nurses. Inevitably, the definition of nursing in all nursing practice acts is stated in terms that are quite broad. This is generally frustrating to nurses who turn to the definition to determine if they are practicing legally, because it does not spell out

---

*Nurse-midwives and nurse anesthetists may be included within a nursing practice act, a medical practice act, separately, or totally ignored legislatively. If mentioned, certification is usually a prerequisite for legal practice. In 1983, nurse-midwives were covered in the nursing practice act of twenty-seven states, nurse anethetists in thirty-one.

specific procedures or activities. Often such activities are not even spelled out in the regulations of the laws. However, a broad definition is usually preferable because of the problems of including specific activities in a law. Changes in health care and nursing practice often move more rapidly than a law can be changed, and the amending process can be long and complex. If particular activities were named, the nurse would be limited to just those listed. Not only would the list be overwhelmingly long, but it is conceivable that any new technique easily and, perhaps necessarily, performed by a nurse would require an amendment to the law. An occasional state law does specify certain procedures, but always includes the phrase "not limited to."

A practicing nurse soon finds that the nursing functions taught in an educational program may differ from those expected by an employer. The differences may be small and caused by variations in the settings of nursing care. Nursing in a medical center may require knowing more sophisticated techniques or assuming more comprehensive responsibilities in nursing care. Sometimes, whether in a large or small agency, there are procedures performed that the nurse has not learned. If the nurse has not practiced for some time, this is even more likely to happen. In other cases, the responsibilities expected in the nursing role are not in nursing care but in clerical and administrative tasks. Although this may not be desirable, it is not illegal. What concerns the nurse is whether the patient-oriented care expected in the employment situation is legal or in the domain of another health profession. Many of the activities in health care overlap. A common example might be the administration of drugs, which could be done by the physician, RN, LPN, and various technicians in other hospital departments if related to a diagnostic procedure or treatment. Yet dispensing a drug from the hospital pharmacy, so commonly done by hospital supervisors at night when no pharmacist is on duty, is in most states a violation of the pharmacy licensing law.

Obviously, one of the greatest concerns for nurses is the possible violation of the Medical Practice Act. Nurses have gradually been performing more and more of the technical procedures that once belonged exclusively to medicine, but often these are delegated willingly by physicians. Whether nurses are always properly prepared to understand and perform them well is seldom questioned. However, as some nurses have assumed more comprehensive overall responsibilities in the care, cure, and coordination of patient care, questions have been raised by both nurses and physicians. Some are resistant to such changes; others are supportive but concerned about the legality of such acts.

In a 1970 position statement on nursing, AMA supported the expanding role of the nurse in providing patient care. In this paper, as in the DHEW report *Extending the Scope of Nursing Practice*, there is a statement that the identical act or procedure "may be the practice of medicine when carried out by a physician and the practice of nursing when carried out by the nurse."[38,39] The AMA statement appears to allude particularly to technical procedures, but the DHEW report looked at the situation more broadly.

> There is an ever-widening area of independent nursing practice entailing nursing judgment, procedures, and techniques. This is due to natural evolution, commencing with the nurse's assumption of certain activities carried out under medical direction, and the subsequent relaxation or removal of that direction.
> Concomitant with increasingly complex nursing practice is the continual realignment of the functions of the professional nurse and physician. The boundaries of responsibility for nurses are not shifting more rapidly simply because of increased demands for health services. The functions of nurses are changing primarily because nurses have demonstrated their competence to perform a greater variety of functions and have been willing to discontinue performing less important functions that were once performed only by nurses.[40]

The same report stated that there are no legal barriers to extending the scope of practice because the statutory laws governing nursing practice (the licensing law) are broad enough to permit such extension, providing that the nurse has the proper skills and necessary knowledge of the underlying science. It did acknowledge that at times common law, essentially judge-made law, has made interpretations of nursing practice not specifically defined by statute through legal decisions and stated that the profession must then look at these decisions to determine the need to change the statutory law. After reviewing some of the problems concerned with specific acts in changing nursing practice, the report concluded that as nursing changes, both nursing and the law must evaluate these changes and make the necessary adaptations to meet society's changing needs.[41]

Until 1974 the nursing practice acts of most states had as their definition of nursing one similar to a model* suggested by ANA in 1955:

> The practice of professional nursing means the performance for compensation of any act in the observation, care, and counsel of the ill, injured, or infirm, or in the maintenance of health or prevention of illness of others, or in the supervision and teaching of other personnel, or the administration of medications and treatments as prescribed by a licensed physician or dentist; requiring substantial specialized judgment and skill and based on knowledge and application of the principles of biological, physical, and social science. (The foregoing shall not be deemed to include acts of diagnosis or prescription of therapeutic or corrective measures.)[42]

The definition distinguished between independent acts that the nurse might perform, but also identified certain dependent acts and pro-

---

*Until the NCSBN developed a model not congruent with ANA's "guidelines," it was generally accepted that it was the professional organization that developed a model licensure law usually introduced into the state legislature by the state nurses' association (SNA).

hibited diagnosis and treatment (not preceded by the word *medical*). In the 1970s, with expanded functions being assumed by nursing, state nurses' associations (SNAs) increasingly became concerned about the adequacy of this definition. Therefore, the first states to change their laws concentrated on broadening the definition to encompass these roles.

Professional nursing literature had been distinguishing between the independent acts that a nurse must undertake and the dependent acts that must be carried out under the supervision or "orders" of the physician, such as administration of medications and treatments. The problem in the 1955 definition, in terms of the needs of the 1970s, was that although the first sentence did not *prohibit* the nurse from carrying out medical acts or making diagnoses, the last sentence effectively prohibited a broad interpretation by the courts.

As nurses in their expanded role seemed to be moving into the gray areas between medicine and nursing, it was evident that, if a state had a licensure law with a dependent clause, nurses might be seen as practicing medicine. The 1971 and 1973 credentialing reports suggested extending delegation of authority in all fields, but nursing was concerned that such delegation might mean including nurses specifically in the exception clause of medical practice acts, thus permitting the practice, but placing control totally in the hands of physicians. Perhaps as a compromise or in the hope that medicine and nursing could work together as they should in providing new health care options to the public, ANA counsel suggested that a new clause be added to the ANA model definition:

A professional nurse may also perform such additional acts, under emergency or other special conditions, which may include special training, as are recognized by the medical and nursing professions as proper to be performed by a professional nurse under such conditions, even though such acts might otherwise be considered diagnosis and prescription.[43]

Later, after various states had amended their laws with this phrase or changed it altogether, with varying success, an ANA ad hoc committee revised the definition entirely in 1976. This model law, recommending one nursing practice law with provisions for licensing practitioners of nursing, used the terms *registered nurse* and *practical/vocational nurse.*

The practice of nursing as performed by a registered nurse is a process in which substantial specialized knowledge derived from the biological, physical, and behavioral sciences is applied to the care, treatment, counsel, and health teaching of persons who are experiencing changes in the normal health processes; or who require assistance in the maintenance of health or the management of illness, injury, or infirmity, or in the achievement of a dignified death; and such additional acts as are recognized by the nursing profession as proper to be performed by a registered nurse.

Practical/vocational nursing means the performance under the supervision of a registered nurse of those services required in observing and caring for the ill, injured, or infirm, in promoting preventive measures in community health, in acting to safeguard life and health, in administering treatment and medication prescribed by a physician or dentist, or in performing other acts not requiring the skill, judgment, and knowledge of a registered nurse.[44]

The new definition differentiated between the independence of the RN's functions and the dependence of the LPN/LVN. It also placed the responsibility for what the RN can legally do in the hands of the nursing profession, always considered a hallmark of professionalism.

The 1980 ANA document on nurse practice acts was introduced as "suggested" legislation (as differentiated from the NCSBN model act), using the Council of State Governments definition:

A model bill is a piece of legislation, which

seeks to address, in comprehensive fashion, a determined need. Model bills are often reform legislation intended to provide order in an area where existing legislation is out of date, internally inconsistent, too broad or too narrow, or for some other reason inadequate to implement current state policy.

On the other hand, suggested legislation, although in appropriate legislative form, is designed to bring to the attention of policymakers some of the critical issues which need to be addressed.[45]

The ANA Ad Hoc Committee on Legal Aspects of Nursing Practice that developed the document noted that not all states would enact this legislation, but that some provisions might be appropriate solutions for a particular state's problems. However, the committee did clearly state the principles considered essential in nurse licensure legislation incorporated in the ANA document. These were:

1. The primary purpose of a licensing law for the regulation of the practice of nursing is to protect the public health and welfare by establishing legal qualifications for the practice of nursing. Such legal standards are recognized as minimum standards that are determined adequate to provide safe and effective nursing practice.

2. All persons practicing or offering to practice nursing or practical nursing should be licensed. Protection of the public is accomplished only if all who practice or offer to practice nursing are licensed. The public should not be expected to differentiate between incompetent and competent practitioners.

3. Since nursing is one occupational field, there should be one nursing practice act that licenses both registered nurses and licensed practical nurses. The public and the practitioners may be confused when there is more than one law regulating the practice of nursing and the practice of practical nursing.

4. The enactment of one nursing practice act necessitates only one licensing board for nursing in a state. The board of nursing should be composed of nurses whose practice is regulated by the licensure law and by a representative or representatives of the public.

5. Candidates for licensure should complete an educational program approved by the board and pass the licensing examination before a license to practice is granted.

6. The nursing practice act should provide for the legal regulation of nursing without reference to a specialized area of practice. It is the function of the professional association to establish the scope and desirable qualifications required for each area of practice, and to certify individuals as competent to engage in specific areas of nursing practice. It is also the function of the professional association to upgrade practice above the minimum standards set by law. The law should not provide for identifying clinical specialists in nursing or require certification or other recognition for practice beyond the minimum qualifications established for the legal regulation of nursing.[46]

The 1980 definition (Exhibit 20-2) speaks of professional services for the RN and technical services for the PN (vocational), probably as a manifestation of the professional/technical differentiation presented in the 1965 ANA position paper and reaffirmed by the House of Delegates in 1978. Direct accountability to the public is also a part of the definition; again, differentiation between the two types of nurses is made. In the commentary section, it was noted that the definition should recognize "the singular element that distinguishes the nurse from other nursing personnel—the breadth and depth of educational preparation that justify entrusting overall responsibility for nursing services to the judgment of the registered nurse."

The NCSBN model act is different in format and, to some extent, content (Exhibit 20-2). In relation to the definition, the language is considerably broader than that of

EXHIBIT 20-2

Comparison of ANA and NCSBN Suggested Definitions of Nursing

PRACTICE OF NURSING

The practice of nursing means the performance for compensation of professional services requiring substantial specialized knowledge of the biological, physical, behavioral, psychological, and sociological sciences and of nursing theory as the basis for assessment, diagnosis, planning, intervention, and evaluation in the promotion and maintenance of health; the casefinding and management of illness, injury, or infirmity; the restoration of optimum function; or the achievement of a dignified death. Nursing practice includes but is not limited to administration, teaching, counseling, supervision, delegation, and evaluation of practice and execution of the medical regimen, including the administration of medications and treatments prescribed by any person authorized by state law to prescribe. Each registered nurse is directly accountable and responsible to the consumer for the quality of nursing care rendered.

The practice of practical nursing means the performance for compensation of technical services requiring basic knowledge of the biological, physical, behavioral, psychological, and sociological sciences and of nursing procedures. These services are performed under the supervision of a registered nurse and utilize standardized procedures leading to predictable outcomes in the observation and care of the ill, injured and infirm; in the maintenance of health, in action to safeguard life and health; and in the administration of medications and treatments

PRACTICE OF NURSING

The "Practice of Nursing" means assisting individuals or groups to maintain or attain optimal health throughout the life process by assessing their health status, establishing a diagnosis, planning and implementing a strategy of care to accomplish defined goals, and evaluating responses to care and treatment.

Registered Nurse. "Registered Nurse" means a person who practices professional nursing by:

(a) Assessing the health status of individuals and groups;
(b) Establishing a nursing diagnosis;
(c) Establishing goals to meet identified health care needs;
(d) Planning a strategy of care;
(e) Prescribing nursing interventions to implement the strategy of care;
(f) Implementing the strategy of care;
(g) Authorizing nursing interventions that may be performed by others and that do not conflict with this Act;
(h) Maintaining safe and effective nursing care rendered directly or indirectly;
(i) Evaluating responses to interventions;
(j) Teaching the theory and practice of nursing;
(k) Managing the practice of nursing, and;
(l) Collaborating with other health professionals in the management of health care.

Licensed Practical Nurse. "Licensed Practical Nurse" means a person who practices nursing by:

(a) Contributing to the assessment of the health status of individuals and groups;
(b) Participating in the development and modification of the strategy of care;
(c) Implementing the appropriate aspects of the strategy of care as defined by the Board;
(d) Maintaining safe and effective nursing care rendered directly or indirectly;
(e) Participating in the evaluation of responses to interventions, and;

prescribed by any person authorized by state law to prescribe.

(f) Delegating nursing interventions that may be performed by others and that do not conflict with this Act.

The Licensed Practical Nurse functions at the direction of the Registered Nurse, licensed physician, or licensed dentist in the performance of activities delegated by that health care professional.

American Nurses' Association 1980.

National Council of State Boards of Nursing 1982.

Source: American Nurses' Association, *The Nursing Practice Act: Suggested State Legislation*, (Kansas City, Mo.: The Association, 1980) p. 6.

Source: The Model Nursing Practice Act, (Chicago, Ill.: National Council of State Boards of Nursing, 1982) pp. 2–3.

ANA, although both support a broad definition. The NCSBN definition is based on information found in an NCSBN research project on "critical requirements for safe/effective nursing practice." It does not deal with the educational preparation or responsibilities common to all health professions. Nor does it consider execution of the medical regimen (carrying out the doctor's orders), because other definitions do so. On the other hand, it is interesting to note that the ANA definition refers to carrying out the medical regimen as prescribed by any person authorized by state law to prescribe. This could certainly include the NP, but like it or not, it might also include the PA since there have already been court rulings for and against the nurse's obligation to follow PA orders. Another big difference is that the LPN is to be directed only by the RN in the ANA statement, but physicians and dentists are added in the NCSBN definition. This concerns ANA, since this type of wording puts a licensed nursing person under the control of another profession. Finally, the NCSBN adds interdisciplinary collaboration as a nursing responsibility. NCSBN noted that this definition "describes the responsibilities and scope of practice of professional nurses and entrusts them with overall responsibility for nursing care" and "clearly distinguishes between a Registered Nurse's practice and the practice of others within the field of nurs-

ing."[47] Most states have not followed either format or content as such.

Just how varied the state licensure laws are was revealed by a 1983 ANA analysis of fifty-one nursing practice acts.[48] Definitions of nursing were looked at in light of the nursing process, that is, assessment, diagnosis, planning, intervention, and evaluation. ANA found that even when the concepts of the process were identifiable in the various laws, the language varied considerably. Terms such as *diagnosis of human responses, nursing diagnosis, problem* or *need identification, nursing analysis*, and *diagnosis of disease* were all used.

A major concern was how states legislated for advanced nursing practice, which is related to both definition and regulations. This was reported in 1983 in considerable detail, including the practice of nurse-midwives and nurse anesthetists.[49]

Up to now, state legislatures have chosen three general means of dealing with expanded nursing practice in the legal definition of the licensure law.[50] The first could be called the use of nonamended statutes. These states either have made no changes from the 1955 ANA model and allow for a liberal interpretation of the definition by the state board or have made minor changes. In some, the word *medical* has been inserted to describe prohibited acts. Thus, certain acts of diagnosis and treatment would presumably be identified as nursing. Other states have retained portions of the traditional definition but omitted or substituted certain other phrases. Although all these states maintain that their acts allow expanded practice, interpretation is the key, so a change in attitude or political/medical pressures could bring a rapid about-face. In 1980, fifteen states had retained this traditional definition.[51]

The second trend, and by far the largest, is the use of administrative statutes. These permit nurses to perform expanded duties, as authorized by the professional licensing boards: nursing alone, nursing and medicine, or medicine alone. Regulations are an integral part of that mechanism. The first to use such statutes was Idaho, (1971); New Hampshire enacted a slightly different version shortly thereafter. Both were similar to the ANA interim suggestion (now disapproved).

Various reasons (with positive and negative connotations) are given for this approach: regulations can spell out specific criteria and protect the public from incompetents and promote the use of NPs by increasing competence and awareness; nursing can limit the role to nurses and exclude others; physicians can extend some control over nurse expansion; nurses and physicians can respond rapidly to changing needs and patterns of practice, because regulations do not go through the legislative process; state professional boards, familiar with both fields as well as the idiosyncrasies of regulation formulation, can act rapidly and effectively. All have some legitimacy. Some states, such as Idaho, found that at first, cooperation between the two boards went well, regulations were formulated rapidly, and nurse practitioners were able to practice freely at a time when they were badly needed. Then, physicians decided to pull back, and legal obstacles were put in the way of such practice. (The law required *joint* agreement.) In some states, regulations could not be agreed upon, even by nurses alone, or there was considerable internal group pres-

sure, and legal practice stayed in limbo. Others had no major problems.

The ANA survey found twenty-four states using this additional acts clause, and four other states have added the language to a definition of advanced practitioners.[52] Two ANA concerns have been, first, that recognition of specialized practice is the function of the professional organization (through certification) and not the law, and second, that the additional acts clauses frequently require at least some medical approval for NP practice. This not only means that another profession can determine the scope of nursing's practice, but it does little to advance the concept of nurses and physicians as equal, collaborating professionals. Both La Bar and the Trandel-Korenchuks have observed a trend of increased physician involvement in the practice of NPs, as shown in the language defining advanced practice. The latter noted some indications:

- the determination and promulgation of rules and regulations by joint boards (medicine and nursing).
- the requirement that certain practices be performed within the scope of protocols, policies and procedures, standing orders, and standardized procedures written in accord with the supervising physician or employment agency.
- the necessity of a written agreement between the physician(s) and the nurse regarding the details of the supervision of the nurse. This agreement is submitted to the board of nursing.[53]

Another problem is that the specificity of the language regarding the practices that can be performed is restrictive and potentially harmful to the expansion or evaluation of these practice areas.

Whether or not the additional acts clause is part of the law, the majority of state boards have now been granted the right to develop administrative rules and regulations for the NP, and forty have developed such rules. The primary method of authorizing advanced practice is certification by an organization approved by the state board. (In a sense, this makes voluntary certification a mandatory legal process.) Second is separate licensure, using a term such as *advanced nurse practitioner*. With the exception of nurse-midwives and nurse anesthetists, this identification and the specific requirements are part of the general nursing practice act. A few states require a bachelor's or master's degree for NPs and various clinical nurse specialists (CNSs). Some states, like Florida, have general rules for NP practice as a whole, but then delineate each specialty and what is required for that particular practitioner. The most common requirement besides certification is a postbasic educational program.

The last category of nursing definitions is termed *authorization*, chosen by the fewest number of states. These states have developed a new definition of nursing that is intended to cover expanded or advanced practice as well as what might be considered ordinary practice at this time. The first of these states was New York (1972), which pioneered the use of the phrase "diagnosing and treating human responses to actual or potential health problems." A number of other states copied this terminology almost verbatim. California (1977) chose a unique definition that is unusually specific. The law permits the performance of basic health care procedures "according to standardized procedures," later defined as policies and protocols developed by health administrators in conjunction with nurses and physicians at a health care facility.[54]

While the New York law was thought to be quite daring at the time, it is now considered rather conservative, because it has no provision for independent acts of treatment. As happens in many cases, this limitation is due in part to the compromises necessary to get the law passed. Although some say that everything NPs do is nursing because they are nurses, this argument is not always accepted legally. If a practice is challenged, its legitimacy may depend on the ruling of a state attorney general or a court. For some states, challenge is not a major issue, and their nurses have done well with the authorization approach.

However, nurses in other states that adopted the New York model (including New York) have had serious problems in achieving acceptance of the overall definitions as adequate to authorize NP practice, because it included no educational training requirements or delineation of practice. Organized medicine in those states has generally insisted that medical diagnosing and treating are off limits. This has caused a schism between NPs, who are willing to accept a more limiting law in order to be able to practice without constant fear of being deemed to be illegally practicing medicine, and the SNA, which usually holds that the general definition protects them.

A breakthrough may have occurred when the Missouri Supreme Court ruled in 1983 that that particular general definition did indeed allow advanced nurse practice.[55] This landmark case, *Sermchief* v. *Gonzales*, was the outcome of a threat by the Missouri Board of Registration for the Healing Arts, which licenses physicians and osteopaths, to initiate proceedings against nurses in a family planning clinic. (Physicians in the area had lodged a complaint.) The nurses, working under standing orders and protocols signed by the clinic physicians, performed a variety of diagnostic and treatment functions, including breast and pelvic examinations; pregnancy testing; Pap smears; gonorrhea cultures and blood serology; the administration of all kinds of contraceptive measures, including oral contraceptives and intrauterine devices; as well as the usual teaching and counseling. The trial court judgment was that the nurses were practicing medicine without a license,[56] but the Missouri Supreme Court judge ruled that the acts of the nurses were "precisely the types of acts the legislature had contemplated when it granted nurses the right to make assessments and nursing diagnoses."[57] The 1975 Missouri law is similar to the ANA guidelines but uses the phrase "including, but not limited to." The nursing board had not promulgated any rules and regulations regarding advanced practice, so the case stood on the interpretation of the definition alone. Although the judgment is limited to Missouri, it is considered a victory for NP practice, with the focus on how clearly a general definition can legally determine whether a nurse is practicing nursing in performing what was once considered the exclusive function of medicine.[58]

It is clear that advanced nurse practice is still in legal flux. Short of a state supreme court ruling, the legality of certain practices can change in that very state with attorney general appointments, the attitude of a judge, or simply the political climate. Health care facility lawyers can only advise on how they interpret the practice act (and they may be influenced by physicians' attitudes or advice). A strong statement for or against advanced practice made by a voluntary professional association (medicine or nursing, for instance) is quite common but has no legal authority; it *can* help mold public opinion.

The doctrines of common practice or custom and usage may also be invoked. This means basically that the act is performed in that particular community or at that current time and is accepted as being within the responsibility of the nurse by the individuals' employer and/or physicians in the area. It usually assumes appropriate training for that function. Although this has been considered acceptable in some courts, it has been denied in others. Practically speaking, statutes cannot be changed informally by mass violation, although they may be changed through the legislative process eventually, because of evidence that a nurse has been taught to perform such a function and is capable of carrying it out safely.

In another approach, joint statements of practice (or function) have been issued by state professional organizations concerning a specific function performed by the nurse, for example, intravenous therapy, inoculations, closed-chest cardiac resuscitation, cardiac de-

fibrillation, and drawing blood. These statements are usually jointly agreed upon by the nurses' association, medical association, and hospital association, and occasionally other professional groups. They are not intended to tell nurses how to practice nursing, but set criteria that attorneys believe would make it possible for them to defend a nurse if legal defense were necessary in relation to emerging, questioned areas of nursing practice.

When joint agreement is reached after a meeting of representatives and attorneys of the concerned associations, the statement is published and distributed by each group and often by the state medical licensing board and nursing licensing board. The statement usually includes specific criteria for performance of the acts concerned and always includes the need for appropriate education and training. Frequently there is a preliminary statement advocating the formation, in each health care institution, of a committee of medicine, nursing, and administration to state responsibilities of doctors and nurses and to set criteria for determining the role and responsibility of each, considering newer developments in health care and education.

Because these organizations do not have legal status in relation to changing the law (although they can initiate such changes), these statements, in a way, only formalize the custom and usage doctrine. The chances of prosecution of the nurse by the medical licensure board are slight, for usually the board has been involved in issuing the statement. However, these statements do not have the effect of law unless the groups are given the legal authority to make them. Theoretically, a case could still be made against the nurse, particularly if a civil malpractice suit is involved. To remedy this situation, some states have taken action to legalize the statements. A number of states have developed and used joint statements without legal sanction.

It is not always easy for nurses of any kind to determine immediately which or how many of these alternatives are operative in the state where they practice. Except for those practices that may be limited to a particular hospital or agency, the State Board of Nursing can usually provide information as to whether a certain activity is permitted or specifically prohibited. When this information is not available, it is essential to remember that whatever nurses do, they must be competent in their performance, which implies education, training, and current competence.

Creighton, writing about the enlarged scope of nursing practice, predicted accurately:

> . . . the professional nurse will become more of an independent practitioner directly involved in decision making. Legally she will be responsible for her decisions. The more independent she becomes as a practitioner, the greater her unshared legal responsibility.[59]

Creation of a Board of Nursing Examiners

The name of the state administrative agency varies from state to state, as does the number of members. Traditionally, this board has been made up entirely of nurses, who may or may not be designated as to area of practice and education. In most states, members are appointed by the governor from a list of names submitted by the SNA and others. In recent years there has been some public outcry against control by professionals, with the result that gradually the addition of non-nurses, either public members or other health professionals, has been legally required. Although some nurses have considered this a danger to the profession, it can be to the advantage of nursing to have the input and support of the public and others on the health team, for these public members can be educated to understand and appreciate the problems of the profession. The danger exists when political pressure seeks to force the creation of a board with a majority of nonnurses, so that nursing practice and education can be totally controlled by others. The majority of states had consumers or other professionals as members in 1977. The ANA guidelines support consumer participation. Board size ranges from five to nineteen appointed members, who make policy. Staff employed by the board carry out the day-to-day activities.[60]

Responsibilities of the Board of Nurse Examiners

The major responsibility of a board is to see that the nursing practice act is carried out. This involves establishing rules and regulations to implement the broad terms in the law itself and setting minimum standards of practice. Usual responsibilities include approval of programs of nursing and development of criteria for approval (minimum standards) such as facilities, curriculum, faculty, and so on; evaluating the personal and educational qualifications of applicants for licensure; determining by examination applicants' competence to practice nursing; issuing licenses to qualified applicants; and disciplining those who violate the law or are found to be unfit to practice nursing, sometimes holding hearings. Recently added responsibilities include developing standards for continuing competency of licensed practitioners and issuing a limited license (for someone who cannot practice the full scope of nursing, perhaps due to a handicap).

Nursing boards may also hold educational programs, collect certain data, and cooperate in various ways with other nursing boards or the boards of other disciplines. If they operate under an overall board, certain administrative responsibilities will be carried out on a central level.

Requirements for Licensure as a Nurse

Licensure is based on fulfilling certain requirements. The following points are usually included.

1. The applicant must have completed an educational program in a state-approved school of nursing and received a diploma or degree from that program; usually the school must send the student's transcript. Some states ask for evidence of high school education. There is increasing legislative pressure that the applicant not be required

to have completed the program, particularly if the uncompleted courses are in a nonnursing area such as liberal arts. This is now true in California. In at least California and West Virginia, an amendment permits military corpsmen to take the examination, providing that there have been certain components in their military courses. Some former corpsmen have passed the state board examinations and become licensed in California, but find it difficult to become licensed in other states or to find employment in agencies that require graduation from an approved school. Other states have bills pending with the same amendment.

2. The applicant must pass an examination given by the board. This examination is currently the NCLEX-RN, developed under the aegis of the NCSBN and given in every state. The NCSBN's recommended passing score is 1600.

3. Some states require evidence of good physical and mental health, but this is not recommended by either ANA or NCSBN.

4. Most states maintain a statement that the applicant must be of good moral character, as determined by the licensing board, but this too is impractical. The model act suggests terminology that refers to acts which are grounds for board disciplinary action if the nurse is licensed.

5. A fee must be paid for admission to the examination. This varies considerably among states.

6. A temporary license may be issued to a graduate of an approved program pending the results of the first licensure exam.

It has been declared unconstitutional to make requirements of age, citizenship, and residence.

Provisions for Endorsement of Persons Licensed in Other States

Nurses have more mobility than any other licensed health professionals because of the use of a national standardized examination.

However, usually the individual must still fulfill the other requirements in the state in which he or she seeks licensure and must submit proof that the license has not been revoked. The nurse's nursing school record is usually evaluated to determine whether the program is generally equivalent to this state's program requirements of the same time period. If it is not, the nurse may be required to take the courses lacking and the examination.

If all requirements are satisfactorily fulfilled, the nurse is granted a license without retaking the state board examination. A fee is also required for this process of endorsement. Endorsement is not the same as reciprocity; the latter means acceptance of a licensee by one state only if the other state does likewise.

Renewal of Licensure

Until the early 1970s, nursing licenses were renewed simply by sending in the renewal fee when notified, usually every two years. For nurses licensed in more than one state, as long as the license was not revoked in any state, the process was the same. Usually the form asked for information about employment and the highest degree (and still does), but no attempt was made to determine if the nurse was competent. At about that time (also the time of the credentialing reports), there was increased concern about the current competency of practicing health professionals, and an estimate was made that perhaps 5 percent of all health professionals were not competent for some reason. Moreover, there was some question as to whether the professions made any real effort to either rehabilitate these people or to revoke their licenses. The credentialing reports emphasized the need for CE as a requirement for relicensure. One outcome was the enactment of a mandatory CE clause in a number of licensure laws; that is, a practitioner's license would not be renewed unless she or he showed evidence of CE. A number of health disciplines have such legislation. By 1977, a number of states had made mandatory CE a requirement for relicensure (or a legal practice requirement) for audiologists, chiropractors, dental hygienists, dentists, emergency medical personnel, nursing home administrators, nurses (RN and PN), opticians optometrists, physicians (MD and DO), pharmacists, physicians' assistants, podiatrists, psychologists, social workers, speech pathologists, and veterinarians. Not all were well enforced. Some states also had permissive legislation for possible later implementation. In addition, some national associations and state medical societies require continuing education for renewal of certification.[61]

In nursing, the California licensure law was amended in 1971 to require evidence of continuing education by RNs and LVNs for relicensure, beginning in 1975, and it was again amended in 1972 to postpone compliance until 1977. It finally went into effect in 1978. There was some feeling that the postponements resulted from the immense complexity and expense of instituting a mandatory system for California's thousands of nurses, and by 1979, there was already some talk of rescinding the requirement.

In 1972 New Mexico also supported mandatory continuing education, in this instance by amending the Nurse Practice Act's regulations, which had the same effect as enactment of a law. Actually, according to DHEW, any state could use regulations to require CE without changing the law because all practice acts give the licensing boards the authority to determine standards of competence, and these are usually delineated in the regulations. Nevertheless, in the 1970s, a number of SNAs introduced legislation either requiring CE or specifically directing the state board to study or plan such a requirement. Realistically, this action may have been attributable as much to the fear of externally introduced legislation that might remove control of the measure from nursing as to the conviction that this was a necessary amendment. Some of these states recognize only CE offerings approved by their boards or given by an agency, group, or institution that has been given a provider (or approval) number. This may create problems for those licensed in more than one state or living in a state other than where licensed. In the latter situation, some states permit the nurse to maintain the license on an inactive status, which can be reactivated when evidence of continuing education is shown.

Forms of CE accepted by states include various formal academic studies in institutions of higher learning converted to CEU credit; college extension courses and studies; grand rounds in the health care setting; home study programs; inservice education; institutes; lectures; seminars; workshops; audiovisual learning systems, including educational television, audiovisual cassettes, tapes, and records with self-study packets; challenge examinations for a course or program; self-learning systems such as community service, controlled independent study, delivery of a paper, preparation and participation in a panel; preparation and publication of articles, monographs, books and so on; and special research. The required number of hours of continuing education, or CEUs varies considerably among states.

No law requires formal education directed toward advanced degrees. In fact, although additional formal education is acceptable, the emphasis is on continuous, *updated competence in practice.* The fears and anger of many nurses have been misdirected because they assumed that advanced degrees would be required. Obviously, there are innumerable ways in which an individual can maintain competence and increase knowledge and skills. How to measure achievement for the large number of nurses concerned is the real problem.

Objections to mandatory CE focus on the difficulty of assessing true learning; the question of whether learning can be forced (attendance does not mean retention or change in behavior); the danger of breeding mediocrity; the lack of research on the effectiveness of CE in relation to performance; limitation of resources, particularly in rural areas; the cost to nurses; the cost to government; the usual rigidity of governmental regulations; the problems in record keeping; and the lack of accreditation or evaluation procedures for many CE programs.[62]

On the other hand, many nursing leaders have advocated the mandatory route. Early on, NLN stated, "In the belief that a continuing education requirement as a requisite for renewal of licensure of nurses will promote the delivery of optimum nursing care, the NLN Board of Directors supports the *gradual and carefully planned* implementation of such a requirement."[63] ANA later agreed.

The reasons for a mandatory approach are clear, but rather depressing; there appears to be considerable evidence that RNs *do not* continue in professional learning, particularly if they are not employed. Even if they are employed, there appears to be a prevalent notion in nursing that working in itself equals learning and subsequent competence. Unfortunately, this is not necessarily true. Yet their nursing license gives these nurses the right to practice. The hope that nurses will take advantage of the educational opportunities offered by their professional organization is dimmed when one realizes that less than 10 percent belong to ANA.

The entire issue is far from resolved. The trend toward mandatory CE slowed considerably in the early 1980's for all occupations, although the call for continued competence did not. It is possible that another trend, peer evaluation, and other kinds of performance evaluation may provide a more effective answer to continued competence.

Exemptions from Licensure*

Generally exempted from RN licensure are basic students in a nursing program; anyone employed previously in a domestic capacity, not as a nurse, and administering family remedies; anyone furnishing nursing assistance in an emergency; anyone licensed in another state and caring for a patient temporarily in

---

*This may also be called an *exception clause*.

the state involved; anyone employed by the U.S. government as a nurse (Veterans Administration, public health, or armed services); any legally qualified nurse recruited by the Red Cross during a disaster; and anyone caring for the sick if care is performed in connection with the practice of religious tenets of any church. In all these cases, the person cannot claim to be an RN of the state concerned. Over strong nursing protests, some states have also incorporated in the exemptions nursing services of attendants in state institutions, if supervised by nurses or doctors, as well as other kinds of nursing assistants under various circumstances. This, of course, weakens the mandatory aspect of the law.

An interesting development is that the NCSBN model act suggests for this clause statements that permit the establishment of an independent practice and fee-for-service reimbursement.

Grounds for Revocation of Licensure

The board has the right to revoke or suspend any nurse's license or otherwise discipline the licensee. The reasons most commonly found in practice acts for revoking a license are acts that might directly endanger the public, such as practicing while one's ability is impaired by alcohol, drugs, or physical or mental disability; being addicted to or dependent on alcohol or other habit-forming drugs or a habitual user of certain drugs; and practicing with incompetence or negligence or beyond the scope of practice. Other reasons are obtaining a license fraudulently, being convicted of a felony or crime involving moral turpitude (or accepting a plea of *nolo contendere*); practicing while the license is suspended or revoked; aiding and abetting a nonlicensed person to perform activities requiring a license; and committing unprofessional conduct or immoral acts as defined by the board. The refusal to provide service to a person because of race, color, creed, or national origin may also have been added in some states.

The most common reasons that nurses lose their licenses are the same as those that apply to physicians—drug use, abuse, or theft. Not all states specify incompetence as a reason for professional discipline, and only a tiny fraction of a percentage of nurses lose their licenses for this reason. In some states, incompetence is subsumed under unprofessional conduct "as defined by the board," but often this phrase was not defined in public rules and regulations. A turning point was the Tuma case. In Idaho in 1977, Jolene Tuma, an instructor in an associate degree program, went with a student to the bedside of a terminally ill woman to start chemotherapy after obtaining the patient's informed consent. When the patient asked Ms. Tuma about alternate treatments for cancer, she was told about several. Her son, upset because his mother stopped the chemotherapy, told the physician, who brought charges against Ms. Tuma. Subsequently, she was not only fired, but her license was suspended for six months by the Idaho board of nursing for unprofessional conduct, because her actions "disrupted the physician-patient relationship."[64] The case aroused a national nursing furor.[65] Ms. Tuma took her case through the courts, and on April 17, 1979, the Idaho Supreme Court handed down a decision that Ms. Tuma could not be found guilty of unprofessional conduct because the Idaho Nurse Practice Act neither defined unprofessional conduct nor set guidelines for providing warnings. The judge also questioned the ability of the hearing officer, who lacked the "personal knowledge and experience" of nursing to determine if Ms. Tuma's behavior was unprofessional.[66] Unfortunately, the court did not address itself to Ms. Tuma's actions, which leaves the nurse's right to inform the patient in some question—at least in Idaho.

While a number of states already had regulations defining unprofessional conduct, this court ruling spurred on those that did not. Depending on how licensure laws are structured, the regulations may apply to all licensed health professions (New York) or may be written into each separate law. Statements in the various laws are pretty much alike, but the regulations promulgated by Utah early on are especially clear and are given as an example. *Unprofessional conduct* is defined as nursing behavior that "fails to conform to the accepted standards of the nursing profession and which could jeopardize the health and welfare of the people." Some of the statements are:

- Failing to utilize appropriate judgment in administering safe nursing practice based upon the level of nursing for which the individual is licensed.
- Failing to exercise technical competence in carrying out nursing care.
- Failing to follow policies or procedures defined in the practice situation to safeguard patient care.
- Failing to safeguard the patient's dignity and right to privacy.
- Violating the confidentiality of information or knowledge concerning the patient.
- Verbally or physically abusing patients.
- Performing any nursing techniques or procedures without proper education and preparation.
- Performing procedures beyond the authorized scope of the level of nursing and/or health care for which the individual is licensed.
- Intentional manipulation or misuse of drug supplies, narcotics, or patients' records.
- Falsifying patients' records or intentionally charting incorrectly.
- Appropriating medications, supplies or personal items of the patient or agency.
- Violating state or federal laws relative to drugs.
- Falsifying records submitted to a government agency.
- Intentionally committing any act that adversely affects the physical or psychosocial welfare of the patient.
- Delegating nursing care, functions, tasks and/or responsibilities to others contrary to the laws governing nursing and/or to the detriment of patient safety.
- Failing to exercise appropriate supervision over persons who are authorized to practice

only under the supervision of the licensed professional.

- Leaving a nursing assignment without properly notifying appropriate personnel.
- Failing to report, through the proper channels facts known to the individual regarding the incompetent, unethical, or illegal practice of any licensed health care professional.

Regulatory language concerning unprofessional conduct is not always so specific and is almost never so in the statutes, because this might forclose action in unanticipated types of behavior. This problem is sometimes resolved by using the phrase "not limited to," but if the legislature has a particular concern, this may be written into the law, such as California's statutes on drug abuse and Florida's prohibition of sexual misconduct in the practice of nursing.[67] (Florida also has a statement in its regulations on failure to conform to minimal standards of "acceptable prevailing nursing practice," whether or not the patient was injured.) Another interesting point is the possibility of unprofessional kinds of nursing conduct once considered specific to medicine, such as fee splitting.

A particular problem in both statutory and regulating language relates to such terms as *moral*, *ethical*, and *moral turpitude*, since these can be interpreted in various ways. The model act uses phrases such as "has engaged in any act inconsistent with standards of nursing practice as defined by Board Rules and Regulations" and "a crime in any jurisdiction that relates adversely to the practice of nursing or to the ability to practice nursing."

Another issue is what a nurse should do about reporting incompetence or unprofessional conduct on the part of physicians or other health professionals. Because the nurses' code of ethics requires that she or he safeguard the patient, incompetent or unprofessional practitioners should be reported. One survey indicated that a large percentage of nurses would take some sort of action, usually speaking with the doctor, head nurse, or supervisor, if the patient was endangered by

medical action. Few would report the physician to a peer review or licensing board.[68] In part, this is because they fear a lawsuit. All but a few states have laws giving immunity from civil action to any person who reports to a peer review board if there is no malice, but this does not preclude being sued, even though legally the accused must be cleared. (Malice is very difficult to prove.) In New York, a statute was enacted in 1977 requiring physicians to report other physicians' misconduct on penalty of being cited for unprofessional conduct themselves; nurses and others are also encouraged to report such misconduct.[69] (Some have interpreted the law as *requiring* such reporting by all licensed professionals.) Other states have similar statutes.[70] There is another problem: some nurses who have reported a physician have either been dismissed from their jobs or harassed, a problem difficult to combat.

Although the law seems to protect the public, data show that relatively few nurses have had licenses revoked or suspended. In part, the reason is believed to be the reluctance of other nurses to report and consequently testify to these acts by their colleagues before either the nursing board or a court of law.[71] Nursing associations and state boards are now emphasizing the responsibility of professional nurses to report incompetent practice. They are also assisting impaired nurses.[72] The model act makes nonreporting a disciplinary offense, as does the law of Florida. (A problem with the latter is that now nurses are reporting even minor one-time events of negligence or error.)

When a report is filed with the state board, charging a nurse with violation of any of the grounds of disciplinary action, he or she is entitled to certain procedural safeguards (due process). After investigation, the nurse must receive notice of the charges and be given time to prepare a defense. A hearing is set and subpoenas are issued (by the board, attorney general, or a hearing officer). The accused has the right to appear personally or be represented by counsel, who may cross-examine witnesses. If the license is revoked or suspended, it may be reissued at the discretion of the board. (Sometimes the individual is only censured or reprimanded.)

Penalties for Practicing Without a License

Penalties for practicing without a license are included only in the mandatory laws. Penalties vary from a minimum fine to a large fine and/or imprisonment. Usually legal action is taken. Penalties are being strengthened to deter illegal practice.

Other Components

In recent years, it has become increasingly popular to add a "good samaritan" clause to medical and nursing laws, although it is not always a part of the licensure law. This clause protects the professional from liability for damages for alleged injuries or death after rendering first aid or emergency treatment in an emergency situation away from proper medical equipment unless there is proven gross negligence.[73] Although such laws exist in all fifty states, there is some feeling that they are really counterproductive.[74]

Another recent addition has been the requirement that equivalency and proficiency exams be used to determine the qualifications of those wishing to enter RN schools. Again, California has been the front runner in enacting this legislation.

Licensing laws for PNs have a similar format. It is a good idea for a nurse who is expected to supervise PNs to also become familiar with laws concerning them.

PROCEDURE FOR OBTAINING A LICENSE

Almost all new graduates of a nursing program apply for RN licensure, because it is otherwise impossible to practice.

Although there is nothing to prohibit you from postponing licensure, it is generally more difficult psychologically and because of lack of clinical practice to take the state board examination (NCLEX) much later.

As a rule, your school makes available all the data and even the application forms necessary for beginning the licensure procedure. Should you wish to become licensed in another state, because of planned relocation, request an application from that nursing board. Correct titles and addresses of the nursing boards of all states are found in the directory issues of the *American Journal of Nursing*. The board advises you of the proper procedure, the cost, and the data needed. For this initial licensing, you must take the state board examination in the state where licensure is sought.

After receiving the completed necessary data, fee, and application, the appropriate state board notifies you of the time and place of the examination. These are given at least once but usually twice a year; examinations are now given simultaneously throughout the nation.

For some years, the examination for licensure as an RN consisted of one or more tests in the following areas: medical nursing, surgical nursing, obstetric nursing, nursing of children, and psychiatric nursing. Each was an integrated test (but scored separately) and included questions in areas such as the physical and social sciences, nutrition and diet therapy, and pharmacology in relation to the particular clinical nursing subject.

In 1979 NCSBN voted to adopt a new test plan, effective July 1982. The new examination, titled NCLEX (RN),* is based on the nursing process and is intended to test primarily for application of knowledge, not just recall of facts. The new test plan states that

> nursing is perceived as deliberate action of a personal and assisting nature. The practice of nursing requires knowledge of: 1) normal growth and development; 2) basic human needs; 3) coping mechanisms; 4) actual or potential health problems; 5) effects of age, sex, culture, ethnicity and/or religion on health needs; and 6) ways by which nursing can assist individuals to maintain health and cope with

---

*NCLEX (LPN) is a separate examination.

health problems. Embodied in these six categories of nursing knowledge are concepts considered relevant to nursing practice, including management, accountability, life cycle and client environment.[75]

One other major difference is that although the exam is divided into four equal parts, only one score is given and failure means that the entire exam must be retaken. NCLEX is also criterion referenced instead of norm referenced, as the previous exam was. That is, the passing score is determined according to a consistent standard or criterion determined by nursing experts to represent acceptable nursing competence.[76] In the norm-referenced approach, a minimally acceptable level of nursing competence is established through the performance of a "norming group," a sample of individuals for whom the test is intended. Using this method, there is always a percentage of candidates that fail because they fall at the end of the normal curve.

The tests are the same for all nurses seeking an RN, whether graduating from a diploma, associate degree, or baccalaureate program. This has been the subject of considerable criticism, because the stated goals of all three programs are different. However, proponents of a single licensing exam state that the purpose is to determine safe and effective practice at a minimal level, and that this criterion applies to all levels of nurses.

Great precautions are taken to preserve the security of the tests. Teachers in schools of nursing do not know the specific questions on the examination, but they are familiar with the types of questions with which the applicant will be confronted, and this type of test is often used in the classroom. Although review books and special review classes or courses are available to assist the nurse to study for the examinations, the best preparation is, of course, a sound educational background. Currently, there are no "practical" examinations, that is, testing proficiency in real patient care situations or laboratories.

Nurses who pass the licensing examination receive a certificate bearing a registration number which remains the same as long as they are registered in that state. The certificate (or registration card) will also carry the expiration date—usually one, two, or three years hence—an important date to keep in mind, for failure to renew promptly may mean that you must pay a special fee to be reinstated.

It is advisable to keep your registration in effect, whether actively engaged in nursing or not. The expense is nominal, and more and more nurses who "retire" temporarily to have families return to nursing. These nurses do have the responsibility (and sometimes the legal requirement) to keep their nursing knowledge updated through CE.

To become licensed or registered by endorsement, applicants must already be registered in one state, territory, or foreign country. They must apply to the state board of nursing in the new state and present credentials, as requested, to prove that they have completed preparation equal to that required. A temporary permit is usually issued to allow the nurse to work until the new license is issued.

Nurses who wish to be reregistered after allowing their licenses to lapse should contact their state board for directions. An RN wishing to practice nursing in another country also needs to investigate its legal requirements for practice. Members of the armed forces or the Peace Corps, or those under the auspices of an organization such as the World Health Organization or a religious denomination will be advised by the sponsoring group. Registration in one state is usually sufficient.

Nurses from other countries are expected to meet the same qualifications for licensure as graduates of schools of nursing in the United States. The procedure for obtaining a license is the same as for graduates of schools here. However, nurses from other countries are now expected to take the CGFNS Qualifying Examination, which screens and examines foreign nursing school graduates while they are still in their own countries to determine their eligibility for professional practice in the

United States (see Chapter 27). The one-day examination covers proficiency in both nursing practice and English comprehension; both exams are given in English. If the applicant passes, she or he is given a CGFNS certificate, which is presented to the U.S. embassy or consulate when applying for a visa and to the SBNE in the state where the nurse wishes to practice. The nurse still must take the state board examination and otherwise fulfill the licensing requirements for that state. Specific information about requirements for licensure must be obtained directly from the board of nursing in the state in which the foreign nurse wishes to be licensed.

ISSUES, DEVELOPMENTS, PREDICTIONS

It seems that almost every month brings information about changes in nurse practice acts or challenges as to what they permit. The scope of practice issue will not go away for quite a while. Whether or not a nurse can diagnose and what the diagnosis is, continues to be argued. Some time ago, a nurse-lawyer made a still pertinent observation:

> The ability for critical thinking and to make decisions, either deliberately or with great speed, has ever been a part of the standard of conduct of the practitioner of professional nursing. This function shifts in complexity with scientific advancement in health care, for to do critical thinking and take appropriate action the nurse must be able to draw from the biological and physical sciences that are continually feeding new knowledge into the field of medical science. The function has long been recognized as an indisputable part of nursing practice, but selection of the proper word to describe the function is a controversial issue.[77]

Although for years the observational function of the nurse included only observing, recording, and reporting the results, research shows the modern function to be more complex. It is conceived to include "observation—recognition of signs and symptoms presented by the patient, inference—making the judgment about the state of the patient and/or nursing needs of the patient, and decision making—determining the action to be taken that will be of optimal benefit to the patient."[78] One definition of *diagnosis* as "the utilization of intelligence to interpret known facts, and acting upon the decision reached from this interpretation"[79] appears to bring into context these more modern functions. In differentiating between medical and nursing diagnosis, one study sees medical diagnosis as determining the cause of disease and seeking to eradicate it through specifics, and nursing diagnosis as making a determination of a symptom and its alleviation.[80]

Because the nurse's actions based on professional inferences do involve the risk of error, there can be serious consequences for the patient, for which the nurse must take responsibility. There is certainly no question that some of these inferences and subsequent actions are being taken almost instantly in today's nursing practice, for example, a coronary-care nurse's action (treatment) to recognize and terminate a potentially fatal heart arrhythmia. It is ironic and anachronistic that some nursing practice acts specifically forbid diagnosing, whereas at the same time some court decisions have held nurses negligent because they have *not* made a diagnosis.[81]

As to nurses prescribing, the law, as usual, varies. By 1983, eighteen states had formally given prescription-writing authority to certain categories of nurses. The regulating body was usually the nursing board, but in four states it was the board of medicine.[82] Both statutory and regulatory law set the criteria. Usually a nurse must have some sort of postbasic education or training, and sometimes special application must be made to the nursing or medical board for permission to prescribe. The substances that can be prescribed are always regulated—by lists, categories, or protocols. However, Cohn notes that NPs without legal prescription-writing authority often manage to prescribe for their patients anyway, which can create legal problems at any point.[83] The trend seems to be toward some legal regulation.

In the ANA study, other trends were predicted based on recent legislation. New Jersey has already enacted a provision that allows nurses to pronounce death. The District of Columbia passed a law giving hospital privileges to NPs, nurse-midwives, and nurse anesthetists; Colorado has added RNs to the list of those who may determine that a person may be admitted for a seventy-two-hour mental health evaluation. Also predicted was that the involvement of the medical profession in board of nursing rules for NPs would decrease and that their challenges to the nursing boards would be debated more often. However, some MDs will still battle against NP practice. It was also expected that as the NCSBN model act indicates, the statement that nurses carry out the medical regimen may also fall by the wayside. Antitrust actions to preserve the competitive market are expected to continue.[84] One trend not mentioned is California's challenge to the NCSBN as to whether the licensing exams have an "adverse impact" on groups protected by the state (usually minorities) because they are not adequately "job related." California was rescoring the exam after elimination of certain questions. This may have enabled those who passed under that system to practice in California, but not elsewhere. The California Board of Registered Nursing (BRN) was funded in 1984 to do a study of entry-level nursing practice. The analysis was to be used, among other things, to evaluate the BRN's curriculum standards for basic education and alternative routes to licensure, such as medic training, and to evaluate NCLEX.

Finally, it should be recognized that the credentialing problems in the health field are not yet resolved. The moratorium on licensing new health personnel is over, according to the calendar, but the problems that instigated the moratorium remain. Even if individual licensure is improved, what of the unlicensed worker? Will certification provide the answer or simply duplicate the problems of licensure with no legal recourse? Has the geometric increase in the number of health care workers improved patient care? Is there another answer? Resolution of the problems posed could well result in helping to resolve some of the other problems of health care delivery. And if some one must take the lead in initiating cooperative action, it may well be nursing.

REFERENCES

1. Study of Accreditation of Selected Health Education Programs, *Part I: Staff Working Papers: Accreditation of Health Educational Programs* (Washington, D.C.: National Committee on Accrediting, 1972), p. A-6.
2. U.S. Department of Health, Education, and Welfare, *Report of the National Advisory Commission on Health Manpower, Vol. 1.* (Washington, D.C.: U.S. Government Printing Office, 1967).
3. _____, *Report. Vol. 2* (Washington, D.C.: U.S. Government Printing Office, 1968).
4. U.S. Department of Labor, *Occupational Licensing and the Supply of Nonprofessional Manpower,* by Karen Green. Manpower Research Monograph No. 11 (Washington, D.C.: U.S. Government Printing Office, 1969).
5. U.S. Department of Health, Education, and Welfare, *Report on Licensure and Related Health Personnel Credentialing* (DHEW Publ. No. (HSM) 72-11), 1971.
6. _____, *Developments in Health Manpower Licensure.* (DHEW Publ. No. (HRA) 74-3000), 1973.
7. _____, *Credentialing Health Manpower.* (DHEW Publ. No. (OS) 77-50057), 1977.
8. Carnegie Commission on Higher Education, *Higher Education and the Nation's Health: Policies for Medical and Dental Education. Special Report and Recommendations* (New York; McGraw-Hill Book Company, 1970).
9. _____, *Less Time, More Options: Education Beyond the High School, Special Report and Recommendations* (New

York: McGraw-Hill Book Company, 1971).

10. *Study of Accreditation of Selected Health Education Programs Commission Report* (Washington, D.C.: National Committee on Accrediting, 1972).

11. *Licensure and Related Health Personnel Credentialing*, op. cit., p. 71.

12. Ibid., p. 7.

13. Edward Forgotson, *"Licensure, Accreditation and Certification as Assurance of High Quality Health Care,"* paper presented at the National Health Forum meeting Los Angeles, March 1968.

14. *Licensure and Related Health Personnel Credentialing*, op. cit., p. 43.

15. Ibid., p. 77.

16. Jane Tollett, "The Issue of Licensure—Institutional vs. Individual," *Nurs. Leadership*, **5**:8–31 (Sept. 1982).

17. Laurence Miike, "Institutional Licensure: An Experimental Model, Not a Solution," paper presented at the New Jersey League for Nursing Symposium on Institutional Licensure: What It Means to You, Mimeographed, Feb. 27, 1973.

18. Nathan Hershey, "Alternative to Mandatory Licensure of Health Professionals," *Hosp. Prog.,* **50**:73(Mar. 1969).

19. Ibid., p. 74.

20. DHEW, 1971, op. cit., pp. 65–70.

21. Lucie Kelly, "Institutional Licensure," *Nurs. Outlook*, **21**:566–572 (Sept. 1973).

22. Randolph Tucker and B. Wetterau, *Credentialing Health Personnel by Licensed Hospitals: The Report of a Study of Institutional Licensure*, Vol. I (Chicago: Rush-Presbyterian-St. Lukes Medical Center, 1975), p. 63.

23. *Credentialing Health Manpower*, p. 6.

24. Lucie Kelly, "End Paper: Danger: Creeping Institutional Licensure," *Nurs. Outlook*, **27**:624(Sept. 1979).

25. Benjamin Shimberg, "Licensing in the Year 2000," *Issues*, **5**:1, 8 (Summer 1984).

26. Clark Havighurst and Nancy King, "Private Credentialing of Health Care Personnel: An Antitrust Perspective," Part One, *Am. J. Law and Med.*, **9**:140 (Summer 1983).

27. Ibid., 133.

28. Ibid., 135.

29. Clark Havighurst and Nancy King, "Private Credentialing of Health Care Personnel: An Antitrust Perspective," Part Two, *Am. J. Law and Med.*, **9**:263–334 (Feb. 1983).

30. American Nurses' Association, *Nursing: A Social Policy Statement* (Kansas City, Mo.: The Association, 1980), p. 24.

31. Neil Weisfeld and Dennis Falk, "Professional Credentials Required," *Hospitals*, **57**:74–79 (Feb. 1983).

32. Susan Grobe, "Sunset Laws, " *Am. J. Nurs.*, **81**:1355–1359 (July 1981).

33. Courtney Thomas, "Sunset: What and Why," *Nurse Practitioner*, **7**:10 (Mar. 1982).

34. Courtney Thomas, "Sunset: How and When," *Nurse Practitioner*, **7**:10–11 (Apr. 1982).

35. *The Study of Credentialing in Nursing: A New Approach*, Vol. 1. The Report of the Committee (Milwaukee, Wisc.: 1979), Vol. 2, Staff Working Papers,has excellent background.

36. American Nurses' Association, *The Nursing Practice Act: Suggested State Legislation* (Kansas City, Mo.: The Association, 1980).

37. *The Model Nursing Practice Act* (Chicago, Ill: National Council of State Boards of Nursing, 1982).

38. AMA Committee on Nursing, *Medicine and Nursing in the 1970s, a Position Statement* (Chicago: American Medical Association, June 1970), p. 2.

39. Department of Health, Education, and Welfare, *Extending the Scope of Nursing Practice* (Washington, D.C.: The Department, Nov. 1971), p. 12.

40. Ibid., p. 12.

41. Ibid., p. 13–14.

42. American Nurses' Association, *Suggestions for Major Provisions to Be Included in a Nursing Practice Act*, Unpublished (New York: The Association, 1955).

43. Lucie Kelly, "Nursing Practice Acts," *Am. J. Nurs.*, **74**:1314–1315 (July 1974).

44. American Nurses' Association, *Model Practice Act*, Unpublished (Kanas City, Mo.: The Association, 1976).

45. Council of State Governments, National Task Force on State Dental Policies, *State Regulatory Policies: Dentistry and the*

Health Professions (Lexington, Ky.: The Council, 1979), p. 3.

46. *The Nursing Practice Act: Suggested State Legislation*, op. cit., pp. 2–3.

47. *The Model Nursing Practice Act*, op. cit., p. 21.

48. Marie Snyder and Clare LaBar, *Nursing: Legal Authority for Practice* (Kansas City, Mo.: American Nurses' Association, 1984).

49. Clare LaBar, *The Regulation of Advanced Nursing Practice as Provided for in Nursing Practice Acts and Administrative Rules* (Kansas City, Mo.: American Nurses' Association, 1983).

50. Darlene Trandel-Korenchuk and Keith Trandel-Korenchuk, "How State Laws Recognize Advanced Nursing Practice," *Nurs. Outlook*, **66**:713–719 (Nov. 1978).

51. Darlene Trandel-Korenchuk and Keith Trandel-Korenchuk, "State Nursing Laws," *Nurse Practitioner*, **5**:39 (Nov.–Dec. 1980).

52. Snyder and LaBar, op. cit., p. 8.

53. Darlene Trandel-Korenchuk and Keith Trandel-Korenchuk, "Current Legal Issues Facing Nursing Practice," *Nurs. Admin. Q.*, **5**:38 (Fall 1980).

54. Trandel Korenchuk, "How State Laws Recognize Advanced Practice," op. cit., 714–716.

55. Michael Wolff, "Court Upholds Expanded Practice Roles for Nurses," *Law, Med. and Health Care*, **12**:26–29 (Feb. 1984).

56. Elaine Doyle and Jeanne Meurer, "Practicing Medicine without a License," *Nurse Practitioner*, **8**:41–44 (June 1983).

57. Margaret Hunter, "These Nurses Weren't Practicing Medicine After All," *RN*, **47**:69 (Jan. 1984).

58. Jane Greenlaw, "*Sermchief* v. *Gonzales* and the Debate Over Advanced Nursing Practice Legislation," *Law, Med. and Health Care*, **12**:30–31, 36 (Feb. 1984).

59. Helen Creighton, "Changes in the Legal Aspects of Nursing," *Hosp. Progress*, **52**:89 (Sept. 1971).

60. Doris McDowell, "How Well Do You Know Your Board of Nursing?" *Nurs. and Health Care*, **2**:557–563 (Dec. 1981).

61. United States Department of Health, Education and Welfare: *State Regulation of Health Manpower* (DHEW Pub. No. (HRA)77–49, 1977), pp. 9–10.

62. *Report on Licensure and Related Health Personnel Credentialing*, op. cit., pp. 57–63.

63. National League for Nursing, *NLN's Role in Continuing Education in Nursing* (New York: The League, 1974.)

64. "Professional Misconduct?" Letters. *Nurs. Outlook*, **25**:546 (Sept. 1977). See also the editorial, p. 561.

65. Follow-up letters in Dec. 1977 issue, pp. 738–743; Jan. 1978 issue, pp. 8–9; Feb. 1978, p. 78; Mar. 1978 issue, pp. 142–143.

66. "Jolene Tuma Wins: Court Rules Practice Act Did Not Define Unprofessional Conduct," *Nurs. Outlook*, **27**:376 (June 1979).

67. Sarah Cohn, "Revocation of Nurses' Licenses: How Does It Happen?" *Law, Med. and Health Care*, **11**:22–24 (Feb. 1983).

68. Linda Stanley, "Dangerous Doctors: What To Do When the MD is Wrong." *RN*, **42**:22–27, 29–30 (Mar. 1979).

69. "Going Beyond the Hospital," *RN*, **42**:28 (Mar. 1979).

70. Andrew Fama, "Reporting Incompetent Physicians: A Comparison of Requirements in Three States," *Law, Med. and Health Care*, **11**:111–117. (June 1983).

71. David Price and Patricia Murphy, "How—and When—to Blow the Whistle on Unsafe Practices," *Nurs. Life*, **3**:51–54 (Jan.–Feb. 1983.)

72. "Help for the Helper," *Am. J. Nurs.*, **82**:572–587 (Apr. 1982).

73. Miles Zarenski, "Good Samaritan Statutes: Do They Protect the Emergency Care Provider?" *Medicolegal News*, **7**:5–7, 14 (Spring 1979).

74. George Annas, "Negligent Samaritans Are No Good," *Medicolegal News*, **7**:4 (Spring 1979).

75. "A New Licensing Exam for Nurses," *Am. J. Nurs.*, **80**:723–725 (Apr. 1980).

76. "Developing, Constructing, and Scoring the National Council Licensure Examination," *Issues*, **4**:1, 6 (Summer 1983).

77. Irene Murchison and Thomas Nichols, *Legal Foundations of Nursing Practice* (New York: Macmillan Publishing Company, Inc., 1970), p. 89.

78. Ibid., p. 90.
79. Ibid., p. 92.
80. Ibid., p. 90.
81. Ibid., pp. 90–99.
82. Clare LaBar, *Prescribing Privileges for Nurses: A Review of Current Law* (Kansas City, Mo.: American Nurses' Association, 1984).
83. Sarah Cohn, "Prescriptive Authority for Nurses," *Law, Med. and Health Care*, **12**:72–75 (Apr. 1984).
84. Snyder and LaBar, op. cit., 17–19.

Nursing Practice and the Law

United States citizens who enter schools of nursing of any type take with them all of the citizen's legal rights and responsibilities. As nursing students, however, they gradually take on duties and responsibilities that may involve them in litigation, directly or indirectly, trivial or serious, that would not concern them as citizens only. Upon graduation and licensure they may be held liable for actions that apply only to RNs, as well as for other acts of a more general nature. With nursing experience and knowledge, responsibilities will increase still further, because a court of law takes these facts into consideration.

There are numerous ways in which nurses become involved with the law in their practice. The impact of statutory law has been previously discussed. In this chapter, other legal aspects will be considered, primarily within the common law of torts, that is, an intentional or unintentional civil wrong.* This is the kind of law that relates to the daily practice of most nurses. When cases are used to illustrate a legal principle, it is important to remember that even a landmark decision may be overturned.

---

*See Chapter 17 for a review of common and civil law and the judicial process.

The law . . . is not rigidly fixed, but a composite of court decisions, state and federal statutes, regulations and procedures. There are no final answers. Law is dynamic—it lives, grows and changes. . . . No book, . . . no lawyer or teacher can tell you with complete assurance what is right or wrong or what the final outcome of any case will be.[1]

BASIC LEGAL CONCEPTS AND TERMS

As in any profession, law has its own terminology. Short definitions and illustrations of key words and phrases used in tort law follow.

Borrowed servant—an employee temporarily under the control of someone other than the employer (a hospital OR scrub nurse placed under the direction of a surgeon).
Breach of duty—under the law of torts, not behaving in a reasonable manner; in the legal sense, causing injury to someone. (Example: careless administration of drugs.)[2]
Captain of the ship doctrine—similar to the borrowed servant concept that physicians are responsible for all those presumably under their supervision. Courts have ruled both for and against this doctrine, but the

trend is to hold the individual responsible for that individual's own acts. (Example: incorrect sponge count done by nurses.) However, this does not preclude the hospital's being sued under the doctrine of *respondeat superior*.[3]

Charitable immunity—originating in English common law, holds that a hospital will not be held liable for negligence to a patient receiving care on a charitable basis. In 1969, the Massachusetts Supreme Court abolished prospectively the immunity of charitable institutions. In other states it varies, but the trend is toward recognizing the liability of charitable institutions. However, some states put a limit on how much money can be recovered from a hospital, and the plaintiff can collect the difference in the award from the negligent nurse.[4] For government hospitals, the old *doctrine of sovereign immunity* granted them freedom from liability ("the government can't be sued" concept). However, the Federal Tort Claims Act (1946) partially waived sovereign immunity of the federal government, and a U.S. Supreme Court ruling in 1950 made the government liable for harm inflicted by its employees. Immunity of state and municipal hospitals varies, but the trend is toward liability. Immunity does not include the individual's liability.[5,6]

Damages or monetary damages—redress sought by plaintiff for injury or loss. *Nominal damages* (usually $1) are token damages when the plaintiff has proven his case but actual injury or loss could not be proven. *Compensatory damages* are the *actual damages,* with amounts awarded for proven loss. These include *general damages* (pain, suffering, loss of limb) and *special damages* which must be proven (wage loss, medical expenses). *Punitive* or *exemplary damages* way be awarded when the defendant has acted with "wanton, reckless disregard."

Defendant—person accused in a court trial.

Employee—someone who works for a person, institution, or company for pay.

Employer—one who selects, pays, can dismiss the employee, and controls his or her conduct during working hours.

Expert witness—Someone with special training, knowledge, skill, or experience who is permitted to offer an opinion in court. The expert witness gives "expert testimony."

Foreseeability—holds the individual liable for all consequences of any negligent act which could or should have been foreseen under the circumstances. (Example: a suicidal patient is left unattended by an open window and jumps).[7]

Indemnification—if the employer is blameless in a negligence case but must pay the plaintiff under *respondeat superior,* the employer may recover the amount of damage paid from the employee in a separate action. *Subrogation* means that the employer can sue the employee for the amount of damages paid because of the employee's negligence.

Liability—being held legally responsible for negligent acts. The *rule or doctrine of personal liability* means that everyone is responsible for his or her own acts, even though someone else may also be held legally liable under another rule of law.
Vicarious liability—liability imposed without personal fault or without a causal relationship between the actions of the one held liable and the injury (usually a case of *respondeat superior*).

Locality rule or community rule—first enunciated in 1880 in *Small* v. *Howard,* in which a small-town doctor unsuccessfully performed complex surgery and was held not liable. The rationale was that a physician in a small or rural community lacks the opportunity to keep abreast of professional advances. Gradually, courts took into account such facts as accessibility of medical facilities and experience. Beginning in the 1950s, various state supreme courts abandoned the locality rule on the basis that modern communications, including availability of professional journals, TV, and rapid transportation, made the rule outdated. The proper standard considered is whether the practitioner is exercising the care and skill of the average qualified practitioner, taking into account advances in the profession.[8]

Long tail—the lag between the time when an injury occurs and the claim is settled. Insurance companies say that because of this lag, it is difficult to determine reasonable premiums for a malpractice insurance risk.

Malpractice—"any *professional* misconduct, unreasonable lack of skill or fidelity in professional or judiciary duties, evil practice or invalid conduct"; also, as related to physicians, "bad, wrong, or injudicious treatment resulting in injury, unnecessary suffering, or death to the patient, and proceeding from carelessness, ignorance, lack of professional skill, disregard of established rules or principles, neglect, malicious or criminal intent."[9] (Note that malpractice refers only to professionals.)

Negligence—failing to conduct oneself in a prescribed manner, with due care, thereby doing harm to another,[10] or doing something that a reasonably prudent person would not do in like circumstances. *Criminal negligence and gross negligence* are sometimes used interchangeably and refer to the commission or omission of an act, lawfully or unlawfully, in which such a degree of negligence exists as may cause a serious wrong to another. Almost any act of negligence resulting in the death of a patient would be considered criminal negligence.

Comparative negligence—takes into consideration the degree of negligence of both the defendant and the plaintiff. This allows the possibility of the plaintiff having some redress, which often is not possible if there has been contributory negligence.

Contributory negligence—a rather misleading expression used when the plaintiff has contributed to his own injury through personal negligence. This he may do accidentally or deliberately. Some authorities assert that a plaintiff who is guilty of contributory negligence cannot collect damages; others state that he may collect under certain conditions. As in most legal matters, decisions vary widely. Because contributory negligence must be proven by the defendant, as much written evidence as possible is needed. *Corporate negligence**—the health care facility or an entity is negligent.[11]

Outrageous conduct doctrine or tort of emotional distress—allows the plaintiff to base his case on intentional or negligent emotional distress caused by the defendant. (Example: a patient gave birth to a premature stillborn child; later, when she asked about burial, the nurse brought the fetus floating in a gallon jug of formaldehyde.)[12]

Plaintiff—party bringing a civil suit, seeking damages or other legal relief.

Proximate cause—the immediate or direct cause of an injury in a malpractice case. The plaintiff must prove that the defendant's malpractice caused, precipitated, or aggravated his condition.

Reasonably prudent man theory—standard that requires an individual to perform a task as any "reasonably prudent man of ordinary prudence, with comparable education, skills, and training under similar circumstances," would perform that same function. It is often described as requiring a person of ordinary sense to use ordinary care and skill.[13] This concept is the key to determination of the standard of care.

Res gestae—all of the related events in a particular legal situation, which may then be admitted into evidence.

Res ipsa loquitor—"The thing speaks for itself," a legal doctrine that gets around the need for expert testimony or the need for the plaintiff to prove the defendant's liability because the situation (harm) is self-evident to even a lay person. The defendant must prove, instead, that he is not responsible for the harm done. Before the rule of *res*

---

*This is a new concept based on the landmark decision *Darling* v. *Charleston Community Memorial Hospital,* discussed later.

ipsa loquitor can be applied, three conditions must be present: the injury would not ordinarily occur unless there were negligence; whatever caused the injury at the time was under the exclusive control of the defendant; the injured person had not contributed to the negligence or voluntarily assumed the risk.[14] A common example involving nurses occurs when sponges have been left inside an abdomen after surgery, and the nurse had made an inaccurate sponge count and did not alert the operating team.

Respondeat superior—"Let the master answer." The employer is responsible for what employees do within the scope of their employment.[15] Independent contractors such as private duty nurses may or may not be included.

Standard of care*—simply defined as the skill and learning commonly possessed by members of the profession.

Standard of reasonableness—liability is based on conduct that is socially unreasonable. Although there is no exact answer, the standard of reasonableness for health care practitioners could be defined as "that degree of skill and knowledge customarily used by a competent health practitioner of similar education and experience in treating and caring for the sick and injured in the community in which the individual is practicing or learning his profession."[16]

Stare decises—"Let the decision stand." The legal principle that previous decisions made by the court should be applied to new cases. Also called *precedent*. The decisions cited are usually made at the appellate level, including the state supreme court or the U.S. Supreme Court, highest appellate court in the land.

Statute of limitations—legal limit on the time a person has to file a suit in a civil matter. The statutory period usually begins when an injury occurs, but, in some cases, as with a sponge left in the abdomen, it starts when the injured person discovers the injury (*discovery*). In the case of an injury done to a minor, the statute will usually not "toll" (begin to run) until the child has reached age eighteen. The statute of limitations that relates to malpractice actions has commonly not been applied to nurses[17]; instead, the longer periods for statutes of limitations for negligence applied to them (thus not considering them as professionals). However, along with other new legislation related to the NP and PA, several states have revised their statutes of limitations to include nurses.[18] Court decisions about the inclusion of nurses in malpractice statutes of limitations have varied, with a previous but changing tendency to hold them liable for negligence, not malpractice, because they were seen as performing under specific directions. The shorter time is intended to ensure a professional a "fair chance to defend on merit and not find his defenses eroded by lapse of time." This apparently was not seen as necessary for anything less than "professional negligence." Although the length of time involved varies from state to state, it is about two years for malpractice, and four years or more for negligence by "others."

Tort—civil wrong against an individual. In order to have a cause of action based on malpractice or negligence, four elements must be present:

1. There was a duty owed to the plaintiff by the defendant to use due care (reasonable care under the circumstances).
2. The duty was breached (the defendant was negligent).
3. The plaintiff was injured or damaged in some way.
4. The plaintiff's injury was caused by the defendant's negligence (proximate cause).

No matter how negligent the health provider was, if there was no injury, there is no case. The plaintiff must also establish that a health practitioner–patient relationship existed and that the practitioner violated the standard of care.

---

*How the standard of care is determined is discussed in detail later.

APPLICATION OF LEGAL PRINCIPLES*

Most civil cases involving malpractice and negligence do not involve only one concept or legal doctrine. Some examples, based on real cases, follow.

A first-year student nurse was assigned by the instructor to care for a patient who later went into shock. Among other things, the student applied hot water bottles around the patient. The patient survived but was badly burned and sued the doctor, hospital, head nurse, faculty members, and school of nursing. This was a case of *res ipsa loquitor*. The student was clearly negligent, perhaps grossly negligent, because she should have known the correct temperature and procedure for applying a hot water bottle to anyone and should have taken special precautions with an unconscious patient. (Whether the hot water bottle was ordered by the doctor or not was immaterial, for the action, properly carried out, was appropriate for a patient in shock.) The student is held to the standards of care (*standards of reasonableness*) of an RN if she is performing RN functions. If the student is not capable of functioning safely unsupervised, she should not be carrying out those functions. The doctor may or may not be held liable, depending on that court's notion about the *captain of the ship doctrine,* or perhaps on whether the doctor saw and/or felt the hot water bottles. The hospital will probably be held liable under *respondeat superior,* because students, even if not employed, are usually treated legally as employees. In addition, because the head nurse is responsible for all patients on the floor and presumably should have been involved in or should have assigned an RN in such an emergency, she too would be liable (and again, the hospital, under *respondeat superior*).

The instructor might be found liable, not on the basis of *respondeat superior*—just as the head nurse or supervisor would not be liable if

---

*Other cases are found in the bibliography. All nursing law textbooks include case examples.

the student had been an RN, because none of these nurses are employers in the legal sense— but on the basis of inadequate supervision. The same would have been true of an RN who had assigned a new nurse's aide to apply the hot water bottles, unless she was sure that the aide knew how to do so and was capable of carrying out that function. If a supervisor or other nurse assigns a task to someone not competent to perform that task and a patient is injured because of that individual's incompetent performance, the supervising nurse can be held personally liable because it is part of her or his responsibility to know the competence and scope of practice of those being supervised.[19] Although theoretically this nurse could rely on the subordinate's licensure, certification, or registration, if any, as an indication of competence, if there is reason to believe that that individual would nevertheless perform carelessly or incompetently and the nurse still assigns that person to the task, the nurse is held accountable (as is the employer under the doctrine of *respondeat superior*). The school might be found liable in the case of the student, if the court believed the director had not used good judgment in employing or assigning the faculty member carrying out those teaching responsibilities.

In another situation, the outcome would be different. A student gave an electric heating pad, per the doctor's order, to a patient who was alert and mentally competent and demonstrated to the nurse her ability to adjust the temperature and her knowledge of the potential hazards. The patient fell asleep on the pad, set at a high temperature, and burned her abdomen. In this case, there would seem to be sufficient evidence of *contributory negligence* on the part of the patient, with the student having good reason to assume that the patient was capable of managing the heating pad. Therefore, even if the patient sued, her case would be weak. If the court used the doctrine of *comparative negligence,* some liability might be assigned to the student, if for instance she or he did not check on the patient in a reasonable time. If the heating pad were faulty, the hospital would probably be liable, not the nurse.

A particularly useful example from many points of view is the landmark decision of *Darling* v. *Charleston Community Memorial Hospital* (211 N.E. 2nd 53, Ill., 1965). A minor broke his leg playing football and was taken to Charleston Community Memorial Hospital, a JCAH-accredited hospital. There a cast was put on the leg in the emergency room, and he was sent to a regular nursing unit. The nurses noted that the toes became cold and blue, charted this, and called the physician, who did not come. Over a period of days, they continued to note and chart deterioration of the condition of the exposed toes and continually notified the physician, who came once but did not remedy the situation. The mother then took the boy to another hospital, where an orthopedist was forced to amputate the leg because of advanced gangrene. The family sued the first doctor, the hospital, and the nurses involved. The physician settled out of court; he admitted he had set few legs and had not looked at a book on orthopedics in forty years. The hospital's defense was that the care provided was in accordance with standard practice of like hospitals, that it had no control over the physician, and that it was not liable for the nurses' conduct because they were acting under the order of a physician. However, the appellate court, upholding the decision of the lower court, said that the hospital could be found liable either for breach of its own duty or for breach of duty of its nurses. The new hospital standards of care set by that ruling were in reference to the hospital by-laws, regulations based on state statutes governing hospital licensure and criteria for JCAH accreditation. The court reasoned that these constituted a commitment that the hospital did not fulfill. In addition, the court held that the hospital had failed in its duties to review the work of the physician or to require consultation when the patient's condition clearly indicated the necessity for such action.

For nurses, the crucial point was the newly defined duty to inform hospital administra-tion of any deviation in proper medical care that poses a threat to the well-being of the patients. (The hospital was also expected to have a sufficient number of trained nurses capable of recognizing unattended problems in a patient's condition and reporting them.) Specifically, the court said:

> . . . the jury could reasonably have concluded that the nurses did not test for circulation in the leg as frequently as necessary, that skilled nurses would have promptly recognized the conditions that signalled a dangerous impairment of circulation in the plaintiff's leg, and would have known that the condition would become irreversible in a matter of hours. At that point, it became the nurses' duty to inform the attending physician, and if he failed to act, to advise the hospital authorities so that appropriate action might be taken (211 N.E. 2d at 258).[20]

Because Darling-type situations are not rare, it is essential for nurses to know their legal responsibilities (and rights) in such cases, so that they can act accordingly.[21]

STANDARD OF CARE

The standard of care basically determines nurses' liability for negligent acts. If this standard is based on what the "reasonably prudent" nurse would do, who makes that judgment?[22] In litigation, it is the judge or jury, based on testimony that could include the following:

1. *Expert witness.* Did the nurse do what was necessary? A nurse with special or appropriate knowledge testifies on what would be expected of a nurse in the defendant's position in like circumstances. The expert witness would have the credentials to validate his or her expertise, but because the opposing side would also produce an equally prestigious expert witness to say what was useful to them, the credibility of that witness on testifying is critical.[23]

2. *Professional literature.* Was the nurse's practice current? The *most current* nursing literature would be examined and perhaps quoted to validate (or invalidate) that the nurse's practice in the situation was totally up-to-date.

3. *Hospital or agency policies.* Were hospital policies, especially nursing policies (in-house law), followed? Example: If side rails were or were not used, was the nurse's action according to hospital policy?*[24]

4. *Manuals or procedure books.* Did the nurse follow accurately the usual procedure? Example: If the nurse gave an injection that was alleged to have injured the patient, was it given correctly according to the procedure manual?[25]

5. *Drug enclosures or drug reference books.* Did the nurse check for the latest information? Example: If the patient suffered from a drug reaction that the nurse did not perceive, was the information about the potential reaction in a drug reference book, such as the *PDR* (*Physicians' Desk Reference*) or a drug insert?[26]

6. *The profession's standards.* Did the nurse behave according to the published ANA standards, both general and in the specialty, if any?[27]

7. *Licensure.* Did the nurse fulfill her responsibilities according to the legal definition of nursing in the licensure law or the law's rules and regulations? Example: Did she teach a diabetic patient about foot care?

If the judge or jury is satisfied that the standards were met satisfactorily, even if the patient has been injured, the injury that occurred would not be considered the result of the nurse's negligence. Different judgments in different jurisdictions must be expected. For instance, in one case, an occupational health nurse, not recognizing the signs and symptoms of a coronary occlusion, sent the patient

home unattended. When he died and she was sued, she was found not liable because having such knowledge was not seen as being a nursing responsibility. In an almost identical situation elsewhere, the nurse was found liable. Nevertheless, a nurse who knows the profession's standards and practices accordingly is in a much firmer position legally than one who does not.

LITIGATION INVOLVING NURSES

A study on litigation that involved nurses between 1967 and 1977 presents some interesting information,[28] although as the nurse assumes increasing responsibility and autonomy, litigation may go in other directions. In fact, the researchers noted major differences from an incident that had occurred in 1944, when nurses were seen as handmaidens, to the 1970s, when the specialist role took hold and the care settings were much more complex. In addition, an increase in the number of cases was noted.

In the period studied, of the cases involving the health care field that were heard at the appellate level, 390 out of 1,696 specifically involved nurses. Although the time lapse from the date of the incident to the final decision varied from one to twenty-five years, most had a lapse of two to eight years, with the largest number having a four-year lapse. This indicates not only that concern about such an incident can affect a nurse for some time, but also that after such a lapse, it is difficult to remember exactly what happened.

The greatest number of suits occurred in Louisiana, Florida, Texas, Georgia, and Alabama; Hawaii, Maine, New Hampshire, and Rhode Island had none. Almost 88 percent of the incidents occurred in general hospitals, followed, in order, by nursing homes, psychiatric hospitals, and doctors' offices. Over half of these suits involved administration of treatments, communications (observing, charting, recording), and supervision of patients; other categories were administration of medicines, foreign objects left in the abdomen during

---

*On the other hand, if a nurse followed an outdated policy or followed policy without using nursing judgment (according to the expert witness), it could be held against her or him.

surgery, postoperative injuries and infection, anesthesia given by nurse anesthetists, and assisting with ambulation or movement. About 5 percent did not fit into any distinct category of nursing practice. Twenty-three of the suits involved injury or death from acts by incompetent patients. In about 45 percent of the cases, someone in nursing service was directly responsible for the alleged negligence but third parties were charged, a situation that is already changing. In most cases, the person in nursing was not solely responsible for the injury. Only in five cases was a nurse the first-named defendant; in forty-one cases, she or he was co-defendant. In at least half of the cases, the incident prompting litigation involved a doctor and a nurse, primarily in errors of communication, medications, and foreign objects left in patients during surgery. Of the categories of nursing practice, nurse anesthetists giving anesthesia were the most often named.

In eighteen of the forty-six cases in which the nurse was first named defendant or co-defendant, the courts ruled in favor of the nurse. In seven, nursing personnel were held financially responsible, with awards ranging from $400 to over $100,000, and with the sum usually paid by several defendants. One of the highest awards went to a teenage girl with a knee injury. A nursing student with three months' experience helped her to the bathroom and the patient fell, injuring her sacrum. However, the highest percentage of financial awards were made when foreign objects were left in the patient after surgery.

An analysis of the cases showed that the court often set parameters of care that patients could expect. For instance, the hospital owes a special duty to its patients arising from the special knowledge of the practitioners; a greater standard of care should be exercised in the treatment of the very young and the very old; reasonable care must be used that can prevent forseeable injuries. Some of the other principles derived are especially related to the concept of the reasonably prudent person. Review of these specific cases reinforces what

has generally been deemed to be the most common acts of negligence in which a nurse might be involved.

MAJOR CAUSES OF LITIGATION

The kinds of incidents reported by Campazzi as most prevalent in causing litigation still continue to be problems. Sometimes they are caused by lack of knowledge, as when a nurse simply does not know the most current use or dangers of a drug or treatment or how to respond to a complication.[29] Sometimes it's simply a matter of carelessness—doing something in a hurry or neglecting to do something routine because one is busy.[30] Often problems result from poor nursing judgment, as when a nurse in the emergency room sends away a patient without consulting with or calling a physician,[31] or does not question a doctor's order, or behavior despite having doubts that the action is correct.[32] The amount of responsibility now put on nurses to judge the physician and to stop and/or report his action was unheard of several years ago. Some cases are frankly amazing and were appealed. For instance, in one case, in which the physician removed nineteen feet of small intestine through a perforation in a woman's uterus, the nurses were held liable for not stopping him because they should have known he was harming the patient.[33] Nevertheless, it shows a trend toward increased legal accountability for nurses. A vast number of the cases are the result of poor physician–nurse communication.

Physician–Nurse Communication Problems

Do you have a responsibility to take action when a doctor writes an order that you think is incorrect or unclear? When he does not respond to a patient's worsening condition? When he does not come to see a patient even if you think it's urgent? When he does not follow accepted precautions in giving a treatment? What if he becomes angry and abusive? What if he was right? According to court decisions in the last few years, the answer to all these questions is that it *is* the nurse's responsibility to take action. Medications seem to be a major problem. When an order is incomplete or written illegibly and the nurse does not question it, the results can be tragic.

A classic case* is that of a nursing supervisor who thought she would help out in a pediatrics unit when it was short-staffed, even though she was not familiar with current pediatric nursing practice. An order for a medication for an infant did not state the appropriate route of administration and, after asking nearby physicians whether the dose was appropriate (not the route), the nurse gave it by injection. By this route, the amount given was a massive overdose and the child died. The nurse was not aware that the drug came in an oral solution and had not called the physician who wrote the order. Both were found liable. (This case also demonstrates the dangers of not having updated knowledge.)

A nurse who follows a physician's orders is just as liable as the physician if the patient is injured because, for instance, a medication was the wrong dose, given by the wrong route, or was actually the wrong drug.[34] If the order is illegible or incomplete, it is necessary to clarify that order with the physician who wrote it. If you doubt its appropriateness, check with a reference source or the pharmacist, and always with the physician who wrote the order.

You have a right to question the physician when in doubt about any aspect of an order, and the nursing service administration should support any nurse who does so. In fact, there should be a written policy on the nurse's rights and responsibility in such matters, so that there is no confusion on anyone's part and no danger of retribution to a justifiably questioning nurse faced with an irate physician.[35] What if the physician refuses to change the order? You should not simply refuse to carry out an

order, for you may not have the most recent medical information and could injure the patient by *not* following the order. You should report your concern promptly to your administrative supervisor. The supervisor or other nurse administrator is often expected to act as an intermediary if there is a problem. However, a good collegial relationship and mutual courtesy can prevent or ease a doctor–nurse confrontation, and should be cultivated by both.

Verbal or telephone orders are another part of this problem.[36] Although they are considered legal, the dangers are evident. In case of patient injury, either the doctor, or the nurse, or both will be held responsible. There frequently are or should be hospital, sometimes legal, policies to serve as guides. If telephone orders are forbidden and a patient is injured through confused orders, the situation could be considered negligence. If telephone orders are acceptable, precautions should be taken that they are clearly understood (and questioned if necessary), with the doctor required to confirm the orders in writing as soon as possible. Some hospital policies require a repetition of the order; it is not unheard of to have two nurses listen together to a telephone order. In states where PAs' orders have been declared legal (as an extension of the physician), the same precautions must be taken, with the physician again confirming the order as quickly as possible.

Another incident that repeatedly shows up in litigation is the failure of a physician to see a patient either on the unit or in the emergency room.[37] Often the nurse is held liable for not following through. More and more often, it is suggested that a system (or a policy) be set up specifying who the nurse then contacts.[38] If you neglect to call a doctor when the patient needs help or simply because you are not aware of the seriousness of the patient's condition, simply charting is not enough. This was clearly demonstrated in the *Darling* case.[39] In another frequently cited case, the nurse did not call the physician when a pregnant woman continued to bleed excessively, "because he

Norton v. Argonaut Insurance Co., 144 S. 2nd 249 (La. 1962), is cited in almost every nursing law text in detail.

wouldn't come.''* The patient died, and the hospital was held vicariously liable because of the nurse's negligence.

Another failure in communication occurs when a nurse does not report a situation because she or he doesn't fully investigate or fully assess it.[40] Still other judgments against the nurse have been given when a doctor has not followed through on appropriate technical procedures, such as the timely removal of an endotracheal tube.[41] If you know that a particular procedure is being done incorrectly (because it's within the scope of your knowledge) and do nothing about it, you can be held liable as well as the physician. Nurses have also been held liable in cases involving the suicide of psychiatric patients. For instance, although a psychiatrist and a psychologist declared that suicide precautions were not necessary for a patient who showed suicidal tendencies, the nurse was held responsible when the patient drowned herself. She had not used nursing judgment and supervised the patient closely enough.[42]

These examples reinforce the need for nurses to recognize their accountability to the patient, even if it means disagreeing with physicians and reporting them if the patient appears to be endangered. Some hospitals that appreciate how difficult the nurses' situation can be in such a potential confrontation have set policies that clarify everyone's responsibilities.[43]

Legal Problems in Record Keeping

It is almost impossible to overemphasize the importance of records in legal action, especially nurses' notes. They hold the only evidence that orders were carried out and what the results were; they are the only notes written with both the time and date in chronological order; they offer the most detailed information on the patient.[44] Nurses' notes, like the rest of the chart, can be subpoenaed. No mat-

ter how skillfully you practice your profession, if your actions and observations are not documented accurately and completely, the jury can judge only by what is recorded. If you are subpoenaed, comprehensive notes will not only give weight to your testimony, but will help you remember what happened. A case may not come up for years, and unless there was a severe problem at the time, it is difficult to remember exact details about one patient. General, broad phrases such as "resting comfortably," "good night," "feeling better," are totally inadequate. How could a jury interpret them? How could even another professional who did not know that patient interpret them?

The correct way to chart, with legal aspects in mind, is probably charting as you were taught and following good nursing practice: write what you see, hear, smell, feel; don't make flip or derogatory remarks.[45] Be as accurate as possible, but if a mistake is made, recopy or cross out with the original attached.[46] Never alter a record in another way; this has been shown to influence a jury negatively.[47] Every good malpractice attorney calls on experts to examine charts for alterations, erasures, and additions. All too often, the nurse makes a change or an omission in the chart to protect a physician or the hospital. This can lead to criminal charges, as in the case of the OR nurse who did not record the illegal participation of an equipment salesman in surgery and who was cited for falsification of records.[48] This practice is always dangerous.

Some of the most serious problems arising from poor charting concern lack of data, such as omission of a temperature reading or other vital signs, lack of observations about a patient's condition, or no record of oxygen liter flow in a newborn infant; these and others have resulted in liability judgments against nurses and hospitals, although in each it was contended that the "right" thing had been done.[49] Moreover, there are instances when a patient might be legally harmed by inaccurate reporting, as in child or adult abuse or rape.[50-52]

---

*Goff v. Doctor's General Hospital of San Jose, 333 P. 2nd 29, (CA 1958).

Information in the patient's record that is particularly important from a legal point of view includes names and signatures of the patient, nurses, and doctors; notations of the patient's condition on admission, with progress notes on changes for the better or worse while in the hospital; accounts of injuries sustained accidentally while in the hospital, if any; a description of the patient's attitude toward the treatment and personnel; medications and other treatments given (what, when, how); vital signs; visits of doctors, consultants, and specialists; receiving the patient's permission for therapy and all special procedures such as surgery. Gaps in documentation can be as dangerous as errors.[53] Another potentially dangerous practice occurs when a nurse must chart what an aide says he or she did or what occurred when the nurse has not personally seen it (as is usual). Some lawyers advise adding a statement that clarifies the facts to protect yourself.[54]

In case of patient injury, most hospitals and health agencies require completion of an ''incident report.'' The purpose is to document the incident accurately for remedial and correctional use by the hospital or agency, for insurance information, and sometimes for legal reasons. The wording should be chosen to avoid the implication of blame and should be totally objective and complete: what happened to the patient; what was done; what his condition is.[55] The incident report may or may not be discoverable, depending on the state's law. It is considered a business record, not part of the patient's chart, but some courts rule that it is not privileged information.[56] The incident *must* be just as accurately recorded in the patient's chart. This kind of omission casts doubt on the nurse's honesty if litigation occurs. However, the fact that an incident report was filed should not be charted.

Appropriate behavior by nurses and other personnel is often a key factor as to whether or not the patient or family sues after an incident, regardless of injury. Maintaining a good rapport and giving honest explanations as needed is very important.[57]

Other Common Acts of Negligence

Among the acts of negligence a nurse is most likely to commit in the practice of nursing are the following (not in order of importance):

1. *Failure to respond or to ask someone else to respond promptly to a patient's call light or signal* if, because of such failure, a patient attempts to take care of his own needs and is injured. This might happen when he attempts to get out of bed to go the bathroom or reaches for a bedpan in the bedside stand.[58]

2. *Failure to use adequate precautions to protect the patient against injury.* As a nurse, you know that drugs, or hot liquids, or potentially harmful implements, such as scissors, must be kept out of the reach of a young child or a delirious or confused patient. You know the necessity of staying with—or having someone else stay with—a patient on a stretcher or narrow treatment table to keep him from falling, or with a helpless or irresponsible person at any time.

   As a student you learn what to do to avoid harming the patient. You learn that the water used to fill a hot water bottle must be a given temperature and no hotter; that certain patients' temperatures should not be taken by mouth lest they bite the thermometers and injure themselves with glass, mercury, or both; that every medicine must be given accurately to the right patient, whether it is five grains of aspirin or an injection of a highly potent drug; that a sponge count is a very important step in certain surgical operations and must never be neglected; that sterility of equipment is essential for safety in giving hypodermics or doing sterile dressings as well as for use during surgery; that particular care must be exercised when performing treatments such as an eye irrigation, bladder instillation, or others involving very delicate tissues; that strict precautions must be observed to prevent infections and cross-infections, such as diarrhea in the nursery for newborn babies; that injections and other procedures must be done with care;[59-61] and that restraints, siderails, and other protective measures should be used with appropriate nursing judgment.[62]

Medication errors are a particularly serious problem. A 1981 study showed that drugs were the major cause of iatrogenic illness and injury to patients in hospitals, 20 percent of which caused a serious disability. The major errors, in order, are wrong dose, wrong drug, omission of a dose, wrong rate of administration, wrong route, and wrong time.[63] Nurses who are imprudent and take unsafe shortcuts or otherwise fail to adhere to what they know is competent nursing practice are being negligent. If harm to a patient or co-worker can be traced to a nurse, and it often can, she or he may be held liable. Negligence tends to involve carelessness as much as lack of knowledge.

3. *Inadequate or dated nursing knowledge.* Since having current knowledge is a professional responsibility, there seems to be little excuse for this kind of negligence. However, on occasion, even the most competent nurse has a problem. If an entirely new type of treatment or piece of equipment is introduced on your unit, it is your responsibility, as well as that of the head nurse or supervisor, to get the appropriate information on it.[64] Further problems can come from "floating" and short staffing. In these cases, you may be placed in a specialty area with which you are not familiar, with or without a more experienced nurse. There is no clear answer to this dilemma, since some courts have ruled that shifting staff is the employer's privilege and refusal can be considered insubordination. The supervisor, of course, is also responsible for any damage done because he or she is supposed to delegate safely. The float nurse must be especially careful and report any change in a patient's condition. Cushing notes that perhaps the best defense if injury occurs is to be able to document that you recognized your knowledge gap, but did not know that specialty and had asked for help. Meanwhile, some union contracts and some individual agreements in hospitals specify that a nurse is not to be floated to an unfamiliar unit without some training in that specialty.[65]

4. *Abandoning a patient. Abandonment* simply means leaving a patient when your duty is to be with him. One example would be leaving a child or incompetent adult without the protection you would have offered. The results can be fatal. In one case, a circulating nurse went, at a doctor's demand, to assist in another operating room, while the OR technician was removing the surgical drapes at the end of a patient's surgery. No one else was in that OR, and when the patient went into cardiac arrest, the technician could not handle the situation alone. The patient became permanently paralyzed and semicomatose. Although the physician and anesthesiologist were also held liable, the court focused on the duty of the circulating nurse, as spelled out in the hospital procedure book. The jury concluded that the nurse was negligent for leaving the unconscious patient's side.[66]

5. *Failure to teach a patient.* Nurses sometimes neglect to teach a patient in preparation for discharge, either because of the time it takes or because the physician objects. An increasing number of suits are being filed because such teaching was not done or not done thoroughly or understandably. Written instructions are often considered necessary to help the patient and family remember the information.[67]

6. *Failure to make sure that faulty equipment is removed* from use, that crowded corridors or hallways adjacent to the nursing unit are cleared, that slippery or unclean floors are taken care of, and that fire hazards are eliminated.

This is an area of negligence that, in most instances, would implicate others just as much as, or more than, the professional nurse. For example, the hospital administration would certainly share responsibility for fire hazards and dangerously crowded corridors, and the housekeeping and maintenance departments would not be blameless either. This does not lessen your responsibility for reporting unsafe conditions and following up on them, or in checking equipment you use.[68] Report persistent hazards in writing and keep a copy for personal protection.

7. *Careless attention to a patient's personal belongings,* resulting in the loss of valuable or necessary property, such as expensive jewelry, money, prostheses, or dentures.[69]

GOOD SAMARITAN LAWS

As noted in Chapter 20, the enactment of good samaritan laws in many states exempts doctors and nurses (and sometimes others) from civil liability when they give emergency care in "good faith" with "due care" or without "gross negligence." The first state to pass such a law was California in 1959; in 1963 California enacted such legislation specifically for nurses. By 1979 all states and the District of Columbia had good samaritan laws, not all including nurses in the coverage. No court has yet interpreted these statutes, and prior to their enactment, no case held a doctor or nurse liable for negligence in care at the site of an emergency. The law is intended to encourage assistance without fear of legal liability. As far as the law in concerned, there is no obligation or duty to render aid or assistance in an emergency. Only by statutory law can the rendering of such assistance be made obligatory.

RNs engaged in occupational health nursing are likely to be called upon to give first-aid treatment to patients with wounds and other injuries as part of their job responsibility. Such emergency treatment in a health care setting is not covered under the good samaritan laws. These nurses, just like nurses in an emergency room, should take every precaution to make sure they are operating within the bounds of legally authorized practice for nurses in their position.

Because of the lack of clarity of terms and the many differences in the law from state to state, many health professionals are still reluctant to give emergency assistance.[70] One lawyer gives this advice: don't give aid unless you know what you're doing; stick to the basics of first aid; offer to help, but make it clear that you won't interfere if the victim or family prefers to wait for other help; don't draw any medical or diagnostic conclusions; don't leave a victim you've begun to assist until you can turn his care over to an equally competent person; whether you do or do not volunteer your services, be absolutely certain to call or have someone else call for a physician or emergency medical service immediately.[71]

SPECIALTY NURSING

As nurses assume more responsibility in nursing, particularly in specialty areas, they often seek help in determining their legal status. Frequently their concern has to do with the scope of practice: are they performing within legal bounds? Negligence, whether in a highly specialized unit, an emergency, or a self-care unit, is still a question of what the reasonably prudent nurse would do. Therefore, although a nurse might look for a specific answer to a specific question, the legal dangers lie in the same set of instances described earlier, simply transposed to another setting.[72-75]

DRUG CONTROL

In 1914, the United States adopted an antinarcotic law—the *Harrison Narcotic Act,* to be administered by a bureau of narcotics within the Department of the Treasury. It was amended frequently to meet the demands of changing times. For example, in 1956 a strong *Narcotic Control Act* was passed, and in 1961 a new law gave federal authorities broader control of drug preparations containing small amounts of narcotics. This came about largely because teenagers were reported to have become addicted by taking preparations such as cough medicines containing a small percentage of narcotics, which they could obtain without a prescription. As noted in Chapter 19, the *Comprehensive Drug Abuse and Control Act* of 1970 *(Controlled Substance Act)* replaced virtually all earlier federal laws dealing with narcotics, stimulants, depressants, and hallucinogens. Sections in the law prohibit nurses from prescribing controlled substances, but they may administer drugs at the direction of legalized practitioners (who are registered). All registrants must follow strict controls and procedures against theft and diversion of controlled substances.[76] New state laws are based on the federal law, although there are variations.

Among the other drugs subject to federal or state control, or both, are poisons, caustics, and corrosives, methyl or wood alcohol, drugs for treatment of venereal disease, and amphetamines. Marijuana has been subject to changing legal patterns. In many states, its use but not its sale has been decriminalized. Barbiturates, principally used therapeutically as sedatives, but also a part of the illegal drug scene, have been state regulated through the so-called lullaby laws—aimed originally at the legitimate user, not the addict. New drugs are also being given closer scrutiny because of misuse and consequent dangerous effects.

Knowledge of the laws controlling the use of drugs will help you to understand the reasons for the policies and procedures established by an institution or agency for the mutual welfare of the employer, employee, and patient. It also helps you to keep free of legal involvements and to intelligently direct and advise others whom you may supervise or who may look to you for guidance in such matters. Nurses should all be alert to changes in drug laws on either the state or national level.

OTHER TORTS AND CRIMES

The average nurse probably will not get involved in criminal offenses, although in the last few years, a number of nurses have been accused of murder.[77] Nurses, like anyone else, may steal, murder, or break other serious laws. Crimes most often committed are criminal assault and battery (striking or otherwise physically mistreating or threatening a patient); murder (sometimes in relation to right-to-live principles); and drug offenses. If found guilty of a felony, the nurse will probably also lose her or his license.

Sometimes nurses will be involved in litigation as *accessories;* that is, they are connected with the commission of a crime but did not actually do it themselves, although present and promoting the crime or near enough to assist if necessary.

An *abettor* encourages the commission of a crime but is absent when it is actually committed. The term *accomplice* is similar in meaning to both *accessory* and *abettor,* although a distinction may be made in some jurisdictions. A nurse (or anyone else for that matter) found guilty of any of these crimes may be held equally guilty with the person who commits the crime. However, whether the nurse is a perpetrator, a victim, or simply has to deal with people who are, it is useful to know the definition and scope of the most common criminal offenses. These can be found in most nursing law texts.[78] Several will be discussed here. Not discussed but worth noting are some torts and crimes in which nurses occasionally are involved in their professional lives: *forgery*—fraudulently making or altering a written document or item, such as a will, chart, or check; *kidnapping*—stealing and carrying off a human being; *rape*—illegal or forcible sexual intercourse; and *bribery*—an offer of a reward for doing wrong or for influencing conduct.

Assault and Battery

In general, every time one person touches another in an angry, rude, or insolent manner and every blow or push that is delivered with an intent to injure, or to put the person in fear of injury, constitutes an assault and a battery in the context of criminal law. Legal action can result from any of these acts unless they can be justified or excused.

Also, every attempt to use force and violence with an intent to injure, or put one in fear of injury, constitutes an *assault*, such as striking at a person with or without a weapon; holding up a fist in a threatening attitude near enough to be able to strike; or advancing with a hand uplifted in a threatening manner with intent to strike or put one in fear of being struck, even if the person is stopped before he gets near enough to carry the intention into effect.

A *battery,* as distinguished from an assault, is the actual striking or touching of the body of a man or woman in a violent, angry, rude, or insolent manner. But every laying on of hands is not a battery. The person's intention must be considered. If someone slaps a person on the back in fun or as an act of friendship, for example, it does not constitute a battery, for there is no intent to injure or put the person in fear of injury. To constitute a battery, intent to injure or put one in fear of injury must be accompanied by "unlawful violence." However, the slightest degree of force may constitute violence in the eyes of the law.

As in so many legal matters, the terms used to describe the acts are much less important than the acts themselves as far as the nonlegal public is concerned. In legal proceedings, however, terminology has a significant bearing on the outcome of a case. For example, should a nurse be either the plaintiff or defendant in a case of assault or battery, or both, the terms used might influence considerably the conduct of the case and the settlement made. In day-to-day practice, however, the nurse need only be aware of the acts related to nursing that might conceivably be considered as assault or battery, or both, and therefore subject to legal action. Assault and battery in the context of civil law is discussed in Chapter 22.

Defamation, Slander, Libel

As is true of so many legal terms, there is some overlapping of meaning and interpretation of the terms *defamation, slander,* and *libel.* In general, however, it is correct to consider *defamation* as the most inclusive because it covers any communication that is seriously detrimental to another person's reputation. If the communication is oral, it is technically called *slander*; if written or shown in pictures, effigies, or signs (without just cause or excuse), it is called *libel.* All three are considered wrongful acts (torts) under the law, and a person convicted of one or more of these in criminal or civil court is ordered to make amends, usually by paying the defamed person a compensatory fee.

In both slander and libel, a third person must be involved. For example, one person can make all kinds of derogatory statements directly to another without getting in trouble with the law *unless* overheard by a third person. Then the remarks become slanderous. Moreover, the third person must be able to understand what has been said. If it is spoken in an unfamiliar language, for example, it is not slanderous under the law. Likewise a person can write anything she or he wishes to another, and the communication will not be considered libelous unless it is read and understood by a third person. A malicious and false statement made by one person to another about a third person also comprises slander.

Statements of a strong and uncomplimentary nature are not necessarily slanderous or libelous. They must be false, damaging to the offended person's reputation, and tending to subject him to public contempt and ridicule. The best and often the only defense allowed for the person accused of slander or libel—under the law—is proof that she or he told the truth in whatever type of communication used.

It is evident that there are many "if's," "and's," and "but's," associated with defamation, slander, and libel. Wise nurses avoid becoming embroiled in such litigations by being extremely careful in what they say or write about anyone.[79] They also proceed with caution when they are the victims of slander and libel, knowing that litigation is expensive and time-consuming and, in many instances, hardly worth the trouble. On the other hand, they should not be overly meek in accepting unfair and untrue statements about them that are likely to adversely affect their reputations and future in nursing, as well as the good name of nursing in the community. There have been documented cases in which nurses were slandered by a physician, for instance, and collected damages.

Homicide and Suicide

Homicide means killing a person by any means whatsoever. It is not necessarily a crime. If it is unquestionably an accident, it is called *excusable homicide*. If it is done in self-defense or in discharging a legal duty, such as taking a prisoner, putting a condemned person to death, or preserving the peace, it is termed *justifiable homicide*. The accused must be able to prove justification, however.

Criminal homicide is either murder or manslaughter. *Murder* means the unlawful killing of one person by another of sound mind and with malice aforethought. It may be by direct violence, such as shooting or strangling, or by indirect violence, such as slow poisoning. Murder is usually divided into two degrees: *first degree* when it is premeditated and carried out deliberately; and *second degree* when it is not planned beforehand, but is nonetheless performed with an intent to kill. In both, there must be a design to effect death.

Suicide is considered criminal if the person is sane and of an age of discretion at the time of his action. An unsuccessful attempt to commit suicide is a misdemeanor under the law. If there is doubt as to whether a person has committed suicide, a court of law usually presumes that he has not, although this judgment may be reversed by evidence to the contrary. A person who encourages another to commit suicide is guilty of murder if the suicide is effected. Statutes vary from state to state.

As a professional person, it is not unusual for a nurse to become implicated in cases of murder and suicide, usually associated with patients. Following are a few suggestions for keeping as free of legal involvement as possible:

1. Any indication on the part of any patient or employee that she or he has suicidal tendencies should be taken seriously and reported to the appropriate person.
2. Generally, a patient with known suicidal inclinations should not be left alone unless completely protected from self-harm by restraints or confinement.
3. Items that a depressed person might use for suicidal purposes should be kept out of reach.
4. Observations should be accurately reported on the patient's chart.
5. Help should be sought for nurses or their families immediately upon becoming aware of suicidal tendencies.
6. Cooperation with the police and hospital authorities guarding a patient who is accused of homicide is important.
7. Unethical discussions of a homicide case involving a patient or employee should be avoided.
8. Complete and accurate records of all facts that might have a bearing on the legal aspects of the case should be kept.

MALPRACTICE (LIABILITY) INSURANCE

Almost all lawyers in the health field now agree that nurses should carry their own malpractice or professional liability insurance, whether or not their employer's insurance includes them. The employer's insurance is intended primarily to protect the employer; the nurse is protected only to the extent needed for that primary purpose. It is quite conceivable that the employer might settle out of court, without consulting the nurse, to the nurse's disadvantage. The nurse has no control and no choice of lawyer.[80] There are a number of other limitations. The nurse is not covered for anything beyond the job in the place of employment during the hours of employment. If the nurse alone is sued and the hospital is not, the hospital has no obligation to provide legal protection (and may choose not to). Moreover, if the nurse carries no personal liability insurance, there is the possibility of subrogation.[81] Should there be criminal charges, the employer or insurance carrier may choose to deny legal assistance, or the kind offered could be inadequate.[82] A nurse must remember that no matter how trivial, how unfounded a charge might be, a legal defense is necessary and often costly, aside from the possibility of being found liable and having to pay damages.

Malpractice insurance should be bought with some care so that adequate coverage is provided. The most important distinction to be made in selecting insurance is whether it is on an "occurrence based" or a "claims made" basis. If the insurance policy is allowed to lapse, an incident that occurred at the time of coverage will be covered in an occurrence based policy, but not on a claims made policy. The latter may be less expensive, but will require almost continuous coverage, which might be a problem for a nurse planning to take time out for child rearing or for one close to retirement. Benefits usually include paying any sum awarded as damages, including medical costs, paying the cost of attorneys, and paying the bond required if appealing an adverse decision. Some policies also pay damages for injury arising out of acts of the insured as a member of an accreditation board or committee of a hospital or professional society, personal liability (such as slander, assault, libel), and personal injury and medical payments (not related to the individual's professional practice).[83]

Except for nurse anesthetists, and sometimes nurse-midwives, who occasionally have difficulty in finding insurance and who pay higher premiums, nurses have had no problems getting malpractice insurance. The 1984 designated liability for an ANA policy is $1 million per occurrence and $3 million aggregate. The average cost per year is about $45. State associations vary in this, as well as in the additional benefits that might be offered. Insurance bought elsewhere is usually more costly, and does not always cover NPs as the ANA insurance does. For the careful nurse, professional liability insurance is a good investment, as well as being tax deductible.

IN COURT: THE DUE PROCESS OF LAW

Yes, you can be sued. What happens if you become involved in litigation? What steps should you take to try to make sure that the case will be handled to the best advantage throughout? The answers to these questions will depend upon (1) whether you are accused of committing the tort or crime; (2) whether you are an accessory, through actual participation or observance; (3) whether you are the person against whom the act was committed; or (4) whether you appear as an expert witness.

Assuming that this is a civil case, five distinct steps are taken:*

(1) the filing of a document called a complaint by a person called the *plaintiff* who contends that his legal rights have been infringed by the conduct of one or more other persons called *defendants*; (2) the written response of the defendants accused of having violated the legal rights of the plaintiff, termed an *answer*; (3) pretrial activities of both parties designed to elicit all the facts of the situation, termed *discovery*; (4) the *trial* of the case, in which all the relevant facts are presented to the judge or jury for decisions; and (5) *appeal* from a decision by a party who contends that the decision was wrongly made.[84]

*Springer gives a detailed explanation of the trial process; others give less detailed versions.

The majority of persons who are asked to appear as witnesses during a hearing accept voluntarily. Others refuse and must be subpoenaed. A *subpoena* is a writ or order in the name of the court, referee, or other person authorized by law to issue the same, which requires the attendance of a witness at a trial or hearing under a penalty for failure. Cases involving the care of patients often necessitate producing hospital records, x-rays, and photographs as evidence. A subpoena requiring a witness to bring this type of evidence with him contains a clause to that effect and is termed a *subpoena duces tecum.*

The plaintiff, defendant, and witnesses may be asked to make a *deposition,* an oral interrogation answering various questions about the issue concerned. It is given under oath and taken in writing before a judicial officer or attorney.[85] A witness has certain rights, including the right to refuse to testify as to privileged communication (extended to the nurse in only a few states) and the protection against self-incrimination afforded by the Fifth Amendment to the Constitution. The judge and jury usually do not expect a person on trial or serving as a witness to remember all of the details of a situation. Witnesses in malpractice suits are permitted to refer to the patient's record, which, of course, they should have reviewed with the attorney before the trial.

Only under serious circumstances is someone accused (and convicted) of *perjury,* which means making a false statement under oath or one that she or he neither knows nor believes to be true.

There are certain guidelines on testifying that are the same whether serving as an expert or other witness or if the nurse is the defendant:[86]

1. Be prepared; review the deposition, the chart, technical and clinical knowledge of the disease or condition; discuss with the lawyer potential questions; educate the lawyer as to what points should be made. Trials are adversary procedures that are intended to probe, question, and explore all aspects of the issue.
2. Dress appropriately.
3. Behave appropriately: keep calm, be courteous, even if insulted; don't be sarcastic or angry; take your time (a cross-examiner attorney may try to put you in a poor light[87]).
4. Give adequate and appropriate information: if you can't remember, notes or the data source, such as the chart, can be checked. Answer fully, but don't volunteer additional information not asked for.
5. Don't use technical terminology, or, if use is necessary, translate it into lay terms.
6. Don't feel incompetent; don't get on the defensive; be decisive.
7. Don't be obviously partisan (unless you're the defendant).
8. Keep all materials; the decision may be appealed.

In the expert witness role,[88,89] the same precepts hold, but in addition the nurse should present her or his credentials, degrees, research, honors, whatever else is pertinent, without modesty; the opposing expert witness will certainly do so.

Expert witnesses are paid for preparation time, pretrial conferences, consultations, and testifying. Nurses are just beginning to act officially in this capacity, and several state nurses' associations (SNAs) accept applications for those interested in placement on an expert witness panel, screen applicants in a given field for a specific case, submit a choice of names to attorneys requesting such information, and have developed guidelines and CE for nurse expert witnesses.

LITIGATION TRENDS IN HEALTH CARE

Part of the doctrine of common law is that anyone can sue anyone if she or he can get a lawyer to take the case or is able to handle it personally (such as is common in a small claims court). This does not necessarily mean that there is just cause or that the person suing (plaintiff) has a good chance of winning; in fact, the defendant might be protected by law from being found liable, as when someone, in good faith, reports child abuse.

Most people are reasonably decent in their dealings with others, and unless a person sustains a serious injury or his property is badly damaged or stolen, they will not institute legal proceedings. Sometimes this is because legal services are expensive, perhaps more so than the cost of repairing the damage or paying the medical bills, and the offended person is realistic enough to know this. Often the person inflicting the injury is also realistic and prefers to settle the matter out of court, knowing that it will be less costly in the long run; or insurance may pay for the damage inflicted. One or both parties may settle their difficulties out of court because one or the other or both wants to avoid publicity and does not want to have a court record of any kind.

Once people seemed particularly reluctant to "make trouble" for nurses, doctors, or health agencies such as certain nonprofit or voluntary hospitals, either out of respect for the services offered and/or because they presumably had so little money that it seemed unfair or pointless. The latter was probably always an inaccurate generality, but today patients and families who are or feel aggrieved are considerably more likely to sue any or all concerned, sometimes for enormous sums. Health care is big business. The number of claims and the severity of awards began to increase in the 1930s, declined during World War II, and then rose again.

A number of reasons have been cited: the "litigant spirit" of the general public, what seems to be a "sue if possible; I'm entitled" attitude;[90] changing medical technology that brought new risks, with a potential for exceptional severity of injury; sometimes high, unrealistic public expectations; the increase in specialization that has resulted in a deterioration of the physician–patient relationship; and patient resentment of depersonalized care and sometimes rude treatment in hospitals.

At the height of the malpractice crisis, a specially appointed interdisciplinary committee reported that the prime factor in malpractice was malpractice. However, because there are so many more medical injuries than medical claims, a major factor might be interpersonal problems between the provider and patient and frustration with the way specific complaints were handled or not handled.[91]

Most suits are settled out of court. The dramatic multi-million-dollar suits seldom result in awards anywhere near the original figure; sometimes they are not won at all. The largest awards have the largest elements of compensation for pain and suffering, almost exclusively occurring after some negligently caused catastrophic injury, such as severe brain damage or paralysis, which obviously has an enormous effect on the victim's life.[92] The frequent suits and large awards were part of the reason for the mid-1970s' malpractice crisis, when many physicians could not get malpractice insurance, and neither hospitals not physicians felt that they could afford it if they could get it.[93]

The vast majority of malpractice cases are against physicians or hospitals. Don't nurses get sued? Absolutely. A good percentage of hospital and physician suits include nurses and may be based on the nurse's negligence. Because of the various legal doctrines, explained earlier, the aggrieved patient has the option of suing multiple defendants. The *deep pocket* theory of naming those who can pay has become traditional tort law strategy, as has the *fishnet theory* of suing every defendant available. Thus, the likelihood of recovery from one or more defendants is greater, and a favorite defense of admitting negligence but blaming an absent party, the so-called empty chair defense, is defeated.[94] Because presumably either or both the physician or the hospital has more money than the nurse, either may have to pay the award even if it is the nurse who is clearly at fault. Particularly in the case of the hospital whose liability and responsibility may be only secondary (vicarious liability), it may recover damages from the employee primarily responsible for the loss.

The possibilities of pretrial arbitration and no-fault insurance have been considered. Some states use an arbitration procedure that makes preliminary recommendations on the viability of a suit. The attraction of no-fault insurance is the increasing public tendency to believe that if someone is hurt, someone must pay, whether or not negligence is clearly evident. How costly this would be remains to be seen; no-fault auto insurance has been much more costly than ever contemplated. To get to the root of the problem—quality of care—government and health providers are looking at the impact of quality assurance techniques. It has also been noted that physicians, through self-owned insurance companies, are more stringently controlling the practice of their peers.[95] In addition, many hospitals have now adopted risk management programs in which nurses are very much involved, focusing on the review and improvement of employee guidelines, personnel policies, incident reports, physician–nurse relationships, safety policies, patient records, research guidelines and anything else that might be a factor in legal suits.[96-98]

All of this involves nurses. For individual nurses who have specific concerns about the legal aspects of their practice, it may be possible to get some information from the employing agency's legal counsel or state licensing board. Keeping abreast of legal trends is always necessary. Observing some basic principles will also help to avert problems:

1. Know your licensure law.
2. Don't do what you don't know how to do. (Learn how, if necessary.)
3. Keep your practice updated; CE is essential.
4. Use self-assessment, peer evaluation, audits, and supervisor's evaluations as guidelines for improving practice and follow up on criticisms and knowledge/skill gaps.
5. Don't be careless.
6. Practice interdependently; communicate with others.
7. Record accurately, objectively, and completely; don't erase.
8. Delegate safely and legally; know the preparation and abilities of those you supervise.
9. Help develop appropriate policies and procedures (in-house law).
10. Carry malpractice insurance.

Alford notes that there are "nurse defenders" who defend their patients from harm and "nurse defendants" whose substandard practices make them a target for litigation.[99] Professional nurses can never forget that licensure is a privilege and a responsibility mandating accountability to the consumer it is intended to protect; therefore, nurses have a legal and moral obligation to practice safely.

REFERENCES

1. Mary Hemelt and Mary Ellen Mackert, *Dynamics of Law in Nursing and Health Care* (Reston, Va.: Reston Publishing Company, 1978), p. 3.
2. Carl DeMarco, "Breach of Duty," *Nurs. 76,* **6**:103–106 (Apr. 1976).
3. Jane Greenlaw, "Liability for Nursing Negligence in the Operating Room," *Law, Med. and Health Care,* **10**:222–224 (Oct. 1982).
4. Donna Lee Guarriello, "Can You Be Sued Without Cause?" *RN,* **47**:19–23 (Feb. 1984).
5. Health Law Center, *Problems in Hospital Law* (Rockville, Md.: Aspen Systems Corp., 1974), pp. 47–54.
6. Helen Creighton, *Law Every Nurse Should Know,* 4th ed. (Philadelphia: W.b. Saunders Company, 1981), pp. 81–83.
7. Hemelt and Mackert, op. cit., pp. 36–38.
8. David Sharpe et al., *Cases and Materials on Law and Medicine* (St. Paul, Minn.: West Publishing Company, 1978), pp. 74–76.
9. Creighton, op. cit., p. 154.
10. Hemelt and Mackert, op. cit., p. 11.
11. Ibid., pp. 31–34.

12. Ibid., pp. 39–40.

13. Ibid., pp. 28–31.

14. Irene Murchison, Thomas Nichols, and Rachel Hanson, *Legal Accountability in the Nursing Process,* 2nd ed. (St. Louis: C. V. Mosby Company, 1977), pp. 94–96.

15. Darlene Trandel-Korenchuk and Keith Trandel Korenchuk, "Nursing Liability and Respondeat Superior," *Nurse Practitioner,* **7**:46–48 (Jan. 1982).

16. Hemelt and Mackert, op. cit., pp. 10–11.

17. Charles Kramer, *Medical Malpractice,* 4th ed. (New York: Practicing Law Institute, 1976), p. 44.

18. Walter Eccard, "A Revolution in White—New Approaches to Treating Nurses as Professionals," *Vanderbilt Law Rev.,* **39**:839–879 (1977).

19. Susan Viles, "Liability for the Negligence of Hospital Nursing Personnel," *Nurs. Admin. Q.,* **5**:83–93 (Fall 1980).

20. Irene Murchison and Thomas Nichols, *Legal Foundations of Nursing Practice* (New York: Macmillan Publishing Company, Inc., 1970), pp. 139–143.

21. William Roach, "Responsible Intervention: A Legal Duty to Act," *J. Nurs. Admin.,* **10**:18–24 (July 1980) .

22. Murchison, Nicholas, and Hanson, op. cit., pp. 63–73.

23. Helen Creighton, "The Expert Winess," *Sup. Nurse,* **11**:71–72 (Apr. 1980).

24. Jane Greenlaw, "When Leaving Siderails Down Can Bring You Up on Charges," *RN,* **45**:75–78 (Dec. 1982).

25. Helen Creighton, "Injections and the Law," *Sup. Nurse,* **10**:68–71 (June 1979).

26. Helen Creighton, "Legal Value of Pharmaceutical Inserts," *Sup. Nurse,* **11**:13–14 (Feb. 1980).

27. Donna Lee Guarriello, "The Legal Boobytraps in Nursing Standards," *RN,* **47**:19–21 (June 1984).

28. Betty Campazzi, "Nurses, Nursing and Malpractice Litigation: 1967–1977," *Nurs. Admin. Q.,* **5**:1–18 (Fall 1980).

29. Helen Creighton, "Nursing Assessment," *Nurs. Mgt.,* **12**:65–69 (Nov. 1981).

30. Frances Herrman, "Four Kinds of Carelessness That Can Send You to Court," *Nurs. Life,* **2**:63 (May–June 1982).

31. Maureen Cushing, "A Matter of Judgment," *Am. J. Nurs.,* **82**:990–992, (June 1982).

32. Helen Creighton, "Nursing Judgment," *Nurs. Mgt.,* **13**:15, 60–63 (May 1982).

33. Cushing, op. cit., p. 992.

34. Mary Mayers, "Legal Guidelines," *Geriatric Nurs.,* **2**:417–421 (Nov.–Dec. 1981).

35. Thomas Rubbert, "Lawyer on Call," *Nurs. 81,* **11**:321 (Nov. 1981).

36. William Regan, "Verbal Orders: Invitations to Disaster," *RN,* **43**:61–62 (July 1980).

37. Helen Creighton, "Refusal to Treat Patient," *Sup. Nurse,* **12**:67–68 (Apr. 1981).

38. William Regan, "How to Force That On-Call MD to Respond," *RN,* **45**:77–78 (Feb. 1982).

39. Jane Greenlaw, "The Deadly Toll of Communication Failure," *RN,* **45**:81–84 (Nov. 1982).

40. Maureen Cushing, "Failure to Communicate," *Am. J. Nus.,* **83**:1597–1598, (Oct. 1982).

41. William Regan, "When in Doubt, Check It Out," *RN,* **46**:87–88, (May 1983).

42. "Does the Doctor Know Best?" *Nurs. 82,* **12**:18 (Jan. 1982).

43. Barbara Katz, "Reporting and Review of Patient Care: The Nurse's Responsibility," *Law, Med. and Health Care,* **11**:76–79 (Apr. 1983).

44. Avice Kerr, "Nurses' Notes: That's Where the Goodies Are," *Nurs. 75,* **5**:34 (Feb. 1975).

45. Marguerite Mancini, "Documenting Clinical Records," *Am. J. Nurs.,* **78**:1556, 1561 (Sept. 1978).

46. Jane Greenlaw, "Documentation of Patient Care: An Often Underestimated Responsibility," *Law, Med. and Health Care,* **10**:172–174 (Sept. 1982).

47. Nathan Hershey and Roger Lawrence, "The Influence of Charting upon Liability Determinations," *J. Nurs. Admin.,* **6**:35–37 (Mar.–Apr. 1976).

48. Jean Greenlaw, "What to Do If Your Supervisor Orders a 'Cover-up'," *RN,* **45**:81–82 (Oct. 1982).

49. Hershey and Lawrence, op. cit.

50. Ann Burgess and Anna Laszlo, "Court-

room Use of Hospital Records in Sexual Assault Cases," *Am. J. Nurse.,* **77**:64–68 (Jan. 1977).

51. June Helberg, "Documentation in Child Abuse," *Am. J. Nurs.,* **83**:234–239 (Feb. 1983).
52. Margaret Mancini, "Adult Abuse Laws," *Am. J. Nurs.,* **80**:739–740 (Apr. 1980).
53. Maureen Cushing, "Gaps in Documentation," *Am. J. Nurs.,* **82**:1899–1900 (Dec. 1982).
54. Mary Hemelt and Mary Mackert, "Your Legal Guide to Nursing Practice," Part I, *Nurs. 79,* **9**:59 (Oct. 1979).
55. Jean Rabinow, "Patient Injury in the Hospital: How to Protect Yourself," *Nurs. Life,* **2**:44–48 (Jan.–Feb. 1982).
56. Helen Creighton, "Incident Reports Subject to Discovery," *Nurs. Mgt.,* **14**:55, 57 (Feb. 1983).
57. Anne Doll, "What to Do After an Incident," *Nurs. 80,* **10**:73–79 (Jan. 1980).
58. Hemelt and Mackert, op. cit., 29–30.
59. Helen Creighton, "Nosocomial Infections," *Sup. Nurse,* **12**:60–62 (Aug. 1981).
60. Helen Creighton, "Injections and the Law," *Sup. Nurse,* **10**:64–68 (May 1979).
61. William Regan, "$30,000 Worth of Trouble Over an Ice Pack," *RN,* **42**:81 (Apr. 1979).
62. Jane Greenlaw, "Failure to Use Siderails: When Is It Negligence?" *Law, Med. and Health Care,* **10**:125–128 (June 1982).
63. Joseph Fink, "Preventing Lawsuits: Medication Errors to Avoid," *Nurs. Life,* **3**:26–29 (Mar.–Apr. 1983).
64. Murchison, Nichols, and Hanson, op. cit., pp. 69–73.
65. Maureen Cushing, "Fears of a Float Nurse," *Am. J. Nurs,* **83**:297–298 (Feb. 1983).
66. William Regan, "The Risks of Abandoning a Patient," *RN,* **46**:297–298 (Feb. 1983).
67. Maureen Cushing, "Legal Lessons on Patient Teaching," *Am. J. Nurs.,* **84**:721–722 (June, 1984).
68. Hermann, op. cit., p. 63
69. Creighton, *Law Every Nurse Should Know,* p. 173.

70. Ardyce Leighton, "Be a Good Samaritan? Better Weigh the Risks," *Nurs. Life,* **2**:61–68 (Mar.–Apr. 1982).
71. Jack Horsley, "You Can't Escape the Good Samaritan Role—Or Its Risks," *RN,* **44**:87–92 (May 1981).
72. Jack Horsley, "Caution: Home Visits Can Be Hazardous to Your License," *RN,* **45**:89–96 (Sept. 1982).
73. Jane Greenlaw, "Nursing Negligence in the Hospital Emergency Department," *Law, Med., and Health Care,* **12**:118–121, 132 (June 1984).
74. Maureen Cushing, "An Occupational Nurse's Liability," *Am. J. Nurs.,* **81**:2207–2208 (Dec. 1981).
75. Helen Creighton, "Your Legal Risks in Nursing Coronary Patients," *Nurs. 77,* **7**:65–71 (Jan. 1977).
76. Mary Cazalas, *Nursing and the Law,* 3rd ed., (Germantown, Md.: Aspen Systems Corp. 1978), pp. 59–67.
77. Beatrice Kalisch et al., "When Nurses Are Accused of Murder," *Nurs. Life,* **2**:45–47 (Sept.–Oct. 1982).
78. Helen Creighton, *Law Every Nurse Should Know,* pp. 234–253.
79. William Regan, "Leave Detective Work to the Cops," *RN,* **43**:78, 85–86 (May 1980).
80. Ronnie Sandroff, "Why You Really Ought to Have Your *Own* Malpractice Policy," *RN,* **46**:29–33 (June 1983).
81. Marguerite Mancini, "What You Should Know About Malpractice Insurance," *Am. J. Nurs.,* **79**:729–730 (Apr. 1979).
82. Joseph Manta, "Malpractice Insurance: Don't Get Caught Without It," *Nurs. Life,* **2**:44–47 (Mar.–Apr. 1982).
83. Maureen Cushing, "Malpractice: Are You Covered?" *Am. J. Nurs.,* **84**:985–986 (Aug. 1984).

84. Murchison and Nichols, op. cit., p. 20.
85. Eric Springer, ed., *Nursing and the Law,* (Pittsburgh, Pa.: Aspen Systems Corp. 1970) p. 155.
86. Marilyn McCartney, "In the Witness Box: How to Give Nursing Testimony," *Nurs. 77,* **7**:89–93 (Apr. 1977).
87. Charles Kramer, "Cross-Examination of

the Medical Expert,'' *Trial,* **13**:26–30 (Dec. 1977).

88. Rose Mary Shannon, ''Testifying as an Expert Witness on Behalf of Your Patient,'' *MCN,* **4**:281–284 (Oct. 1977).

89. Helen Creighton, ''The Expert Witness,'' *Sup. Nurse,* **11**:71–72 (Apr. 1980).

90. Frank Trippet, ''Of Hazards, Risks, and Culprits,'' *Time,* Aug. 28, 1978, p. 76.

91. Department of Health, Education and Welfare, *Medical Malpractice: Report of the Secretary's Commission on Medical Malpractice* (Washington, D.C.: The Department, 1973), pp. 24–25.

92. William Schwartz and Neil Komesar, ''Doctors, Damages and Deterrence: An Economic View of Medical Malpractice,'' *N. Engl. J. Med.,* **298**:1282–1289 (June 1978).

93. Cynthia Northrup, ''Responding to the Malpractice Crisis,'' *Am. J. Nurs.,* **80**:2245–2246 (Dec. 1980).

94. Donna Lee Guarriello, ''Can You Be Sued Without Cause?'' *RN,* **47**:19 (Feb. 1984).

95. James Cooper and Sharman Stephens, ''The Malpractice Crisis—What Was It All About?'' *Inquiry,* **14**:243–253 (Sept. 1977).

96. Shannon Perry, ''Managing to Avoid Malpractice,'' Parts I and II. *J. Nurs. Admin.,* **8**:43–47 (Aug. 1978) and **8**:16–22 (Sept. 1978).

97. Barbara Rubin, ''Medical Malpractice Suits Can Be Avoided,'' *Hospitals,* **52**:86–88 (Nov. 1978).

98. Judith Ann Spaulding, ''Risk Management: A Hospital-Wide Approach'' *Nurs. Mgt.,* **13**:29–31 (Apr. 1982).

99. Dolores Alford, ''Are You Courting Disaster?'' *Nurs. Life,* **1**:44–48 (Nov.–Dec. 1981).

Health Care and the Rights of People

Whether it is a consequence of the civil rights movement, the consumer movement (described in Chapter 6), or simply a new era in society, everyone now seems to be concerned with people's rights. As might be expected, health care has also been affected.

Until recently, people have felt helpless in their patient role—and small wonder. Stripped of their individuality as well as their belongings, they are thrust into an alien environment with little control over what happens to them. They are surrounded by unidentified faces and unidentifiable equipment. Their privacy is invaded. Their dignity is lost. They hesitate to complain or criticize for fear of reprisals from the staff. They are reluctant to press for answers to their questions because a "busy" message is communicated loud and clear. Underlying all is fear for their health, and even their lives.

There is evidence, however, that consumers are no longer willing to put up with this state of affairs, will no longer accept the traditional role of "good" patient: the one who does as he's told and asks no awkward questions. The frequent denial of their fundamental rights—among them, to courtesy, privacy, and, most of all, information—has brought about the ul-

timate form of patient rebellion—malpractice suits. As the DHEW Secretary's Commission on Medical Malpractice noted, the quality of the relationship between the patient, on the one hand, and the doctor or hospital, on the other, may make the difference between filing or not filing a malpractice suit. The Commission adds that it "believes that to ignore these and other rights of the patient is both to betray simple humanity and to invite dissatisfaction that may lead to malpractice suits."[1] The more recent President's Commission for the Study of Ethical Problems in Medicine and Biomedical and Behavioral Research (hereafter called the President's Commission) made equally strong statements and recommendations.*

PATIENTS' RIGHTS

Most of the rights about which patients are concerned are theirs legally as well as morally and have been so established by common law. They are also stated in the codes of ethics of both physicians and nurses (although, to be

---

*All these reports are listed in the bibliography.

EXHIBIT 22-1

STATEMENT ON A PATIENT'S BILL OF RIGHTS
AMERICAN HOSPITAL ASSOCIATION, 1972.

The American Hospital Association presents a Patient's Bill of Rights with the expectation that observance of these rights will contribute to more effective patient care and greater satisfaction for the patient, his physician, and the hospital organization. Further, the Association presents these rights in the expectation that they will be supported by the hospital on behalf of its patients, as an integral part of the healing process. It is recognized that a personal relationship between the physician and the patient is essential for the provision of proper medical care. The traditional physician-patient relationship takes on a new dimension when care is rendered within an organizational structure. Legal precedent has established that the institution itself also has a responsibility to the patient. It is in recognition of these factors that these rights are affirmed.

1. The patient has the right to considerate and respectful care.

2. The patient has the right to obtain from his physician complete current information concerning his diagnosis, treatment, and prognosis in terms the patient can be reasonably expected to understand. When it is not medically advisable to give such information to the patient, the information should be made available to an appropriate person in his behalf. He has the right to know by name, the physician responsible for coordinating his care.

3. The patient has the right to receive from his physician information necessary to give informed consent prior to the start of any procedure and/or treatment. Except in emergencies, such information for informed consent, should include but not necessarily be limited to the specific procedure and/or treatment, the medically significant risks involved, and the probable duration of incapacitation. Where medically significant alternatives for care or treatment exist, or when the patient requests information concerning medical alternatives, the patient has the right to such information. The patient also has the right to know the name of the person responsible for the procedures and/or treatment.

4. The patient has the right to refuse treatment to the extent permitted by law, and to be informed of the medical consequences of his action.

5. The patient has the right to every consideration of his privacy concerning his own medical care program. Case discussion, consultation, examination, and treatment are confidential and should be conducted discreetly. Those not directly involved in his care must have the permission of the patient to be present.

6. The patient has the right to expect that all communications and records pertaining to his care should be treated as confidential.

7. The patient has the right to expect that within its capacity a hospital must make reasonable response to the request of a patient for services. The hospital must provide evaluation, service, and/or referral as indicated by the urgency of the case. When medically permissible a patient may be transferred to another facility only after he has received complete information and explanation concerning the needs for and alternatives to such a transfer. The institution to which the patient is to be transferred must first have accepted the patient for transfer.

8. The patient has the right to obtain information as to any relationship of his hospital to other health care and educational institutions insofar as his care is concerned. The patient has the right to obtain information as to the existence of any professional relationships among individuals, by name, who are treating him.

9. The patient has the right to be advised if the hospital proposes to engage in or perform human experimentation affecting his care or treatment. The patient has the right to refuse to participate in such research projects.

10. The patient has the right to expect reasonable continuity of care. He has the right to know in advance what appointment times and physicians are available and where. The patient has the right to expect that the hospital will provide a mechanism whereby he is informed by his physician or a delegate of the physician of the patient's continuing health care requirements following discharge.

11. The patient has the right to examine and receive an explanation of his bill regardless of source of payment.

12. The patient has the right to know what hospital rules and regulations apply to his conduct as a patient.

No catalogue of rights can guarantee for the patient the kind of treatment he has a right to expect. A hospital has many functions to perform, including the prevention and treatment of disease, the education of both health professionals and patients, and the conduct of clinical research. All these activities must be conducted with an overriding concern for the patient, and, above all, the recognition of his dignity as a human being. Success in achieving this recognition assures success in the defense of the rights of the patient.

honest, much is stated by implication and thus open to considerable personal interpretation). Moreover, they closely reiterate the four basic consumer rights President John F. Kennedy enunciated in his consumer message to Congress in 1962:

1. The right to safety
2. The right to be informed
3. The right to choose
4. The right to be heard

Since the well-publicized American Hospital Association's (AHA) "A Patient's Bill of Rights" was presented in 1972 (Exhibit 22-1), a spate of such "rights" statements has followed: for the disabled, the mentally ill, the retarded, the old, the young, the pregnant, the handicapped, and the dying.

In some cases, these statements have been the basis for new statutory law. The first was the Minnesota legislature's adoption of a variation of the AHA Patient's Bill of Rights. A follow-up by the Minnesota Hospital Association on the effectiveness of this legislation one year later indicated that several of the hospitals and nursing homes surveyed reported that

patients' rights and the importance of confidentiality had been heightened, and that in some cases patient advocates had been appointed. However, a major flouting of the law was noted in relation to patient consent to observation of care by nonessential personnel; more than half of the respondents did not obtain such consent.

The vagueness of the AHA statement and the inability to force compliance without legal intervention have made it a butt for some bitter humor. Annas, an attorney in the health field, quotes a commentator who likened the document to a fox telling the chickens what their rights are. Nevertheless, commenting on the required posting in hospitals of the Minnesota bill, Annas notes that the "trend toward publishing rights is important because it not only reminds people that they have rights, it also encourages them to assert them and to make further demands."[2] It might also remind the staff, for there is some evidence that they, too, are often unaware of the patient's rights, even legal rights.

By the end of the 1970s, variations of the Patient's Bill of Rights became law in many states. Some legislatures passed specific bills incorporating either the AHA statements or a

---

Source: Reprinted with the permission of the American Hospital Association, copyright 1972.

similar version; state or municipal hospital codes took similar action, sometimes including mental institutions and nursing homes. In 1974, new Medicare regulations for skilled nursing facilities included a section on patients' rights. Just how disgraceful the violation of rights of this captive group was might be judged when reviewing the rights: the right to send and receive mail; the right to have spouses share rooms if both are patients, or allow privacy for visits; the right to have restraints used only if authorized by the physician and only for a limited time; the right to use one's own clothes and possessions, as space permits; and the right to require both written permission by the patient, and accounting, for management of his/her funds. And, as in other laws, patients had to be told what their rights were.

Now Annas suggests a "patients' rights agenda for the 1980s":

1. No routine procedures
2. Open access to medical records
3. Full experience disclosure
4. Twenty-four-hour-a-day visiting rights
5. Effective patient advocates[3]

INFORMED CONSENT

For years, when patients have been admitted to hospitals, they signed a frequently unread, universal consent form that almost literally gave the physician, his associates, and the hospital carte blanche in determining the patient's care. There was some rationale for this because civil suits for battery (unlawful touching) could theoretically be filed as a result of giving routine care such as baths. Patients undergoing surgery or some complex, dangerous treatment were asked to sign a separate form, usually stating something to the effect that permission was granted to the physician and/or his colleagues to perform the operation or treatment. Just how much the patient knew about the hows and whys of the surgery, the dangers and the alternatives, depended on the patient's assertiveness in asking questions and demanding answers and the physician's willingness to provide information. Nurses were taught *never* to answer those questions, or few others, but to suggest, "Ask your doctor." Health professionals, and especially physicians, took the attitude, "We know best and will decide for you."

Many patients probably still enter treatment and undergo a variety of tests and even surgery without a clear understanding of the nature of the condition they have and what can be done about it. Although they may very well be receiving care that is medically acceptable, they have no real part in deciding what that care should be. Most physicians have believed that anything more than a superficial explanation is unnecessary, for the patient should "trust" the doctor. Kalisch has elaborated this point, calling it *Aesculapian authority*.[4] Yet the patient has always had the right to make decisions about his own body. A case was heard as early as 1905 on surgery without consent, and the classic legal decision is that of Judge Cardoza (*Schloendorff* vs. *The Society of New York Hospital*, 211 NY.125, 129–130, 105 NE 92, 93–1914): "Every human being of adult years and sound mind has a right to determine what shall be done with his own body."

A noted hospital law book also states:

> It is an established principle of law that every human being of adult years and sound mind has the right to determine what shall be done with his own body. He may choose whether to be treated or not and to what extent, no matter how necessary the medical care, nor how imminent the danger to his life or health if he fails to submit to treatment.[5]

The patient's need for and right to this kind of knowledge is highlighted by the increasing number of malpractice suits that involve an element of informed consent.* For many years, in such suits, courts have tended to rule that the physician must provide only as much in-

---

*Some lawyers are advocating the use of the term *authorization for treatment,* implying patient control.

formation as is general practice among his colleagues in the area, as determined by their expert testimony. Some recent decisions, however, are changing this attitude, most of them hinging on informed consent.

The landmark decisions have involved situations in which the surgery was not done ineffectively but in which patients sued because of complications or results about which they had not been warned. In one such case, a patient who had numerous complications after surgery for a duodenal ulcer had been informed of the risks of the anesthesia but not the surgery. He received a verdict against both hospital and surgeon.[6] In another case, a woman of Korean ancestry won because the physician had not explained that with the dermabrasion she agreed to, the risk of hyperpigmentation (which she developed) was greater in those of Oriental background.[7]

In these and other cases, judges disallowed the right of the medical profession to determine how much the patient should be told; rather, they said, the patient should be told enough, in understandable lay language, to make a decision. The materiality of the risk or facts to be disclosed by the physician "is to be determined by applying the standards of a reasonable man, not a reasonable medical practitioner."[8]

There continue to be similar judgments and some legislation supporting the same concept. The trend now is for the courts to view the doctor–patient relationship as a partnership in decision making. They are expected to pay increased attention to the "physician's fiduciary duty to disclose fully to his patients the condition of their bodies" even where this is caused by the physician's own negligence.[9]

Principles of Informed Consent

Consent is defined as a free, rational act which presupposes knowledge of the thing to which consent is given by a person who is legally capable of consent. *Informed consent* is not expected to include minutiae but to delineate the essential nature of the procedure and the consequences. The disclosure is to be "reasonable," without details which might unnecessarily frighten the patient. The patient may, of course, waive the right to such explanation, or any teaching.[10] Consents are *not* needed for emergency care if there is an immediate threat to life and health, if experts agree that it is an emergency, if the patient is unable to consent and a legally authorized person can't be reached, and when the patient submits voluntarily.

Criteria for a valid consent are: written (unless oral consent can be proved in court); signed by the patient or person legally responsible for him or her (a person cannot give consent for a spouse in a nonemergency situation); the procedure performed is the one consented to; and the presence of essential elements of an informed consent.[11] These include (1) an explanation of the condition; (2) a fair explanation of the procedures to be used and the consequences; (3) a description of alternative treatments or procedures; (4) a description of the benefits to be expected; (5) an offer to answer the patient's inquiries; and (6) freedom from coercion or unfair persuasions and inducements.

The last has special significance, because the concept of informed consent really became viable with the Nuremberg Code, originating from the trials of Nazi physicians who were convicted of experimenting on prisoners without their consent. The principles were then formalized in the Declaration of Helsinki, adopted by the Eighteenth World Medical Assembly in 1964, and revised in 1975. HHS accepts the same principles and requires their adherence in human research.[12]

Trends in Informed Consent

The right to consent or not is one of the evolving issues in informed consent. The competent patient has the right to refuse consent, but a hospital can request, under certain circumstances, a court order to act if the refusal endangers the patient's life. If a patient is considered physically unable, legally incompetent, or a minor, a guardian has the right to give or withhold consent. The trend in court decisions seems to be that the patient, unless proven totally incompetent, has the right to refuse. For example, a Jehovah's Witness refuses a blood transfusion, even though it might mean his life, because taking such transfusions are against his religious beliefs.[13] The rulings have been in favor of allowing him to make his own decision; in fact, the Witnesses and AMA in 1979 agreed upon a consent form requesting that no blood or blood derivative* be administered and releasing medical personnel and the hospital for responsibility for untoward results because of that refusal. If a minor child of a Witness needs the blood and the parent refuses, a court order requested by the hospital usually permits the transfusion. This is based on a 1944 legal precedent when the Supreme Court ruled that parents had a right to be martyrs, if they wished, but had no right to make martyrs of their children.[14] On the other hand, if the child is deemed a "mature minor," able to make an intelligent decision, regardless of chronological age, the child has been allowed to refuse the treatment.

In another type of case, a seventy-nine-year-old diabetic refused to consent to a leg amputation. Her daughter petitioned to be her legal guardian so that she (the daughter) could sign the consent. The judge ruled that the woman was old but not senile, and had a right to make her own decision. In a slightly different situation, an alcoholic derelict was found unconscious on the street and taken to a hospital. When he became conscious, he refused to have his legs amputated for severe frostbite. The court order sought by the hospital was denied because, although the man was alcoholic, he was competent at the time of making his decision. (As it happened, he lost only a few toes from his frostbite.) In still another case, a young man on permanent kidney dialysis decided he did not want to live that way and refused continued treatment. He was allowed to do so and died within a short time.

_____

*This particular problem has been lessened to some extent as better blood substitutes have become available.

Other cases can also be cited. The right of a competent patient to refuse treatment seems more firmly established than ever, but when the patient is unconscious or in certain other situations, difficult legal questions arise.

Is Informed Consent Practical?

Some physicians do not believe that it is feasible to obtain an informed consent because of such factors as lack of interest or education and high anxiety level, in which case a patient might refuse a "necessary treatment or operation."[15] The physician may invoke "therapeutic privilege," in which disclosure is not required because it might be detrimental to the patient.[16] Just what that means is not clear. Or information about certain alternatives may be withheld because the physician feels that they are too risky, unproven, or not appropriate. There are physicians and others who believe that despite the increasing number of rulings favoring patients' right to full knowledge, most patients are not given information so that they really understand (and the courts don't do enough about it).[17]

Although the President's Commission avoided recommending *legal* alternatives, the members came out in unequivocal support of "shared decision-making" and full disclosure to patients except in unusual circumstances.[18] Their surveys (like others before) indicated that people *do* want full information even when they trust their doctor completely and will probably go along with his recommendations. They may not always remember the details later, but with a full explanation, given in lay terms, and with enough time for questions and answers, they can understand.[19] However, many patients are still reluctant to ask for fear of appearing stupid or "bothering the doctor." The written consent form that is generally accepted as the legal affirmation that the patient has agreed to a particular test or treatment has undergone a number of changes in the last few years. The patient's rights movement has moved hospitals, especially, to review and revise their consent forms. The catchall admissions consent has already been ruled as "almost completely worthless" for anything other than avoiding battery complaints, because it does not designate the nature of the treatment to be given.[20] What has emerged are forms that contain all the required elements for the informed consent process, usually individualized by the physician for each patient, somewhat similar to those developed earlier by Alfidi[21] and Hershey.[22] Often they are available in the foreign languages most prevalent in the area. One of the key points is having a form that avoids unnecessary technical terms or compound-complex sentences. Communications specialists who have developed and tested such forms conclude, "A comprehensible consent form is not, of course, a guarantee that physician and patient have communicated to either's satisfaction. It is, however, at least an indication of good faith and a reflection of the physician's sincere attempt not only to enable the patient to understand, but also to educate the patient."[23]

Although many people think of informed consent only in terms of hospitalization, there are already some court cases that indicate that the concept embraces the continuum of health care, such as a clinic or doctor's office. An interesting aspect of one of these cases[24] was that the physician was held to have breached his duty by failing to inform the patient of the risks of *not* consenting to a diagnostic procedure, in this case a Pap smear. The patient died of advanced cervical cancer.

The Nurse's Role in Informed Consent

What is the nurse's role in informed consent? To provide or add information before or after the doctor's explanation has been given? To refer the patient to the doctor? To avoid any participation? The advice given varies. Some suggest that getting involved in informed consent is simply not your business and is best left to the doctor; others consider it a professional responsibility.[25]

It is generally agreed that nurses do not have the primary responsibility for getting informed consent. However, the President's Commission noted that "nurses as a practical matter, typically have a central role in the process of providing patients with information,"[26] and that NPs, including nurse-midwives, have *full* responsibility for informing patients about their conditions, tests, and treatment, and obtaining consent. There was also at least one serious court case in which a patient sued, because the physician *and* nurses withheld information about his condition. Both were held liable.[27] Nevertheless, the question asked by most nurses is how much can be told, especially if the physician chooses not to reveal further information. The Tuma case (Chapter 20) did not resolve the nurse's right to supply the missing information, and the nurse may be taking a personal risk. Greenlaw suggests that patients' questions may range over a variety of topics, including what you are doing to the patient and your qualifications (if so, answer honestly) to interpretation of what the doctor said (explain in lay terms) to "What's wrong with me?" (don't answer directly) or "Is my doctor any good?" (tell the patient that he has a right to ask his doctor for his qualifications and experience or to get a second opinion).[28] A variety of other opinions are offered,[29] but a point that is always made is that the patient's lack of information should always be discussed with the doctor (tactfully) and, if there is no response, with administrative superiors. There is nothing wrong with questioning the patient to see what he or she really understands and clarifying points, providing you know what you are talking about. If you decide to give further information, it should be totally accurate and carefully recorded, and the fact that it was given should be shared with the physician and others. Nurses have found ways to make the patient aware of knowledge gaps so that they ask the right questions, but it's unfortunate that most are still employed in situations in which it could be detrimental to them to be the patient's advocate.[30] More nurses are taking the risk, however, as some polls indicate.*

---

*See Chapters 10 and 11.

Of course, if the patient is coaxed or coerced into signing without such an explanation, the consent is invalid. Moreover, if the patient withdraws consent, even verbally, the nurse is responsible for reporting this and ensuring that the patient is not treated. This is a legal responsibility not only to the patient but also to the hospital, which can be held liable.[31]

Hospitals are beginning to use a clerk to witness the consent form, after the physician provides an explanation, on the theory that only the signature is being witnessed, not the accuracy or depth of the explanation. Other hospitals ask the physician to bring another physician, presumably to validate the explanation. Where nurses still witness the form, it should be clear *what* they are witnessing—the signature or the explanation.[32] Hospital policy can clarify this.

The nurse's specific responsibility is to explain nursing care, including the whys and hows. An interesting idea to contemplate is whether you should tell patients about the risks of the *nursing* procedures you do, even though this is not a legal requirement. (Nor does it prevent you from doing so.) The answer seems to be—maybe, but carefully.[33]

THE RIGHT TO DIE

Perhaps because improved technology has succeeded in artificially maintaining both respiratory and cardiac functions when a person can no longer do so, the definition of *clinical death* as the irrevocable cessation of heartbeat and breathing is no longer pertinent.* What of irreversible coma? In 1968, a faculty committee of the Harvard Medical School identified certain characteristics of a permanently nonfunctioning brain: (1) unreceptivity and unresponsivity, (2) no movements of breathing, (3) no reflexes, (4) flat electroencephalo-

gram. Others developed variations of this definition.[34]

In common law, there had been a strongly entrenched cardiac definition of death until, in 1977, in Massachusetts, the Supreme Judicial Court officially recognized the use of brain death criteria.[35] In 1970, Kansas was the first state to adopt a brain death statute, using the same Harvard-type criteria, thus offering two alternative definitions of death to be used at the discretion of the attending physician. More than half of the states have passed similar legislation. Various types of criteria have been adopted by state legislatures, but all are based on cessation of brain functioning. Black notes an important aspect of brain death:

> Patients with brain death are not merely perpetually unresponsive: they are patients whose brain destruction, including loss of respiratory and cardiovascular control, means that life of all kind is soon to be lost as well.[36]

Currently, the AMA, the Bar Association, the President's Commission and others are suggesting that states adopt the following statute:

> An individual who has sustained either (1) irreversible cessation of circulatory and respiratory functions, or (2) irreversible cessation of all functions of the entire brain, including the brain stem, is dead. A determination of death must be made in accordance with accepted medical standards.[37]

Still, there are many lay people and health professionals who do not feel that brain death is an adequate definition of physiological death. (On the other hand, a variety of surveys indicate that most people are beginning to favor euthanasia if there is a terminal illness.) In states that still use the classic definition, questions arise about the status of patients maintained on respirators.

Two important rulings on the terminally ill, incompetent patient, made by two different state supreme courts, were the Saikewicz[38] and Quinlan[39] cases. In the first, the court upheld a decision not to give a severely retarded sixty-

---

*Physicians have had the sole authority and responsibility to pronounce a patient dead, even though a nurse may quite accurately do so. The law has not caught up with reality, except in New Jersey, where nurses can now pronounce death.

seven-year-old more chemotherapy that would be unpleasant for the sake of a short, extended life span. (He died a month later of pneumonia.) However, such a decision was seen to be a court's responsibility, after an adjudicatory hearing. In the Quinlan case, a twenty-two-year-old woman received severe and irreversible brain damage that reduced her to a vegetative state, and the father petitioned the court to be made her guardian with the intention of having all extraordinary medical procedures sustaining her life removed. The New Jersey Supreme Court ruled that the father could be the guardian and have the life support systems discontinued with the concurrence of her family, the attending physicians, who might be chosen by the father, and the hospital ethics committee.[40] (After disconnection of the respirator, Karen Quinlan continued to live, sustained by fluids and other maintenance measures, and was transferred to a nursing home.) Health law experts debate the congruity of these and similar cases, and it is expected that other supreme courts faced by other unique circumstances will make separate rulings.[41] This has proven to be an accurate prediction, as in the case of Brother Fox, Peter Cinque, Earle Spring, and others.[42]

Some of the judges' comments in the Quinlan case and others related to the belief that the person would have made a similar choice, if able to do so. Until 1977, a person could not be assured that she or he would be allowed to die if brain death existed. The Euthanasia Educational Council (now called Concern for Dying) has made available a "living will" (Exhibit 22-2) that directs the family, physician, and friends to withhold artificial means in a case of inevitable death.[43] It also has space for specific directions about treatments that the individual may refuse, such as "electrical or mechanical resuscitation of my heart when it has stopped beating"; "nasogastric tube feedings when I am paralyzed or unable to take nourishment by mouth"; "mechanical respiration if I am no longer able to sustain my own breathing." Other versions also exist.[44]

The will itself, which can be revoked at any time, has no legal power, although presumably, if the writer's intention were followed, those involved would not be judged guilty of murder. How much the will influences action (legally) when the patient is unconscious has been tested only a few times, with a trend toward its acceptance but also, after a slow start, toward legislation.

In 1977, California enacted a *Natural Death Act,* with carefully delineated and protective living will components. The next year, Arkansas, Idaho, Nevada, New Mexico, North Carolina, Oregon, and Texas followed with similar statutes.[45,46] By 1984, twenty-one laws had been passed and others were being debated. All granted civil and criminal immunity for those carrying out living will requests. Although there were no reported difficulties, some believe that because the right to refuse treatment already exists, such legislation only creates problems.[47] In 1984, California also enacted a law entitled the *Durable Power of Attorney for Health Care,* the first of its kind. It allows terminally ill patients to designate another individual to make life-or-death decisions in the event that the patient is unable to do so. The agreement conveys the authority to consent, refuse, or withdraw consent "to any care, treatment, service or procedure to maintain, diagnose, or treat a mental or physical condition." (This is also an optional statement in the living will.) A model act, *Right to Refuse Treatment,* developed by Concern for Dying legal advisors, is being studied by states considering this type of legislation.[48]

The right-to-die issue is related to the concept of *euthanasia,* a word of Greek origin meaning painless, easy, gentle, or good death. It is now commonly used to signify a killing that is promoted by some humanitarian motive, such as the relief of intolerable pain. There are two major categories of euthanasia: voluntary and involuntary. The first usually involves two parties: the competent adult patient and a doctor, nurse, or both, or an adult friend or relative. (The patient could commit suicide alone.) It is voluntary euthanasia that

EXHIBIT 22-2

My Living Will
To My Family, My Physician, My Lawyer
and All Others Whom It May Concern

Death is as much a reality as birth, growth, maturity and old age—it is the one certainty of life. If the time comes when I can no longer take part in decisions for my own future, let this statement stand as an expression of my wishes and directions, while I am still of sound mind.

If at such a time the situation should arise in which there is no reasonable expectation of my recovery from extreme physical or mental disability, I direct that I be allowed to die and not be kept alive by medications, artificial means or "heroic measures". I do, however, ask that medication be mercifully administered to me to alleviate suffering even though this may shorten my remaining life.

This statement is made after careful consideration and is in accordance with my strong convictions and beliefs. I want the wishes and directions here expressed carried out to the extent permitted by law. Insofar as they are not legally enforceable, I hope that those to whom this Will is addressed will regard themselves as morally bound by these provisions.

(Optional specific provisions to be made in this space)

DURABLE POWER OF ATTORNEY (optional)

I hereby designate _____ to serve as my attorney-in-fact for the purpose of making medical treatment decisions. This power of attorney shall remain effective in the event that I become incompetent or otherwise unable to make such decisions for myself.

Optional Notarization: Signed_____

"Sworn and subscribed to   Date _____

before me this _____ day   Witness _____
of _____, 19_____."
                                             _____
                                                              Address
_____   Witness _____
         Notary Public
           (seal)   _____
                                                              Address
Copies of this request have been given to _____

_____   _____

(Optional)   My Living Will is registered with Concern for Dying (No. _____)

Source: Distributed by Concern for Dying, 250 W. 57th Street, New York, NY 10017.

the natural death laws seek to serve. Involuntary euthanasia, sometimes called *mercy killing,* is performed by someone other than the patient without the patient's consent, possibly because of unconsciousness. There are many pros and cons of euthanasia, with arguments usually falling into secular or religious categories.[49,50] Nevertheless, according to the law, euthanasia is murder. In cases where a physician, nurse, or family have "pulled the plug" or otherwise carried out involuntary euthanasia, and there appeared to be no ulterior motive, the jury has usually freed the individual, often on the basis of temporary insanity. In 1979, however, a Maryland nurse was indicted for murder for discontinuing life support systems of brain dead patients. She did not deny that she had done so, but based her not guilty pleas on the fact that the patients were brain dead GORKs (God only really knows), according to local terminology.[51] She was acquitted but lost her license. (Although she was termed compassionate by her nursing colleagues, they felt obligated to report her actions when she would not stop.)

Orders Not to Resuscitate

Patients in irreversible coma may have orders not to resuscitate (*no code, code blue,* or other terms), with or without the consent and knowledge of the family. Are nurses in legal jeopardy if they obey? Are they in trouble if they choose not to? To a great extent, these questions remain unanswered, because families may choose to let the patient die but do not want to say so, and many codes have been carried out with little discussion after the decision was made. Nurses who object on moral or religious grounds cannot be forced to participate (but for some people, it is just as wrong to resuscitate). However, without a specific hospital protocol, *not resuscitating* could be considered malpractice.

Nonwritten orders are a special problem for the nurse. Some physicians believe, wrongly, that their liability is dispelled by not writing a "do not resuscitate (DNR)" order, or cloaking the intent with words such as "comfort nursing measures only." Sometimes a *slow code* is understood or carried out by nurses when a terminally ill patient is not put on DNR. This means that they do not hurry to alert the emergency team. Again, the fear is that the doctor or hospital would be criminally or civilly liable. Even when the family agrees with the decision—and they should always be involved—there are times when both physicians and hospitals are hesitant to act. This does not seem reasonable when cardiopulmonary resuscitation (CPR) procedures were never intended for "cases of terminal irreversible illness where death is not unexpected."[52]

DNR orders are generally the responsibility of the attending physician. If a nurse carries out a verbal DNR or a slow code order, she assumes the risk that it will be disclaimed by the physician. An important AHA publication[53] reiterates that having nurses or other staff solely responsible for making DNR decisions is inappropriate and probably illegal. DNR orders are legally valid, provided that they are in accordance with accepted medical standards. Development of hospital policy on the matter is recommended, including review mechanisms. If there is continuing disagreement about resuscitation, the statement says, the case should be brought to court.

One of the mechanisms mentioned is an ethics committee, similar to what was mandated by the judge in the Quinlan case. The President's Commission, although concluding that the courts should only be a last resort as the decision makers for incompetent individuals, suggested that some form of review and consultation mechanism such as an ethics committee, should be considered. An ethics committee, in this context, is a "multidisciplinary group of health professionals within a health care situation that has been specifically established to address the ethical dilemmas that occur within the institution, such as those relating to the treatment or non-treatment of patients who lack decision-making capacities."[54] (Nurses are expected to be part of this group.)

Not many ethics committees had been

formed since the Quinlan case (that ruling was binding only in New Jersey), but the case of Infant Doe, discussed later, created a new impetus for their establishment. An AMA official predicted that soon all hospitals would have ethics committees. Suggested functions are education, development of policies and guidelines, consultation, and case review. Some hospitals are following the Massachusetts General Hospital model, in which some critically ill patients are put into four categories ranging from "maximal therapeutic effort" to "all therapy can be discontinued," with definitive protocols for each.[55] The arguments are strong that some policy should be set as a safeguard for all, including the patient.[56]

Greenlaw and other nurse attorneys are all in agreement that nurses should not be involved in slow codes or verbal orders, but there is no doubt that the nurse is intimately involved when a DNR decision must be considered. In some cases, as in long-term care facilities, the responsibility for review of DNR orders will fall on the nurse.[57] If there are no policies, nurses can be instrumental in the development of appropriate guidelines and procedures.

Current Issues

Considering the fact that it appears to be a person's basic legal right to make decisions about his or her own body, the proliferation of court cases on that issue may seem surprising. The lack of consistency in rulings is even more so as illustrated in these 1984 cases. When someone wants to discontinue kidney dialysis today because the quality of life is unacceptable, there is relatively little objection. But that may be because the patient is ambulatory and may simply choose not to come back for treatment. Yet when a competent seventy-year-old California man with multiple serious ailments, but not at the point of dying, wanted the right to have his respirator turned off because *he* found the quality of life unbearable, neither the hospital, nor the doctors, nor the court would allow him to do so,

and no other hospital or doctor would accept him. (He had signed a living will and other documents.) His arms were restrained to prevent any action on his part; the hospital said he continued to "live a useful life." His medical and hospital expenses were by then almost $500,000.[58] William Bartling died the day before the state appeals court heard his case. Six weeks later the court ruled that he did have the constitutional right to refuse medical treatment, including the respirator.

Also in California, a twenty-six-year-old woman almost totally paralyzed from cerebral palsy found the quality of her life intolerable and had herself admitted to a hospital and asked the staff to keep her comfortable and pain-free, but to let her starve herself to death. They refused, and a court supported that decision. She was described by psychiatrists as "mentally stable," not clinically depressed. She finally signed herself out to a nursing home in Mexico, but found that she would have been force-fed there also and consented to eat.[59] Later that year Elizabeth Bouvia returned to California and by early 1985 was being cared for in a "sanctuary" described as something like a half-way house. It is reported that she has not changed her mind about wanting to die and is waiting until she acquires a serious illness for which she can legally refuse treatment. On the other hand, an elderly man with multiple conditions who was in a nursing home was permitted to fast until he died.

Two California physicians were charged with murder because they discontinued the intravenous feedings on a fifty-five-year-old man who had a "severe anoxic cerebral injury" and was comatose. The family had requested no further treatment. These charges were dropped, but a civil suit was pending for some time. In New Jersey, at the same time, a lower court agreed to removal of a nasogastric tube on an eighty-four-year-old incompetent (but not brain-dead) woman, Ms. Conroy, at the request of her nephew. The case was appealed, but the patient died before a final appellate decision was reached.[60] In both cases, nurses were involved. One or more nurses reported the California physicians to a right-to-life group. The nurse who had cared for Ms. Conroy testified in the case, in detail, as to Ms. Conroy's condition; she thought that the tube should not have been removed. In all of these cases, the nurses were the ones in intimate contact with the patient, and if the decision was to let the patient die, it was their responsibility to keep the patient as comfortable as possible.[61]

What will happen now? In what is probably the most comprehensive part of their 1983 report, *Deciding to Forego Life-Sustaining Treatment,* the President's Commission supported the patient's right to die[62] and the right of the patient and, secondly, the family to make that decision with the physician. (The data presented are unusually detailed.) The next year, a group of experienced physicians from various disciplines and institutions came to the conclusion that in relation to these issues, "the patient's role in decision-making is paramount, and a decrease in aggressive treatment when such treatment would only prolong a difficult and uncomfortable process of dying" is acceptable.[63] In summary, several important points were made. In dealing with a competent patient, the treatment should "reflect an understanding between patient and physician and should be reassessed from time to time." Patients who are determined to be brain-dead require no treatment. With patients in a persistent vegetative state, "it is morally justifiable to withhold antibiotics and artificial nutrition and hydration, as well as other forms of life-sustaining treatment, allowing the patient to die. (This requires family agreement and an attempt to ascertain what would have been the patient's wishes.)" Severely demented and irreversibly demented patients need only care to make them comfortable. It is ethically appropriate not to treat intercurrent illness. Again, the patient's previous desires and the family's wishes must be considered. With elderly patients who have permanent mild impairment of competence, the "pleasantly senile," emergency resuscita-

tion and intensive care should be provided "sparingly." The group did not touch on the impaired child or infant, but their care is perhaps among the most controversial right-to-live or right-to-die issues.

THE RIGHTS OF THE HELPLESS

Children, the mentally ill, the mentally retarded, and certain patients in nursing homes are often seen as relatively helpless, because they have been termed legally incompetent to make decisions about their health care for many years. Often the rights overlap, as when a child or elderly person is mentally retarded (as in the Saikewicz case). Some of the rights of the elderly are being protected by a legalized bill of rights.

The Mentally Disabled

For mental patients, state laws and some high court decisions have served the same purpose. Both have focused on mental patients' rights in the areas of voluntary and involuntary admissions; kind and length of restraints, including seclusion; informed consent to treatment, especially sterilization and psychosurgery; the rights of citizenship (voting); right of privacy, especially in relation to records; rights in research; and especially, the right to treatment.[64-66] Although rulings have varied, the trend is toward the protection of rights. The landmark decision of *Wyatt* v. *Stickney* (325 Federal Supplement, Alabama, 1972) clearly defined the purposes of commitment to a public hospital and the constitutional right to adequate treatment.[67]

More recently, an Oklahoma court's decision in *Rogers* v. *Okin* that gives a voluntary mental patient the right to refuse psychiatric medication created a furor.[68] The appeals court modified the ruling, holding that voluntary patients could be forced to choose between leaving the hospital or accepting the prescribed treatment. (Or physicians could modify the treatment.)[69] Later, a Massachusetts court ruled that an *incompetent* person could refuse medication if he was able to express a "sensible" opinion, unless there was a proven danger to the public. For certain extraordinary medical treatments, the courts would have the ultimate authority to decide whether treatment is given.[70]

In later situations, a structured internal review system in which patients could appeal treatment decisions has seemed to work. On the other hand, follow-up on patients who refused treatment showed a deterioration in their functioning when they were released to the community.[71]

In issues of informed consent, other rulings have determined that if the mentally incompetent cannot understand the benefits or dangers of treatment, the family must be fully informed and allowed to make the decision.[72] Some legal decisions relate to sterilization of the retarded, which came to a head when it was found that retarded adolescent black girls were being sterilized with neither the girls nor their mothers apparently having a clear notion of what that meant. Restraints were increasingly put on sterilization until, in 1979, DHEW tightened the regulations for federal participation in funding of sterilization procedures. Regulations included requirements of written and oral explanations of the operation, advice about alternate forms of birth control to be given in understandable language, and a waiting period. In addition, no federal funding was allowed for sterilization of those under twenty-one, mentally incompetent, or institutionalized in correctional facilities or mental hospitals. However, this does not mean that a parent cannot have a retarded girl sterilized; it means that more precautions are being taken by the courts and the government to ensure that the child's rights are not violated.[73] There is general concern for the rights of young people in the mental health system,[74] but parents maintain considerable control. In 1979, the Supreme Court upheld the constitutionality of state laws that allow parents to commit their minor children to state mental institutions; thirty-six states have such laws.[75]

Other Rights of Children and Adolescents*

The other rights of young people and children relate primarily to consent for treatment or research and protection against abuse. It is a general rule that a parent or guardian must give consent for the medical or surgical treatment of a minor except in an emergency when it is imperative to give immediate care to save the minor's life. Legally, however, anyone who is capable of understanding what he is doing may give consent, because age is not always an exact criterion of maturity or intelligence. Many minors are perfectly capable of deciding for themselves whether to accept or reject recommended therapy and, in cases involving simple procedures, the courts have refused to invoke the rule requiring the consent of a parent or guardian. If the minor is married or has been otherwise emancipated from his or her parents, there is likely to be little question legally. In addition, states cite different ages and situations in which parental permission is needed for medical treatment. The almost universal exception is allowing minors to consent to treatment for venereal disease, drug abuse, and pregnancy-related care.[76] Although it has been understood that health professionals have no legal obligation to report to parents that the minor has sought such treatment, a few states are beginning to add statutes that say that the minor does not need parental permission, but that parents must be notified. In 1983, the Reagan Administration issued a rule that would require parents to be notified whenever children under eighteen received any contraceptives from federally funded family planning clinics. After a number of court challenges, this was overruled as infringing on a woman's right to privacy.

The entire question of permission for contraception, abortion, and sterilization is in flux. The key appears to be a designation of *mature minor;* emancipated minors are treated as adults. As recently as 1972, the Supreme Court ruled that state statutes prohibit-

---

*Child abuse laws are discussed later.

ing the prescription of contraceptives to unmarried persons were unconstitutional because they interfere with the right of privacy of those desiring them.[77] However, it did not rule on a minor's right to privacy in seeking or buying contraceptives. This was left to the states, and a number still set age limitations from fourteen to twenty-one. In many, however, doctors and other health professionals may provide birth control information and prescribe contraceptives to patients of any age without parental consent.[78] Changes in federal and state laws also frequently require welfare agencies to offer family planning services and supplies to sexually active minors. In general, there has been a national trend toward granting minors the right to contraceptive advice and devices, but the political power of conservative groups who oppose this trend is being felt.

An even more dramatic change has occurred in relation to abortion. In 1976 the Supreme Court held that states may not constitutionally require the consent of a girl's parents for an abortion during the first twelve weeks of pregnancy. In addition, parents cannot either prevent or force an abortion on the daughter who, in the eyes of the Court, is now "a competent minor mature enough to have become pregnant." In the words of one federal court that overturned a parental consent statute:

> It is not they (the parents) who have to bear the child. . . . It is difficult to think of any self-interest that a parent would have that compares with those significant interests of the pregnant minor.[79]

Should the young woman decide against an abortion and elect to bear the child, she can receive care related to her pregnancy without parental consent in almost every state. An unwed mature minor may also consent to treatment of her child.[80]

Groups such as the American Academy of Pediatrics, the Society for Adolescent Medicine, and the National Association of Children's Hospitals and Related Institutions have taken stands on protecting the rights of minors in health care. For example, the AAP Committee on Youth has presented a model act for consent of minors for health services, recommended for enactment in all states.[81] The Pediatric Bill of Rights may also be a forerunner to legal action, as was the AHA Patient's Bill of Rights. (Unless such a statement is incorporated into law, the effect is only moral, a guideline to encourage protection of rights, with no enforcement powers.) The Pediatric Bill of Rights deals with the rights of young people in the areas of counseling and treatment for birth control, abortion, pregnancy, drug or alcohol dependency, venereal disease, confidentiality, and information about her or his condition, as well as protection if a parent refuses consent for needed treatment.[82] A psychologist suggested an extension to the Pediatric Bill of Rights, believing that "children will be as competent as society allows them to be."[83] Actually, cases in which mature minors are being permitted to make life-and-death decisions are increasing. An example is the case of a thirteen-year-old who chose not to have a bone marrow transplant because of religious beliefs and potential danger to her donor sister.

The question of whether parents may make a decision for a child if the child's well-being is their prime consideration, as in giving Laetrile to a leukemic child, has not been decided with any consistency. (For that matter, neither has the legality of Laetrile.)[84] Two very diverse cases are often cited in relation to these issues.[85] Chad Green's parents refused life-prolonging treatment for this cancer patient, choosing instead various unorthodox treatments like Laetrile. When ordered by the court to allow the child to be given cancer therapy, they fled with him to Mexico. He died shortly thereafter. Phillip Becker was an institutionalized retarded child who had been diagnosed as having Down's syndrome. His parents never established any parental bonding relationship with him and seldom visited. When it was discovered that he had a congenital heart defect, his parents refused consent for cardiac catheterization or surgery. The court upheld the decision. Shortly thereafter, a volunteer couple who had been attracted to him petitioned for guardianship, which was granted. Phillip later had the surgery and recovered.

The legal principles involved are *parental autonomy,* a constitutionally protected right; *parens patriae,* the state's right and duty to protect the child; the *best interest doctrine,* which requires the court to determine what is best for the child; and the *substituted judgment doctrine,* in which the court determines what choice an incompetent individual would make if he or she were competent. (The last could also apply to other mentally incompetent and unconscious individuals discussed earlier.)

Another unresolved issue is whether the grossly deformed neonate should be allowed to live. Few judges will rule to let it die, but often the decision is quietly made by parents and health personnel.[86] These situations are especially difficult for a nurse who may see the infant simply starve to death. More nurses and others are reporting such situations, but as in the right-to-die issue, ethical and moral considerations weigh strongly.

Several landmark cases occurred in the early 1980s. In Illinois, newborn Siamese twins joined below the waist and sharing an intestinal track and three legs were not expected to live. "Do not feed, in accordance with parents' wishes" was written on the chart. However, several nurses did feed the babies, and someone reported the situation to a government agency. A court order was obtained to gain temporary custody of the children, and a neglect petition was filed. The parents (a doctor and nurse) and the doctor were charged with attempted murder, a charge which was later dismissed. Four months later, they regained custody of the children, whose care had mounted to several hundred thousand dollars. They were also in danger of losing their licenses.[87]

In Indiana, about a year later, a Baby Doe was born with Down's syndrome and a correctable esophageal fistula. The parents refused surgery, and their decision was upheld by the courts. The child was deprived of artificial nutritional life support and died. Although similar action had been taken in other Baby Doe cases, this one came to the attention of President Reagan. It resulted in an HHS regulation that threatened hospitals that neglected such children with loss of funds under Section 504 of the Rehabilitation Act of 1973 (which protects the handicapped). Large signs had to be posted alerting people to a "hot line" number to call to report such incidents. After a series of legal challenges, this regulation was ruled unconstitutional—"arbitrary and capricious," among other things. Eventually, an alternative suggestion by the American Academy of Pediatrics was agreed on: establishment of infant bioethics committees (IBC) with diverse membership whose responsibility, in part, would be to advise about decisions to withhold or withdraw life-sustaining measures.[88,89] It was later reported that the hot line saved the lives of three unidentified infants.

Finally, in 1983, Baby Jane Doe was born in New York with multiple serious congenital conditions, one of which required immediate surgery. The family was told that even if she lived, she would be in a vegetative state, so after consultation with a physician and a religious advisor, they opted for conservative treatment. A right-to-life attorney from Vermont learned of the case and managed to be appointed guardian by a like-minded judge, but this was overruled by an appeals court. Other right-to-life groups attempted to intervene; so did the federal government, which demanded the child's medical records to see if Section 504 was being violated. After considerable time, effort, and money had been spent, the government finally gave up.[90] The child survived on conservative treatment and went home, where she requires constant care because of her paralysis and lack of mental development. The parents, who would like to have another child, feel that they cannot do so because of the cost and time involved in this child's care.

Many questions are raised by these cases, and all are concerns of nursing. Creighton discusses a number of similar cases, as well as a Yale study in which some malformed infants were allowed to die with parental and physician consent. She notes how a nurse can influence a family to accept their deformed baby by emphasizing the normal.[91] Such cases will certainly continue, and the issue is not easily resolved; it is not just the rights of the infant that must be considered, but also those of the family and society. However, it appears that the federal government is setting a pattern for intervention. In late 1984, the ''Baby Doe'' bill, the Child Abuse Amendments of 1984, was signed into law. PL 98–45 made federal funding for a state's child protective services agency contingent on the establishment of procedures for reporting instances of medical neglect of newborns including ''withholding of medically indicated treatment from disabled infants with life threatening conditions.'' Some exceptions were indicated and establishment of IBCs was encouraged.

RIGHTS OF PATIENTS IN RESEARCH

The use of new, experimental drugs and treatments in hospitals, nursing homes, and other institutions that have a captive population—for example, prisons or homes for the mentally retarded—has been extensive. Nurses are often involved in giving the treatment or drugs. As noted earlier, DHHS regulations now require specific informed consent for any human research carried out under DHHS auspices, with strong emphasis on the need for a clear explanation of the experiment, possible dangers, and the subject's complete freedom to refuse or withdraw at any time.

In addition, the National Research Act of 1974 established a commission to, among other things, ''identify the requirements for informed consent procedures for children, prisoners, and the mentally disabled and determine the need for a mechanism to assure that human subjects not covered by HEW regulations are protected.''[92] (Part of that Commission report was cited previously.)

An interesting trend is toward including very young children in making decisions about research in which they are asked to participate. In the past, as a rule, parents were asked whether they consented to their child's participation in research—medical, educational, psychological, or other. There has always been some concern as to whether the child should be subjected to such research if it was not at least potentially beneficial to him (such as the use of a new drug for a leukemic child). The child was seldom given the opportunity to decide whether or not to participate. New knowledge of the potential harm that could be done to the child, however innocuous the experiment, and appreciation of the child as a human being with individual rights have now resulted in recommendations that even a very young child be given a simple explanation of the proposed research and allowed to participate or not, or even to withdraw later, without any form of coercion.[93-95] Given that choice, some children have decided not to participate.[96] Overall, though, the support for using healthy children in research or being volunteered for procedures not beneficial to themselves is eroding. A recent development is that in 1983 DHHS published rules requiring children's consent to participate in research.[97]

Nurses were in the forefront of the move to protect subjects, with a statement in the ANA Code of Ethics, ''The nurse participates in research activities when assured that the rights of individual subjects are protected,'' as well as an extensive ANA document on research guidelines.* When the nurse is participating in

---

*See Chapter 10.

research, at whatever level, ensuring that the rights of patients are honored is both an ethical and a legal responsibility. Nurses should know the patients' rights: self-determination to choose to participate; to have full information; to terminate participation without penalty; privacy and dignity; conservation of personal resources; freedom from arbitrary hurt and intrinsic risk of injury; as well as the special rights of minor and incompetent persons previously discussed.[98] For instance, nurses have been ordered to begin an experimental drug knowing that the patient has not given an informed consent. The nurse is then obligated to see that that patient does have the appropriate explanation. This is one more case in which institutional policy that sets an administrative protocol for the nurse in such a situation is helpful.[99]

If the nurse is the investigator, she or he must observe all the usual requirements, such as informed consent and confidentiality. An interesting phenomenon that has been uncovered is that because nurses are generally trusted by patients, subjects will participate "for the nurse," but either refuse to sign the consent or not listen to an explanation, as being unnecessary.[100,101] The quality of research in which human subjects are involved is particularly important. Peer review, such as that offered by a hospital review board, can be helpful.[102] Although sometimes there are no nurses on the board, nurses present bring a useful perspective to the review.[103]

Unfortunately, these boards, required if the research is DHHS funded, have been found to be less protective of patients' rights than they should be, especially in the area of informed consent. There is usually no follow-up to determine whether the plans to preserve subjects' rights that are presented in the proposals are really carried through. There is also criticism about lack of consistency in proposal approval.[104] The nurse, as a primary investigator or participant, is in a position to see that these rights are not abrogated.

PATIENT RECORDS: CONFIDENTIALITY AND AVAILABILITY

There is some evidence that in situations other than these legally required ones, confidentiality of patients' records is frequently violated. Everyone has access except the patient.

"The tremendous growth of computerized health data, the development of huge data banks, and the advancements in record linkage pose an enormous threat to the privacy of medical information," says a position paper on confidentiality adopted by the American Medical Records Association. "The public is generally unaware of this threat or of the serious consequences of a loss of confidentiality in the health care system. Adequate measures to control medical privacy in the light of electronic information processing can and must be established . . .."[105]

A national study pointed out that from birth certificate to death certificate, the health and medical records of most Americans are part of a system that allows access by insurance companies, student researchers, and governmental agencies, to name a few, and that the information is often shared illegally with others such as employers. The report's author, Alan Westin, recommended that:

Health data systems should be created, altered and periodically audited through public rather than closed procedures.

Every health data system should put limits on relevance and social propriety of the personal information it collects and records.

Every health data system should have clear rules and procedures to insure citizen rights.

Health data system managers should take special measures to protect the accuracy and the security of the data they keep.

Managers should follow special procedures to allow medical research, health care evaluation and public oversight without impairing citizens' rights.[106]

Many states have enacted laws to protect medical records, and the federal Freedom of Information Act (FOIA) denies access to an individual's medical record without that person's consent. Still, there are practical problems: if certain data are needed, as in following through on occupational health hazards, can exceptions be made for research that would be beneficial to the well-being of people? The problem is not in aggregate figures, but occurs when individual records must be scrutinized.[107] Researchers were quite concerned with enactment of the 1974 Privacy Act* because DHEW-funded research projects involving human subjects would be available to anyone, including participating subjects, by filing a request. Some of these cases are and will continue to go to court, but there seems to be a definite legislative and judicial trend toward safeguarding medical records and, in addition, giving patients access to their own records.

Most physicians and health administrators, however, have been hostile toward the concept of sharing the record with the patient. Some attorneys serving health care facilities tend to share that feeling, one group of authors writing that "it is undesirable to allow patient or family to inspect the chart. [They] might find comments . . . which may be considered uncomplimentary or incorrect. The patient may then attempt to have the record changed or cause annoyance to the administration or the medical staff."[108] The writer was also concerned about the possibility of libel suits and suggested the omission of "characterizations or other remarks which may offend" in the chart abstract (which could be given to the patient).

The time when there is a choice in the matter of sharing the record may be ending. Whereas it is legally recognized that the patient's record is the property of the hospital or physician (in his office), the information that the record contains is not similarly protected. Both states and the federal government are legislating access—either direct patient access, with or without a right to copy or indirect access (physician, attorney, or provision of a summary only). In 1979, nineteen states allowed patients direct access to their records; others are following. States may differentiate between doctors' and hospital records and have other idiosyncratic qualifications.[109] Of course, one certain way in which the patient can get access is through a malpractice suit in which the record is subpoenaed, a costly process for both provider and consumer. Westin's study recommended giving patients access, and he anticipated that this was an inevitability.[110] The Privacy Protection Study Commission, created by the 1974 Privacy Act, also included recommendations on patient access. One federal step in this direction was the same FOIA and Privacy Act that prevented unauthorized access. Included are any records under the control of any agency of the federal government that contain an individual's name or any other identifying information. Medical records are specifically cited and include those of patients in the Veterans Administration and other federal hospitals. Whether patients receiving medical care under Medicare are included is a subject of debate.

Although perhaps the majority of physicians and hospitals still object to the open record concept because of the notion that patients wouldn't understand, would be frightened, or might choose to treat themselves, a new philosophy is developing to share the record with the patient so that both provider and consumer have an open relationship and decide on the needed care together. A health care center associated with the University of Vermont stated in its "Principles of Practice":

> The best care of the patient is assured when the patient is part of the team and he shares his medical records with the providers of care. This is best effected by assuring that the rec-

---

*See Chapter 19.

ord is complete, well organized, and available to the patient so that he can review the record for reliability, the subjective data and clarity of plans for treatment and education.[111]

Annas and others suggest that if the record is too technical, a knowledgeable patient advocate could be of assistance.[112] (Patient advocates are also recommended for other supportive purposes.) Does the nurse have any legal responsibility to be that intermediary? The answer is more complex than just yes or no. Certainly, a nurse would not hand a patient the chart at request, for that would be inappropriate. Most states, as well as health care agencies, that permit access to records have a protocol to be followed. This usually involves providing both privacy and an opportunity for the physician and/or another person to explain the content. Many hospitals are now willing to have the patient see the record, because the administration realizes that if the patient is concerned enough to demand his chart and it is withheld, the next step is probably a malpractice suit;[113] others agree that access is a right, or at least a trend, and are not waiting for legislation. Both Annas[114] and Auerbach[115] give specific directions for obtaining records.

Privacy

Nurses and others who work with patients must be especially careful to avoid invading the patient's right to privacy, which is identical to that of any other person. There are a number of special concerns. With the advent of computerized records, the patient's privacy might easily be violated.[116] Consent to treatment does not cover the use of a picture without specific permission, nor does it mean that the patient can be subjected to repeated examinations not necessary to therapy without express consent.

Exceptions to respect for the patient's privacy are related to legal reporting obligations. All states have laws requiring hospitals, doctors, nurses, and sometimes other health workers to report on certain kinds of situations, because the patient may be unwilling or unable to do so. The nurse often has responsibility in these matters because, although it may be the physician's legal obligation, the nurse may be the only one actually aware of the situation. Even if such reporting is not required by a law per se, regulations of various state agencies may require such a report. Common reporting requirements are for communicable diseases, diseases in newborn babies, gunshot wounds, and criminal acts, including rape. More recently, reporting a physically abused or neglected child (battered child)* has been given legal attention, and every state and the District of Columbia has such a law.[117] Although other kinds of reporting are relatively objective, there are problems in reporting abused children because of the varying definitions of *child* and the question of whether there was abuse or an accident, with the consequent fear of parents suing. Usually, however, the person reporting is protected if good faith exists. In some states, there are penalties for *not* reporting such situations. The nurse may also be obligated to testify about otherwise confidential information in criminal cases.

Ethical practice prohibits the professional person from divulging any confidential information to anyone else, unless possibly to another physician or nurse who serves as a consultant. Neither does the ethical person engage in gossip based on this information, trivial and harmless though it may seem at the time. Moreover, the professional nurse has an obligation to set a good example for others in nonprofessional groups who may be less aware of their responsibilities in this respect.

Confidential information obtained through professional relationships is not the same as *privileged communication,* which is a legal concept providing that a physician and patient, attorney and client, and priest and penitent have a special privilege. Should any court action arise in which the person (or persons) involved is called to testify, the law (in many

---

*Wife abuse and parent abuse are also becoming reportable.

states) will not require that such information be divulged. Not all states acknowledge that nurses can be recipients of privileged communication, but there are specific cases in which the nurse–patient privilege has been accepted.[118] A relatively new issue is that psychiatric nurses, like other psychotherapists, have a responsibility to warn potential victims about their homicidal clients.[119]

ASSAULT AND BATTERY

Assault and battery, although often discussed with emphasis on the criminal interpretation, also has a patients' rights aspect that is related to everyday nursing practice, especially when dealing with certain types of patients.[120] Grounds for civil action might include the following:

1. Forcing a patient to submit to a treatment for which he has not given his consent either expressly in writing, orally, or by implication. Whether or not a consent was signed, a patient should not be forced, for resistance implies a withdrawal of consent.
2. Forcefully handling an unconscious patient.
3. Lifting a protesting patient from his bed to a wheelchair or stretcher.
4. Threatening to strike or actually striking an unruly child or adult, except in self-defense.
5. Forcing a patient out of bed to walk post-operatively.
6. In some states, performing alcohol, blood, urine, or health tests for presumed drunken driving without consent. There are some "implied consent" statutes in motor vehicle codes that provide that a person, for the privilege of being allowed to drive, gives an implied consent to furnishing a sample of blood, urine, or breath for chemical analysis when charged with driving while intoxicated. However, if the person objects and is forced, it might still be considered battery. Several states, ac-

knowledging this, have enacted legislation to insulate hospital employees and health professionals from liability.[121]

As a rule, intentional torts, such as assault and battery, are not covered by malpractice insurance.

FALSE IMPRISONMENT

As the term implies, *false imprisonment* means "restraining a person's liberty without the sanction of the law, or imprisonment of a person who is later found to be innocent of the crime for which he was imprisoned." The term also applies to many procedures that actually or conceivably are performed in hospital and nursing situations *if they are performed without the consent of the patient or his legal representative.*[122] In most instances, the nurse or other employee would not be held liable if it can be proved that what was done was necessary to protect others.

Among the most common nursing situations that might be considered false imprisonment are the following:

1. Restraining a patient by physical force or using appliances without written consent, especially in procedures where the use of restraints is not usually necessary. This is, or may be, a delicate situation because if you do not use a restraint, such as siderails, to protect a patient, you may be accused of negligence, and if you use them without consent, you may be accused of false imprisonment. This is a typical example of the need for prudent and reasonable action that a court of law would undoubtedly uphold.
2. Restraining a mentally ill patient who is neither dangerous to himself nor to others. For example, patients who wander about the hospital division making a nuisance of themselves usually cannot legally be locked in a room unless they show signs of violence.

3. Using arm, leg, or body restraints to keep a patient quiet while administering an intravenous infusion may be considered false imprisonment. If this risk is involved—that is, if the patient objects to the treatment and refuses to consent to it—the physician should be called. Should the doctor order restraints for the patient, make sure that the order is given in writing before allowing anyone to proceed with the treatment. It is much better to assign someone to stay with the patient throughout a procedure than to use restraint without authorization.

4. Detaining an unwilling patient in the hospital. If a patient insists on going home, or a parent or guardian insists on taking a minor or other dependent person out of the hospital before his condition warrants it, hospital authorities cannot legally require him to remain. In such instances, the doctor should write an order permitting the hospital to allow the patient to go home "against advice," and the hospital's representative should see that the patient or guardian signs an official form absolving the hospital, medical staff, and nursing staff of all responsibility should the patient's early departure be detrimental to his health and welfare. If the patient refuses to sign, a record should be made on the chart of exactly what occurred, and an incident report probably should be filed. Take the patient to the hospital entrance in the usual manner.

5. Detaining for an unreasonable period of time a patient who is medically ready to be discharged. The delay may be due to the patient's inability to pay his bill or to an inordinate wait, at his expense, for the delivery of an orthopedic appliance or other service. In such instances, the nurse or nursing department may or may not be directly involved, but it is always wise to know the possibility of legal developments and to exercise sound judgment in order to be completely fair to the patient and avoid trouble.

LEGAL ISSUES RELATED TO REPRODUCTION

Laws permitting abortion* have varied greatly from state to state over the years. In early 1973, the Supreme Court ruled that no state can interfere with a woman's right to obtain an abortion during the first trimester (twelve weeks) of pregnancy. During the second trimester, the state may interfere only to the extent of imposing regulations to safeguard the health of women seeking abortions. During the last trimester of pregnancy, a state may prohibit abortions except when the mother's life is at stake (*Doe* v. *Bolton* and *Roe* v. *Wade*).

Theoretically, all hospitals are required to perform abortions within these guidelines, and it is legal to assist with such a procedure; actually, the right cannot be withheld. However, because of religious and moral reasons, some institutions are exempted from complying with the law, and individual doctors and nurses have refused to participate in abortions. Individual professionals or other health workers may make that choice, and there is legal support for them (conscience clause).[123] This does not preclude the right of the hospital to dismiss a nurse for refusing to carry out an assigned responsibility or to transfer her to another unit. There have been some suits by nurses objecting to transfer, but rulings have varied.

The Supreme Court has also addressed the issue of the spouse's consent and found that such consent was not necessary. As mentioned earlier, the courts are also moving in the direction of not distinguishing between adult and minor females on abortion rights.[124]

More than ten years after the *Roe* v. *Wade* decision, opinions are still strong on abortion issues.[125,126] The major court cases have been in relation to legislation attempting to outlaw or limit abortion. In one major case, the Su-

---

*Legislation relating to abortion is discussed in Chapter 19; other aspects are covered in Chapter 6.

preme Court struck down an Akron, Ohio, ordinance that placed numerous obstacles in the way of a woman who chose abortion.[127] In several others, it supported the Hyde Amendment, which declares that states have no constitutional obligation to pay for abortions.[128]

Sterilization means "termination of the ability to produce offspring." Both laws and regulations have been in the process of change. If the life of a woman may be jeopardized if she becomes pregnant, a therapeutic sterilization may be performed with consent of the patient and sometimes her husband, although the latter rule is being challenged. If no statutes or judicial decisions state a policy against therapeutic sterilization, such operations may be considered medically necessary. If there is no medical necessity, the operation is termed *sterilization of convenience* or *contraceptive sterilization*. In some states, this is illegal; in others, arguable. Only a few states regulate therapeutic sterilization. Here too, consents are often required from the individual and spouse, and there may be a mandatory waiting period. The consequences of the operation must be made clear to all concerned, and often a special consent form is required. There seems to be little legal concern about male sterilization, *vasectomy*, which is being done with increasing frequency. The legal consequences of unsuccessful sterilization, both male and female, have resulted in suits. Called *wrongful birth*, these suits usually seek to recover the costs of raising an unplanned or unwanted child, normal or abnormal—but usually the latter. Judgments have varied, but are more likely to favor the plaintiff if the child is abnormal.[129]

Eugenic sterilization is the attempt to eliminate specific hereditary defects by sterilizing individuals who could pass on such defects to their offspring. Once, approximately half the states authorized eugenic sterilization of the mentally deficient, mentally ill, and others, but since the case mentioned earlier, only a few do so.[130] Legality where no law exists is questionable. Civil or criminal liability for assault and battery may be imposed on anyone

sterilizing another without following legal procedure or specific legal guidelines.

Laws on *family planning,* in general, also vary greatly. Some laws appear to be absolute prohibitions against information about contraceptive materials, but courts usually allow considerable freedom. The Economic Opportunity Amendments of 1967 made family planning one of the eight national emphasis efforts and funded it accordingly. Family planning programs are growing under federal, state, and private aegis, because many individuals and groups see family planning as a basic human right. Nurses are particularly involved, for they do much of this counselling, either as specialists or as part of their general nursing role. Because there are still some state limitations and, as noted earlier, the federal government is becoming more involved, it is important for the nurse to keep up to date in this area.

Artificial insemination, the injection of seminal fluid by instrument into a female to induce pregnancy, is evolving into an acceptable medical procedure used by childless couples. (Consent by the husband and wife is generally required.) Homologous artificial insemination (AIH) uses the semen of the husband and appears to present no legal dangers for doctors or nurses. Heterologous artificial insemination (AID) uses the semen of someone other than the husband and does raise the question of the child's legitimacy. On occasion, the question of adultery also arises in the courts if the husband's consent has not been obtained. Few states have enacted statutes to deal with the AID situation.[131] When a woman, for a fee, is artificially inseminated with a man's sperm and bears a child, who is then turned over to the man and his wife, this is termed *surrogate motherhood*. It has already created some legal problems, once when the woman decided not to give up the child and again when neither wanted a baby born with a birth defect. Even the legality of the process is in doubt.[132]

Among the most controversial legal concerns related to reproduction are *in vitro fer-*

tilization and *surrogate embryo transfer,* each of which is intended to enhance the fertility of infertile couples. Just one of the issues is related to patenting the process. Annas suggests that such commercial patenting should be rejected unless the patent holder can assure quality control and reproductive privacy.[133]

One relatively new legal aspect of human reproduction concerns the field of *genetics,* with which nurses, physicians, and lay genetic counselors must be concerned. Some of the issues have to do with AID, human genetic disease, genetic screening, *in vitro* fertilization (IVF), and genetic data banks. In addition, legislation, such as the National Sickle Cell Anemia, Cooley's Anemia, Tay-Sachs, and Genetic Diseases Act, has encouraged or forced states to expand genetic screening to cover other disorders. Neonatal screening, for instance, will probably be expanded considerably and offers new opportunities and responsibilities for nurses. But with what is still a relatively new science, many legal questions will be evolving.[134] Confidentiality is of major importance. If a genetic disease is discovered, the counselor should not contact other relatives, even if it would benefit those relatives, without the screenee's consent. One emerging problem is *wrongful life,* which occurs when a deformed baby is born, although abortion was an option, because the physician or other counselor neglected to tell parents of the risk.[135] Informed consent that enables the patient to make such serious decisions as having an abortion, sterilization, or artificial insemination is also vital.

TRANSPLANTS AND ARTIFICIAL PARTS

Since Dr. Christian Barnard performed the first human heart transplant in 1967, the question of tissue and organ *transplants* has become a point of controversy. Tissue may be obtained from living persons or a dead body. With the living person, the major legal impli-cations relate to negligence and informed consent.[136]

The greatest legal problems arise from procurement of tissue and organs from a dead body. The major question is, "When is an individual dead?" When the definition of death as brain death has not been clarified, there have been suits against doctors and hospitals concerning removal of organs before "death," as seen by the family, even if it was a desire of the patient.

Common law once prevented the decedent from donating his own body or individual organs if the next of kin objected and statutes prohibited mutilation of bodies. However, now, most states have adopted, in one form or another, the *Uniform Anatomical Gift Act,* approved in 1968 by the National Conference of Commissioners on Uniform State Laws. The basic purposes are to permit an individual to control the disposition of his own body after death, to encourage such donations, to eliminate unnecessary and complicated formalities regarding the donation of human tissues and organs, to provide the necessary safeguards to protect the varied interests involved, and to define clearly the rights of the next of kin, the physician, the health institution, and the public (as represented by the medical examiner) in relation to the dead body. The act provides that "any person who has attained majority may give all or any part of his body for research, transplantation, education, or for the general advancement of medical science, and may designate as the donee any hospital, surgeon, physician, medical or dental school or anatomical board."[137] The anatomical gift must be made in writing at least fifteen days prior to the donor's death. There is no obligation for the donee to accept the gift.

An autopsy (postmortem examination) by a licensed physician may be authorized by the deceased during his lifetime or after his death by the surviving spouse. In some states, the nearest living kin, who claims the body, may give the authorization. Physicians have the responsibility of getting the family's permission, although the nurses may be asked to witness the form. Sometimes they are also asked to encourage the family to agree to autopsy; there is no legal obligation one way or the other. In most states, an unclaimed body falls under the jurisdiction of the state's anatomical board and may be used for any legitimate purpose. Usually, unattended deaths or deaths of suspicious origin must be autopsied by a city (or other official) medical examiner.

A word should be said about the future legal implications of artificial parts. One concern is whether these will be paid for by government funds. Another is whether an individual, such as Barney Clark, who received the first artificial heart, would have the right to disconnect the equipment if the quality of life was found to be untenable.

NURSES' RIGHTS

Nurses may have more legal responsibilities because of their RN status, but they have the same rights as any other citizen. In relation to a nurse's profession, Fagin lists seven basic rights:

1. The right to find dignity in self-expression and self-enhancement through the use of our special abilities and educational background.
2. The right to recognition for our contribution through the provision of an environment for its practice, and proper, professional economic rewards.
3. The right to a work environment which will minimize physical and emotional stress and health risks.
4. The right to control what is professional practice within the limits of the law.
5. The right to set standards for excellence in nursing.
6. The right to participate in policy making affecting nursing.
7. The right to social and political action in behalf of nursing and health care.[138]

In addition is the human/professional right to participate in professional decision making.

Many of the legal rights of nurses are delineated in the nurse practice acts (Chapter 20), an indication of the power and privilege given by society. Nevertheless, some of the rights nurses may assume they have, such as being patient advocates, may conflict with the rights other professionals see as theirs or what employers see as inappropriate for employees.[139] There are those who believe that nurses should want no rights, because the concept of rights is interpreted as being given only to the powerless.[140]

Employment Rights

Since most working nurses are employees, knowing their rights in that respect is very important. One common worry is being fired, particularly when positions are hard to find. Can you be fired without reason? The answer is yes, if you have no contract.[141] (This will be discussed later.) The law allows an employee to sue for wrongful discharge when the discharge is contrary to public policy or well-being, such as when a nurse is fired for refusing to carry out an illegal act (perhaps contrary to the nursing practice act). Nurses have sued for reinstatement on similar grounds, as when a head nurse was fired for failing to reduce staff overtime. She argued that this would endanger patient welfare, introducing the nursing practice act as support. However, the court ruled against her.[142] She did not cite the ANA code, although another nurse did when she gave information to JCAH investigators about substandard conditions and was fired. In this case, the National Labor Relations Board supported her, although she was not a union member. Whistle blowing, which frequently results in being fired, is usually supported by the courts.[143]

Due process—that is, an orderly way to ensure that the employee has had adequate foreknowledge of the possible consequences of an act, that an effort was made to discover whether that employee did indeed violate a rule or order, that the investigation was held fairly and objectively, that the application of rules was even-handed, and that the penalty was in line with the offense[144]—is an important protection.

Another point to check in order to determine whether you have a case is whether your civil rights were violated. One recent case concerned the rights of a pregnant woman who was fired rather than given a leave because she was exposed to hazardous materials.[145]

Whether you can safely refuse an assignment is not clear. Employers are usually required to offer an alternate position if the refusal is on the basis of a conscience clause. However, if you refuse that assignment, you have little recourse.[146] One situation that has been gaining attention is fair treatment for nurses who cannot work on certain days for religious reasons. As might be expected, rulings have differed, so further Equal Employment Opportunity Commission (EEOC) and/ or legal suits can be expected. A factor is whether the nurse is offered and is willing to accept alternatives, such as working other holidays or Sundays. Other areas of discrimination are related to racial discrimination[147] and, increasingly, discrimination against male nurses. In a major case, a woman judge in Arkansas upheld a ban on male RNs in the delivery room, ruling that "Due to the intimate touching required in labor and delivery, services of all male nurses are very inappropriate."[148] (What about the services of the male doctor?) Similar cases were lost for a male nurse doing private duty who had never been assigned a woman patient and one in a nursing home who was not permitted to care for women. Here the judge ruled that it might upset the elderly women. A landmark case was heard by the Supreme Court, which ruled that an all-women's nursing school could not refuse to admit a male student.[149]

Other nurses have fought sex discrimination on the job, such as the Denver nurses who fought for comparable worth,[150] and nursing faculty who have suffered rank and salary discrimination. These are still open issues with varying results. For instance, the Supreme Court refused to hear the Denver case; it also ruled against the faculty at the University of Washington in another comparable worth case.[151] Rank and salary discrimination cases have been won, on occasion, but not always.

An unusual case was that of two nurses who were fired for having "outside interests," their private practice carried on outside of their hospital working hours. The nurses knew that it was common practice for men employed by the hospital to have second jobs or private patients. Sixteen months later, an EEOC investigation found "reasonable cause" to believe that they were victims of sex discrimination. When the hospital would not accept this finding, the nurses brought suit. Finally, the hospital settled out of court.[152]

Another type of civil rights violation, discrimination against the handicapped, has also resulted in contradictory judgments, usually because the situation was not clear-cut.[153] In one case related to a partially deaf PN student who wanted to enter an RN program, the Supreme Court ruled against her on the basis of her inability to function adequately at that level.[154]

A number of other rights came into play in the job situation. One is related to on-the-job safety,[155] another to sexual harassment, which has become a more visible problem for women.[156] Action is gradually being taken in support of these women, with not only the harassers but also the employer considered liable.[157]

Does it pay to stand up for your patients? A nurse, acting as a patient advocate, who speaks up for the patient can have a problem; some nurses have been fired. At least one won a dramatic victory. She publicly criticized the care of patients in a state mental hospital, after leaving there in frustration because the administration neither listened to her nor made an effort to improve conditions. She was hired by another state institution but dismissed shortly afterwards because of "incompetence." A newspaper had printed her complaints about the first hospital, and this caused "staff anxiety." There was no grievance procedure, so eventually she instituted a lawsuit. Both the American Civil Liberties

Union and the Pennsylvania Nurses' Association joined as *amicus curiae.* The court ruled in her favor, noting that incompetence was unproven and also an afterthought in her discharge, and that the employer simply wanted to get rid of an outspoken employee; the nurse's First Amendment rights had been violated. She was reinstated and awarded back pay.[158] In another case, a head nurse who reported that a patient's rights were being violated was fired after refusing to be demoted to a staff nurse job. The court held for her because she had not been deficient in her work. However, an appellate court, although agreeing that she had been unlawfully fired, reversed the reinstatement to head nurse because of her "insubordinate and critical attitude."[159]

Collective Bargaining

Some employment issues are resolved by collective bargaining. Since the enactment of PL 93-360 in 1974, employees of nonprofit institutions have joined the ranks of other workers who have collective bargaining rights. Labor laws are discussed in Chapter 19, but nurses' rights in the bargaining process are pertinent here.

The process of collective bargaining, because it is set by law, is similar regardless of who the bargaining agent is, and details can be found in any book on labor relations. In the context of ANA, that is, state nurses' associations (SNAs) as collective bargaining agents, the following is presented as a brief overview.

1. The nurses (or group of nurses) in an institution, discontented with a situation or conditions, and having exhausted the usual channels for correction or improvement, ask the SNA for assistance.
2. A meeting is held outside the premises of the institution and always on off-duty time. SNA staff and the nurses explore the problems, and the nurses are given advice about reasonable, negotiable issues and how to form a unit; for instance, they are told who can be included in a unit.

Administrative nurses are excluded, but the question of supervisors is still being debated in some places.

3. Authorization cards, which authorize the SNA to act as the nurses' bargaining representative, must be signed by at least 30 percent of the group to be represented. Membership forms are also suggested because the SNA cannot provide service without funds. All collective bargaining activity must be carried out in nonwork areas where the employee is protected from employer interference. (There are a series of NLRB rules governing employee distribution and solicitation.)
4. If sufficient cards are signed, the SNA notifies the employer that organization is going on, calling attention to the fact that the activity is protected. Copies of the notice are distributed to the nurses so that they know they are protected.
5. An informational meeting is held for all nurses and SNA staff.
6. If it is agreed that the SNA will represent the nurses, a bargaining unit is formed and officers are elected.
7. To seek voluntary recognition of the unit by the employer, a majority of the nurses must sign designation cards; this will probably be checked by a mutually accepted third party.
8. If the employer chooses not to recognize the unit, or if the designation is challenged by another union, a series of actions takes place, including an NLRB-conducted election. To petition for election, any union must have designation cards signed by 30 percent of the nurses in the proposed unit. The election is won or lost by the majority of nurses *voting.* They may vote for a particular union or specify none at all. The NLRB then certifies the winner as the exclusive bargaining agent. If the majority of nurses vote against *any* bargaining agent, the NLRB certifies this as well.
9. Assuming that the SNA wins the election, the SNA representative, at the direction

of the unit, attempts to settle the problems and complaints of the nurses by negotiating with administration. There are specific rules about what is negotiable. *Mandatory* subjects include salaries, fringe benefits, and conditions of employment, and both sides must bargain in good faith about these issues. *Voluntary* subjects can be almost anything else that *both* sides want to discuss, except for *prohibited* or illegal subjects such as a requirement that all workers become members of a union before being employed for thirty days. It should be remembered that the director of nursing, both through position and under law, is an administrator. Even though the director may be in complete support of the nurses' demands, he or she cannot join them. Quite often the director has previously tried unsuccessfully to help them achieve their goals.[160]

10. An agreement may or may not be reached, probably with some compromise on both sides. If there is agreement, a contract is signed outlining agreed-upon conditions and the responsibilities of each group. Contracts are renegotiated at set time periods, usually of several years. If no agreement can be reached, the dispute may be referred to binding or nonbinding arbitration by an outside group, or some job action such as picketing or a strike may occur. Picketing may be merely informational, to communicate the issues to the community, or it may be intended to prevent other employees or services from entering the institution. The latter, combined with a strike, is the very last resort, to be used when all other efforts fail. If such action is decided upon, sufficient notice is given to allow for disposition of patient care. Even if strikes are successful, there is often a lingering, unpleasant feeling between participants and nonparticipants. However, as ANA members agreed as they gradually removed no-strike clauses from ANA and SNA policies, the strike is an ultimate weapon that may be

necessary when the employer refuses any attempt to resolve the issues.

Once a labor contract is in place, there are times when individual nurses are in dispute with the employer. A grievance procedure is generally used to resolve the problem. A grievance may be caused by "an alleged violation of a contract provision, a change in a past practice, or an employer decision that is considered arbitrary, capricious, unreasonable, unfair, or discriminatory."[161] Simple complaints are not considered grievances. If informed discussion does not resolve the issue, a grievance procedure is followed. The steps include (1) written notice of the grievance, with a written response within a set time; (2) if the response is not satisfactory, an appeal to the director of nursing follows; (3) the employee, SNA representative, grievance chairman, and/or delegate, director of nursing, and director of personnel meet; (4) if no resolution occurs, the final step is arbitration by a neutral third party selected by both parties involved.[162] The technique for carrying out the process involves interpersonal, adversary, and negotiating skills.[163]

Whether or not a union is the answer to some of the problems of nurse employees,[164,165] the right to bargain is a valuable economic tool, as more nurses are beginning to realize.[166] There are alternatives to collective bargaining, and some have worked,[167] but sometimes it is the most useful tool for conflict resolution.[168] Nevertheless, there is still disagreement about whether collective bargaining is the solution to nursing's problems.[169] It is one way of controlling professional practice.[170]

Other Contracts

Whether or not nurses are unionized, a good contract is useful in defining employer–employee and patient–nurse agreements. Fewer problems arise when both parties understand the rights and responsibilities of each. Although sometimes not realizing it, nurses are continually making contracts, whether as employees or as independent practitioners. A *contract* is defined as a legally enforceable promise between two or more persons to do or not to do something. The essential elements of a contract are mutual assent, promises or considerations, two or more parties of competent legal capacity, and an agreement that is a lawful act and not against public policy. Contracts can be oral (verbally entered into) or written (all elements in writing). *Expressed contracts* are those in which specific terms have been agreed upon in writing or orally; *implied contracts* give rise to contractual obligations by some action or inaction without verbalization of terms. A *breach of contract* is the unjustified failure to fulfill the terms of the contract as agreed upon or when due. Three legal remedies are recognized: money damages, specific performance (what was promised must be carried out), and injunction (stopping a party from performing the act under other circumstances).

Several examples of nurse contracts can be given. A nurse seeks employment, and in the interview, employer and employee come to certain understandings. The nurse will perform the job safely, competently, and in accordance with the standards and policies of the institution (hours, dress, behavior). The employer will pay for those services (salary, fringes), will provide needed equipment to perform the services, and will maintain the facilities and equipment properly. (It might be noted at this point that if the nurse is hurt in an accident on the job, whether or not safe equipment or facilities were lacking, she or he is covered by workmen's compensation.) The contract may be oral, but it is expressed. A written contract has many advantages; it prevents later misunderstandings about such common problems as rotations, shifts, and opportunities for transfer. If the nurse chooses not to come to that institution after agreeing to do so, that is breach of contract, but the employer probably would not find it worthwhile to seek damages. If the employee had falsified references or other credentials, the contract would be void, because that is illegal. If the employee with a written contract

found that the employer was violating it, she or he could seek redress, either damages or the fulfillment of the clause, for example, transfer to a specialty unit at the next vacancy.

A written employment contract ideally follows a more or less standard form, setting forth the terms of agreement in understandable language, in logical sequence, and in readable form. Every written employment contract—both individual and group—should contain the following items. Some will be even more inclusive.

1. *Hours.* This refers to the length of the working day and week and, preferably, includes a statement about what will constitute overtime, for which the employee will be entitled to extra pay at a higher rate.
2. *Salary.* The beginning salary should be set for the position the employee is accepting, as well as the amounts of periodic increases, when they are due, and the criteria for salary increase and/or promotion. Differentials for evening and night shifts and the rate and conditions of overtime pay should also be stipulated.
3. *Vacation.* The number of days or weeks allowed should be stated, along with the time when the employee will be entitled to take his or her first vacation. Any details of vacation earnings should be clearly stated, such as: "Vacation for the first year of employment is given on the basis of one day per month. The nurse is entitled to take earned vacation days after she has completed six months of service. For the next two years, she is allowed two weeks of vacation per calendar year; three weeks thereafter."*
4. *Sick leave.* The number of days allowed should be stated as well as the basis on which they are earned. The date on which the benefit begins should be included. If cumulative sick leave is allowed, this should be stated, with any limitations clearly defined. Special regulations should

---

*The figures given here are intended only as examples.

be itemized, such as the necessity for presenting a health certificate from a physician when returning after sick leave. If a hospital requires nurses to carry hospitalization insurance, or takes care of them when they are ill or gives special rates, this should also be included. (The last is seldom done now.)

5. *Holidays.* The holidays allowed should be listed and any fixed regulations regarding time off in lieu of a holiday should be stated, as well as agreements related to tours of duty on holidays.

6. *Social Security coverage.* If the employing agency participates in the federal Social Security program, the contract should carry a statement to that effect and specify when salary deductions will be made.

7. *Pension plan.* If the employing agency has a retirement or pension plan, eligibility requirements should be mentioned in the contract, although details of the plan will not be included, of course.

8. *Duration of contract.* The contract should state the period of its duration, under what conditions it can be terminated by either the employee or employer, and what the length of notice will be.

Information about rest periods or breaks, meal hours, and so on may be included in the contract if either the employing agency or the employee so desires.

Nurses wishing to pursue their education while employed might be wise to have the conditions under which they may do so stipulated in the contract or at least verified in a letter or memorandum—for example, whether they will be able to enroll in daytime courses or be excused from evening duty while taking an evening course. If the hospital offers an in-service education program, it is advisable for both the institution and the employed nurse to have a written agreement about obligations for attending sessions in on- or off-duty hours. Regulations about extended leaves of absence for any reason, including maternity leave, should be clearly spelled out.

Over and above the specific details of the contract and the way it is phrased is the fact that nurses should be sure they understand it and the terms to which they are agreeing. They should also be sure that the person with whom they make the contract has the authority to do so. If a formal contract is not used, ask for a letter of appointment covering the most important points listed and others of importance in that particular situation.[171]

Contracts between patients and an independent NP might be just as clear-cut if it is an employer–employee situation. Even if the patient comes to the primary care nurse, the situation is the same: service and payment. More complex is the nurse–patient relationship in the therapeutic situation. Assuming that their contract is related to improvement of the patient's health, is there also a patient responsibility? There are some doctors and nurses who now plan with their patient to develop a contract in which the responsibilities of each are spelled out. This is a new area in contractual relationships.

Another type of contract affects the education of nurses. The contract between schools and clinical facilities includes such important aspects as mutual agreements on autonomy and the rights of each party, as well as cooperation, nondiscrimination, staffing (not to be altered because of the presence of students), provision and reimbursement for equipment, fees or exchange of services (faculty practice), responsibilities and rights of faculty and students, and faculty–student ratios.[172] Well-thought-out contracts will not only improve learning opportunities, but help avoid legal problems.

Rights and Responsibilities of Students

When students of nursing begin their course of study, they in effect, if not in writing, enter into a contract with the school that does not expire until they graduate. It is understood that both the students and the school will assume certain responsibilities, many of which have legal implications. Most legal cases related to education have involved institutions of higher education (junior and senior colleges, universities) or general education. In one case, students of a diploma program that closed threatened to sue for breach of contract because no arrangements had been made for continuation of their education, but the situation was resolved.

Most legislation and judicial decisions affecting education, however, probably can be applied to nursing education as well. Every approved school of professional nursing must meet the criteria for approval set by the state board of nursing, a legally appointed body found in every state, sometimes under a different name. The state-approved school must conduct an educational program that will prepare its graduates to take state board examinations and become licensed to practice as RNs. No matter where the students receive education and experience, the nursing school is still responsible for the content of the course of study. The board's minimum standards require the school to provide a faculty competent to teach students to practice nursing skillfully and safely. Students are expected to be under the supervision of a faculty member who is also an RN, and the school and teacher are responsible, with the student, for the student's errors. As discussed in Chapter 21, most legal experts hold that when students give patient care, they are, for legal purposes, considered employees of the hospital or agency. They are liable for their own negligence if injury results, and the institution will also be liable for the harm suffered under the doctrine of *respondeat superior.*

The student nurse is held to the standard of a competent professional nurse in the performance of nursing duties. In several judicial decisions, it was determined that those performing duties customarily performed by professional nurses are held to professional standards of care. Faculty supervising students are particularly liable if negligence occurs while the student is performing a task that he or she is not yet capable of performing in a manner consistent with proper standards of care. Such judgments are related not only to physical tasks or techniques performed, but also to knowledge and judgment in relation to the patient's care. If, for instance, a student does not take appropriate action, either personally or through correct reporting of an incipient injury to the patient, negligence is equally present. Carrying malpractice insurance is a wise precaution, and many schools recommend or require its purchase by all students. Many state student nurses' associations offer low-cost insurance with membership.

Whether it is wise educationally and practically for a nursing student to perform nursing functions as a regular, paid employee is debatable, because a student can legally function in only those capacities not restricted to licensed nursing personnel. State laws governing the practice of nursing vary widely and are subject to misinterpretation by the employing agency. Most laws classify students working part time as employees. In this capacity, students performing tasks requiring more judgment and skill than the position for which they are employed are subject not only to civil suits, but also to criminal charges for practicing without a license.

Traditionally, the relationship of institutions of higher education to a student under twenty-one years of age had been that of *in loco parentis,* which means that the school stands "in the place of the parent" and has the right to exercise similar authority over the student's physical, intellectual, and moral training. Since the early 1960s, courts have overturned this concept, and it is no longer considered to have much legal validity. However, the student's enrollment in a particular college generally is an implied contract, which requires that the student live up to the reasonable academic and moral standards of the college, with the school also having certain responsibilities. For instance, if the student lives in a dormitory connected with the school, it must meet safety and sanitation standards established by local regulations. However, the school rarely assumes responsibility for the student's loss of personal property.

Undesirable student conduct may result in

some discipline, including suspension or expulsion, and there has been considerable disagreement on the school's power in such circumstances. Generally, it is expected that the school's rules of conduct are made public and that the student has the right to a public hearing and due process. Legal rulings may be different when applied to private or public universities. Private universities have greater power in many ways.

Constitutional rights are most frequently cited by students in complaints: the First Amendment (freedom of speech, religion, association, expression); the Fourth Amendment (freedom from illegal search and seizure); and the Fifth and Fourteenth amendments (due process of law). The courts recognize the student first as a citizen, so that they will consider possible infringements of these rights. Most commonly, First Amendment rights involve dress codes and personal appearance. Although schools do not possess absolute authority over students in this sense, some lower court rulings have approved the establishment of dress codes necessary for cleanliness, safety, and health.[173] Beginning with *Dixon* v. *Alabama State Board of Education* in 1961, random, unannounced searches that schools had carried out previously were no longer allowed without student permission or a search warrant; otherwise, evidence found is inadmissible in court. If material uncovered is proscribed by *written* institutional policy, it may be used in institutional proceedings.[174]

Due process has been a major issue of legal contention. In essence, this term means that the purpose of the rule or law must be examined for fairness and reasonableness. Are the student and faculty understanding of the rule the same? Did the student have the opportunity to know about the rule and its implications? What is the relationship between the rule and the objectives of the school? A decade ago, few schools had a grievance procedure, and this situation was believed by students to be a serious violation of rights. In 1975, the National Student Nurses' Association (NSNA) developed grievance procedure

guidelines as part of a bill of rights for students.* Besides suggesting the makeup of the committee and general procedures, such issues as allowing sufficient time, access to information and appropriate records, presentation of evidence and use of witnesses were included.[175] The usual steps in any grievance process are also followed for academic grievances: an informal process first, consisting of a written complaint and suggested remedy by the student grievant, a written reply, a hearing with presentation of evidence on both sides, a decision by the committee within a specific time, right of appeal, and sometimes arbitration. With students, the right to continue with classwork during the total process is considered necessary.

Due process is considered crucial for students who are expelled or suspended for disciplinary reasons or who feel that they are discriminated against in their extracurricular activities because of race, religion, sex, or sexual preference. However, there seem to be an increasing number of grievances filed or legal complaints made because of academic concerns, especially grades. The courts have been reluctant to enter this area of academic freedom. There has yet to be a definitive ruling on curriculum and degree requirements. The attitude is demonstrated by a highly significant statement made by one court (45 Federal Rules Decisions, 133[1968], 136):

> Education is the living and growing source of our progressive civilization, of our open repository of increasing knowledge, culture and our salutory democratic traditions. As such, education deserves the highest respect and the fullest protection of the courts in the performance of its lawful missions. . . . Only when erroneous and unwise actions in the field of education deprive students of federally protected rights or privileges does a federal court have power to intervene in the educational process. . . .[176]

This statement has a number of counterparts in other jurisdictions, such as the affirmation

---

*See Chapter 24.

of a U.S. District Court (*Connelly* v. *University of Vermont and State Agricultural College,* 1965):

> in matters of scholarship, the school authorities are uniquely qualified by training and experience to judge the qualifications of a student. . . . The court is in a poor position indeed to substitute its judgments for that of the university. . . .[177]

The academic issues have almost always been settled by due process; therefore, schools are developing grievance procedures to resolve academic disputes between students and schools.[178] The process can create a number of tensions, but it may also bring to light school and teacher problems that should have been and can be resolved to avoid serious student complaints.[179]

Most colleges now have grievance procedures for students who think that they have received unfair grades, and these procedures must be followed first before any lawsuit can be filed. It is generally advised that before the student wages an all-out battle, the situation should be considered practically. It must be proved that the grade is arbitrary, capricious, and manifestly unjust, which is generally very difficult. Furthermore, unless that particular grade is extremely important to a student's career, the cost and time involved are greater than even a favorable result might warrant. This advice is borne out by more recent cases involving nurses. In one case, a nurse who refused to take a predoctoral exam she had failed twice was terminated as a student of the university and not permitted to enter the doctoral program. She sued. The Court could find no showing of bad motive or ill will on the part of the faculty, "which would warrant reviewing academic records based upon academic standards that are within the peculiar knowledge, experience, and expertise of the academicians."[180]

A major case involved a female fourth-year medical student who, after receiving many documented warnings, was dismissed because of her attitude in the clinical area, her unac-

ceptable personal hygiene, inappropriate bedside manner, and tardiness. However, she had an excellent academic record. She fought this issue to the Supreme Court,* charging violation of her constitutional rights to liberty and property. She lost, in part because her clinical evaluations had been consistently unsatisfactory and she had been given sufficient warning,[181] and the court accepted the faculty's judgment. This was considered an "academic" case, as opposed to a dismissal for disciplinary reasons.

Cases in which the results have been more favorable to the student are related to inadequate program advisement[182] and the school catalog as a written contract.[183] The school had to deal with the nursing student according to the statements in the catalog the year she entered, not the later, more restrictive requirements.

Another type of student right involves school records. The types of student records kept by schools vary. They may consist of only the academic transcript, or may include extracurricular activities and problem situations, which are kept in an informal file. The enactment of the Buckley Amendment, described in Chapter 19, has clarified the issue of student access to records. The individual loses the right to confidentiality by waiving the right or by disclosing the information to a third person. A student's academic transcript is the most common document released, particularly to other schools and employers.

As more student activists, most of whom are now voting citizens, request or demand certain rights as part of the academic community, more legal decisions are made.† But

---

Board of Curators of the University of Missouri v. *Horowitz.*

†One example is the "truth in testing" laws, the first of which was passed in New York State in 1979. It required manufacturers of standardized admission tests, such as the Scholastic Aptitude Test and the Graduate Record Examination, to file test questions and correct answers with the New York Commissioner of Education after student scores are released. A federal version also allowed the students to see their answers and the correct answers after release of scores.

school rules that were once ironclad have become flexible, even without legal intervention. Students can often bring about desirable changes through participation in committees intended for this purpose. Nevertheless, it is also helpful to know one's basic legal rights as an individual and a student.

The concept of rights need not be seen as an adversary proceeding. Both the student and the school have a new accountability. In the long run, it might be more meaningful to look at certain student rights as freedoms and responsibilities. The following have been suggested:

1. Freedom to disagree.
2. Freedom to explore ideas.
3. Freedom to help choose educational goals.
4. Freedom to study independently.
5. Freedom to experiment.
6. Freedom to know faculty.[184]

These freedoms are based on mutual respect and commitment by faculty and students, and enhance not only the educational process, but also nursing professionalism.

REFERENCES

1. U.S. Department of Health, Education and Welfare, *Secretary's Commission on Medical Malpractice* Report, DHEW Pub.No. (OS) 73-88 (Washington, D.C.: U.S. Government Printing Office, 1973), p. 71.
2. George Annas, "The Hospital: A Human Rights Wasteland," *Civil Liberties Rep.,* **9**:20 (Fall 1974).
3. George Annas, "The Emerging Stowaway: Patients' Rights in the 1980s," *Law, Med. and Health Care,* **10**:32-35, 46 (Feb. 1982).
4. Beatrice Kalisch, "Of Half Gods and Mortals: Aesculapian Authority," *Nurs. Outlook,* **23**:22-28 (Jan. 1975).
5. Emanuel Hayt, Lillian Hayt, and August Groeschel, *Law of Hospital, Physician and Patient,* 3rd ed. (Berwyn, Ill: Physicians' Record Co., 1972), p. 479.
6. Helen Creighton, "Law for the Nurse Supervisor: Informed Consent," *Superv. Nurs.,* **6**:9, 48-49 (Jan. 1975).
7. Ibid, 9.
8. Ibid, 48.
9. Theodore LeBlang, "Disclosure of Injury and Illness: Responsibilities in the Physician-Patient Relationship," *Law, Med. and Health Care,* **9**:4-7 (Sept. 1981).
10. Mae McWeeny, "The Patient's Right to Learn or Not to Learn" *Nurs. Admin. Q.,* **4**:83-87 (Winter 1980).
11. David Warren, *Problems in Hospital Law,* 3rd ed. (Germantown, Md.: Aspen Systems Corp., 1978), pp. 95, 138-141, 178.
12. Linda Besch, "Informed Consent: A Patient's Right," *Nurs. Outlook,* **27**:33 (Jan. 1979).
13. Martha Barry, "The Life of Every Creature . . . a Case of Patients' Rights," *Am. J. Nurs.,* **82**:1440-1441 (Sept. 1982).
14. Terence Ackerman, "The Limits of Beneficence: Jehovah's Witnesses and Childhood Cancer," *Hasting's Center Rep.,* **4**:13-18 (Aug. 1980).
15. H. L. Hirsch, "Informed Consent—Fact or Fiction," *J. Leg. Med.,* **5**:28 (Jan. 1977).
16. Margaret Somerville, "Therapeutic Privilege: Variation on the Theme of Informed Consent," *Law, Med. and Health Care,* **12**:4-12 (Feb. 1984).
17. Jay Katz, "Informed Consent—A Fairy Tale? Law's Vision," *University of Pittsburgh Law Rev.* **39**:137-174 (Winter 1977).
18. Lucie Kelly, "The Patient's Right to Know—a Reprise," *Nurs. Outlook,* **31**:6-8,9 (Jan.–Feb. 1983).
19. Sheila Taub, "Cancer and the Law of Informed Consent," *Law, Med. and Health Care,* **10**:62 (Apr. 1982).
20. Nathan Hershey and S. H. Bushkoff, *Informed Consent Study* (Pittsburgh: Aspen Systems Corp., 1969), p. 3.
21. R. J. Alfidi, "Informed Consent: A Study of Patient Reaction," *J. Am. Med. Assn.,* **216**:1225-1329, (May 1971).
22. Hershey and Bushkoff, op. cit.
23. David Kaufer et al., "Revising Medical Consent Forms: An Empirical Model

and Test," *Law, Med. and Health Care,* **11**:155–162 (Sept. 1983).

24. Helen Creighton, "The Right of Informed Refusal," *Nurs. Mgt.,* **13**:48 (Sept. 1982).

25. Lucie Kelly, "Neither Maverick Nor Martyr," *Nurs. Outlook,* **28**:644 (Oct. 1980).

26. President's Commission for the Study of Ethical Problems in Medicine and Biomedical and Behavioral Research, *Making Health Care Decisions* (Washington, D.C.: President's Commission, 1982), p. 147.

27. "Court Case: What Went Wrong?" *Nurs. Life,* **2**:88 (Mar.–Apr. 1982).

28. Jane Greenlaw, "When Patients' Questions Put You on the Spot," *RN,* **46**:79–80 (Mar. 1983).

29. "A Question of Ethics: The Patient's Right to Know," *Nurs. Life,* **2**:56–59 (Mar.–Apr. 1982).

30. Elsie Bandman, "How Much Dare You Tell Your Patient?" *RN,* **41**:39–41 (Aug. 1978).

31. William Regan, "Informed Consent: Must You Double-Check the MD?" *RN,* **46**:19–20 (Aug. 1983).

32. Maureen Cushing, "Informed Consent: An MD Responsibility?" *Am. J. Nurs.,* **84**:437–438 (Apr. 1984).

33. Loretta Trimberger, et al., "Should You Tell Your Patients About the Risks of Nursing Procedures?" *Nurs. Life,* **3**:26–32 (Nov.–Dec. 1983).

34. Helen Creighton, "What Is Death and Who Determines It? *Sup. Nurse,* **10**:17–75 (Sept. 1979).

35. Peter Black, "Brain Death," *New Engl. J. Med.,* **299**:398 (Aug. 1978).

36. Ibid., 399.

37. James Bernat et al., "Defining Death in Theory and Practice," *Hastings Center Rep.,* **12**:5–9 (Feb. 1982).

38. *Belchertown State School* v. *Saikewcz,* 1977 Mass. Adv. Sh. 2461, 370 N.E. 2nd 417 (1977).

39. *In re Karen Quinlan* 69 N.J. 399 (1976).

40. Daniel Rothman and Nancy Rothman, *The Professional Nurse and the Law* (Boston: Little, Brown and Company, 1977), pp. 139–140.

41. George Annas, "Reconciling 'Quinlan' and 'Saikewicz': Decision Making for the Terminally Ill Incompetent," *Am. J. of Law and Med.,* **4**:367–396 (Winter 1979).

42. Helen Creighton, "Termination of Life-Sustaining Treatment," *Nurs. Mgt.,* **14**:14–15 (Aug. 1983).

43. Sara Cohn, "The Living Will from the Nurse's Perspective," *Law, Med. and Health Care,* **11**:121–124, 180 (June 1983).

44. Sissela Bok, "Personal Directions for Care at the End of Life," *New Engl. J. Med.,* **295**:367–369 (Aug. 1976).

45. Jane Raible, "The Right to Refuse Treatment and Natural Death Legislation," *Medicological News,* **5**:6–8 (Fall 1977).

46. Emily Friedman, "'Natural Death' Laws Cause Hospitals Few Problems," *Hospitals,* **52**:124–148 (May 1978).

47. Stuart Eisendrath and Albert Jonsen, "The Living Will: Help or Hindrance?" *J. Am. Med. Assn.,* **249**:2054–2058 (Apr. 1983).

48. "The Right to Refuse Treatment: A Model Act," *Am. J. Pub. Health,* **73**:918–921 (Aug. 1983).

49. Joyce Beauchamp, "Euthanasia and the Nurse Practitioner," *Nurs. Forum,* **14**(1):56–73 (1975).

50. Marya Mannes, *Last Rights* (New York: William Morrow & Co., Inc., 1974).

51. "Nurse, on Trial for Murder, Called Compassionate," *New York Times,* Mar. 14, 1979, p. A17.

52. Maureen Cushing, "Verbal No-Code Orders," *Am. J. Nurs.,* **81**:1215–1216 (June 1981).

53. William Read, *Hospital's Role in Resuscitation Decisions* (Chicago: Hospital Research and Educational Fund, 1983).

54. Ronald Cranford and A. Edward Doudera, "The Emergence of Institutional Ethics Committees," *Law, Med. and Health Care,* **12**:13–20 (Feb. 1984).

55. "Optimum Care for Hopelessly Ill Patients," *N. Engl. J. Med.,* **295**:362–364 (Aug. 1976).

56. Mitchell Rabkin et al., "Orders Not to Resuscitate," *N. Engl. J. Med.,* **295**:364–366 (Aug. 12, 1976).

57. Jane Greenlaw, "Orders Not to Resusci-

tate: Dilemma for Acute Care as Well as Long Term Care," *Law, Med. and Health Care,* **10**:29–31, 45 (Feb. 1982).

58. "70-Year-Old Man Fights Enforced Life-Support in California Hospital" *Concern for Dying Newsletter,* **19**:3–4 (Summer 1984).

59. George Annas, "When Suicide Prevention Becomes Brutality: The Case of Elizabeth Bouvia," *Hastings Center Rep.,* **14**:20–21 (Apr. 1984).

60. Maureen Cushing, "The Implications of Withdrawing Nutritional Devices," *Am. J. Nurs.,* **84**:191–192, 194 (Feb. 1984).

61. Helen Creighton, "Decisions on Food and Fluid in Life-Sustaining Measures," Part I, *Nurs. Mgt.,* **15**:47–48 (June, 1984).

62. Carolyn Williams, "Deciding to Forego Life-Sustaining Treatment: Recommendations on Ethics," *Nurs. Outlook,* **31**:294–295 (Nov.–Dec. 1983).

63. Sidney Wanzer et al., "The Physician's Responsibility Toward Hopelessly Ill Patients," *N. Engl. J. Med.,* **310**:955–959 (Apr. 1984).

64. A. H. Bernstein, "Legal Rights of Mental Patients," *Hosp.,* **53**:49–52, 92 (Mar. 1979).

65. E. Parker and G. Tennent, "The 1959 Mental Health Act and Mentally Abnormal Offenders: A Comparative Study," *Med. Science and the Law,* **19**:29–38 (Jan. 1979).

66. Walter Barton and Charlotte Sandborn, *Law and the Mental Health Professions* (New York: International Universities Press, 1978).

67. Charles Prigmore and Paul Davis, *"Wyatt* v. *Stickney:* Rights of the Committed," *Nurs. Dig.,* **3**:70–77 (Summer 1974).

68. Daryl Matthews, "The Right to Refuse Psychiatric Medication," *Medicolegal News,* **8**:4–6, 16 (Apr. 1980).

69. Richard Cole, "The Patient's Right to Refuse Anti-Psychotic Drugs: The Court of Appeals Decision in *Rogers* v. *Okin,*" *Medicolegal News,* **9**:10–13 (Feb. 1981).

70. Richard Cole, "Patients' Rights to Refuse Antipsychotic Drugs," *Law, Med. and Health Care,* **9**:19–22, 38 (Sept. 1981).

71. Paul Appelbaum, "Can Mental Patients Say No to Drugs?" *New York Times Magazine,* Mar. 21, 1982, pp. 46, 51–56.

72. Darlene Trandel-Korenchuck and Keith Trandel-Korenchuck, "Informed Consent and Mental Incompetency," *Nurs. Admin. Q.,* **7**:76–78 (Fall 1983).

73. George Annas, "Sterilization of the Mentally Retarded: A Decision for the Courts," *Hastings Center Rep.,* **11**:18–19 (Aug. 1981).

74. John Wilson, *The Rights of Adolescents in the Mental Health System* (Lexington, Mass.: Lexington Books, 1978).

75. Linda Tiano, *"Parham* v. *J. R.:* 'Voluntary' Commitment of Minors to Mental Institutions," *Am. J. of Law and Med.,* **6**:125–149 (Apr. 1980).

76. Marguerite Mancini, "Nursing, Minors, and the Law," *Am. J. Nurs.,* **78**:124, 126 (Jan. 1978).

77. Alan Sussman, *The Rights of Young People,* An American Civil Liberties Union Handbook (New York: Avon Books, 1977), p. 26.

78. Ibid., pp. 224–226.

79. Ibid., p. 29.

80. Ibid., pp. 30–31.

81. "A Model Act Providing for Consent of Minors For Health Services," *Pediatrics,* **59**:293–296 (Feb. 1973).

82. The National Association of Children's Hospitals and Related Institutions, Inc., *The Pediatric Bill of Rights,* (Wilmington, Del.: The Association, 1974).

83. Nancy Medenwald, "Children's Liberation—in a Hospital," *MCN,* **5**:231–232 (July–Aug. 1980).

84. George Annas, "Legalizing Laetrile for the Terminally Ill," *Hastings Center Rep.,* **7**:19–20 (Dec. 1977).

85. Maureen Cushing, "Whose Best Interest? Parents vs. Child Rights," *Am. J. Nurs.,* **82**:313–314 (Feb. 1982).

86. John Kahring, "Conference Report: Seeking a Judicial Determination That Treatment May Be Withheld from a Seriously Ill Newborn," *Medicolegal News,* **7**:10–11 (Summer 1979).

87. Maureen Cushing, "Do Not Feed . . . ," *Am. J. Nurs.,* **83**:602–604 (Apr. 1983).

88. Leah Curtin, "Should We Feed Baby

Doe,?'' *Nurs. Mgt.,* **15**:22–28 (Aug. 1984).

89. Sheila Taub, "Withholding Treatment from Defective Newborns," *Law, Med. and Health Care,* **10**:4–10 (Feb. 1982).

90. Helen Creighton, "Shall We Choose Life or Let Die?" *Nurs. Mgt.,* **15**:16–18 (Aug. 1984).

91. Ibid.

92. R. S. Stone, "The Rights of Human Beings Participating as Subjects in Biochemical Research," guest editorial, *J. Lab. Clin. Med.,* **85**:184 (Feb. 1975).

93. Ida Moore, "Nontherapeutic Research Using Children as Subjects," *MCN,* **7**:285–289ff. (Sept.–Oct. 1982).

94. A. R. Jonesen, "Research Involving Children: Recommendations of the National Commission for the Protection of Human Subjects of Biomedical and Behavioral Research," *Pediatrics,* **62**:131–137 (1978).

95. "The Age of Consent," editorial *Am. J. Pub. Health,* **68**:1071–1072 (Nov. 1978).

96. Charles Lewis et al., "Informed Consent by Children and Participation in an Influenza Vaccine Trial," *Am. J. Pub. Health,* **63**:1079–1082 (Nov. 1978).

97. Cheryl Fields, "Children Must Consent to Taking Part in Experiments, New Rules Specify," *Nation's Health,* **13**:9, 14 (Mar. 1983).

98. "Protecting Research Subjects," *Am. J. Nurs.,* **79**:1139–1140 (June 1979).

99. Lisa Marchette, "Experimental Drugs: Where Do You Stand Legally?" *RN,* **47**:23–24 (Mar. 1984).

100. Katharyn May, "The Nurse as Researcher: Impediment to Informed Consent," *Nurs. Outlook,* **27**:36–39 (Jan. 1979).

101. Kathleen Kelly and Eleanor McClelland, "Signed Consent: Protection or Constraint?" *Nurs. Outlook,* **27**:40–42 (Jan. 1979).

102. Ruth MacKay and John Soule, "Nurses as Investigators: Some Ethical and Legal Issues," *Nurs Digest,* **5**:7–9 (Spring 1977).

103. Susanne Robb, "Nurse Involvement in Institutional Review Boards: The Service Setting Perspective," *Nurs. Res.,* **39**:27–29 (Jan.–Feb. 1981).

104. Susan Gortner et al. "The Institutional Review Board: A Case Study of No-Risk Decisions in Health Related Research." *Nurs. Res.* **30**:21–24 (Jan.–Feb. 1981).

105. Marcia Opp, "The Confidentiality Dilemma," *Nurs. Digest,* **4**:17–19 (Fall 1976).

106. Harold Schmeck, Jr., "Medical Records Privacy Violated, Government-Backed Study Finds," *New York Times,* Jan. 13, 1977, p. 42. (The Westin report is cited in the bibliography of this chapter.)

107. Carol Levine, "Sharing Secrets: Health Records and Health Hazards," *Hastings Center Rep.,* **7**:13–15 (Dec. 1977).

108. Hayt et al., op. cit., p. 1094.

109. Melissa Auerbach and Ted Bogue, *Getting Yours: A Consumer's Guide to Obtaining Your Medical Record* (Washington, D.C.: Public Citizen's Health Research Group, 1978).

110. Alan Westin, "New Era in Medical Records," *Hastings Center Rep.,* **7**:23–28 (Dec. 1977).

111. Given Health Care Center, *Principles of Practice* (Burlington, Vt.: University of Vermont, mimeographed), 1974 p. 1.

112. George Annas and Joseph Healey, "The Patient's Rights Advocate," *J. Nurs. Admin.,* **4**:25–31 (May–June 1974).

113. John Altman et al., "Patients Who Read Their Charts," *New Engl. J. Med.,* **302**:169–171 (Jan. 1980).

114. George Annas, *The Rights of Hospital Patients,* ACLU Handbook, (New York: Avon Books, 1975), pp. 112–120.

115. Auerbach and Bogue, op. cit., pp. 10–17.

116. Marc Hiller and Vivian Beyda, "Computers, Medical Records, and the Right to Privacy," *J. Health, Politics, Policy and Law,* **6**:463–487 (Fall 1981).

117. Donald Brass, "Professional and Agency Liability for Negligence in Child Protection," *Law, Med. and Health Care,* **11**:71–75 (Apr. 1983).

118. Ann O'Sullivan, "Privileged Communication," *Am. J. Nurs.,* **80**:947–950 (May 1980).

119. Diane Kjervik, "The Psychiatric Nurse's Duty to Warn Potential Victims of Homicidal Psychotherapy Outpatients,"

Law, Med. and Health Care, **9**:11–16, 39 (Dec. 1981).

120. Cathy Klein, "Assault and Battery," *Nurse Practitioner,* **9**:47–55 (July 1984).

121. Helen Creighton, *Law Every Nurse Should Know*, 4th ed. (Philadelphia: W. B. Saunder Company, 1981), p. 205.

122. Cathy Klein, "False Imprisonment," *Nurse Practitioner,* **9**:41–44 (Sept. 1984).

123. William Regan, "Assisting at Abortions: Can You Really Say No?" *RN,* **45**:71 (June 1982).

124. Leonard Glantz, "Limiting State Regulation of Reproductive Decisions," *Am. J. Pub. Health,* **74**:168–169 (Feb. 1984).

125. Larry Churchill and Jose Jorge Siman, "Abortion and the Rhetoric of Individual Rights," *Hastings Center Rep.,* **12**:9–12 (Feb. 1982).

126. Gloria Steinem, "The Ultimate Invasion of Privacy," *Ms,* **9**:43–46ff. (Feb. 1981).

127. George Annas, "*Roe* v. *Wade* Reaffirmed," *Hastings Center Rep.,* **13**:21–22 (Aug. 1983).

128. George Annas, Leonard Glantz, and Barbara Katz, *The Rights of Doctors, Nurses and Allied Health Professionals* (New York: Avon Books, 1981), pp. 206–207.

129. Creighton, *Law Every Nurse Should Know,* pp. 220–223.

130. Ibid.

131. Ibid., pp. 252–253.

132. George Annas, "Contracts to Bear a Child: Compassion or Commercialism?" *Hastings Center Rep.,* **11**:23–24 (Apr. 1981).

133. George Annas, "Surrogate Embryo Transfer: The Perils of Patenting," *Hastings Center Rep.,* **14**:25–26 (June 1984).

134. Philip Reilly, *Genetics, Law and Social Policy* (Cambridge, Mass.: Harvard University Press, 1977).

135. Helen Creighton, "Wrongful Life," *Nurs. Mgt.,* **14**:54–56 (Apr. 1983).

136. Creighton, *Law Every Nurse Should Know,* pp. 226–229.

137. Daniel Rothman and Nancy Rothman, *The Professional Nurse and the Law* (Boston: Little, Brown and Company, 1977), pp. 149–150.

138. Claire Fagin, "Nurses' Rights," *Am. J. Nurs.,* **75**:84 (Jan. 1975).

139. Elsie Bandman, "Do Nurses Have Rights? Yes," *Am. J. Nurs.,* **78**:84–86 (Jan. 1978).

140. Bertram Bandman, "Do Nurses Have Rights? No," *Am. J. Nurs.,* **78**:84–86 (Jan. 1978).

141. Seymour Moskowitz and Linda Moskowitz, "Protecting Your Job," *Am. J. Nurs.,* **84**:55–58 (Jan. 1984).

142. Keith Trandel-Korenchuk and Darlene Trandel-Korenchuk, "Conflicting Loyalties of the Nurse," *Nurs. Admin. Q.,* **6**:63–66 (Winter 1982).

143. "The Risk of Whistle Blowing," *Am. J. Nurs.,* **83**:1387 (Oct. 1983).

144. Beatrice Iho, "Due Process in Termination," *Michigan Nurse,* **57**:8–9 (July-Aug. 1984).

145. Moskowitz and Moskowitz, op. cit., 57.

146. Jack Horsley, "When You Can Safely Refuse an Assignment," *RN,* **43**:93–96 (Feb. 1980).

147. Helen Creighton, "Hospital Guilty of Racial Discrimination," *Nurs. Mgt.,* **14**:20–21 (Mar. 1983).

148. Jane Greenlaw, "A Sexist Judgment Threatens All of Nursing," *RN,* **45**:69–70 (July 1982).

149. "Supreme Court Rules Against All-Woman Nursing School," *Am. J. Nurs.,* **82**:1187, 1283 (Aug. 1982).

150. Bonnie Bullough, "The Struggle for Women's Rights in Denver: A Personal Account," *Nurs. Outlook,* **25**:535–536 (Sept. 1978).

151. "New Ruling Said to Make Job Bias Harder to Prove," *Chron. Higher Ed.* **28**:1, 9 (Aug. 1984).

152. "Two Tenacious RNs Fight Hospital Over Sex Discrimination and Make It Pay," *RN,* **42**:15–16 (Mar. 1979).

153. Kent Hull, "Fourth Circuit Limits Section 504 Employment Rights of the Handicapped," *Medicolegal News,* **8**:8–9, 24 (June 1980).

154. Marlene Strader, "Schools of Nursing and the Handicapped Applicant: Status of the Law," *Nurs. and Health Care,* **4**:322–326 (June 1983).

155. Moskowitz and Moskowitz, op. cit., 56–57.

156. Bonnie Duldt, "Sexual Harrassment in Nursing," *Nurs. Outlook,* **30**:336–343 (June 1982).

157. Moskowitz and Moskowitz, op. cit., p. 58.

158. Helen Creighton, "A Nurse's Freedom of Speech," *Sup. Nurs.,* **5**:45–48 (Apr. 1974).

159. "She Stuck Up For Her Patient—And Got Fired," *Nurs. Life,* **4**:72 (July–Aug. 1984).

160. Pamela Atkinson and Linda Goodwin, "The Role of the Nursing Administrator in Collective Bargaining," *Nurs. Cl. of North America,* **13**:111–118 (Mar. 1978).

161. Elaine Beletz and Mary Meng, "The Grievance Process," *Am. J. Nurs.,* **77**:265 (Feb. 1977).

162. Ibid., 257–260.

163. Elaine Beletz, "Some Pointers for Grievance Handlers," *Sup. Nurs.,* **8**:12–14 (Aug. 1977).

164. Debra Wynne, "A Union Contract Was the Only Language Our Hospital Would Understand," *RN,* **41**:66–68 (May 1978).

165. Jan Natonski, "Why a Union Contract Didn't Work at Our Hospital," *RN* **41**:69–71 (May 1978).

166. Anthony Lee, "A Wary New Welcome for Unions," *RN,* **45**:35–40 (Nov. 1982).

167. Neil Sorrentino, "An Alternative to Collective Bargaining," *Nurs. Admin. Q.,* **6**:81–84 (Winter 1982).

168. Eve Stern "Collective Bargaining: A Means of Conflict Resolution," *Nurs. Admin. Q.,* **6**:9–20 (Winter 1982).

169. Laurel Eisenhauer and Virginia Cleland, "Is Collective Bargaining the Solution?" *Nurs. Outlook,* **31**:150–153 (May–June 1983).

170. Irene Eldridge and Margaret Levi, "Collective Bargaining as a Power Resource for Professional Goals," *Nurs. Admin. Q.,* **6**:29–40 (Winter 1982).

171. Gail Wolf, "Negotiating an Employment Contract," *Nurse Practitioner,* **5**:55, 60 (Jan.–Feb. 1980).

172. Rosemary Dale, "Contracting for Student Clinical Experience," *Nurse Educator,* **1**:22–25 (May–June 1965).

173. Clementine Pollok et al., "Students' Rights," *Am. J. Nurs.,* **76**:601 (Apr. 1976).

174. Ibid., 601.

175. National Student Nurses' Association, *The Bill of Rights for Students of Nursing* (New York: The Association 1975).

176. Clementine Pollok et al., "Faculties Have Rights, Too," *Am. J. Nurs.,* **77**:636 (Apr. 1977).

177. Ibid., 637.

178. Jann Logsdon et al., "The Development of an Academic Grievance Procedure," *Nurs. Outlook,* **27**:184–190 (Mar. 1979).

179. Karen Robinson and Sharon Bridgewater, "Named in a Grievance: It Happened to Us," *Nurs. Outlook,* **27**:191–194 (Mar. 1979).

180. Helen Creighton, "Right of Nursing Student to Pursue Higher Degree," *Nurs. Mgt.,* **14**:16–17 (Dec. 1983).

181. Linda Niedringhaus and Dorothy O'Driscoll, "Staying within the Law—Academic Probation and Dismissal," *Nurs. Outlook,* **31**:156–159 (May–June 1983).

182. Joyce Jones, "University Liability in Program Advisement," *Nurs. and Health Care,* **4**:83–84 (Feb. 1983).

183. Helen Creighton, "Nursing School Catalog Is Written Contract," *Nurs. Mgt.,* **15**:68–69 (Feb. 1984).

184. Rothman and Rothman, op cit., pp. 90–91.

III

PROFESSIONAL COMPONENTS AND CAREER DEVELOPMENT

ORGANIZATIONS AND PUBLICATIONS

23

Organizational Procedures and Issues

The more complex and highly organized society becomes, the harder it is for a single individual to exert any significant influence or power. There are exceptions to this rule, of course. There will always be pioneers and crusaders—individuals who, through sheer force of personality, conviction, and determination succeed in making an impact. But by and large, the concerted effort of a group of people working in an organized manner is necessary today to accomplish a given purpose, to effect a change in the status quo.

This is as true in nursing as in any other field on both student and graduate levels. One student alone, for instance, can do little to change what may seem to be the out-of-date or autocratic practices of the nursing school administration, but working through the student association in the school or through a unit of the National Student Nurses' Association (NSNA), she or he may very well bring about the desired improvements. Similarly, one nurse, no matter how dedicated or determined, would never have been able to make it easier and less expensive for our older citizens to obtain needed hospital and medical care. Yet the strong voice of the ANA, speaking out in favor of health insurance coverage for the aging under the Social Security system, was one of the factors that brought about what is now known as Medicare. And it must be remembered that the ANA took this stand because the majority of its members indicated that this was what *they* wanted. So, working through the professional organization, the individual *was* heard, *did* have influence, *did* help to bring about change.

There are many persons who are inclined to do nothing more than grumble to themselves and their colleagues about what they don't like or, on the other hand, what they would like to see accomplished. But so long as these individuals do no more than complain and unless they join with their colleagues to act in an organized, effective way, they will in all probability continue to be powerless and dissatisfied. This is not to say that a person should simply become a "joiner"—someone who seems to become a member of almost any organization for which she or he is eligible. Such a process only scatters one's interests and energies in many directions and provides no focus. But there are many organizations concerned with health and nursing that a nursing student or RN will want to either join, support, or at least be familiar with. By joining some of them, individuals will be able to work with colleagues in advancing their own nursing interests or those of nursing as a whole; in others, they will find the companionship of those with the same, perhaps more specific, concerns; and in still others, they will be able to keep abreast of the many forces that are influencing nursing and health care today.

The nature and purpose of these nursing and health organizations will be discussed in succeeding chapters. Of concern here, however, is the nurse's role—or anyone's role, for that matter—as an organization member. Presumably, one has joined the organization because its concerns and goals are the same as one's own. Joining is not enough, however; full realization of one's own and the organization's objectives demands active and informed participation. For whatever an association's purposes may be, its success depends on intelligent, industrious, and conscientious leadership; a willing, enthusiastic, and well-informed membership; adequate financial support; and sound business organization and administration. It is the responsibility of each member to help make all of these things realities.

MEMBERSHIP RESPONSIBILITIES

Members of any organization should feel responsible for learning as much as possible about it—its history, purposes, the number and composition of its membership, and its principal activities. They should study the constitution and bylaws, the code of ethics if there is one, and subscribe to its official publication. They should learn the names of the organization's principal current officers and preferably their background. When attending meetings, they should listen carefully to the discussion, and become familiar with the most important issues under consideration and the conditions and facts that influence the decisions to be taken. This will take time, but just a few hours spent on such matters can eventually prepare new members for productive and personally rewarding participation in the organization's work.

As soon as the individual is ready to take a more active part in the meetings, he or she can enter into discussions, ask relevant questions, help clarify issues by presenting a fresh and knowledgeable point of view, accept appointments to committees, and volunteer to help as time and ability dictate. Restraint, diplomacy, and a sense of good timing should guide new members as they find their place in any group.

Individuals who hold or aspire to hold office should have a copy of authoritative rules of order for organizing and conducting an organization's business and should become familiar enough with the publication so that they can readily find the information needed. The individual who holds the president's office or presides over formal business meetings in any other capacity must know how to do so efficiently, without recourse to the book of rules, except for an answer to unusually difficult questions. The rules of order used by a particular association are usually named in its bylaws.

The average member does not need to be as conversant as an officer with the minute details of parliamentary procedure, but should know how to address the presiding officer; formulate, present, and vote on a motion; and be familiar with other basic procedures that facilitate the progress of the meeting. This knowledge will enhance his or her ability to express views and contribute to the discussion without embarrassment or lack of confidence. On the other hand, it would be naive not to recognize that parliamentary procedure can be used as a manipulative tool to bring about certain action or lack of action. For instance, if an item is not placed on the agenda by the presider, other officers, or members, it is not likely to be discussed and certainly not acted on. If the item is placed in an unfavorable position—at the end of a long session when people are less alert, at a point when a certain voting constituency is present for a short time (some bylaws allow any member present to vote), or at a point when certain information is not yet available, or after a controversial, emotional, related item—the action taken might be quite different than it would be if the topic were discussed at another time. There are also those who misuse the intricacies of parliamentary procedure by complex motions to amend, substitute, or amend the amendment of a motion repeatedly so that the members may be totally confused about the real issue in the motion to be voted on. Those speaking to a motion may also be deliberately or inadvertently obscure, incorrect, or inappropriate in their statements, which, if the usual procedure in speaking from the floor is observed, may make the point difficult to correct and clarify. (And then there are always those who like to be heard whether or not what they say is pertinent.) Therefore, the average member should be alert to these machinations and learn how to combat them. If a motion seems to have been railroaded through, it is particularly useful to know how that action can be reversed before the final adjournment.* Because any organization has its political aspects, those who are interested in seeing that a certain action is taken seldom take a chance on this simply occurring during a business meeting. An effort is made to sell individuals or subgroups within the organization on the idea before formal action is taken—that is, lobbying. The formal action can be orchestrated: who makes the motion, who speaks to it, what supporting information must be introduced, is it best referred to a task force or committee, and, most important of all, are the votes there? A politically astute member tries to estimate at what point the issue is more likely to be voted in the desired direction, delaying the vote by some form of postponement if necessary.

WHO DOES THE WORK?

Even the most careful plans and the finest constitution and bylaws do not ensure a healthy, productive organization. The plans and directions must be implemented. Who

does this? Every officer, every committee member, every member at large shares the responsibility for knowing what that person as an individual can do for the good of the entire membership and for doing it—unless health or some other serious problem is a deterrent.

An incapacitated officer should resign promptly and give the organization the opportunity and privilege of deciding whether or not it needs and wants him or her to continue in office in spite of the handicap. Members who accept an appointment to a committee and later find themselves unable to assist with its work should withdraw, leaving the chairman or other authorized person free to appoint another, more productive member.

The ideal members of any organization unquestionably are those who pay their dues promptly, attend meetings whenever possible, keep abreast of developments, support and help advance the association's programs, speak intelligently at meetings, offer constructive suggestions, volunteer their services and talents, accept committee appointments, and promote the goals that have been adopted by the association, even though they may occasionally have some personal reservations about them.

Such paragons, of course, do not come in large numbers, but most of an association's active members have at least some of these attributes. Even the members who do no more than pay their dues regularly make some contribution, because by so doing, they provide both moral and financial support for the organization's programs. The general rule, however, is that the more actively individuals participate in the functioning of their association, the more benefit and satisfaction they will derive from their membership. By the same token, the more active, articulate, and informed members an association has, the better its chances of accomplishing the objectives for which it was formed.

President, Chairperson,* Moderator

Although the elected or appointed head of an association does a great deal of work be-

---

*See later section on motions.

hind the scenes day after day throughout a term of office, the membership thinks of this person most frequently as the one who presides at meetings. This is one of the most important responsibilities for which a leader needs particular skills, talents, and personality assets.

The individual should be in complete control of emotions; avoid distracting mannerisms and loquacity; speak in a clear, well-modulated voice; be discreet, impartial, and courteous; have considerable stamina; and be businesslike. However, a good sense of humor and the ability to laugh at oneself is a decided asset. A good leader should be able to sense the atmosphere of a meeting and prevent it from becoming explosive or detrimental to productive progress. It is even important to be sensitive to the physical comfort of the assembly and to do what is possible to improve ventilation, lighting, seating arrangements, or whatever else is indicated to keep everyone alert and interested. The presiding officer should be prompt for every meeting, ready to function at the appointed time, and, as soon as a quorum is present, call the meeting to order. This encourages habitual latecomers to be on time and helps to assure prompt adjournment also.

The president must have a thorough knowledge of the history of the organization, what it has done in the past, and what it plans to do in the future. Rarely should a question find this person completely unprepared; if the president does not know the answer, he or she should know on whom to call for it or where it can be found. Sometimes, of course, the questions are referred to someone else even if the chair knows the answer. This might happen when a query is raised about the organization's finances, and the president asks the treasurer to answer. Any officer must know

when it is appropriate to withhold information as well as when to disclose it. It is important always to be in control of the situation and to keep the assembled audience informed about the discussion before the house to avoid the confusion that results when members do not understand the issue.

Rarely should the presiding officer express a personal opinion on an issue. This is because of the need to maintain a neutral attitude and because one of the chief duties of a leader is to encourage others to participate. It is a good policy to subtly encourage the less assertive member to speak up and discourage the individuals who always want to express their views at length. In doing this, the presiding head must be eminently fair and unbiased, allowing all the right to air their views.

The chair must be thoroughly familiar with the agenda of every meeting over which she or he presides and know how to complete it expeditiously and in accordance with the rules of procedure adopted by the organization. This is learned through studying the rules, observing other presiding officers in action, and experience. Every meeting will bring confidence and learning from successes and failures.

A president may have exhibited considerable ability to lead discussions, but may not have had extensive practice in handling motions, one of the major responsibilities of a presiding officer. Sometimes this is a simple procedure, but it can become involved. The chair who understands the intricacies guides the action deftly and gains the respect of the group; the one who gets confused about what step takes precedence over another, for example, may create a chaotic situation that will leave the members dissatisfied and possibly highly critical.

It is vital to be acquainted with as many members of the organization as possible and to become familiar with their interests and abilities. This will help in making appointments to committees and selecting members for other assignments. If the organization is widespread, visits to several different areas or

---

*The current trend is to use the term *chairperson* instead of *chairman*. However, some organizations may use *chairman* or *chairwoman,* or simply, *chair*.

constituent associations each year, giving necessary help, often stimulate the members in their work. On social occasions the president should mingle with members; this will establish rapport with the various groups and will tend to promote interest and enthusiasm.

The president must keep in touch with the work and progress of other officers and the committees in the organization and cooperate amicably and constructively with them. Democratic principles must be observed, allowing each person to use the initiative and authority necessary to discharge assigned duties and responsibilities without interference while, at the same time, demanding first-rate performance. If the organization has a paid executive secretary or director and a headquarters staff, the officers must observe the same principles and practices, carrying the appropriate responsibilities but never usurping prerogatives that are rightfully those of the staff.

It is clear that the head of any organization needs leadership qualities in large measure. Although every individual elected to such an office probably will not possess all of them, there will be innumerable opportunities to develop them.

Vice President

Although, theoretically, a vice president—particularly a first vice president—is as capable as the president, because she or he must be prepared to function in the president's absence or in an emergency, the qualifications tend to be less exacting. Many persons with outstanding leadership ability are unwilling to accept the relatively inactive post of the vice presidency. This happens in organizations of all sizes and types, from a local volunteer group to the federal government.

To make the office more challenging, some associations declare in their bylaws that the vice presidents shall also be heads of committees or assume other responsibilities. Among the most common are chairperson of the program, policy development, or bylaws committees. Vice presidents may also represent the organization in meetings, interorganizational committees, or task forces. This gives the vice president an opportunity to make a specific contribution to the organization and also gives visibility. Sometimes large organizations have more than one vice president, all with specific responsibilities.

One trend that seems to be occurring is to include a president-elect on the board, preparing that person for assumption of the presidential office with minimal orientation. There are some disadvantages: a double-term commitment on the part of that individual and probable inability to prevent that person from succeeding to the presidency if she or he proves to be ineffectual at the board level.

Secretary

Some organizations have two secretaries: the recording secretary, who takes the minutes, and the corresponding secretary, who deals with the correspondence. There is also the secretary-treasurer option. If the organization is large enough to have a professional staff, the actual taking of detailed minutes and handling of correspondence are done by staff, but both are checked and sometimes signed by the secretary, president, or other appropriate person. Nevertheless, the functions of the secretary as spelled out in the bylaws are the responsibility of the elected person.

In a smaller organization, the secretary who thinks and writes clearly, is well informed about the association's business, and has the necessary knowledge and skill to write appropriate minutes is invaluable.[1] The secretary must be able to keep alert throughout meetings that can be both tedious and frustrating, and maintain an outward attitude of equanimity, neutrality, and cooperation regardless of inner conflicts. She or he must be objective and impartial in all reports in spite of the fact that at times it is necessary to "interpret the interpretations" of others when transcribing the notes taken at a meeting. It is important to be methodical, reliable, and prompt in getting out all reports and memoranda. The corresponding secretary needs to be a master of the courteous and appropriate phrase, because these responsibilities have important public relations connotations. Neatness and promptness of response in correspondence are highly desirable.

Treasurer

It is not unusual for the treasurer of an organization to be selected with greater care than the president, and almost as much is expected. The principal qualifications should be honesty, accuracy, and conscientiousness in keeping records, and knowledge of bookkeeping procedures, budgeting, and financial reporting. Business experience is a decided asset. The membership, even when it knows better, often judges the treasurer's ability by the balance on hand in the treasury.

The treasurer of any organization is often chairman of its committee on finance. This post requires the usual skills necessary to conduct a committee meeting well plus additional ability to discuss facts and figures intelligently, often before board members who may not be well versed in financial matters but are vitally interested in the organization's purse strings. The president's work is also facilitated by a competent treasurer because so many of the organization's activities depend on its financial status. Even if the details of the financial management of the organization are carried out by skilled employees, the board has fiduciary responsibility for the association. Budgets cannot be properly developed or adhered to and intelligent financial decisions cannot be made if accurate information is not available. Therefore, board members and especially the treasurer must have at least a basic understanding of financial management.

Councils and Committees

An organization's bylaws usually call for the inclusion of permanent councils and standing committees, with the number depending more on the scope of the activities than on the volume.

The quantity and quality of work done by each special group greatly influence the status and progress of the organization, although sometimes so indirectly that the general membership is unaware of their extent. For example, the nominating committee is responsible for finding persons who are willing and eligible to fill elected offices and who have the qualifications for them. This requires diligence and excellent salesmanship, especially if the prospective candidate is initially reluctant to serve. In large or widely scattered organizations, many members do not know the candidates personally. They must depend on the nominating committee to select the best available people; they then base their voting decisions on whatever information about them is released through official channels.

Members of the nominating committee, therefore, must always seek the best person or persons regardless of friendships, school ties, personal obligations, or any such influencing factor. And it follows logically that the persons responsible for appointing or electing members of this committee must consider integrity to be one of their most important personal qualifications. Their influence on the future of the organization is considerable, for a ballot can be set up in such a way that a certain individual or someone representing a particular constituency is sure to win that election. This is especially true with a mail ballot, where a strong write-in vote is almost impossible to achieve unless it is highly organized.

The work of other permanent councils and committees often is equally important. Some aspects may be obvious; others may need definition and delineation of responsibilities.[2]

PARLIAMENTARY PROCEDURES

The purpose of the business meetings of any organization is to transact business with the greatest possible dispatch while recognizing the rights of individual members, present and absent, and giving minority and opposing groups ample opportunity to air their views, yet assuring that the wishes of the majority prevail. To achieve this purpose, a methodical order of conducting the meetings is essential.

When early American congresses first organized, they naturally borrowed from the British Parliament many practices, which they adapted for their own use. Further changes were made from time to time until a distinctive American system evolved. The terms *parliamentary procedure* and (incorrectly) *parliamentary law* are used, however, in referring to both the American and British systems, which still have a good deal in common.

The procedures that have been used for many years by the United States Senate and House of Representatives developed from four sources:

1. The Constitution of the United States.
2. Jefferson's *Manual of Parliamentary Procedure,* which he prepared while he was vice president and presided over the Senate.
3. Rules that have been adopted by the House since its beginning and that may be changed with each Congress; these rules are sometimes called the *legislative manual.*
4. Decisions rendered by the presiding officer and the chairman of the Committee of the Whole House.

The transactions of less imposing bodies than the United States Congress are governed similarly. Each usually has a constitution and bylaws citing the officers and their duties in general, the order of business, voting regulations, and other matters related to the conduct of business meetings. The presiding officer makes decisions consistent with his or her authority, often with the advice of a parliamentarian employed by the organization. Each major meeting of the membership or house of delegates may produce changes in rules or the formulation of new ones needed to expedite its own activities, and each organization adopts a manual of parliamentary procedure to guide the business transactions.

The most popular guide for formal business procedure is *Robert's Rules of Order, Revised.* This reference work, written by General Henry M. Robert of the United States Army and published originally in 1876, is based upon the rules and practices of Congress. It is generally considered the most authoritative book of its kind, and some organizations attempt to follow it to the letter. Others use it only as a final authority to settle a controversial point. Still others select simpler but equally reliable rules of order to guide their transactions, such as *Sturgis' Standard Code of Parliamentary Procedure* by Alice F. Sturgis, and *Parliamentary Law* by F. M. Gregg.

As stated in *Robert's Rules of Order, Revised:*

> Parliamentary procedure, properly used, provides the means whereby the affairs of an organization or club can be controlled by the general will within the whole membership. The "general will" in this sense does not always imply even near unanimity or "consensus" but rather the right of the deliberate majority to decide. Complementary to this is the right of the minority—at least a strong minority—to require the majority to be deliberate—that is—to act according to its considered judgment after a full and fair "working through" of the issues involved.[3]

Although *Robert's Rules of Order* and other such publications include duties of officers and committees and other information, the discussion here will be concerned with the conduct of a business meeting because duties of officers and other details are defined in an organization's constitution and bylaws, which supersede any other rules.

Some of the principles and techniques of parliamentary procedure can perhaps be best presented by following an imaginary annual meeting of the NSNA from beginning to end. This organization, described in the next chapter, is the membership organization for nursing students. When the NSNA bylaws do not specify a procedure, *Robert's Rules of Order, Revised* is used as a guide.

Most formal meetings have an order of business. A classic example follows.

1. Call to order.
2. Minutes of previous meetings.
3. Reports of officers, boards, standing committees.

Executive reports.
Executive announcements.
Order and procedure of reports.
  President.
  Vice president.
  Secretary.
  Treasurer.
  Board of directors.
Standing committees.
4. Reports of special committees.
5. Announcements.
6. Unfinished business.
7. New business.
8. Adjournment.

In this meeting, these steps will be considered one at a time and others, which are often included in the order of business, interpolated.

Although the following discussion implies that the NSNA's business is completed in one session, it usually takes several sessions to finish it. This is usual at convention meetings and may be required in the bylaws by certain wording, such as the need for the nominating committee to report the ticket at a certain time.

An order of business must be flexible enough to be realistic. For example, if there is good reason for having the reports of special committees given ahead of the standing committees, the president is privileged to make that change simply by announcing it from the chair. The president is also privileged to make announcements or have others make them and to invite the headquarters staff members and guests to address the assembly whenever it appears prudent, proper, and helpful to so do. A major reordering of the agenda by the presiding officer or another member may require approval of the total group.

Call to Order

The president* calls the meeting to order by rapping a gavel for attention if necessary and

—————————

*To simplify the use of pronouns, it will be assumed that the president is female.

saying, "Will the meeting please come to order?" or words to that effect. The secretary then presents the agenda for the meeting and the parliamentarian explains the basic rules of parliamentary procedure that will be followed.

To make sure that a quorum (as defined in the NSNA bylaws) is present, the president asks the secretary to call a roll of delegates. If a quorum is present, the president so states; if not, she may declare a recess or fill in the time with matters of a nonbusiness nature until sufficient members arrive.

Minutes of the Preceding Meeting

Although the NSNA's secretary keeps accurate and complete files on all business transacted at every meeting of the association, it is highly improbable that minutes of the association's last meeting will be read, because these would be long, detailed, and time-consuming. So, in lieu of reading the minutes, most large membership organizations distribute mimeographed copies of the previous meeting's minutes.

However, in meetings of smaller groups within the NSNA, such as the executive board or one of the committees, the second step in the order of business could be the reading of the minutes of the preceding meeting. This is done by the secretary at the request of the chairman or silently by the members. It is also possible that minutes will have been distributed and read before the meeting. When this is finished, the chair asks the members if they wish to make any additions or corrections. A member wishing to make a change rises and after being recognized makes a statement that might be something like this: "Madame Chairman, my name is Helen Gibson [or simply "Helen Gibson"], Kentucky. The secretary reported that the president of the New Jersey association moved that the executive board investigate the feasibility of promoting a national student nurse week. The motion was actually made by the president of the New York State association."

Small groups in which members know each

other may not need to identify themselves. Nonetheless, it is correct parliamentary procedure. The chairman and the recording secretary *must* know who is speaking and other members *like* to know.

The president says "Thank you" to the member and asks the secretary to change the record, unless the correction is contradicted by someone. When all requests for additions or corrections have been made, the president states, "The minutes will be accepted as corrected." If no changes are indicated, she says, "The minutes will be accepted as read."

Report of the President

The president usually reads her own report, but has the privilege of asking the secretary or someone else to read it. If reading it personally, she will ask the first vice president to take the chair until the report is completed. This is because correct parliamentary procedure requires that a meeting must always have a presiding officer and the president cannot preside and read a report at the same time.

Although the president's report may contain some facts and figures, it is not usually a business report. Rather it is of a general nature and greatly influenced by the president's personality. Included will be an account of the progress made by the association during the past year, the satisfactions and perhaps the disappointments; some of the things done while president, such as visiting state nurses' associations and speaking at meetings; plans and ambitions for the future with implied and possibly formulated recommendations based on needs as she sees them; and expressions of appreciation to others for their support and assistance.

No formal acceptance procedure of the president's report is indicated. After concluding this address the president gives a copy of it to the secretary for the record and resumes the chair.

Everyone who makes a formal report before the house of delegates will follow the president's example and give the secretary a copy either before or immediately after presenting it to the assembly.

Report of the Secretary

The secretary's report includes information about his or her personal activities in the office, stressing the broad scope of official duties. When the report has been completed, the president accepts it as read without asking for a vote by the delegates.

Report of the Treasurer

The treasurer's report is a statement showing the income and expenses of the association during the past year and its financial status at the end of the fiscal year. When the treasurer has finished reading the report, the president says, "The treasurer's report is accepted as read," and may add, "And it is filed for audit."

Any questions about the treasurer's report should be asked at this time. The president may reply or may ask the treasurer to do so. General discussion is permitted at the president's discretion.

Report of the Committee on Nominations

Much of the work of the nominating committee—deciding upon appropriate candidates for office, securing their permission to be nominated, and compiling their biographies—is done prior to the annual meeting. At the meeting the chairman of the nominating committee, when called upon by the president, reads the slate of officers to the assembly. When finished, she or he says, "Madame Chairman, I move the adoption of this slate of officers." The president then asks the house if there are other nominations. If there are none, a delegate will move that the nominations be closed. This motion will be seconded and voted promptly.

A *nomination from the floor* can be made by any delegate by addressing the chair, naming the proposed candidate, and giving briefly the proposed nominee's qualifications for the post. A special form supplied by the nominating committee, containing detailed information about the candidate, is submitted to the nominating committee if the nomination is seconded. Nominations from the floor are closed by house vote.

Following the meeting, the nominating committee reviews the information about candidates who were nominated from the floor and may post their names and the offices for which they are candidates near the voting place where balloting is done. It is also possible that a convention paper or other form of written communication will be distributed to members with election information and the nominees' names and qualifications. It may or may not be possible to have the new names printed on the ballot in time for the election. If not, the names may be written in by the delegates wishing to vote for them.

Voting is done at a time and place designated by the executive board. Delegates must present credentials before they are allowed to vote. When voting is completed—usually within a few hours—the tellers who were appointed by the president at the first meeting count the ballots and prepare a report to be given at the NSNA's closing business session. A plurality vote (more votes than any other candidate for the same office) is required for election by the NSNA. If a majority vote were required, a candidate would need at least one more than half the votes cast to be elected.

Reports of Other Committees

As the NSNA president calls for reports of the association's other committees, the chairman of each goes to the platform—if invited by the president—or to a microphone or other place where she or he can be seen and heard easily by the entire assembly, addresses the chair, and reads the report. If any action is to be taken (usually recommendations), the committee chairman or someone else says, "Madame Chairman (or President), I move the acceptance of this report" or "adoption of the recommendation." A delegate may second the motion, and the motion is handled like any other. If no action is required on any sections of the report, the preceding step may be omit-

ted and the president will thank the reporting person. At times, reports are presented in a book of reports and are not read if the business of the committee does not appear controversial or call for action. They can still be discussed, however, if members desire.

Unfinished Business

At this point the president makes sure that any items of business left incomplete because of time limitations, absent persons, and so on, are satisfactorily completed.

New Business

New business is often the most interesting and exciting part of the agenda. If the issues are controversial, debate may be heated and lengthy. Even if they're not, the topics discussed indicate the course the association will take during the months ahead.

Resolutions

Resolutions may be one of the most important parts of a major meeting, because they are indications of the organization's position on key issues. Resolutions are submitted by individual members, groups, or committees within the organization to a resolutions committee and/or the board of directors. A resolutions committee, may, usually with the permission of the originators, combine similar resolutions or change some aspect of a resolution.

The board has the privilege of supporting or not supporting the resolution, and in some organizations it can withhold it from the voting body. Some organizations hold preliminary hearings to expedite action and/or agreement without the formality of strict parliamentary procedure. This often clarifies misunderstandings and saves time during the business meeting. Generally, a member whose resolution has been rejected for presentation has the right to introduce it from the floor.

Resolutions, except courtesy resolutions, are often meant to be acted upon by the organization after the meeting. For instance, a resolution may call for a letter to the President of the United States requesting better federal funding of nursing education, or it could direct long-term activities of the organization. Although the wording is often formal, with one or more *whereas* clauses giving the reasons for the resolution preceding the resolution, there is no reason why the wording cannot be clear and concise, so that the message is understood by all. Reviewing the past resolutions of an organization gives an excellent picture of its philosophy and goals and is one means of judging its quality. Therefore, although resolutions frequently come toward the end of a meeting, they should be given thought before voting.

Adjournment

After the amenities have been observed, such as the passing of other resolutions expressing appreciation for services and courtesies, and perhaps introduction of the new officers, the meeting is adjourned by motion and vote.

MANAGING MOTIONS

The work of a business session is greatly facilitated if officers and members know and practice the proper methods of handling motions according to parliamentary procedure. A motion is a proposal or suggestion intended to initiate action, effect progress, or allow the assembly to express itself as holding certain views. It is through these motions—made, seconded, discussed, and approved by a majority of the delegates—that the association is enabled to transact its business, make decisions, and move forward.

Uncomplicated motions may be passed very quickly by *silent assent,* such as accepting the secretary's report as read; or by *viva voce,* which means responding "aye" or "no" ("yea" or "nay") in response to a request from the presiding officer; *viva voce* may also be used in voting on involved issues. However, if the vote is, or is likely to be, close, the chair will ask for a *show of hands* or a *standing vote,* because they permit an actual count.

A *written vote,* or *ballot,* may be indicated and is usually required for elections.

To Make a Motion

A member who wishes to make a motion always:

1. Stands and goes to a microphone when indicated.
2. Waits, if necessary, until the speaker ahead has stopped talking. In general, it is advisable to remain seated until the previous speaker has finished, but if several members have motions to present, it is well to "get in line."
3. Waits for the chair's signal to go ahead. This may be done with a nod of the head or verbally.
4. Addresses the presiding officer as "Madame (or Mister) Chairman," "Chairperson," "President," or "Speaker."
5. Identifies oneself by name and state, as indicated. Sometimes stating the name of the office held, the committee, or some other affiliation is appropriate.
6. States the motion clearly and succinctly. When time permits, it is a good idea to write out a motion before rising to make it. This helps the individual to be sure she or he will say what is intended and also repeat it verbatim, if requested. Frequently, a written motion is given to the secretary to be sure it will be recorded accurately in the minutes.

Most motions require seconding before action. The chair will call for a second, if indicated, particularly when there is likely to be discussion of the motion. The member who does the seconding rises, addresses the chair, and after identification, says, "I second the motion." If no one seconds a motion calling for seconding, the motion is automatically lost and the president so states. No mention of it is made in the official records.

Discussion

Assuming that a motion is seconded, the chair next says, "It has been moved and seconded that . . . Is there any discussion?'' If there is none, she asks for a vote by one of the methods previously mentioned. A member wishing to ask a question or make a comment follows the usual procedure for recognition.

Sometimes discussion is prolonged, heated, and confused, involving proposed amendments to the original motion and perhaps even amendments to the amendment, known as *subsidiary amendments.* The presiding officer must be fair and skillful to permit all persons to express their views and yet not seriously impede the progress of the meeting. The action must then be guided back to the original motion, disposing of the last-mentioned items first.

Discussion of a motion may be terminated if a member calls for ''the question.'' This means that the member feels that the matter has been discussed sufficiently for the members to vote intelligently on it.

Because to terminate the discussion without the approval of the assembly would infringe on the privilege of unlimited debate, the chairman then asks, ''Are you ready for the question?'' If a sufficient number, as predetermined by the association's rules of order, vote in the affirmative, the motion is put to a vote. Otherwise, debate must be reopened or some other method must be used to handle the motion before the house.

Decision

The ultimate disposition of a motion depends on the majority decision of the delegates.* If more than half of them vote, ''yes,'' it is passed; if the majority vote ''no,'' the motion is, of course, defeated. Sometimes a motion is passed ''as amended,'' that is, not in its original form, but with one or more changes in it, or additions to it, as proposed from the floor during the discussion.

When there is obvious conflict or confusion about a particular motion, especially when it

*Some organizations require a two-thirds vote for passage of a motion or of motions in certain areas. These requirements are spelled out in the association's bylaws.

may have become complicated or unclear as a result of several proposed amendments, a motion to *refer it to a committee* may be made. This motion in itself may be debated. If it is passed, then the original motion goes to an appropriate committee for further study and possible presentation at some later date.

It is also possible to vote to *table* a motion; this means that it is set aside temporarily, permitting the chair to progress with the agenda, but will be taken up again later in the same session or meeting. A vote to *postpone* action on the motion until some other time may also be taken. Decisions to table or postpone action on a motion are most likely to be made when the matter at hand is a complicated or hotly debated issue. Any of these actions gives the members more time to clarify their thinking about it. It also permits more time to marshal arguments pro and con and, finally, permits the president, possibly aided by the parliamentarian, to study the motion so that at some later date it may be reviewed lucidly for the delegates. Sometimes a tabled motion never comes for action again, because everyone agrees that it is better not acted on.

Occasionally, members pass a motion that they later regret, either because the decision was made hastily, with incomplete information, or in a state of confusion. To bring that same motion before the assembly again, an individual voting on the prevailing side may move to reconsider. Anyone can second. The motion to reconsider takes precedence over other motions, and therefore is acted on at once, regardless of what else is being discussed. It is debatable, and if passed, the entire issue of the previously passed motion is open for discussion, with the opportunity to clarify or to introduce needed information. It is then handled in the usual manner.

The responsible member and, especially, the officer of any organization will not want to depend on this necessarily brief presentation of parliamentary procedure as the sole guide to informed action. If a meeting is not run expeditiously and fairly, members become rapidly disenchanted with the entire organization. Meetings may be the only way in which members participate in the decision-making process of the organization, and if they see it as disorganized or a setup, many will withdraw completely. The knowledge and skill of both officers and members are required to ensure that meetings are conducted as they should be, so that the voice of the members prevails.

MEMBER–STAFF RELATIONSHIPS

As nursing organizations grow larger, many acquire professional staff, supported by clerical and sometimes technical assistants. Not too long ago, an executive secretary was a retired member of a nursing association, untutored in association management, who learned on the job. Today, the professional executive, still scarce, is seen as essential, for she or he deals with large amounts of money, a complex organization, and, frequently, thousands of volunteers.

Although the professional staff of nursing associations may consist of nurses, members of the same organization, with voting and officeholding rights, the *job* role is different. The members make policy through the volunteer board and officers; the staff carries out policy. Because volunteers are transient—a board of directors inevitably changes after each election—it is often only the staff who have continuity. Yet, should their opinions as to a certain action be in direct opposition to the board's or committee's, unless they can sell their point of view, it is the staff's responsibility to do what the volunteers decide. Staff may try very hard, directly or indirectly, to influence the key members of the organization.

Many members do not have a clear concept of the careful balance needed between board and staff lines of authority and responsibility. Just as volunteers should expect to devote an adequate amount of time to the association and bring to it the same amount of intellectual commitment and judgment used in their professional pursuits, staff members are expected to provide not just services but leadership, and must create confidence in their judgment and in the program. Staff are expected to prepare guidelines and backup material so that volunteers' time is not wasted and they can react to specifics, not generalities. Staff and volunteers should regard each other as valuable colleagues with whom bad news as well as good news is shared. Staff must learn to identify the special abilities of volunteers so that they are put to use.[4]

It is also important that staff identify their roles, responsibilities, and activities, so that expectations are real. Volunteers should not get involved in what is not their responsibility. An executive director (ED) manages the office and personnel. When volunteers attempt to interfere in personnel matters, problems inevitably result. If the ED is incompetent, she or he should be terminated by the board.

Selection of an ED in a large nursing association may be made by an appointed search committee. Criteria for selection should be carefully thought through to meet the needs of that organization. In a study done by the Foundation of the American Society of Association Executives, the qualities considered most important for a successful association executive were listed by both EDs and voluntary leaders. Agreed on by both as most important were (1) interpersonal relationships, empathy, rapport, and (2) dedication, commitment, energy, and hard work. EDs then listed, in order, (1) integrity, (2) organizational/administrative abilities, (3) creativity, innovativeness, and vision; the volunteers preferred (1) organizational/administrative abilities, (2) intelligence, planning, and (3) knowledge of the industry or profession and of association management.[5] The heavy emphasis on management skills by the volunteer leaders is not unexpected when the importance of having a well-run organization is considered. However, perhaps the most significant point to remember in staff–volunteer relationships is that both are presumably working toward the same goals, and when there are unusual tensions between the two, it is often the result of misunderstanding or disagreement on how these goals are to be achieved. As in any other professional and human relationship, good communication is essential.

Issues and Concerns

Probably because of the proliferation of professional associations, there are many more concerns about them. At one time, organizations were run by volunteers in their spare time, typing notices with two fingers or with the help of somebody's sister; now they are a form of big business, including powerful unions and well-funded professional organizations. In 1979, 5,000 major trade and professional associations were identified, with the figure jumping to 40,000 if state and local constituent groups are included. This meant, on the average, one nonprofit association for every two or three for-profit corporations.[6] In 1983, according to Gale's *Encyclopedia of Associations,* there were 16,519 national associations, representing 173 million people. All seek economic and other advantages for their members, as well as the power necessary to succeed. Politicians do not want a strong, organized group against them, and there is no doubt that organizational lobbying gets action, especially if associations cooperate with each other.[7] Still, there is also concern that the power of such organizations is not good for the public, and trade associations and professional organizations have been found subject to the Sherman Act and the Federal Trade Commission Act, which relate to price fixing and restraint of trade.[8] In nursing, this has stopped the setting of fees for private duty nurses and raised questions about certification and accreditation by the professional organizations.

Because of this growth and power, or potential power, the concerns of voluntary organizations have become more and more similar to those of their for-profit counterparts. Recently, for instance, attention has been given to ethical dilemmas of staff and management, whereas previously this was considered more

of a theoretical topic relating to a profession or business in general.[9] However, given special attention is good management, since a voluntary organization, like any business, must be solvent. Few, if any, can expect an automatic increase in members or can retain members without considerable effort. Few people belong to just one organization in the various aspects of their lives, and there comes a time when they may decide that some are of less value and will be dropped. Therefore, some of the more sophisticated associations mount extensive marketing campaigns[10] and search for membership services such as travel, insurance, and health care packages, publications, and even loans that add to the professional benefits of membership. In addition, strengthening both the image of the organization and the group it represents is always part of the marketing picture.

One executive suggested a series of questions which a prospective member may wish to have answered before joining an association:

1. What are your programs and services?
2. Are you legal?
3. How will I be involved in your association?
4. Is the association properly financed?
5. What is the structure of the organization?
6. How well does the association represent the industry or profession?
7. Will I find peer identification in your association?
8. What are your association's relationships with other organizations?
9. Does the association have a competent professional staff?
10. How well does the association communicate with its members?
11. How well does the association create an environment for the industry or profession?[11]

But most critical are the issues of what the president of one professional organization calls the *internal crisis of identity and mission.*[12] The key question asked about this professional organization for university professors is also pertinent to nursing's professional organization: recognizing that the heterogeneity of the professionals generates threatening tensions and divisions within the organization, is there a sufficient residue of *common* concern to justify the creation of one body to bring together all who call themselves professional nurses?

One problem in nursing is that so many nurses do not understand what the functions of a professional association are and therefore have inappropriate expectations. Sociologist Robert Merton has delineated the functions in three categories: functions for individual practitioners, for the profession, and for society. For individuals, the association (1) gives social and moral support to help them perform their roles, especially in terms of economic and general welfare (salary, conditions of work, opportunities for advancement), CE, and working toward legally enforced standards of competence; and (2) develops social and moral ties among its members so that each becomes his brother's keeper. For the profession, the organization must set rigorous standards and help enforce them (quality of those recruited, of education, practice, and research). The profession must always press for higher standards. For society, the organization helps furnish the social bonds through which society coheres, providing unity in action.

> The association mediates between the practitioner and profession on the one hand, and on the other, their social environment, of which the most important parts are allied occupations and professions, the universities, the local community, and the government.[13]

The conclusion for the American Association of University Professors (AAUP) was that it did indeed have common purposes for all, but that it was necessary to work at maintaining and gaining membership and to be selective in the issues and roles that can be reasonably undertaken. The membership of most organizations, however, is and probably always will be made up of people with varying degrees of commitment, with at least half indifferent and the others ranging from the ambitious to the ambivalent/dissident.[14] No association can please them all. But one president concluded, "We are what we are because we are a voice of and for the profession. Without that, we are nothing."[15]

Peplau addressed the same problems: the dilemmas of diversity versus consensus; part versus the whole; wishes of members versus public interest.[16] Both presidents, like Merton, concluded that unless there is one voice for a profession, no one will listen. Adequate numbers of participating members are crucial. "To be able to speak for the profession, the association must be representative of as many of the profession as possible."[17]

In the following chapters, it will be seen how the increasing numbers of organizations that nurses can and do join overlap, compete, and frequently disagree. Add to that the trade unions that some nurses are choosing to represent them, and it is small wonder that the public asks, "Which is nursing's real association? Who speaks for nursing?"

REFERENCES

1. "Meeting Minutes: What They Should Contain," *Leadership,* **1**:59–60 (May 1979).
2. Samuel Shapiro, "A Primer on the Workings of Committees," *Leadership,* **2**:23–25 (Nov. 1979).
3. Henry Robert, *Robert's Rules of Order, Revised* (New York: William Morrow and Co., Inc, 1971), p. iii.
4. "What Should You Expect from Staff and Staff from You?" *Leadership,* **1**:63–64 (Nov. 1978).
5. "Qualities Needed for a Successful Chief Staff Executive," *Leadership,* **1**:54–55 (Nov. 1978).
6. "What Is an Association?" *Leadership,* **2**:51–52 (May 1979).
7. Margo Vanover, "Get Things Done Through Coalitions," *Leadership,* **3**:24–28 (Dec. 1980).
8. Basil Mezines and Steven Fillman, "Anti-

trust Guide for Association Members,'' *Leadership,* **1**:47–49 (Nov. 1978).

9. Margo Vanover Porter, ''The Ethical Dilemma: What's Right? What's Wrong?'' *Assn. Mgt.,* **33**:77–80 (Oct. 1981).

10. ''Seven Ways to a Sound Membership Marketing Strategy,'' *Assn. Mgt.,* **33**:62–63 (May 1981).

11. James Low, ''Ways to Evaluate Your Association Memberships,'' *Leadership,* **3**:14–15 (Dec. 1980).

12. Peter Steiner, ''The Current Crisis of the Association,'' *AAUP Bull.,* **64**:135–141 (Sept. 1978).

13. Robert Merton, ''The Functions of the Professional Association,'' *Am. J. Nurs.,* **58**:50–54 (Jan. 1958).

14. James Low, ''The Public, Your Members, Your Staff: Forces That Shape Your Professional Organization,'' *Leadership,* **1**:9–13 (May 1970).

15. Steiner, op. cit., 138.

16. Hildegard Peplau, ''Dilemmas of Organizing Nurses,'' *Image,* **4**(3):4–8 (1970–1971).

17. Merton, op. cit., 54.

National Student Nurses' Association

The National Student Nurses' Association, Inc. (NSNA), established in 1953, is the national organization for nursing students in the United States and its territories, possessions, and dependencies. NSNA's purpose is "to assume responsibility for contributing to nursing education in order to provide for the highest quality health care; to provide programs representative of fundamental and current professional interests and concerns; and to aid in the development of the whole person, his/her professional role, and his/her responsibility for the health care of people in all walks of life."[1] The functions of the organization, as listed in the bylaws, are as follows:

1. To have direct input into standards of nursing education and influence the educational process.
2. To influence health care, nursing education, and practice through legislative activities, as appropriate.
3. To promote and encourage participation in community affairs and activities toward improved health care and the resolution of related social issues.
4. To represent nursing students to the consumer, to institutions, and other organizations.

5. To promote and encourage students' participation in interdisciplinary activities.
6. To promote and encourage recruitment efforts, participation in student activities, and educational opportunities regardless of a person's race, color, creed, sex, age, life-style, national origin, or economic status
7. To promote and encourage collaborative relationships with ANA, NLN, and the International Council of Nurses, as well as the other nursing and related health organizations.

The NSNA is autonomous, student financed, and student run. It is the voice of all nursing students speaking out on issues of concern to nursing students and nursing.

MEMBERSHIP

Students are eligible for active membership in NSNA if they are enrolled in state-approved programs leading to licensure as an RN or are RNs enrolled in programs leading to a baccalaureate degree in nursing. Students are eligible for associate membership if they are prenursing students enrolled in college or university programs designed to prepare them for programs leading to a degree in nursing. Associate members have all of the privileges of membership except the right to hold office as president and vice president at state and national levels.

Application for membership is made directly to NSNA. Dues* paid to NSNA are a combination of national and state association dues; the latter vary from state to state. The dues structure is decided by a vote of the membership.

NSNA also has two categories of membership not open to students. Sustaining membership is open at the national level to any individual or organization interested in furthering the development and growth of NSNA, upon approval by the board of directors. Sustaining members receive literature and other information from the NSNA office. Dues vary for sustaining members, which may include NSNA alumni, other individuals, local organizations, and national organizations. Honorary membership is conferred by a two-thirds vote of the House of Delegates upon recommendation by the board of directors on persons who have rendered distinguished service or valuable assistance to NSNA. This is the highest honor NSNA can bestow upon an individual.

History

Just when or where the idea of a national association of nursing students originated will probably never be known. But for many years and in increasing numbers, students had been attending the national conventions of ANA and NLN, eager to learn of the activities of these two associations that would soon be affecting them as graduate nurses. Special sessions were arranged at these conventions so that students could meet together and discuss mutual problems. At the same time, some student nurses' organizations had been formed on the state level, giving students an awareness of both the strength and the values of

group association and action. It was inevitable, of course, that sooner or later, the idea of a national association would arise. Once it did, nursing students throughout the United States began to work enthusiastically in that direction.

In June 1952, approximately 1,000 students attending a national nursing convention in Atlantic City, New Jersey, voted to start preparations for the formal organization in 1953 of a national student nurses' association under the sponsorship of the Coordinating Council of the ANA and NLN. In the intervening year, a committee of nursing students and representatives of ANA and NLN worked on organization plans, and in June 1953 the National Student Nurses' Association was officially launched. Bylaws were adopted and NSNA's first officers were elected.

In its first few years, NSNA had little money, a small membership, no real headquarters of its own, and no headquarters staff. Its main assets at the time were the persistence, determination, and dedication of its members, plus financial and moral support from ANA and NLN. A year after NSNA's founding, these two organizations appointed (and paid) a coordinator to help NSNA function; many of the association's activities were transacted through correspondence. Each organization also provided a staff consultant to NSNA and helped finance the association's necessary expenses and publications. Among the latter were the bylaws and a newsletter. The next step was a headquarters office. Today NSNA rents its own office at 555 West 57th St., New York, New York 10019.

Even in its early years, NSNA was able to help finance itself. And year after year, NSNA's share of the costs increased. Membership grew, and annual dues, which had originally been fifteen cents per year, were raised to fifty cents in 1957. Finally, in 1958, only five years after its inception, NSNA became financially independent. The original coordinator appointed in 1954, Frances Tompkins, became the executive secretary (the title was later changed to *executive direc-*

---

*Because dues change, the current figure should be checked with the organization.

tor) and headed a staff of two. In 1959, NSNA became legally incorporated as the National Student Nurses' Association, Inc., a nonprofit association. Today the association pays for headquarters offices, a staff, and all the other expenses incidental to running the business of a large association. It holds and finances its own annual convention. And, at the same time, it has initiated and financed several important projects in the interests not only of its members but of the nursing profession as a whole.

General Plan of Organization

The policies and programs of NSNA are determined by its House of Delegates, whose membership consists of elected representatives from the school and state associations. The delegates at each annual convention elect NSNA's three officers; six nonofficer directors, one of whom will become editor of *Imprint,* the official journal of NSNA; and a four-member nominating committee. Officers serve for one year or until their respective successors are elected.

Two consultants are appointed, one each by the ANA and NLN, in consultation with the NSNA board of directors. They serve for a two-year period or until their respective successors are appointed. According to the bylaws, these consultants are charged with providing an interchange of information between their boards and NSNA. All consultants are expected to serve only as resource persons, consulting with officers, members, and staff and attending meetings of the association. In *Guidelines for Consultants,* published by NSNA, a summary of responsibilities states:

> It is truly the consultant's role to stand and wait for the student organization to grow by providing background information and encouragement, but not by providing decisions. The decisions must come from the students themselves.[2]

The board of directors manages the affairs of the association between the annual meetings of the membership, and an executive committee, consisting of the president, vice president, and secretary/treasurer, transacts emergency business between board meetings. There is only one standing committee (nominating), but the board has the authority to establish other committees as needed.

Constituent organizations may or may not function in a similar manner; their bylaws must be submitted to NSNA for review.

In 1976, the NSNA House of Delegates mandated a change in the structure of the association, giving school chapters the eligibility for constituency status and delegate representation. Under this system, school chapters must submit their bylaws to NSNA for review and must have fifteen members. Delegate representation is based upon the number of students in the school who are members. State associations that have two recognized school chapters and their own bylaws in conformity are recognized as NSNA constituents and are entitled to one voting delegate.

Projects, Activities, Services

NSNA has a wide variety of activities, services, and projects to carry out its purpose and functions. Even in its early years, the association sought participation in ANA and NLN committees and sent representatives to the National Conference on Citizenship and the International Council of Nurses (ICN).

Early projects were the Minority Group Recruitment Project (which has developed into Breakthrough to Nursing) and the Taiwan Project.

The latter project, carried out in cooperation with the American Bureau for Medical Aid to China, grew out of NSNA members' interest in nursing students in other countries, coupled with a desire to assist whenever possible. After a firsthand report about the inadequate, overcrowded living conditions for nursing students at the National Defense Medical Center, Taiwan, delegates to the 1961 NSNA convention voted to raise $25,000 to build and equip a new dormitory for this group. By 1965, through vigorous fund-raising drives carried out at all levels of NSNA, the larger sum of $37,000 had been accumulated.

The completed fifty-student residence, named the NSNA Dormitory, was officially dedicated in March 1966, with American government officials cutting the traditional ribbon at the ceremony and representing both NSNA and the United States government.

Today, NSNA representatives sit on committees of ANA and other health organizations. NSNA is also a leading participant in the student assembly of the ICN, and the NSNA president served as its chairperson during the 1977 ICN in Tokyo. NSNA served as host for the 1981 student assembly.

NSNA members are involved in community health activities such as hypertension screening, health fairs, child abuse, teenage pregnancy, and education on death and dying. Some of these activities are carried out in cooperation with other student health groups.

In addition to health- and nursing-related issues, social, women's, and human rights issues are supported by NSNA. The association is working hard to educate its members about the need for the Equal Rights Amendment (ERA), the dangers of nuclear war, and the importance of registering to vote and voting. In 1984, a Voter Registration Campaign was initiated with students registering voters on their own campuses.

Community health activities receive major emphasis by NSNA, and projects planned and implemented by NSNA members cover a wide variety of community health needs. Community projects are frequently sponsored by local NSNA chapters or in collaboration with other associations or agencies. For example, NSNA members have organized walkathons to raise funds for the March of Dimes Birth Defect Foundation and have held blood pressure screenings and counseling in conjunction with National High Blood Pressure Month.

Breakthrough to Nursing

NSNA has always been involved in recruitment activities designed to interest qualified men and women in undertaking nursing careers. In 1965, however, NSNA launched a nationwide project directed toward the recruitment of blacks, Indians, Spanish-surnamed, Hispanic, and other minority group members into the nursing profession. Known as the National Recruitment Project, this long-term effort grew out of an increasing awareness on the part of nursing students of their collective responsibility for supporting the civil rights movement, for recruiting for nursing, for alerting young men and women in minority groups to the opportunities in a nursing career, and in recognition of the value of such nurses in improving the care of their own ethnic groups.[3]

The national project was proposed at the 1965 NSNA convention by the 1964–1965 NSNA Nursing Recruitment Committee, whose recommendations were based on results of pilot projects conducted in Colorado, Minnesota, and Washington, D.C. The delegates voted to undertake the project on a national scale.

The project was officially defined as

> focusing on the recruitment of Negroes and other minority groups into the nursing profession. Also, this project takes into account that nursing students have a vital interest in improving the position of Negroes and other minority groups in our society. Especially valuable volunteers in this project would be those students of minority groups. Not only would these students help in establishing rapport, but also would serve as an example that the nursing profession is attainable for all. This is truly a project for every NSNA member.[4]

By early 1967 the project was well underway in many different areas of the country, with the different state associations tackling the problem in various ways. In collaboration with other appropriate community groups—the Urban League, those associated with Head Start or other antipoverty programs, and civil rights groups—nursing students throughout the United States worked diligently not only to interest minority group members in nursing but also to help them financially, morally, and educationally to undertake such a career.

In 1971 NSNA set the Breakthrough to Nursing Project,[5] as it is now called, as a priority and sought funds to strengthen and expand the existing program. Later that year, NSNA was awarded a contract for $100,000 by the Division of Nursing, DHEW. In 1974, a three-year grant was received from DHEW that expanded Breakthrough to forty funded target areas. The grant ended in June 1977, but students are still involved in Breakthrough to Nursing on a nonfunded basis.

The objectives of the project were (1) to develop and implement a publicity campaign to inform and interest potential nursing candidates in a nursing career; (2) to coordinate nursing student recruitment efforts with community organizations and schools of nursing in support of the program to reach more minority students; (3) to participate in recruitment program activities such as conferences, workshops, and career days focused on increasing the number of minority students recruited into nursing; (4) to work with public school counselors, teachers, school nurses, and other secondary school personnel to assist with the identification, motivation, and encouragement of disadvantaged and/or minority group students interested in a career in nursing; and (5) to inform the public and the nursing community of the goals of the project.

In order to carry out these objectives, the involvement and support of nursing student volunteers, faculty, and heads of schools of nursing were essential. Student volunteers in Breakthrough areas carried out such activities as career fairs, education of school counselors, work with schools and community groups to provide tutorial and counseling services, development and distribution of brochures, help with the application and registration procedures in colleges, and provision of information about financial resources.

To raise the level of awareness of the need for minority nurses, a publicity campaign was developed using various media. A number of brochures, booklets, and posters are available for distribution nationally. Although there are still problems such as racial polarization, increasingly competitive entrance into crowded nursing programs, and retention of students after recruitment, there is no doubt that the project has had an impact on nursing, on NSNA members, and on the community.

Legislation

One of the most impressive NSNA developments in recent years is the active and knowledgeable participation of NSNA members in legislation. Excellent resources on legislative activities on a national level and assistance and support in legislation provided by NSNA to constituent associations resulted in legislative committees in most states. During the crises of federal funding for health during the 1970s, students testified before congressional committees and supported the passage of the Nurse Training Act by their active participation in the political process. They have also urged passage of the ERA and national health insurance. Students are also encouraged to work with state nurses' associations (SNAs), state political action committees (PACs), and other groups on health legislation on the local and state levels, and to educate members in such areas as state nurse practice acts and political activism.

Interdisciplinary Activities

NSNA has shown a forward-looking interest in the health and social problems of society, often combined with like interest in interdisciplinary cooperation. With the American Medical Student Association, Student American Pharmaceutical Association (SAPhA), and American Student Dental Association (ASDA), individual nursing students have participated in Head Start, Appalachian and Indian health, migrant health, and Job Corps projects. Unfortunately, federal cutbacks have reduced these nationally sponsored summer projects considerably. However, on the local level, involvement in Student Professionals Engaged in Education on Drugs (SPEED) and the OTC (over-the-counter) Drug Project to educate the public to the dangers of over-the-counter drugs continued. NSNA was also one of the sixteen original sponsors of the well-received television film *VD Blues,* carried by the Public Broadcasting Service, and members helped answer phones at the local VD hotline the night of the broadcast.

One major interdisciplinary activity in which NSNA participates is Concern for Dying's Interdisciplinary Collaboration on Death and Dying. This student program recruits representatives from the American Medical Student Association, the Law Student Division of the American Bar Association, and students from social work and theology schools. The Collaboration, begun in 1977, introduces students to a variety of professional perspectives on death and dying and creates a dialogue among future professionals.

Other Professional Activities

Almost since the inception of NSNA, members have been invited to participate in the committees of ANA and NLN. Such participation has increased as NSNA has sought to take an active part in the debates, discussions, and decisions concerning nursing. Usually the resolutions of NSNA support the goals of the ANA and NLN, and, at times, they move ahead of the others in their acceptance of change. The support of both organizations is often asked on issues that require the support of nurse administrators, educators, or others. Some of the issues involved have been in relation to curriculum change, clinical experience opportunities, responsibilities of male students, education for practice, career mobility, and accreditation.

Scholarship Funds

The Foundation of the National Student Nurses' Association administers its own scholarship program, giving scholarships ranging from $1,000 to $2,000 to its members. The Foundation was established in 1969 as the Frances Tompkins Educational Opportunity Fund to enable individuals and organizations to contribute funds to educate nursing students and others to study and understand the scope of present and future community health needs with a view to developing innovative programs. The fund is incorporated and has obtained federal tax exemption. Scholarship monies are obtained from various organizations, and contributors have included both commercial enterprises and professional organizations. Individual contributions are accepted for the Mary Ann Tuft Scholarship Fund and the Alice Robinson Memorial Scholarship Fund. Scholarship applications become available in the fall of each year.

Also under the aegis of NSNA is the Laura D. Smith Scholarship Fund. Each year the NSNA has awarded a $600 scholarship to an RN who plans to matriculate for either a bachelor's or master's degree. The nurse may be a graduate of a diploma, associate degree, baccalaureate degree, or doctor of nursing (ND) program but must have been a member of NSNA while in nursing school. This scholarship was established in 1962 in honor of Laura D. Smith, former senior editor of the *American Journal of Nursing* and NSNA adviser, who died in 1961. Application for the scholarship should be made to its administrator, Nurses' Educational Funds, AJN Company, 555 West 57th Street, New York, N.Y. 10019.

Publications and Resources

Imprint, the official NSNA magazine, came into existence in 1968, and a subscription is given to members. Subscriptions are also available to other interested groups, schools, and individuals. *Imprint,* published five times during the academic year, is the only publication of its kind specifically for students. It is the only nursing magazine written by and for nursing students, and students are encouraged to contribute articles and letters. Students may also take advantage of the annual John-son & Johnson Baby Products Writing Con-test, which offers cash prizes.

Other publications include the *NSNA News,* a newsletter that keeps organization leaders at state and school levels informed of pertinent issues and activities; *The Dean's Notes,* a newsletter for deans and directors of schools of nursing; the *Business Book,* which serves as an annual report and is printed for the annual convention; *Getting the Pieces to Fit*, a yearly handbook for state and school chapters; and informational, supportive mate-rials on students' rights, guidelines for faculty evaluation, and guidelines for clinical evalua-tion. Most states and some schools also pub-lish newsletters.

At the tenth anniversary of its founding, NSNA had accomplished a great deal.[6] Before its thirtieth, it had become an involved group whose activities demonstrated committed pro-fessionalism.[7] Gone were the stunt nights and uniform nights of the early days. "Students learned to conduct meetings and to use parlia-mentary procedure, they showed concern about their education and their future prac-tice, and they showed concern for others."[8] They were involved in many of the same issues as ANA and NLN and often seemed to show more foresight.

Education was of prime interest, and among the issues discussed were curriculum planning, accreditation, entry into practice, and student rights. Perhaps the last two were the most controversial. Since 1963, entry into practice has been discussed at conventions, and in 1967 the NSNA House of Delegates, composed largely of diploma graduates, made the historic decision to support ANA's first position paper on education for nursing, call-ing for a minimum of a baccalaureate degree for entry into practice. This position was rein-forced in 1976 and 1979, but, as early as 1969, NSNA delegates also encouraged the develop-ment and demonstration of nursing education programs that would recognize an individual's previously acquired knowledge and skill. For

the next decade, convention resolutions called for pathways for career mobility for AD and diploma nurses.

As in other fields, nursing students have also fought for their own rights, and NSNA has maintained a commitment to student rights. In 1970, a guideline for a student bill of rights was distributed to all constituents, a mandate of the 1969 delegates. In 1975, a comprehensive bill of rights, responsibilities and grievance procedures was accepted and published.[9] The statement was adopted in schools throughout the country.

In the area of practice, students have taken positive stands on the concept of mandatory licensure, maldistribution of nursing man-power, national standards for practice, substi-tution of unlicensed personnel for nurses, and use of student nurses as a substitute for nurses. They have also supported economic security and in 1966 and 1975 supported the ANA position that in the event of a non-RN strike, students would not substitute for strik-ing workers unless patients were endangered.

Finally, NSNA members have been in-volved in issues affecting the public's health—for instance, by participating in projects to ed-ucate the public about the dangers of smoking. NSNA offers the opportunity for nursing students to be heard, becomes a fo-rum for debates on health and social issues as well as nursing issues, provides opportunities for interdisciplinary contacts, and is a testing ground for leadership skills. Participation and involvement can be a meaningful and valuable part of the nursing student's education.

NSNA members, and students in general, have become more and more aware of their re-sponsibilities and of the impact they can have. As new issues have arisen, especially during the past decade, they have not been afraid to face them and take a stand. They have not only spoken words, they have acted to carry out their beliefs. They have come a long way from the silent generation of the fifties.[10]

REFERENCES

1. "Meeting Minutes: What They Should Contain," *Leadership*, **1**:59–60 (May 1979).
2. Samuel Shapiro, "A Primer on the Workings of Committees," *Leadership*, **2**:23–25 (Nov. 1979).
3. Henry Robert, *Robert's Rules of Order, Revised* (New York: William Morrow and Co., Inc., 1971), p. iii.
4. "What Should You Expect from Staff and Staff from You?" *Leadership*, **1**:63–64 (Nov. 1978).
5. "Qualities Needed for a Successful Chief Staff Executive," *Leadership*, **1**:54–55 (Nov. 1978).
6. "What Is an Association?" *Leadership*, **2**:51–52 (May 1979).
7. Margo Vanover, "Get Things Done Through Coalitions," *Leadership*, **3**:24–28 (Dec. 1980).
8. Basil Mezines and Steven Fillman, "Antitrust Guide for Association Members," *Leadership*, **1**:47–49 (Nov. 1978).
9. Margo Vanover Porter, "The Ethical Dilemma: What's Right? What's Wrong?" *Assn. Mgt.*, **33**:77–80 (Oct. 1981).
10. "Seven Ways to a Sound Membership Marketing Strategy," *Assn. Mgt.*, **33**:62–63 (May 1981).
11. James Low, "Ways to Evaluate Your Association Memberships," *Leadership*, **3**:14–15 (Dec. 1980).
12. Peter Steiner, "The Current Crisis of the Association," *AAUP Bull.*, **64**:135–141 (Sept. 1978).
13. Robert Merton, "The Functions of the Professional Association," *Am. J. Nurs.*, **58**:50–54 (Jan. 1958).
14. James Low, "The Public, Your Members, Your Staff: Forces That Shape Your Professional Organization," *Leadership*, **1**:9–13 (May 1970).
15. Steiner, op. cit., 138.
16. Hildegard Peplau, "Dilemmas of Organizing Nurses," *Image*, **4**(3):4–8 (1970–1971).
17. Merton, op. cit., 54.

American Nurses' Association

The American Nurses' Association (ANA) is nursing's professional organization, with membership in its state constituent associations (SNA's) open only to registered professional nurses. As such, it is the most significant organization to which nurses may belong, because it is the one through which nurses decide upon the functions, activities, and goals of their profession.* ANA serves as spokesman and agent for nurses and nursing, acting in accordance with the expressed wishes of its membership. ANA membership is voluntary and in 1985 totaled more than 165,000 nurses.

The ANA was established in 1897 by a group of nurses who, even then, recognized the need for a membership association within which nurses could work together in concerted action. Its original name was the Nurses' Associated Alumnae of the United States and Canada, but in order to incorporate under the laws of the state of New York, it was necessary to drop the reference to another country in the organization's title. This was done in 1901; however, the name remained Nurses'

Associated Alumnae of the United States until 1911, when it became the American Nurses' Association. The Canadian nurses formed their own membership association.

History shows that ANA's primary concern has always been individual nurses and the public they serve. Thus, in its early years ANA worked diligently for improved and uniform standards of nursing education, for registration and licensure of all nurses educated according to these standards, and for improvement of the welfare of nurses. The need for such actions and the difficulties involved become apparent if one remembers that in the early 1900s many hospitals opened schools for economic reasons only, with no real interest in the education or employment of the nurses, and the public had no guarantee that any nurse gave safe care.[1] ANA's efforts served to protect the public from unsafe nursing care provided by those who might call themselves nurses but who had little or no preparation. In recent years, ANA has continued to give major attention to setting standards of practice and education, although the National League for Nursing (NLN) has retained the accreditation functions for nursing education programs.

---

*For a comprehensive history of ANA, the best source is *One Strong Voice,* cited in Chapter 3.

PURPOSES AND FUNCTIONS

Throughout its existence, ANA's functions and activities have been adapted or expanded in accordance with the changing needs of the profession and the public. As a changed or changing major function becomes crystallized, it is incorporated in the bylaws by vote of the ANA House of Delegates. Thus, the purposes of ANA, as stated in the current bylaws, are to:

1. Work for the improvement of health standards and the availability of health care services for all people.
2. Foster high standards of nursing.
3. Stimulate and promote the professional development of nurses and advance their economic and general welfare.

These purposes are unrestricted by considerations of nationality, race, creed, life-style, color, sex, or age.

ANA's current functions, also as outlined in the bylaws, are to:

- establish standards of nursing practice, nursing education, and nursing services.
- establish a code of ethical conduct for nurses.
- ensure a system of credentialing in nursing.
- initiate and influence legislation, governmental programs, national health policy, and international health policy.
- support systematic study, evaluation, and research in nursing.
- serve as the central agency for the collection, analysis, and dissemination of information relevant to nursing.
- promote and protect the economic and general welfare of nurses.
- provide leadership in national and international nursing.
- provide for the professional development of nurses.
- conduct an affirmative action program.
- ensure a collective bargaining program for nurses.
- provide services to constituent state nurses' associations.

- maintain communication with members through official publications.
- assume an active role as consumer advocate.
- represent and speak for the nursing profession with allied health groups, national and international organizations, governmental bodies, and the public.[2]

MEMBERSHIP AND DUES

ANA is made up of state and territorial associations. The former consist of district nurses' associations, the number within each state varying with its geography, population distribution, and other factors. The state or territorial associations are known as *constituent units,* of which there are at present fifty-three: one in each of the fifty states plus the District of Columbia, the Virgin Islands, and Guam. (State associations are frequently referred to as SNAs; districts, as DNAs.)

From the inception of ANA, individual nurses could become members, usually by joining their district association. They then automatically became members of the SNA and ANA. This began to change in the 1970s, when a number of SNAs began experimental programs (some sanctioned by ANA) allowing members to join at any level without having to join all three—or pay dues for all three. Certain states, especially those with many collective bargaining units, felt that this would attract more members to the SNAs, and perhaps to ANA, since, of course, dues would be less and since a number of nurses were not interested in national professional issues or vice versa. It was also expected that the SNA would then have more power in policy formation. Some of these states did gain a larger membership: few nurses chose only ANA as the level at which to join. Finally, at the 1982 House of Delegates,* after a heated debate,

---

*See the bibliography for information about convention reports.

the bylaws were changed and a new organizational entity was born—the federation. No longer could an individual member become a member of ANA. Now ANA is composed only of qualified member state associations, called *constituent SNAs,* and a nurse can only join an SNA. Qualifications are delineated in the bylaws:

A constituent SNA is an association that—

a. has articles of incorporation and bylaws that govern its members and regulate its affairs.

b. has stated purposes and functions congruent with those of ANA.

c. provides that each of its members either has been granted a license to practice as a registered nurse in at least one state, territory, or possession of the United States and does not have a license under suspension or revocation in any state, or has completed a nursing education program qualifying the individual to take the state-recognized examination for registered nurse licensure as a first-time writer.

d. serves a geographic area such as a state, territory, or possession of the United States where there is no other recognized constituent SNA.

e. maintains a membership that meets the qualifications in these bylaws, unrestricted by consideration of nationality, race, creed, lifestyle, color, sex, or age.

f. is not delinquent in paying dues to ANA.

Responsibilities

a. The bylaws of each constituent SNA shall—

1) provide for the obligation of the constituent SNA to pay dues to ANA in accordance with policies adopted by the House of Delegates.

2) provide for members to elect delegates and alternates to the ANA House of Delegates according to provisions of these bylaws.

3) protect members' right to participate in the constituent SNA.

4) specify the obligations of members.

5) provide for disciplinary action and an appeal procedure for members pursuant to common parliamentary and statutory law.

6) provide for official recognition of constituent associations of the constituent SNA.

b. Each constituent SNA shall—

1) enter into a written agreement with ANA for the collection and forwarding of membership dues and for the verification of the membership base of the constituent SNA, and

2) abide by the terms of such agreement.

3) apprise its members of their right to—

a) receive a constituent SNA/ANA membership card and *The American Nurse.*

b) be a candidate for ANA elective and appointive positions in accordance with these bylaws.

c) participate in the election of constituent SNA delegates to the ANA House of Delegates in accordance with these bylaws.

d) attend the meetings of the ANA House of Delegates, the convention, and other unrestricted ANA activities.

e) attend the congress of the International Council of Nurses.

f) hold membership in ANA councils in accordance with provisions of these bylaws.

4) require that members of the constituent SNA abide by the ANA Code for Nurses.[3]

Dues are set by the House of Delegates and are based on the number of members in the constituent SNAs. To this would be added SNA dues and DNA dues, if the nurse belonged to the latter.

GENERAL PLAN OF ORGANIZATION

From time to time, ANA's organizational structure undergoes some minor or major changes to enable the association to function more efficiently in the light of changing circumstances or needs. The major changes made in 1982 by the House of Delegates meeting in convention are included in the following description of how ANA is organized and how it functions.

House of Delegates, Officers, Board[4]

The business of the association is carried on by its House of Delegates and board of directors. The House of Delegates, made up of a designated number of membership representatives elected by the SNAs, is the highest authority in the association. It meets every year to transact the association's business and to establish policies and programs.* It also elects ANA's board of directors and officers, the majority of the members of its nominating committee, and some members of its cabinets (to be described later). Thus, control of the association remains always in the hands of its membership, the SNAs.

Throughout the years, ANA's House of Delegates has made many important decisions related to nursing and nurses. At many successive conventions, for instance, it went on record as supporting the principle underlying the legislation that eventually brought Medicare into being. As early as 1946, it made several decisions designed to discourage discriminatory policies in regard to nationality, race, religion, or color within the nursing profession. In 1964 it voted to revise the bylaws so that ANA's responsibility for nursing education and nursing services might be more explicitly stated. In 1966 it adopted a national salary goal with a differential for nurses with a baccalaureate degree. In 1968 the Congress on Practice was created, reemphasizing ANA's concern with practice. In 1970, even with the

*Once in two years, it meets at the ANA convention. Until 1985, it had met biennially at conventions.

news that ANA was in a financial crisis because of mismanagement of funds and a consequent cutback of programs, the delegates resolved to recruit more of the disadvantaged into nursing, to help reduce the many threats to the environment, to become more deeply involved in health planning, and to develop closer working relationships with consumers of health care.

In 1972 some of the priorities set were directed toward defining requirements for high-quality nursing services, clarifying the scope of nursing practice, providing for continuing peer review, recognizing excellence and continued competence among practitioners of nursing, expanding and improving all aspects of education, and assisting SNAs with their economic security activities. Also adopted was an affirmative action program, which called for appointment of an ombudsman to the ANA staff.

In 1974, convention action gave major emphasis to national health insurance, nurses' participation in Professional Standards Review Organizations (PSROs), implementation of standards for nursing practice, certification for excellence in practice, reaffirmation of support of individual licensure (as opposed to institutional licensure), support of CE programs and a mandate to the ANA board of directors to establish a system of accreditation of CE programs and to study the possibility of accrediting other nursing education programs, efforts to effect direct fee-for-service reimbursement for NPs, the role of the ANA in collective bargaining, and a series of activities related to foreign nurses to eradicate their exploitation and assist in their becoming qualified to practice.

In 1976, the bicentennial convention year, the House passed resolutions on nurse advocacy for the elderly, responsibilities of nurses in nursing homes, alternatives to hospitalization for the mentally disabled and retarded, and involvement of nurses in health planning. The 1978 and 1980 Houses set as priorities for the next biennium: improving the quality of care provided to the public; advancing the profession so that the health care needs of people are met; enlarging the influence of the nursing profession in the determination and execution of public policy, and strengthening ANA so that it may better serve the needs and interests of the profession. Also approved were major resolutions on national health insurance, quality assurance, human rights, career mobility, and identifying, titling, and developing competency statements for two categories of nursing practice.

In 1982 and 1984, the House adopted the following statement of association priorities for the biennium: "To promote and protect the economic worth, the education and the practice of nurses." Specific goals were related to better communication with the public, standard setting for nursing, influencing health policy, and strengthening ANA's role in credentialing. The action taken in the House and the actions taken by the association throughout the year focused on these efforts. For instance, proposals accepted by the House in 1984 were related to smoking and other hazards of the workplace; the role of nurses within the prospective payment system, in home care, and in long-term care; implementing the goal of entry into practice at the baccalaureate level; supporting ERA; action to improve the economic status of women and children; nurse accountability and ethics; and protection of collective bargaining rights.[5] These are all illustrations of the wide scope of House of Delegates' decisions and ANA activities and the directions in which the efforts of the organization are moving.

In the intervals between the House of Delegate's meetings, the board of directors transacts the general business of the association. This is a fifteen-member body, consisting of ten directors and the association's officers: a president, two vice presidents, secretary, and treasurer. Terms of office are staggered to prevent a complete turnover at any one time and to provide for continuity of programs and action.

Serving to implement ANA policies and programs is the headquarters staff, most of them nurses, and a supporting clerical and secretarial staff. They carry out the day-by-day activities of the association in accordance with the policies adopted by the House of Delegates and ANA's general functions. ANA headquarters, since 1972, is at 2420 Pershing Road, Kansas City, Missouri 64108.

Standing Committees

Like other large organizations, ANA has its standing committees, those that are written into the bylaws and that continue from year to year to assist with specific, continuing programs and functions of the association. There are four such committees of the House of Delegates: bylaws, nominating, reference, and ethics. These standing committees differ from what are called *special committees,* which are appointed on an ad hoc basis to accomplish special purposes. Special committees may be board committees or House of Delegates committees.

Except for the nominating committee and committees of the cabinets and councils, committee members are appointed by the board. The standing committees are accountable to the House and submit reports to the board. The board also appoints its own committees to carry out its work.

Other Organization Entities

In 1982 and 1984, several other entities were created.* The *cabinets* are organized deliberative bodies "to which the House of Delegates assigns specific responsibilities related to fulfilling the functions of ANA. Cabinets are accountable to the Board of Directors and report to the House of Delegates." Members are both elected by the House and appointed by the board. Their major responsibilities are to evaluate trends, developments, and issues in the particular cabinet's area of responsibility and to develop standards and recommend policies and positions. Cabinets established at the

---

*Specific responsibilities of the cabinets, councils, and forums are delineated in the ANA bylaws.

time focused on nursing education, nursing practice, nursing research, nursing service, economic and general welfare, and human rights.

Councils have a clinical or functional focus and are established by the board. In 1984, they included the Council of Clinical Nurse Specialists, Council of Community Health Nurses, Council on Continuing Education, Council on Cultural Diversity in Nursing Practice, Council on Gerontological Nursing, Council on Maternal/Child Nursing, Council on Medical-Surgical Nursing Practice, Council of Nurse Researchers, Council on Nursing Administration, Council of Perinatal Nurses, Council of Primary Health Care Nurse Practitioners, Council on Psychiatric and Mental Health Nursing, and Council on Computer Applications in Nursing. Their primary purpose relates to providing: ''a forum for discussion; continuing education; consultation; and promoting adherence to approved standards of nursing through certification and other appropriate means.''

The *Constituent Forum* is made up of the president and chief administrative officer of each SNA or its designees. The purpose is to discuss nursing affairs of concern to ANA, SNAs, and the profession. *The Nursing Organization Liaison Forum* (NOLF) is made up of duly authorized representatives of ANA and other nursing organizations, who meet for the purpose of discussing issues of concern to the profession and promoting concerted action on them.

Academy of Nursing

A significant action taken by the 1966 House of Delegates was the creation of an Academy of Nursing (AAN) to provide for recognition of professional achievement and excellence. Because of the financial problems of ANA in 1970, the Academy was not established until early 1973. At that time, thirty-six nationally prominent nurses were selected as charter fellows of the Academy by the ANA board of directors. Included were practitioners, researchers, academicians, and adminis-

trators from thirty-four states. Criteria for selection of the charter fellows took into account:

1. Evidence of ability to contribute creatively to the advancement of nursing education, administration, clinical practice, or research.
2. Evidence of ability to perceive nursing in its broadest social and cultural aspects.
3. Evidence of ability to analyze facts, ideas, trends, and problems, to generalize and draw conclusions.
4. Evidence of ability to develop, evolve, and test theory.[6]

Within its first year, the Academy members developed bylaws, elected a ten-member governing council, set criteria for admission of additional fellows, initiated a publication, took a stand on the differences between medical care and health care, explored the roles of nursing and other professions in health care delivery, the political influence of nursing, female identity, patient rights versus professional rights and power, and also urged that the effects of the ANA Standards of Nursing Practice be spelled out in quantifiable terms.[7]

The objectives of the AAN are to

Advance new concepts in nursing and health care.

Identify and explore issues in health, in the professions, and in society as they affect and are affected by nurses and nursing.

Examine the dynamics within nursing, the interrelationships among the segments within nursing, and examine the interaction among nurses as all these affect the development of the nursing profession.

Identify and propose resolutions to issues and problems confronting nursing and health.[8]

The members, designated as Fellows of the American Academy of Nursing, are entitled to use the initials FAAN following their names.

Potential Fellows may be nominated by a Fellow in good standing (except during service on the Governing Council). After screening by the elected AAN Governing Council, a confidential ballot of names of candidates judged to fulfill the membership criteria is sent to all Fellows. The Governing Council then lists the candidates according to votes cast and declares as newly elected Fellows those receiving affirmative votes from at least two thirds of the Fellows voting.

Criteria for selection of Fellows are as follows:

1. Member in good standing in ANA.
2. Five years of professional experience, exclusive of educational preparation.
3. Evidence of outstanding contributions to nursing, such as:
   a. Pioneering efforts that contribute information useful in surmounting barriers to effective nursing practice or facilitating excellence in nursing practice.
   b. Successful implementation of creative approaches to curriculum development, definition of specialized areas for practice, or development of specialized training programs.
   c. Research or demonstration projects that contribute to improvement in nursing and health service delivery.
   d. Creative development, utilization, or evaluation of specific concepts or principles in nursing education, nursing practice, or health services.
   e. Authorship of books, papers, or other works that have significant implications for nursing.
4. Evidence of potential to continue to make contributions to nursing, such as:
   a. Efforts and projects that relate to contemporary problems.
   b. Efforts and projects that reflect a broad perspective on nursing, including social, cultural and political considerations.

The Governing Council may also recommend and the Academy approve the admission of Honorary Fellows in recognition of outstanding past contributions to nursing. There is a limit (500) to the number of Fellows that comprise the Academy. Those who attain the age of sixty-five may elect emeritus status which allows for participation but not election to the Governing Council. Since 1973, the Academy has held a yearly Scientific Session combined with business meetings. The focus of these sessions has been on such topics as models for health care delivery, long-term care, primary care, nursing image, prospective reimbursement, health economics, and nursing's influence on health policy. The published papers are available from ANA and are included in the ANA Publications List.

Other major activities in the 1980s have been the Magnet Hospital Study,* the Teaching Nursing Home program,[9] the Nursing Faculty Practice Symposia to showcase and discuss effective concepts of nursing faculty practice, and a Nursing Classics Study to identify and analyze classics in various areas of nursing for their contributions to nursing and society.

MAJOR ANA PROGRAMS AND SERVICES

The programs and services of ANA represent the total results of the efforts of members and staff, elected officers, committees, forums, cabinets, and councils. These include meeting with members of other groups and disciplines; planning or attending institutes, workshops, conventions, or committee meetings; developing and writing brochures, manuals, position papers, standards, or testimony to be presented to Congress; and implementing ongoing programs, planning new ones, or trying to solve the problem of how to serve the members best within the limitations of the budget. Every issue of the *American Journal of Nursing* and of *The American Nurse* carries reports of these many and varied activities. Presented here are brief descriptions of some (but not all) of the major ANA programs and services.

---

*See Chapter 5.

Nursing Service and Practice

ANA works continually and in many ways to improve the quality of nursing care available to the public. In its role as the professional association for RNs, it assumes responsibility for the competence of its members and defines and interprets principles and standards of nursing practice and education. These publications are available from ANA.

The formation of the Council, now Division, of Nurse Administrators, first called the Council of Nursing Service Facilitators, increased the ability of ANA to serve the needs of this key group. (Because of ANA's involvement in collective bargaining through the SNAs, some nurse administrators have felt a conflict of interest and have chosen to belong to the NLN or AHA administrator groups.) In 1979, a two-level certification program for nurse administrators was initiated—one for those at the executive level and the other for those in middle management nursing positions.

ANA's concern for quality nursing care is clearly manifested by the practice standards, with their implications for peer review, and the consequent action of ANA and many state associations to assist nurses to implement the standards. The *General Standards of Nursing Practice** and standards in areas of nursing specialty are general enough to encompass the variety of practitioners within each division. They are intended as models to measure the quality of nursing performance, another assurance to the public that quality care will be delivered. As the need for standards in highly specialized areas of practice was identified, various ANA divisions cooperated with specialty organizations to formulate standards. The many excellent publications are part of the overall plan to assist SNAs and individuals in the utilization of the standards of practice. Many workshops, seminars, and other programs were also held to provide nurses with new knowledge to facilitate implementation and thereby improve nursing care. Major pa-

*See Chapter 9.

pers and/or the proceedings of these conferences were made available, particularly for national conferences.

Certification

Probably the most exciting development in recent years is the ANA certification program. This program was originally intended to recognize professional achievement and excellence in practice, both to help practitioners maintain motivation for superior performance and to provide another means to establish and maintain standards of professional practice "to the end that all citizens will have quality nursing care."[10]

This concern for control of standards and improvement of nursing practice was manifested in the adoption by the 1958 House of Delegates of Goal Two: "To establish ways within the ANA to provide formal recognition of personal achievement and superior performance in nursing." In 1968, Interim Certification Boards began work with the Congress for Nursing Practice to establish criteria for certification. Action slowed during the period of financial crisis, but by 1973 ANA was completing arrangements for its certification program. Included was an arrangement with the Educational Testing Service (ETS) of Princeton, New Jersey, to provide technical support in the development of systems for certification, including appropriate examinations. (ANA-appointed groups provided the content for these tests, and ETS the test development expertise.) By 1974, criteria had been fully delineated for geriatric nursing, psychiatric and mental health nursing, pediatric NPs in ambulatory care, and community health nursing. Any currently licensed RN who could demonstrate currency of knowledge and excellence in practice, regardless of the basic program from which the nurse graduated, was eligible to take the examinations.

The first examinations were taken by approximately 300 pediatric and geriatric nurses in May 1973, but more than 5,000 applications had been received, attesting to the significance members attached to the program. Until then, the nurse had rarely been recognized or rewarded for excellent patient care; monetary rewards, prestige, and promotion had been via the administrative route or through educational achievement.

However, almost immediately, several problems arose. Not everyone agreed that ANA was the best group to certify nurses. For example, both the American Association of Nurse Anesthetists and the American College of Nurse Midwives expected to continue to certify in their specialties (although this is for admission into the specialty field). Other specialty nursing organizations also planned their own certification program. Most of these certifications were for a different purpose from that of ANA, which was for excellence in practice.

In 1976, the ANA announced that it would certify at two levels: (1) certification for *competence* in specialized areas of practice with distinctive eligibility requirements, and (2) certification for *excellence in practice,* with diplomate status in a proposed American College of Nursing Practice for certified nurses who met additional criteria.[11] This proposal was given a hostile reception at that year's convention, largely because the new diplomate status called for a master's degree, and many of those certified for excellence had no degree at all and little hope of acquiring a master's in the near future. With protests mounting, the diplomate proposal was put in abeyance, and although those nurses who were already certified for excellence maintained that certification, emphasis for the new clinical certification programs was on advanced specialty practice. Certification, then, was described as based on assessment of knowledge, demonstration of current clinical practice, and endorsement of colleagues, and was seen as a tangible acknowledgement of achievement in a specific area of nursing practice.

By 1984, certification examinations were being offered in seventeen specialty areas: adult NP; clinical specialist in adult psychiatric and mental health nursing; clinical special-

ist in child and adolescent psychiatric and mental health nursing; clinical specialist in medical-surgical nursing; family NP; gerontological nurse; gerontological NP; medical-surgical nursing; child and adolescent nurse; high-risk perinatal nurse; maternal and child health nurse; pediatric NP; psychiatric and mental health nurse; community health nurse; school NP; and two levels of nursing administration. More programs are planned.

Criteria for certification vary to some extent for the various specialties, but may include an examination and evaluation of specified documents submitted by the nurse such as pilot studies, projects, case studies, abstracts representing the candidate's case load, other evidence of continuing growth as a practitioner, statement of a philosophy of practice, references, and biographical data. In all cases, currency in practice beyond the requirements of licensure must be shown, and the candidate must be licensed in the United States. Past practice experience is no longer required. (There must have been a practice component in the program of study.) Specific details on each certification, including eligibility criteria and cost, are available from ANA. Certification is granted for five years, at the end of which time the individual has the option of submitting evidence and credentials for renewal. As of 1984, some 22,000 nurses had been certified by ANA.

Since 1979, ANA and some of the specialty nursing organizations have been making efforts to cooperate in the certification process. Because certification is intended as a protection of the public, certification of the same type by several organizations is confusing. Various alternatives include joint sponsorship of a certification process or endorsement of each other's certification.

Nursing Education

The important ANA function of setting standards and policies for nursing education has been demonstrated in many ways. The 1965 Position Paper was the beginning of a series of specific actions toward implementing the position that education for entry into professional nursing practice should be at the baccalaureate level.* ANA has made a number of other important educational statements in the last few years; these are available from ANA.

The topic of CE has also been given considerable attention by ANA, gaining impetus in 1971 with the establishment of the Council on Continuing Education and the awarding of a grant for a project entitled "Identification of Need for Continuing Education for Nurses by the National Professional Organization."†

ANA endorsed the concept of CE for all nurses as one of the means by which they can maintain competence. ANA believes that maintaining competence is primarily the responsibility of the practitioner. Because of a practical and philosophical reluctance to transfer this responsibility to government, the association, by a vote of its 1972 House of Delegates, opposed mandatory CE as a condition for renewal of a license to practice. This was reversed by the ANA House in 1974, and particular emphasis was put on SNA control rather than government control. The House directed ANA to provide support to those states that choose to establish CE as one prerequisite for relicensure, as well as to those states that choose to encourage CE through a voluntary program. By 1979, most SNAs had some sort of CE approved programs. However, as NP programs continued to proliferate on a CE basis, some type of accreditation of these educational programs was also adjudged essential. Extensive planning was done, with the result that since 1975, the association has provided a mechanism for voluntary national accreditation of continuing education in nursing. Through that mechanism, the National Accreditation Board and regional accrediting committees grant accreditation to various providers and approvers of continuing education in nursing. They also grant approval of spe-

cific continuing education programs and offerings.

Legislation and Legal Activities

ANA's legislative program is an important one that often affects, directly and indirectly, the welfare of both nurses and the public.* The association's legislative endeavors are concentrated on matters affecting nurses, nursing, and health, but in today's society these matters represent an extremely broad area of activity, ranging from child care to gun control.[12]

ANA's legislative program comprises three main endeavors: (1) to help SNAs promote effective nursing practice acts in their states in order to protect the public and the nursing profession from unqualified practitioners; (2) to offer consultation on other legislative measures that affect nurses; and (3) to speak for nursing in relation to federal legislation for health, education, labor, and welfare, and for social programs such as civil rights.

The first ANA Committee on Legislation was established in 1923, with the responsibility of watching federal legislation affecting nursing and representing ANA in such matters. The ANA board also determined at that time to confine the association legislatively to matters of health, nurses, and nursing. Until 1970, when it was disbanded by House action, the committee formulated policy and recommended action. Since that time, the various ANA organizational entities have developed legislative policies, which are then referred to the staff and the board for action. Legislative decisions are based on these policy statements, House resolutions, and, of course, the ANA platform.

The major responsibility for coordinating legislative information and action lies with the ANA governmental affairs arm. It was not until late 1951 that ANA opened an office in Washington, with one staff person to act as full-time lobbyist, and even then direction for

---

*This is discussed in some detail in Chapter 12.

†See Chapters 12 and 13 for discussion of issues in CE, as well as information on CE units and accreditation.

---

*For more information regarding legislation, see Chapters 18 and 19.

the legislative program emanated from ANA headquarters in New York. From that time on, the Washington staff has expanded considerably, and their responsibilities have increased and broadened to include lobbying (through its registered lobbyists); development of relationships with congressional members and their staffs and committee staffs; contacts with key figures in the administrative branch of government; maintaining relations with other national organizations; preparing most of the statements and information presented to congressional committees; drafting letters to government officials; presenting testimony; acting as backup for members presenting testimony; and representing ANA in many capacities.

Over the years, ANA has represented nursing in the capital on a number of major issues; funds for nursing education, Social Security amendments to cover nurses, national health insurance, quality of care in nursing homes, collective bargaining rights, health hazards, civil rights, Federal Trade Commission authority and regulations, problems of nurses in the federal service, tax revision, higher education, problems of health manpower, prospective reimbursement, and general support for improvement of health care. In addition, ANA lobbies for or against legislation that may affect nursing directly and immediately, such as funding for nursing education, collective bargaining, and reimbursement for nurses. For instance, ANA has always monitored the status of the Nurse Training Act (NTA), which has funded so much of nursing education and research.

Major newspapers and journals have commented on nursing's clout. It is important to note that as invaluable as the ANA Washington staff is, with its behind-the-scenes and visible lobbying activities, there would be no success without the active backup of nurses, as well as consumers, labor, and other health groups. Participation in the legislative process, as described in Chapter 18, is essential for nurses if the profession is to have any impact in influencing health policy.

ANA has often cooperated and coordinated with other health disciplines, but has also faced areas of disagreement (such as early opposition of AMA and other groups to funding for nurse education). Such philosophical differences still occur, but there has been increasing cooperation with both health and social groups to achieve mutual legislative goals.

Communication about legislative matters is particularly important to help members keep abreast of key legislative issues. Beginning in 1955, *Capital Commentary,* first called *Legislation News,* was sent to state associations, schools of nursing, state boards of nursing, state boards of health, chief nurses in federal services, and selected individuals. The demand and the need became so great that now it is incorporated in *American Nurse.* Prepared monthly while Congress is in session, *Capital Commentary* highlights major legislative and related developments. A monthly newsletter *Capital Update,* is sent to over 2,000 individuals and groups, including SNAs.

Legislative information is also provided in the *American Journal of Nursing,* and special communications are sent out from the Washington office when membership support is needed for legislative programs. Periodically, discussion guides and manuals have been developed for the use of SNAs, and the government relations staff frequently participates in state and national conventions and other meetings. For many nurses, the real excitement has occurred on the state level, particularly in the last few years, when issues of health care, health education, and especially new nurse practice acts have been the focus of legislative attention. SNAs have a vital role in providing information and assistance to members on pertinent legislative issues, and, when funds allow, there is often a legislative staff, a lobbyist, and perhaps a separate legislative newsletter at the state level.

In addition to specific legislative action, ANA becomes involved in various legal matters that affect the welfare of nurses. In some cases, ANA acts as a friend of the court, providing information about the issues involved. Since 1973, ANA has filed charges of discrimination in various district offices of the Equal Employment Opportunity Commission (EEOC), some of which it won and some of which are still unsettled. ANA has also presented oral arguments and briefs on various National Labor Relations Board (NLRB) hearings. The attorneys of SNAs also become involved in collective bargaining litigation or, at times, provide support for nurse practitioners cited by a medical board for practice of medicine without a license. The number of such services that ANA offers expands yearly.

Nurses' Coalition for Action in Politics

Important components of nursing lobbying efforts are the nursing political action groups. Most professional organizations have such groups, which are independent of the organization but related to it. This is because a tax-exempt, incorporated professional organization such as ANA (or AMA) is under definite legal constraints as far as partisan political action is concerned. In 1971, a small group of nurses in New York formed the Nurses for Political Action (NPA) to serve as a political arm for ANA by providing financial support for candidates and engaging in other political activities, as well as providing political education to nurses. In 1973, ANA directed an ad hoc committee to explore the possibility of a political action committee (PAC). For various reasons, a new organization evolved: Nurses' Coalition for Action in Politics (N-CAP), which was officially organized in 1974 with a $50,000 ANA grant as a voluntary, unincorporated, nonpartisan political action group. Since the initial grant, ANA has not funded N-CAP, but it does appoint some members of the board of trustees. N-CAP has a single purpose: to promote the improvement of the health care of the people through political action. Its two major functions are education and support. Education is directed toward encouraging nurses and others to take a more active part in governmental affairs, educating them on the political process and political is-

sues relevant to health care, and assisting them in organizing themselves for effective political action. For this purpose, N-CAP has sponsored workshops and prepared educational materials. N-CAP has also encouraged and assisted PACs on the state level. Many states now have active PACs that primarily give attention to state issues but are also able to coordinate collective action on national legislation.

Support is offered to political candidates (regardless of political affiliation) whose acts demonstrate dedication to constructive health care legislation. This support may be in the form of endorsement or include monetary contributions. Endorsements are made in consultation with state PACs whenever possible. State political action coalitions endorse state candidates. The fact that nurses, or at least ANA members, are perhaps more politically active than other citizens was shown by an N-CAP sponsored survey: 91 percent are registered to vote, 75 percent have written a letter to an officeholder expressing an opinion, 58 percent have attended a political meeting or rally, and about 58 percent have contributed money to a candidate.[13]

To support these activities, N-CAP accepts donations from nurses and others. N-CAP is headquartered at ANA's Washington Office: 1101 14th Street, N.W., Washington, D.C. 20005.

Economic and General Welfare

The ways in which ANA has worked to promote the welfare of its membership have varied with the times. When it was first incorporated, it gave as one of its purposes "To distribute relief among such nurses as may become ill, disabled, or destitute." Today, thanks to an economic security program adopted in 1946 and steadily expanded and strengthened since that time, it works actively to ensure that nurses have a voice in determining their employment conditions, that nursing salaries are appropriate to nursing responsibilities, and that employment conditions are of the kind to enable nurses to give high-quality care.

ANA's economic security program promotes the concept that nurses have a right to form a group to choose a representative to negotiate for them with their employer, and to have the mutually agreed-upon provisions put in writing. It endorses the constructive use of collective bargaining techniques in nurses' negotiations with their employers. Although ANA does not serve as bargaining agent for groups of nurses, many SNAs do so. ANA helps to develop the principles and techniques for such employer–employee negotiations and advises and assists the SNAs with their economic security activities as much as possible. In addition, a major role of the ANA and the Cabinet on Economic and General Welfare on the national level is to develop policy positions such as the 1974 statement on third-party reimbursement for services of independent NPs and the 1979 statement on hospital cost containment, and to act as a clearing house for information related to collective bargaining and nurses' economic and general welfare. Because of its status as a collective bargaining organization, ANA must follow the requirements of the Labor-Management Reporting Act of 1959 (Landrum-Griffin Law), which affects voting rights and elections of officers.

ANA has been providing the SNAs with varying degrees of assistance over the years, sometimes to the extent of supporting staff especially employed to work in state economic security programs, but this kind of help tends to be eliminated when the overall budget is limited. However, in November 1973, the president of ANA announced, "The association will commit substantial financial resources to support the constituent nurses' associations to bring about collective bargaining in each health care facility."[14] It was noted that ANA's previous collective bargaining efforts had been focused primarily on improving salaries, fringe benefits, and working conditions, but that now the thrust would be broadened "to improved the quality of nursing care, to assure the public of the individual

and collective accountability of qualified professional nurses, and to increase accessibility of health care services for the public."[15] This was to be accomplished by nurses achieving the right to make decisions affecting them, their practice, and the quality of care.

Although this approach to collective bargaining might be considered new to individuals who think of economic security only in terms of salaries, fringe benefits, and working conditions, job action by nurses has often been in protest of inadequate patient care, which has not been improved by the employer.

The ANA economic security program is often misunderstood by members, nonmembers, and others. Seeing that the economic security of its members is maintained is one of the classic roles of a professional association, and, especially in recent years, economic security has been seen as extending beyond purely monetary matters and conditions of employment to involvement of nurses in the decision-making aspects of nursing care. An example might be that, through an agreed-upon process, perhaps including a formal committee structure, nurses' objections to inadequate staffing or illegal or inappropriate job assignments would be instrumental in bringing about changes that would provide improved care.

In the last few years, the nurse's right to adequate monetary compensation has been recognized almost universally, although in many places, salaries and benefits are still abysmal, and there is still a struggle involved for improvement, with or without ANA representation as a bargaining agent. However, there is even more employer resistance to allowing nurses a voice in policymaking, both because of the possible financial impact and because of fear of loss of control, as well as on the basis of general philosophic disagreement.

One major advantage that employers in nonprofit health care institutions and government agencies have had is that the National Labor Relations Act (NLRA), which provides the legal basis for collective bargaining activities, did not extend its protection to employees of these institutions. This means, basically, that the employer did not need to engage in collective bargaining activities or acknowledge the rights of workers to organize and elect representatives. If employees did organize, they could be dismissed; only if the individual state had passed legislation including these workers would they be protected. Since 1946, when ANA first called on its state constituents to represent nurses in collective bargaining, states have been active in varying degrees, often concentrating first on gaining legal protection.[16] Even so, the degree of SNA activity has varied depending on finances, staff, and the acceptance of the collective bargaining concept in specific communities. From 1963 to 1973, the number of SNAs that have negotiated contracts increased from eight to thirty-two, and the number of nurses covered increased fivefold to 60,000.[17] Also in that time period, the ANA House made several major decisions in relation to economic security issues. In 1968, ANA's eighteen-year-old no-strike policy was rescinded, and in 1970 the twenty-year-old neutrality policy (that nurses maintain a neutral position in labor–management disputes between their employers and nonnurse employees) was also rescinded.

The 1974 passage of the NLRA amendment to include employees of nonprofit health care institutions created a flurry of activity. In 1975, as the result of a legal brief presented by ANA, NLRA ruled that a separate unit of professional RNs is appropriate under the normal unit determination criteria, and by early 1980, the professional organization was the largest collective bargaining representative of RNs employed in the nation. Also in 1975, the ANA board of directors established the Shirley Titus Award in recognition of individual nurses' contributions to the association's economic and general welfare program. Finally, the formation of the Commission of Economic and General Welfare in 1976 was a further indication of increased ANA membership interest and commitment in economic and general welfare issues.

The fact that unions, which have been suc-

cessful in organizing nonprofessional health workers and a number of professionals, will inevitably look toward including nurses in a bargaining package brings some impetus to ANA/SNA activities. There is serious concern that unions, with strong economic backing and single-purpose goals to increasing monetary and working benefits, may prove competitive, for nurses frequently do not see the professional organization as a strong or even appropriate bargaining agent. Because past experience has shown that unions have taken little action to negotiate contracts involving nurses in decisions that could improve patient care, and because many nurses are not even aware that such participation is possible, one of the most worthwhile purposes of collective bargaining could be lost.

In the years following the 1974 NLRA amendments, ANA and SNAs were frequently involved in legal actions regarding various aspects of collective bargaining that are unique to nursing: whether nurses could be in separate units, the status of head nurses and supervisors as management, and whether the fact that supervisors and directors of nursing may sit on the board of directors of an SNA means that the collective bargaining agent (the SNA) is controlled by management. Decisions favoring unions have been fluctuating in the last few years, as unions have lost ground; this also effects ANA. Such cases are not settled with one ruling, and frequently further action is taken through appeal mechanisms or legislation. Litigation on key issues can be long and expensive, but the carefully structured process of forming a unit also takes knowledge, effort, and sometimes legal consultation.*

Because ANA recognizes that other employed groups also have the right to organize, guidelines were developed in the event of a dispute between the employer and these groups. Nurses were urged to continue to per-

---

*The steps in forming a collective bargaining unit are presented in Chapter 22.

form their distinctive nursing duties; press for action in the interest of safe patient care to reduce the patient census; refuse to assume duties normally discharged by other personnel unless a clear and present danger to patients exists; and coordinate their activities and efforts through their local unit organizations and SNAs, using established channels for intercommunications with management and the other employee groups.

It should be noted that concern for the economic security of nurses is not limited to the American scene. In 1973 an unprecedented committee meeting was held jointly by the World Health Organization and the International Labor Organization to discuss urgent and radical measures to alleviate international problems of shortage, maldistribution, and poor utilization of nurses. A major objective of the meeting of health care experts from nineteen nations was to set viable recommendations for an international labor instrument covering factors influencing conditions of life and work in the nursing profession. Among the proposals presented were the right of collective bargaining, a forty-hour basic week, payment for overtime, two consecutive days of rest, and four weeks compulsory paid leave per year. There is a belief that the meeting, initiated by the International Council of Nurses (ICN) will have positive long-range effects on nursing around the world.

But the issues are not easily resolved. At ICN meetings, economic issues are discussed extensively, and in meetings of the Council of National Representatives, the subject of social and economic welfare affecting nurses is a top priority. Reports indicate that unions in many countries are attempting to represent nursing and control the profession.

Although the economic benefits gained through collective bargaining are obvious, the test of nurses' commitment to patient care will come as they acquire the right to become joint decision makers in improvement of patient care—in how well and how fully they participate.

Human Rights Activities

ANA works toward integrating qualified members of all racial and ethnic groups into the nursing profession and tries to achieve sound human rights practices. From the time of its founding, ANA as a national organization has never had any discriminatory policies for membership in the association. Until 1964, however, a few of its constituent associations denied membership to black nurses. In these instances, ANA made provision for black nurses to bypass district and state associations and become members of ANA directly. At that point (1950), the National Association for Colored Graduate Nurses (NACGN) voluntarily went out of existence, on the basis that there was no longer a need for such a specialized membership association. At the same time, strong pressure from ANA and the other state associations was exerted until now all state and district associations have discontinued such discriminatory practices, and minority group nurses are appointed and elected to committees and offices at district, state, and national levels. ANA has also strongly supported every major civil rights bill affecting health, education, public accommodations, nursing, and equal employment opportunities. In 1956, long before most health and professional associations had taken a positive stance on civil rights, ANA's board of directors adopted a statement supporting the principle that health and education should not be supported by tax funds if there are any discriminatory practices. Testimony along these lines was presented at federal hearings.

Even so, there was some feeling that a greater effort was necessary, and in 1972 the House of Delegates passed the Affirmative Action Resolution, calling for a task force to develop and implement a program to correct inequities. The program was defined as "a positive ongoing effort which is results-oriented and specifically designed to transcend neutrality." It was aimed at not only nondiscriminatory programming but action to correct past deficiencies at all levels and in all segments of an organization.[18] An ombudsman was also provided for and appointed.

The program went into action in 1973, and a task force of minority and nonminority members met with ANA units to identify problems and make plans. A minority position statement was developed, recommending methodology for change on such issues as problems of recruitment and retention of minority students, lack of data on career patterns of minority group RNs, and the need to include information in nursing education about the health needs of minority groups. In the years that followed, several regional conferences were held on quality care for ethnic minority clients, and the papers were published. A bibliography, *Minority Groups in Nursing,* was also published by the Task Force in 1973, and an updated bibliography was published in 1976 after the establishment of the Commission on Human Rights. Both were a compilation of the literature on ethnic people of color, men, and people with different life-styles who are in nursing, as well as other pertinent topics relating to minorities and the provision of health care to minorities.

In 1974, ANA was awarded a six-year grant by the Center for Minority Group Mental Health Programs of the National Institutes of Mental Health to establish and administer the Registered Nurse Fellowship Program for Ethnic/Racial Minorities. The program supported a number of minority nurses in doctoral study in psychiatric mental health nursing or a related behavioral or social science. It was funded again, and over half of the fellows have earned doctorates. Most are teaching or doing research on the health needs of minorities.

ANA's Human Rights Commission (now Cabinet) has been extremely active since its formation. Among its activities are human rights conferences and the initiation of a plan to produce monographs on historical and contemporary minority/ethnic nursing leaders. The Cabinet in general is alert to, and makes statements about, potential or actual prob-

lems in human rights, especially in relation to minority groups. Recently, the members formed strategic plans for ANA to address human rights concerns through acceptance of international, national, and organizational responsibilities.

ANA has taken positive legal action on minority rights, such as the Bakke case, and women's rights (salary and pension discrepancies). Since 1974 ANA has taken a position in support of the Equal Rights Amendment (ERA) and participates in various women's rights programs and activities. There is no doubt that activities related to human rights will continue. It is important that the valuable services of all nurses be fully utilized and the nursing needs of the American pluralistic society met.

Research and Studies

ANA has always been involved in various types of research or data-gathering activities. These have increased over the years.

ANA took a definitive step toward developing a distinct and coordinated research program for nursing and fulfilling its role as the source of national data related to the profession with the establishment of the Center for Research in January 1983. The center, one of ANA's administrative units, provides staff resources for the research, statistical and policy analysis functions of ANA and for the programs and activities of the American Nurses' Foundation and the American Academy of Nursing. The center allows for efficient use of resources and coordination of programmatic priorities of ANA and these two affiliate organizations. A Center Coordinating Committee, composed of the presidents of the three organizations, establishes center priorities and reviews and evaluates center operations and effectiveness. . . . A Technical Advisory Committee reviews research proposals for merit and has designed a review process for proposals. The Institutional Review Board reviews projects which involve human subjects and confidentiality of data for compliance with Department of Health and Human Services regulations.[19]

This staff continually collects data about nurses, nursing, and nursing resources. One result of this effort is *Facts About Nursing,* published periodically, a statistical summary of information about nurses, nursing, and related health services and groups. ANA is also the recipient of contracts to carry out specific programs or projects.

The American Nurses' Foundation

The American Nurses' Foundation (ANF) was created by ANA to meet the need for an independent, permanent, nonprofit organization devoted to nursing research. It was an outgrowth of the ANA's expanding research activities, particularly the five-year *Studies of Nursing Function,* which was undertaken by ANA after the 1950 convention, both because of a mandate by membership nationally and as an assumption of the profession's responsibility to determine its own functions.

Initial financing of this project was provided by the SNAs, but by the third year the ANA board of directors decided to finance the program from the association's budget. Between 1950 and 1955, twenty-seven studies were funded. *Nurses Invest in Patient Care,* a preliminary report, was prepared and published by ANA in 1956. *20,000 Nurses Tell Their Story,* by Everett C. Hughes, Helen MacGill Hughes, and Irwin Deutscher, was published in 1958; it was a synthesis of the findings of the studies.

So that such research could be continued and expanded, the ANA board recommended that the 1954 House of Delegates "authorize the incoming board of directors to secure information and to develop a foundation or trust for receiving tax-free funds for desirable charitable, scientific, literary or educational projects in line with the aims and purposes of the American Nurses' Association." After six months of committee study, the establishment of the American Nurses' Foundation was ap-

proved by the new board. It was incorporated in 1955, and its tax-exempt status was approved in 1956. The foundation was organized exclusively for charitable, scientific, literary, and educational purposes.

Between 1955 and 1973, the major objectives of ANF were to provide financial support for research and to disseminate and promote dissemination of research findings through publications, conferences, and other communications media.

In 1979, the ANF board established major new objectives focusing on analysis of health policy issues of priority to nursing, support for the career development of nurses, and assistance to the educational and research activities of ANA.

ANF has continued its Competitive Extramural Grants Program, funded through the contributions of both corporations and individuals. In 1983 in collaboration with ANA and AAN, the ANF Distinguished Scholar Program was established. The purpose of the program is to permit nurse health policy analysts and scholars to analyze selected policy issues related to economics, delivery of nursing services, nursing practice, and nursing education as identified by the nursing profession. Two prominent nurses have been named the first distinguished scholars. In 1980, in collaboration with the American Nurses' Association Council of Nurse Researchers, ANF also established an award to recognize nurse researchers who have made significant contributions to the nursing profession. The Professional Practice for Nurse Administrators in Long-Term Care Facilities Project (NA/LTC) was co-sponsored by ANF and the Foundation of the American College of Health Care Administrators, Inc. (FACHCA), and was supported by a grant from the W. K. Kellogg Foundation. The primary goal of this three-year project (completed in April 1984 and then re-funded) was the continued professional development of nurse administrators/directors of nursing in long-term care. A health education project was also administered by ANF.

The American Nurses' Foundation solicits, receives and/or administers funds for a variety of projects for the American Nurses' Association and the American Academy of Nursing. For the American Nurses' Association, this has included the Teresa E. Christy Grant, sponsored by the ANA Cabinet on Nursing Research and funded by individual contributions, and the newsletter of the ANA Council of Nursing Home Nurses, funded for quarterly publication by [a pharmaceutical company].

For the American Academy of Nursing, the foundation has received and administered funds for three projects: the study resulting in the publication, *Magnet Hospitals: Attraction and Retention of Professional Nurses*; the Career Patterns in Nursing Project from which the publication, *Nursing in the 1980s: Crises, Opportunities, Challenges,* resulted; and the three-year Nursing Faculty Practice Symposia Project.[20]

Obviously, funding is of vital concern to ANF. Unfortunately, the foundation never attained a stable financial base. In 1959, in order to establish a strong base upon which to operate, the foundation launched a nationwide drive for funds, enlisting support from the nursing community, the business community, and the general public. When the campaign closed officially in 1964, $750,000 had been raised. Since then, there have been a number of efforts to reach potential donors, including others in the health field. Many individuals, nursing institutions, and other groups give spontaneously, sometimes in the form of memorial gifts or bequests. All are tax deductible. However, increased funding is necessary to maintain and expand programs, and in 1979 another major fund drive was initiated, spurred by a matching fund offer of the American Journal of Nursing Company.

ANF is governed by its bylaws and directed by a nine-member board of trustees. All trustees are RNs. A finance committee and a research advisory committee report to the board of trustees. The finance committee monitors budget preparation, the investment portfolio, and fund-raising activities. The research advisory committee establishes guidelines for administering the small grant program and recommends recipients to the board for final approval. In 1978, the executive director of ANA was appointed as part-time executive director of ANF. There is also a professional headquarters staff involved in carrying out certain research projects.

Requests for information about completed ANF research projects or applications for grants (which should include an outline of the research question and the proposed design) may be sent to ANF headquarters at 2420 Pershing Road, Kansas City, Missouri 64108.

Communications

ANA's professional journal, the *American Journal of Nursing,* published monthly by the American Journal of Nursing (AJN) Company, which is owned by ANA, is available to SNA members at a reduced rate. Because ANA is the sole stockholder of the AJN Company (see Chapter 29), the ANA board of directors votes the stock to choose the directors of the board of the AJN Company. The association publishes *The American Nurse,* ANA's official organ, which reports ANA activities and happenings important to nursing. Other organizational entities may also publish newsletters as funds permit.

Other publications include *Facts About Nursing*; major reports, its *Reports to the ANA House of Delegates* and *Summary Convention Proceedings*; papers presented at meetings; and certain publications of the AAN and ANF. The association also publishes position statements, guidelines for practice, bulletins, manuals, and brochures for specialized groups within the organization and sends out news releases and announcements concerning activities of interest to the public. Available from the ANA upon request is its periodically revised *Publications.* ANA also conducts an ongoing educational and informational service to interpret ANA's activities, programs, and goals to nurses, allied groups, government, special agencies, and the public, and monitors news and public opinion trends affecting the profession.

ANA Participation with Other Groups

Cooperation and coordination with other groups is an important part of the function of ANA. Conferences, programs, workshops, task forces, and other meetings to share information and learning, or work on mutual problems are ongoing with other nursing, medical, and health organizations, hospital and health professional groups, and many others.

Participation of nurses, usually ANA members, in governmental planning and action groups is the result of concerted ANA efforts and carefully developed relationships with other groups and organizations. Besides such formally established communicating/coordinating groups as those between the Council of State Boards, the AMA, the NSNA,* the NLN,* the NFLPN,* and the AACN,* ANA staff and members relate to or meet with some 200 organizations and groups. ANA, NLN and AACN also form the Tri-Council, where issues of mutual interest are discussed.

Other Activities and Services

Among other ANA benefits for nurses is insurance of various kinds, available at favorable group rates at national and state levels. Many educational programs, seminars, workshops, clinical conferences, scientific sessions, and so on are available at all levels at reduced rates for SNA members. They are geared to current issues and new developments in health and nursing.

Nurses are also increasingly interested in international nursing. ANA was one of the three charter members of the ICN and is an active participant in the work of this international nursing organization. Essentially, ICN is a federation of national associations of professional nurses (one from each country), and ANA is the member association for the United

States (see Chapter 28). ANA also supports United Nations programs.

The Individual Nurse and ANA

A classic article by sociologist Robert Merton cites the functions of any professional organization as including social and moral support for the individual practitioner to help him perform his role as a professional, to set rigorous standards for the profession and help enforce them, to advance and disseminate research and professional knowledge, to help furnish the social bonds through which society coheres, and to speak for the profession.[21] In carrying out some of these functions, the association is seen as a "kind of organizational gadfly, stinging the profession into new and more demanding formulations of purpose."[22] Not all members agree with their organization's goals, and the difficult task of achieving a flexible consensus of values and policies must be accomplished with full two-way communication between the constituencies and the organizational top. However, the key to the success of any organization is the participation of its actual and potential members. This review of the ANA and its activities is at best an overview. As the needs of members and the demands of society require, changes occur, rapidly, inevitably, and, it is hoped, appropriately—but not always easily. The best way for a nurse to keep up with and share in the changes taking place is through active membership. ANA speaks for nurses; nonmembers have no part in that voice and have no right to complain if it is not representing them. The strength in the organization and in nursing lies in thinking, communicating nurses committed to the goal of improving nursing care for the public and working together in an organized fashion to achieve this goal.

REFERENCES

1. Teresa Christy, "The First Fifty Years," *Am. J. Nurs.,***71**:1788 (Sept. 1971).
2. American Nurses' Association, *Bylaws* (Kansas City, Mo.: The Association, 1982), pp. 5,6.

---

*These organizations are described in Chapters 24, 26, and 27.

3. Ibid., pp. 6–7.

4. Ibid., pp. 9–10.

5. "Association Priorities Adopted by House of Delegates," *Am. Nurse,* **16**:5, 8, 15, 16 (July–Aug. 1984).

6. Press release, ANA, "National Academy of Nursing Launched by ANA," Feb. 6, 1973.

7. "Academy President Says Medical, Health Care Differ," *Am. Nurse,* **5**:3 (Dec. 1973).

8. American Academy of Nursing, *Bylaws* (Kansas City, Mo.: The Academy, 1983). p. 1.

9. Mathy Mezey et al., "The Teaching Nursing Home Program," *Nurs. Outlook,* **32**: 146–150 (May–June 1984).

10. American Nurses' Association, *ANA Certification* (Kansas City, Mo.: The Association, 1973).

11. "New Certification Approach to be Initiated," *Am. Nurse,* **8**:1 (June 1976).

12. Julia Thompson, *ANA in Washington* (Kansas City, Mo.: American Nurses' Association, 1972).

13. "Nurses Politically Concerned and Active, Study of Voting Habits Reveals," *Am. J. Nurs.,* **79**:1181, 1194 (July 1979).

14. "Campaign Launched to Organize RNs," *Am. Nurse,* **5**:1 (Dec. 1973).

15. Ibid., 10.

16. Barbara Schutt, "Collective Action for Professional Security," *Am. J. Nurs.,* **73**: 1947 (Nov. 1973).

17. Ibid., 1946–1947.

18. "Affirmative Action Projects Launched," *Am. Nurse,* **5**:1 (May 1973).

19. American Nurses' Association, *Annual Report* (Kansas City, Mo.: The Association, 1984), p. 9.

20. American Nurses' Foundation, *Focus* (Kansas City, Mo.: The Association 1983–84), p. 2.

21. Robert Merton, "The Functions of the Professional Association," *Am. J. Nurs.,* **58**:50–54 (Jan. 1958).

22. Ibid.

National League for Nursing

The main purpose of the National League for Nursing (usually referred to as NLN or the League) is best expressed in this phrase from its certificate of incorporation: "that the nursing needs of the people will be met."[1] ANA is concerned with the same goal, but these two major nursing organizations approach this objective in different ways. ANA, as the membership organization for registered nurses, works primarily through nurses and within the profession. NLN, whose membership includes not only nurses but other members of the health team, interested lay people, and agencies concerned with nursing education and service, works within the community and in association with individuals and groups outside of, but interested in, nursing. In pursuit of the same general end of better nursing care, each organization has its own programs, responsibilities, and functions.

HISTORY

It is easier, perhaps, to understand the distinction between NLN and ANA if the events that led up to the establishment of the NLN in 1952 are reviewed. In many ways, NLN is older than the date suggests, because it grew out of several preexisting nursing organizations and absorbed many of the functions they had carried.*

In the mid-1940s the nursing profession decided to take a long, hard look at its entire organizational structure. At this time there were six national nursing organizations and a host of jointly sponsored committees, activities, and services. This somewhat cumbersome arrangement resulted not only in an overlapping expenditure of time, effort, and resources, but also in confusion in the minds of both nurses and the public as to the purpose and functions of each organization.

Starting in 1944, nurses, under the leadership of the Committee on Structure of National Nursing Organizations, began to study the way in which their profession was organized. The culmination of this long and painstaking self-examination came in 1952. At that time, nurses voted in favor of having two major organizations: a strengthened and reorganized ANA, which would continue to serve as the membership association for RNs, and a new organization, the National League for

_____

*See Chapters 3 and 4.

Nursing, through which nurses and others interested in nursing, along with institutions (both educational and service), could work together to strengthen nursing education and nursing services.

The six organizations prior to the 1952 decision were ANA, the National League of Nursing Education (NLNE), the National Organization for Public Health Nursing (NOPHN), the Association of Collegiate Schools of Nursing (ACSN), the National Association of Colored Graduate Nurses (NACGN), and the American Association of Industrial Nurses (AAIN). NACGN voluntarily went out of existence in 1951, because ANA required all its constituents to admit to membership RNs without discrimination on the basis of color. AAIN decided to continue as a separate organization. The newly created NLN, however, inherited the major functions of the other three organizations—excluding, of course, ANA.

NLNE was the first nursing organization in the United States. Established in 1893 under the formidable title of the American Society of Superintendents of Training Schools for Nurses of the United States and Canada (it became NLNE in 1912), its purpose was to standardize and improve the education of nurses. Originally for nurses only, it broadened its membership policies in 1943 to admit lay members.

NOPHN was established in 1912. As its title implies, it was an organization concerned not only with public health nurses but also with the development of public health nursing services. It provided for both agency and individual membership—the latter, except in NOPHN's very early years, open to nonnurses as well as nurses.

The prime objective of ACSN, started in 1933 when baccalaureate degree education for nurses was just beginning to make headway, was to develop nursing education on a professional and collegiate basis. Membership was open principally to accredited programs offering college degrees in nursing.

PURPOSES AND FUNCTIONS

NLN's original purpose, as described in its certificate of incorporation, remains unchanged: "to foster the development and improvement of hospital, industrial, public health, and other organized nursing service and of nursing education through the coordinated action of nursing, allied professional groups, citizens, agencies, and schools to the end that the nursing needs of the people will be met."[1]

In 1983, a revised statement on the mission of NLN was developed by the task force on long-range planning and approved by the NLN membership:

> The National League for Nursing serves the changing health needs of the nation by promoting quality nursing service and by fostering the effective educational preparation of nursing practitioners through the cooperative efforts of nursing leaders and concerned representatives of agencies and the general public.

To carry out its stated mission, the National League for Nursing, with its diverse constituencies, sets forth the following goals and objectives for the 1983–1985 biennium and beyond:

1. Strengthen current NLN activities in support of nursing services by evaluating and revising these activities to meet identified needs.
2. Identify and encourage research to strengthen the knowledge base for nursing education and practice.
3. Strengthen NLN's activities in support of nursing education by evaluating and revising these activities to meet identified needs.
4. Develop a marketing-oriented approach throughout the organization.
5. Review NLN's organizational structure and alter the structure, as appropriate, to maximize the League's effectiveness and its responsiveness to membership.

6. Develop revenue-producing activities that support NLN's mission.
7. Establish an effective public relations program to increase public understanding and acceptance of, cooperation with, and support for nursing.
8. Explore the need for NLN services in and to alternate health care settings.

In 1984, the newly created long-range planning committee, a standing committee of the board, began work on a statement which set the framework from which a strategic planning process could proceed.

MEMBERSHIP

There are two major classes of membership within NLN: individual and agency. *Individual* membership is open to anyone interested in fostering the development and improvement of nursing service and education. This might include professional nurses, student nurses, LPNs, other workers in nursing, members of allied professions, and lay persons interested in nursing. Top-echelon administrators (directors of nursing) and those persons next in line bearing the title "associate" or "assistant" may join the National Forum for Administrators of Nursing Services (NFANS), formed in 1977 as the first special-interest forum for individual members. *Agency* membership is for organizations or groups providing various nursing services and for the various schools conducting approved educational programs in nursing. Each member agency designates two individuals, with voting rights, to serve as its representatives within NLN.

There is another category of agency membership (allied) for agencies interested in the work of the NLN but not qualifying within the preceding categories. These agencies do not have voting power.

Until 1967, NLN, like ANA, was structured on a local-state-national basis. At that time, however, it was decided that the "constituent units" (formerly state leagues) of NLN need

not necessarily follow state lines. A constituent league may now take in only part of a state (a large metropolitan center, for instance), a whole state, parts of several different states, or several different states as a whole. The emphasis is on organization according to interests and needs in given regions or areas rather than in given states. (This change reflects the emphasis now given in many other fields to regional organization or planning.) Forty-eight constituent leagues for nursing implement national goals and objectives through statewide programming. Many have local units to stimulate community interest in cooperative planning for nursing and health care services and present programs at the local level.

Individual members join NLN and the constituent league in the area in which they reside or work. If there is no league in that area, they may join NLN directly at the national level. Annual dues for each individual combine the national and constituent league dues. Retiree fees are correspondingly lower.

Agency members join NLN directly, not through its constituent units. Dues for NLN member agencies vary with many factors, including available services.

GENERAL PLAN OF ORGANIZATION

Although both individual and agency members are concerned with the "further development and improvement of nursing services and education,"[2] the groups approach this task through different channels.

Accordingly, in NLN's organizational pattern, these two large membership groups are divided into the Division of Individual Members and the Division of Agency Members. The Division of Individual Members is expected to work through the constituent leagues for nursing, the forums, and the Assembly of Constituent Leagues for Nursing. The last is composed of the president of each constituent league and other individuals who may be designated by the Assembly. Among the purposes of the Assembly is to plan and facilitate ways in which the NLN program may be implemented; to serve as a forum for exchange and discussion of ideas, problems, and recommendations; to serve in an advisory capacity to the League; and to present recommendations for action to the board of directors—usually through the executive committee of the Assembly. The Assembly meets annually. There are also four regional assemblies meeting annually and sponsoring forums, conferences, and workshops. Individual members may join any one of the councils in the Division of Agency Members.

Councils of Agency Members

Agency members are expected to work through their respective councils, although, of course, their two representatives also have votes in the general affairs of the organization. There are six councils: Associate Degree Programs (CADP), Baccalaureate and Higher Degree Programs (CBHDP), Diploma Programs (CDP), Practical Nursing Programs (CPNP), Community Health Services (CCHS), and Nursing Services for Hospitals and Related Facilities (CNSHRF). The first four fall into one of the two large categories of agencies represented in NLN membership, programs of nursing education, whereas, the other two represent nursing services. Councils may be dissolved, or new ones created, in the light of changing circumstances.

Each council works within its own readily identifiable field of interest, but there are certain activities in which all engage. All are involved in consultation, and all have CE functions. Workshops and programs are held regionally and nationally. The four education councils also have accreditation as part of their programs. In addition, NLN co-sponsors, with the American Public Health Association, an accreditation program for some health agencies and community nursing services.

Council committees vary according to each council's needs. Each has an executive committee, which guides and administers the affairs of the council under the direction of the

board of directors. The executive committee also determines what meetings other than the biennial meeting are held.

Forums

In 1979, forums were added to the organizational structure. As defined by the bylaws, the word forum means any group of individual members of the League with an identified interest that has been authorized by the board of directors. Forums have executive committees to administer forum affairs.

Board of Directors, Officers, Committees

The NLN's board of directors consists of its five elected officers (president, president elect, first and second vice presidents, and treasurer), the chairmen of the councils, twelve elected directors, the executive committee (four members) of the Assembly of Constituent Leagues for Nursing, and two board-appointed directors. The executive director serves as secretary, but is not a voting member.

The council chairmen and the executive committee of the Assembly of Constituent Leagues are elected by their respective groups. The officers, six directors, and three members of the committee on nominations are elected by the membership every two years.

Balloting is done by mail, with both individual and agency members entitled to vote. All of these offices and elected positions are open to both nurse and nonnurse NLN members. In the 1979–1981 biennium, the first nonnurse president served.

At NLN business sessions held at the biennial conventions, decisions are made by the individual and agency members present, provided there are enough to meet the League's quorum requirements. Each individual member has one vote, and each member agency has two.

The NLN has two types of committees—standing and special—and these may be elected or appointed. The composition and methods of election or appointment and the term of office of committees are spelled out in the bylaws. The Committee on Nominations is currently the only elected committee of the overall organization.

In the appointed category are eight standing committees: executive, constitution and by-laws, finance, perspectives, pension, long-range planning, accreditation, and long-term care. The executive committee, composed of NLN's elected officers, other board members appointed to the committee as representatives of NLN's broad services and programs, and NLN's executive director (without vote), act for the entire board between meetings of that group.

The perspectives committee predicts the societal changes that affect nursing, analyzes issues in the delivery of health services, and examines trends in professional and technical education. It also identifies goals for each biennium.

Also considered standing committees are the Council Executive Committees, the Forum Executive Committees, and the Executive Committee of the Assembly of Constituent Leagues for Nursing, mentioned previously, and the Interdivision Coordinating Committee, which consists of the chairman or appointed alternate of the council executive committees and assembly executive committee. The major purposes of this last committee are primarily communication and coordination.

From time to time the League appoints other special committees to deal with matters of general, and often continuing, concern to the organization as a whole.

SERVICES AND PROGRAMS

More or less permanent components within the League are a variety of services and programs carried out through its organized staff divisions.

Accreditation*

The NLN accrediting service has been a stimulant to the improvement of nursing edu-

*See Chapter 12 for controversial issues in accreditation.

cation since its inception in 1949 under the name of the National Nursing Accrediting Service. Related to nursing education, it is a service that reviews and evaluates nursing education programs of various types such as those preparing PNs; diploma, associate degree, and baccalaureate degree programs for RNs; and programs leading to a master's degree in nursing. Those meeting NLN criteria within each category are granted NLN accreditation.

To operate legally, of course, each school of nursing must have the approval of the state government, as represented by its board of nurse examiners. But standards vary from state to state, despite efforts to standardize them as much as possible; in some, the requirements for school approval are minimal. Criteria for NLN accreditation, however, are nationally determined; they represent the combined thinking of experts in the various kinds of programs. League accreditation, therefore, symbolizes a nursing education program of high quality in all respects—admission and achievement standards, curriculum, faculty preparation, library, laboratory and other facilities, and the like. NLN accreditation is voluntary. The school requests this service and pays for the evaluation. There is no guarantee that the end result will be accreditation.

The published criteria for evaluation of each type of program, determined by the appropriate council, are basic guides, as is the booklet on policies and procedures of accreditation. Most schools conduct a thorough evaluation of all aspects of their program through committees of faculty and students, use of studies, and review of other data. The results of the evaluation are incorporated in a self-evaluation report, which is sent to NLN (previously notified as to the program's intent to seek evaluation). NLN accreditation is a peer evaluation and the visitors who come to the program to amplify, verify, and clarify the data and explore ramifications of the report are faculty and/or faculty administrators of like programs, who have been selected for and especially trained by NLN to review programs. Often NLN visits are made cooperatively with regional or specialty accrediting associations or state board visits. NLN visitors may be able to point out weaknesses in the report, which can be corrected, and also give supplementary information to the board of review, which meets in New York several times a year to review the materials for accreditation that have been sent from the schools and the visitors' reports.

Recommendations for improvement are sent to the school, with or without the granting of accreditation. If a program is accredited, interim reports of the status of the program are sent to NLN at specified intervals before another major accreditation visit. If the program is not accredited, there is an appeal procedure, and, of course, the opportunity to correct the deficiencies and reapply for accreditation. In recent years, there has been greater flexibility in the acceptance of ways to meet accreditation standards, so that programs of greatly varying educational approaches are being accredited. The common denominator is quality. Increasingly, NLN accreditation is sought and worked toward, because of the significance of this accreditation to the prospective student, the faculty member, and the community. In addition, only NLN-accredited schools are eligible for the nursing education funds made available through the Nurse Training Act of 1964 and later amendments. NLN is officially recognized by the Council on Post-Secondary Accreditation and the U.S. Office of Education[3] as the accrediting agency for master's, baccalaureate, associate degree, diploma, and PN programs. A deterring factor has been the resistance to NLN accreditation by some junior colleges that feared requests for accreditation from all other specialty programs. Even so, the number of accredited AD programs has risen to more than one-half of the total number operating. CE programs within the total nursing program seeking accreditation are also accredited.

Each year, a list of NLN-accredited programs of nursing is published in the NLN journal. There are also pamphlets issued listing all state-approved and accredited nursing programs. By 1985, more than 1,350 educational programs held NLN accreditation; over 75 percent of the total of basic RN programs were accredited by the League.

Early in 1966 the NLN inaugurated a second type of accreditation program, in conjunction with the American Public Health Association (APHA), this one for community nursing services. (Although NLN does not accredit nursing services in other institutions, it has developed criteria and other tools for hospitals and nursing homes to use in self-evaluation.) It was initiated because of the interest expressed by the membership of both organizations in a method of evaluating the services being provided by them in the community. The program was made available to all organizations offering nursing services to people outside of hospitals, extended-care facilities, and nursing homes. From 1966 through 1968, agencies applied for and received preliminary accreditation. In 1968, as agencies began to meet the criteria required, the program moved into its second phase of full accreditation. Policies were developed by a joint NLN-APHA policy committee, but the program is administered by the NLN.

In 1971 consideration was given to the possibility of expanding the program to include other disciplines that provide out-of-institution personal care service. Therefore, the American Dietetic Association, American Occupational Therapy Association, American Physical Therapy Association, American Speech, Language and Hearing Association, National Association of Social Workers, and National Home Caring Council now work with the Accreditation Standards and Review Committee. In 1985 the program underwent extensive restructuring aimed at program self-governance. Agencies seeking NLN-APHA accreditation receive a *Guide for Preparing Accreditation Reports,* which is used in the extensive self-study necessary. A site visit is then made by administrators from comparable agencies in other states. The agency's report and site visitors' report are then studied by a peer member board of review. There is a process of appeal if the Board's decision is not acceptable to the agency. A brief interim report is required two years after accreditation, and another report and a site visit at least every five years. More than 120 of these services were accredited in 1984. A list of accredited agencies has appeared yearly in *Nursing and Health Care* and is reported in various NLN publications.

Consultation Services

In connection with its accreditation services, NLN offers consultation to any school of nursing seeking help with its educational program; thus, a school failing to meet accreditation standards may be helped to achieve them, or one just starting or seeking to improve its program can be helped by NLN expertise. Consultation may be given through personal visits to the schools or through regional meetings such as workshops and institutes. Paid staff and appointed NLN members work steadily on this NLN program. It offers similar assistance to community health agencies searching for better and more efficient ways to serve their communities. And with new attention being given to evaluation techniques in all fields of nursing, the testing service offers valuable assistance.

Consultation services to NLN constituencies and other community groups embrace a wide range of interests such as organization and management, financial development, establishing new community health service and education programs, evaluating programs, improving administrative practices, and areas of research and testing.

Test Services

NLN conducts one of the largest professional testing services in the country. Test batteries have been developed by NLN using experts in tests and educational measurements and in nursing. The tests available through NLN fall into several categories: guidance and placement of students for schools of profes-

sional and practical nursing, and achievement of professional and practical nursing students while in nursing school, and, since 1978–1979, the preimmigration screening examination and nursing tests prepared for the Commission on Graduates of Foreign Nursing Schools.* All are objective tests that are machine-scored under the direction of the NLN Test Services. There are separate sets of tests for practical nursing and for professional nursing. Also included are achievement tests for baccalaureate students. In addition, tests have been developed for schools to use in making advanced placement decisions relative to educational mobility.

Depending on the nature and purpose of the tests, they may be given at central locations within a state or the nation, or at individual schools. They are all returned to NLN headquarters for scoring, and the scores are then released to the schools of nursing. Preadmission test results are available directly to the examinees. The League does not make the decision as to whether an individual's score means that she or he is qualified for admission to a school or has a satisfactory achievement in the subjects tested. This judgment is left to the individual schools, although NLN provides national standards as a guide.

The League's testing services are offered on a voluntary basis; no school or state is required to use them. Costs to individual nurses and schools are minimal. The tests undergo almost continual evaluation and revision to maintain their validity and ensure appropriateness of content. League policy stipulates that tests must be current, and they are updated annually or every two to three years, depending on the content area and level of usage.

Information Services

If NLN is to achieve its objective of improving nursing education and service, it must maintain a constant flow of information to both its membership and the general public.

---

*See Chapter 27.

Therefore, it distributes a wide variety of informative materials.

Some of this material is promotional, explaining the nature and purpose of League programs and activities. Other publications are statistical or highly factual, such as school directories, lists of accredited schools of nursing, or reports of conferences and workshops. Still other materials available through the League include accreditation criteria, management guides, evaluation aids, and career guidance materials.

Each year NLN issues a publications catalog that is available on request from its headquarters office and is also sent to all members. The councils prepare and distribute material of interest to their members through memos and newsletters. The official journal, *Nursing and Health Care* is published ten times a year. Members are kept informed of current federal and state legislation and health care issues through some of the publications cited, as well as through position papers on major issues.

Research and Studies

Activities of the Division of Research include data collection (as well as development of the data-gathering instruments), research studies, and special projects. Annually, for instance, NLN collects information on admissions, graduations, and enrollments in programs of practical and professional nursing education. Aspects of these data are reported in various NLN publications. The *NLN Nursing Data Review* is a compilation of statistical information on nursing education and newly licensed nurses. Also published are booklets and directories on state-approved programs preparing students for licensure as RNs or LPNs. The directories indicate types of programs, accreditation status, administrative control, financial support, and data on admissions, enrollments, and graduation. The Nursing Student Census and a Nurse-Faculty Census are also published.

NLN, as need and resources permit, surveys or studies other selected aspects of nursing education or nursing service programs. In addition, it carries on both short-term and long-term research projects. Some of these projects are financed by the League itself; some are financed through grants from other agencies. (NLN, unlike ANA, enjoys tax-exempt status, and funds granted to it are not considered taxable income.)

Interorganizational Relationships

NLN works closely with ANA and AACN (especially as part of the Tri-Council), and NSNA. However, throughout its entire program, NLN also maintains active liaison with many other national agencies, both governmental and voluntary. Among them are APHA, the National Federation of Licensed Practical Nurses, the National Association for Practical Nurse Education and Service, the United States Public Health Service, the American Health Care Association, the American Association of Community and Junior Colleges, the American Hospital Association, the American Medical Association, the American Lung Association and the Joint Commission on Accreditation of Hospitals, as well as several consumer groups and health care coalitions.

Other Services and Activities

Because of its tax-exempt status as an educational and charitable organization, the League (and its constituent leagues) is prohibited from participating in any political campaign on behalf of or in opposition to any particular candidate, and no substantial part of its activities may consist of influencing legislation. Therefore, the League has no lobbyist. However, this prohibition does not extend to dealing with administrative agencies or the executive branch of the government. Hence the NLN's successful suit on behalf of nursing schools against the DHEW secretary and the federal budget director in 1973 to release impounded funds (see Chapter 18), although precedent-breaking, was a suitable activity. The League is also permitted to inform members fully of proposed legislation, engage in nonpartisan analysis or study and disseminate results, and give factual testimony and information. Preferably these presentations are made on request of the legislators. Within this framework, NLN has been involved in legislation affecting nursing and has been helpful in its implementation.

When ANA moved to Kansas City, Missouri, a joint careers program, in which ANA and NLN exchanged daily requests from the public for information about nursing, was terminated. However, the decision was made for the NLN to fulfill its obligation to the public with information and materials about nursing, nursing careers, and nursing education. In late 1973, NLN's Nursing Information Service was granted funds by the National Fund for Graduate Nursing Education to produce two leaflets on nursing careers. Since that time, new brochures have been developed, and NLN's Careers Information Service sends packets of information about nursing as a career to high school counselors each year.

Also in 1973, the NLN chose the National Library of Medicine in Bethesda, Maryland, home of the world's largest collection of health sciences literature, as the official repository of NLN's historical documents and records. These include the history of NLN, old photographs of American nurses, correspondence by Florence Nightingale and other nursing leaders, and the history of NOPHN. League officials also plan to join in a campaign to identify and acquire other nursing memorabilia for the library.[4]

The impact of NLN on nursing does not lie only in the services and activities of the organization and its component groups. It is equally important to look at some of the major pronouncements made by NLN in taking stands on nursing issues. Among these is a 1965 resolution on nursing education that recommended community planning to "implement the orderly movement of nursing education into institutions of higher learning in such a way that the flow of nurses into the community will not be interrupted." A 1970 statement on open curriculum urged changes in programs to aid mobility in nursing without

lowering standards, and in 1976 a new and stronger version was approved by the board of directors. A 1971 statement (revised 1976) about degree programs with no major in nursing was intended, in part, to help RNs who were seeking degrees to make informed choices. In 1972 *Nursing Education in the Seventies* spelled out the needed characteristics of an effective system of nursing education and the actions needed to attain these characteristics. A 1966 statement encouraged continuity of nursing care, and in 1973, the statement on *Quality Review of Health Care Services* urged intra- and interprofessional review of care standards; the updated 1979 version urged greater anticipation of nurses in Professional Standards Review Organizations (PSROs). Other position papers are on national health insurance, nursing's responsibility to minorities and disadvantaged groups, and NLN's role in continuing education in nursing.

A controversial NLN statement was made in 1979, "Preparation for Beginning Practice in Nursing," in which support for all four types of nursing education programs was reiterated, "for the present." Because the League accredits all four types of programs, this position was not surprising to some, although the 1965 NLN resolution that was never rescinded seemed to present a contradictory view. A report of the NLN Task Force on Competencies of Graduates of Nursing Programs, also released in 1979, identified differences in the knowledge base and in minimal expectations of the new graduate of the four types of nursing programs studied (PN, AD, diploma, and baccalaureate), as well as differences in the practice role in terms of structured/unstructured settings, focus of care and accountability.

In February 1982, the NLN board of directors approved a position statement entitled "Nursing Roles—Scope and Preparation," which stated that professional nursing practice requires a minimum of a baccalaureate degree with a major in nursing, that technical nursing practice requires an associate degree or diploma in nursing, and that vocational nursing practice requires a certificate or diploma in vocational/practical nursing. At its 1983 convention, the membership voted to support the board's action, although the vote was preceded by a hot debate.

One of the most successful NLN projects was a service to the community, the League's childhood immunization project, funded for two years by DHEW's Center for Disease Control. NLN coordinated the nation's voluntary sector to join the federal government to immunize 20 million children by October 1, 1979, and to establish a permanent maintenance system to ensure routine protection for all newborns. In addition, at the grass roots level, NLN's constituent leagues worked closely with various community groups to solve special health and education problems, thus helping to fulfill the ultimate purpose of NLN.

The NLN headquarters is located at 10 Columbus Circle, New York, N.Y. 10019. Regional offices are located in Chicago, Atlanta, and San Francisco, California.

REFERENCES

1. National League for Nursing, *Bylaws* (New York: The League, 1983).
2. Ibid., p. 12.
3. Richard Millard, "The Accrediting Community: Its Members and Their Interrelations," *Nurs. and Health Care*, **5**:451–454 (Oct. 1984).
4. "Historical Records Go to Archives," *NLN News*, **21**:2–3 (Nov. 1973).

Other Nursing and Related Organizations in the United States

Within the last ten years, an increasing number of specialty organizations for nurses has been added to those already well established. Although all nurses can find a place for themselves within ANA, some, particularly those in clinical or occupational specialties, have elected to join one of the other nursing organizations instead of, or in addition to, ANA. The aegis of these organizations varies. Some are totally independent; others are part of a medical or educational organization. Some restrict membership to nurses; others include medical-technical personnel employed in the same clinical specialty.

Although there have always been other nursing organizations, ANA has generally been accepted as *the* professional organization that speaks for nursing. Some of the earlier groups later merged into ANA. The first of the specialty organizations that still exists was the American Association of Nurse Anesthetists (1931). In the 1940s and 1950s, the American Association of Industrial Nurses (AAIN),

now the American Association of Occupational Health Nurses (AAOHN), the Association of Operating Room Nurses (AORN), and the American College of Nurse-Midwives (ACNM) followed, but beginning in 1968, literally dozens of others were organized. They were splinter groups that broke off from ANA and either formed their own association or evolved as the profession became more specialized.

Nurses who switched membership often said that ANA did not meet their needs, particularly after ANA directed more of its resources to the economic security program. Few maintained dual membership, either because they could not or would not spare the time or dues money. Special-interest groups seem to have several things in common: they state that they do not intend to get involved in the economic security concerns of their members, and their major concern is to provide a forum for sharing ideas, experiences, and problems related to a particular specialty or interest, including continuing education and standard setting. Most indicate that they plan to remain autonomous organizations.

NATIONAL FEDERATION FOR SPECIALTY ORGANIZATIONS

The proliferation of nursing organizations, although meeting the special needs of some nurses, has also caused some confusion among nurses, other health workers, and the public. Do these organizations speak for nursing in addition to ANA? In place of ANA? Members of the nursing organizations were also concerned. A lack of unity in common health care interests can prohibit the achievement of desired goals. Therefore, in November 1972, ANA hosted a meeting of ten specialty groups and NSNA to "explore how the organizations can work toward more coordination in areas of common interest." It was found that concerns were similar and that such a meeting was generally considered long overdue.[1]

In its second meeting, hosted by the American Association of Critical Care Nurses (AACN) and held at the Western White House in San Clemente, California, in January 1973, federal nurses and representatives from the National Commission on Nursing and Nursing Education were also invited, and the group was asked to consider forming a National Nurses Congress. Although this suggestion was rejected, the participants accepted the importance of the specialty groups, at the same time recognizing the unique role of ANA. They agreed in principle to statements on institutional licensure and continuing education (CE), and reaffirmed that practice was the basic purpose of the nursing profession.[2]

At the third meeting of presidents and executive secretaries of the specialty nursing organizations, ANA, and NSNA, held in June 1973, this group adopted a name—The Federation of Specialty Nursing Organizations and American Nurses' Association. They identi-fied a specialty nursing organization as a "national organization of registered nurses governed by an elected body with bylaws defining purpose and functions for improvement of health care; and a body of knowledge and skill in a defined area of clinical practice." Those attending expressed mutual support and agreed on some of the issues of the times.[3]

Meetings of the group were held on a semi-annual basis in the following years, with the member organizations alternating as hosts, responsible for arranging and conducting the meeting and writing the minutes. The nursing press and auditors were permitted to attend meetings. The focus of the meetings was usually on current issues, but often related to CE accreditation procedures and certification, about which ANA and the other organizations seldom agreed. However, the Federation did support ANA on such issues as membership in JCAH and on various legislative proposals. Resolutions on issues raised by other members were also supported from time to time.

In 1981, the title of the organization was changed to National Federation for Specialty Nursing Organizations (NFSNO), which more clearly defined the membership, not all of whom represented clinical specialties. Accepted for publication were the purpose and functions of the federation:

This organization is a voluntary, unincorporated organization whose purpose is to work toward coordination among participating nursing organizations in matters that relate to nursing practice, education, and other matters of mutual concern. (Social economics and legislation affecting health care were topics deleted in June 1981.)

The functions of the Federation are:

1. To support collective efforts to improve nursing practice
2. To develop statements on matters of national concern for nursing
3. To facilitate cooperation among the member organizations

4. To emphasize nursing's role as patient advocate

Eligibility for membership was limited to those nursing organizations that:

1. Have a specialty nursing focus related to a clinical practice area or role function that is national in scope.
    a. Clinical area is defined as those pathological states or human responses characteristic of adults and children.
    b. Role function is defined as:
        1) administration
        2) education
        3) research
        4) consultation
        5) clinical practice:
            — generalist
            — specialist
            — clinician
            — practitioner
2. Are national in scope of membership.
3. Are composed of a majority of registered nurses.
4. Are governed by an elected body with by-laws defining the purpose and functions for improvement of specialty nursing practice and education.
5. Have a mechanism in place to insure continuity in representation at the National Federation for Specialty Nursing Organizations meetings.

A recurring agenda item was whether the Federation should become more formalized, and incorporation was repeatedly discussed. Two problems in responding to issues were the turnover in officers of the member organizations and the fact that many had no organizational office or staff and had limited finances. There also seemed to be a reluctance about giving up individual organizational autonomy. For instance, almost none of the groups were willing to participate in a freestanding credentialing center (see Chapter 5). A long-range planning committee, a public relations committee, and a finance committee were established to consider some of these concerns.

(A history of NFSNO, *The First Ten Years*, was also written at that time.) Although several proposals for a more formal structure were discussed, none were acceptable. A formal motion for incorporation lost by a narrow margin in 1984. At the same time, it was agreed that there would be a moratorium on accepting new members.

As of 1984, the Federation membership included:

American Association of Critical-Care Nurses (AACN)*
American Association of Occupational Health Nurses (AAOHN)*
American Nephrology Nurses' Association (ANNA)*
American Association of Neurosurgical Nurses (AANN)*
American Association of Nurse Anesthetists (AANA)*
American College of Nurse-Midwives (ACNM)*
American Nurses' Association*
American Urological Association Allied (AUAA)*
Association of Operating Room Nurses (AORN)*
National Association of School Nurses (NASN)*
Emergency Department Nurses Association (EDNA)*
Nurses' Association of the American College of Obstetricians and Gynecologists (NAACOG)*
Public Health Nursing Section, American Public Health Association (PHN/APHA)*
American Organization of Nurse Executives (AONE)
American Society of Ophthalmic Registered Nurses (ASORN)
American Society of Plastic and Reconstructive Surgical Nurses (ASPRSN)
American Society of Post Anesthesia Nurses (ASPAN)

---

*Charter members. (Some organizational names have changed.)

Association of Practitioners in Infection Control (APIC)

Association of Rehabilitation Nurses (ARN)

International Association for Enterostomal Therapy (IAET)

National Association of Orthopaedic Nurses (NAON)

National Association of Pediatric Nurse Associates and Practitioners (NAPNAP)

National Intravenous Therapy Association (NITA)

National League for Nursing (NLN)

National Nurses Society on Alcoholism (NNSA)

Nurse Consultant Association (NCA)

Oncology Nursing Society (ONS)

The mailing address for NFSNO is P.O. Box 23836, L'Enfant Plaza, S.W., Washington, D.C., 20024.

OTHER COOPERATIVE EFFORTS

ANA also made an effort to bring together the various nursing organizations. A change in the 1982 bylaws provided for the formation of a Nursing Organization Liaison Forum (NOLF) to promote unified action as an organization on professional and health policy issues. In December 1983, ANA invited forty-five nursing organizations to Kansas City to explore the possibilities. The meeting was cordial, but the results were somewhat noncommital. There was a question of whether NOLF and NFSO would be duplicative efforts, although ANA indicated that NOLF would focus on broad issues. A particular deterrent to membership was that since NOLF was an advisory body to ANA, there was no guarantee that any recommendations would be accepted as policy. Some organizations also objected to the fact that representatives had to be members of a state nurses' organization (SNA). However, whether NOLF was a factor in the next month's negative vote for NFSO incorporation remains a question.

What does appear to be a successful cooperative effort was initiated when, at about the same time that the specialty groups first met, ANA and NLN developed closer working relationships with the relatively new American Association of Colleges of Nursing (AACN). Many of their mutual interests were in the area of federal legislation for health care, and their first major joint statement noted the need for a system of health maintenance that would allow people to benefit fully from nursing's contributions. Representatives of the three organizations then met to draft plans to implement the proposals in the statement.[4] In January 1974, ANA and AACN formed the Alliance of the American Nurses' Association and the American Association of Colleges of Nursing.[5]

Later, the Tri-Council was formed, consisting of ANA, NLN, and AACN, with the president and executive director of each meeting periodically. From these meetings, joint policy statements were formulated, with joint action taken as deemed appropriate. An example is the decision to support legislation for a national institute of nursing, although this did create internal political problems in each organization.*

Such collaborative activities among nursing organizations show a new maturity in nursing that not only recognizes the importance of joining together on major health issues, but also fosters positive cooperative action. Such action will enable nurses to be a stronger force in the planning and delivery of health care services. As Margretta Styles noted at a meeting of NFSO, "For a profession to be successfully self-regulating, to speak a common language, and to develop and disseminate its science and skill, it is necessary that the education, credentialing, organizational, and practice components of the field develop in substantial synchrony."

The nursing organizations noted in this chapter are not all clinical specialty groups; some exist to serve other needs of nurses, educationally, socially, or spiritually. It is evident

---

*See Chapter 14.

that still more nursing organizations will evolve as nurses assume new health roles and related interests. Those discussed in this chapter appear to be most firmly established and active at this time. All are national organizations, with the exception of the five regional associations: MARNA, NEON, MAIN, SCCEN, and WCHEN. These are presented at the end of the nursing section.

ALPHA TAU DELTA

The Alpha Tau Delta (ATD) Nursing Fraternity, Incorporated, is a professional fraternity that was founded on February 15, 1921, at the University of California, Berkeley. Chapters are established only in schools of nursing where the baccalaureate or higher degree programs are fully accredited by NLN. ATD has twenty active collegiate and alumnae chapters. Membership is based upon scholarship, personality, and character and has no restriction as to race, color, or creed.

The purposes of ATD are to further higher professional and educational standards, to develop character and leadership, to encourage excellence of individual performance, and to organize and maintain an interfraternity spirit of cooperation. Besides the chapter scholarships, financial aid is given annually through the Miriam Fay Furlong National Grant Awards and the PRN Alumni Awards. Other awards are the National Chapter Members of the Year, and award keys and merit awards to individuals for outstanding accomplishments.

The governing body of ATD is its biennial national convention. It is composed of elected delegates from each college and alumnae chapter, and the four national council officers.

The national paper, *Cap'tions of Alpha Tau Delta,* is published in the spring and fall of each year. ATD is a member of the Professional Fraternity Association, and through this organization is represented in the Interfraternity Research and Advisory Council. National headquarters for ATD is located at 14631 N. Second Drive, Phoenix, Arizona 85023.

AMERICAN ASSEMBLY FOR MEN IN NURSING

The American Assembly for Men in Nursing (AAMN) was organized in 1971 under the name National Male Nurse Association. The primary objective of the NMNA was to interest men in the nursing profession. The objectives of AAMN have not changed and remain limited. The objectives and their rationale are as follows:

Men and young men in the United States are encouraged to become nurses and join together with all nurses in strengthening and humanizing health care for Americans.

Rationale: Caring should not be considered a sexual trait. It is a personal, human quality. The public should not be deprived of any segment of caregivers, particularly based on gender.

Men who are now nurses are encouraged to grow professionally and demonstrate to each other and to society the increasing contributions being made by men within the nursing profession.

Rationale: The AAMN provides a vehicle for mutual support and development of interests that exist among men in nursing. Men have made significant contributions to the nursing care of patients and have found rewarding careers in doing so. A broad range of participation within the profession without regard to gender is desirable. The AAMN can serve to disseminate these ideas.

The Assembly intends that its members be full participants in the nursing profession and its organizations and use this assembly for the limited goals stated above.

Rationale: It is not the intent of the AAMN to further fragment the nursing profession, but rather to encourage full participation of all nurses within the profession.

The headquarters of AAMN is at the College of Nursing, Rush University, 600 South Paulina, 474-H, Chicago, Illinois, 60612.

AMERICAN ASSOCIATION OF COLLEGES OF NURSING

The American Association of Colleges of Nursing (AACN) was formed in May 1969 at a meeting attended by forty-four deans and directors of nursing programs located in institutions of higher education. For approximately two years prior to this time, a group of deans of NLN accredited graduate programs in nursing had been meeting together informally to explore the kind of organizational arrangement needed to focus on significant issues influencing higher education in nursing, and to provide a forum for the deans and directors to meet together to debate these issues and to take rapid and concerted action with respect to them. These early meetings culminated in the vote in 1969 to establish an independent Conference of Deans of College and University Schools of Nursing, composed of the deans and directors of NLN accredited baccalaureate and higher degree programs in the United States, and directed toward the purpose of providing knowledgeable leadership in nursing.

The first general meeting of the newly organized group was held in Chicago during October 1969. The association has undergone several changes in names since the initial meeting; its present name, the American Association of Colleges of Nursing, was accepted by the membership at the meeting held in February 1973. AACN meets regularly twice yearly. A headquarters office was established in Washington, D.C., early in 1973, and the association became legally incorporated in Washington, D.C., in March of that year.

The central purpose of the association is to serve the public interest to improve the practice of professional nursing by advancing the quality of baccalaureate and graduate programs in nursing, promoting research in nurs-

ing, and providing for the development of academic leaders. Membership in the association is of one kind: institutional, represented by the key nurse administrative person (or designee) of a baccalaureate and/or graduate program leading to a degree in nursing.

AACN offers baccalaureate and higher degree programs in nursing a framework through which issues critical to nursing can be considered and acted upon expeditiously. The framework is designed to promote academic leadership in nursing; disseminate information concerning the needs and goals of baccalaureate and graduate preparation for nursing to governmental agencies, foundations, other health professions, and consumers; encourage research in nursing; maintain a data bank; and provide continuing education for deans, including programs and forums, at semiannual meetings.

AACN, through its membership, has been involved actively in strengthening and extending the position of collegiate nursing education within institutions of higher learning. Since its inception, the association has been involved in legislation, socialization of deans, and issues pertinent to higher education for nurses. AACN has grown rapidly in membership and has provided active, vigorous leadership for higher education in nursing. As an association and through action by individual deans, it has taken a strong position in influencing legislation for the improvement of health care delivery and for the support of health manpower education.

The association also works closely with both ANA and NLN, meeting periodically as the Tri-Council.

AACN publishes the *AACN Newsletter* ten to twelve times a year, a series of papers on nursing education issues, and extensive reports on subjects such as enrollment in baccalaureate and graduate nursing programs and salaries of nursing faculty and administration based on data from the organization's Institutional Data System. In 1985, a bimonthly journal, *The Journal of Professional Nursing,* was launched.

AACN is located at Eleven Dupont Circle, Suite 430, Washington, D.C. 20036.

AMERICAN ASSOCIATION OF CRITICAL-CARE NURSES

The American Association of Critical-Care Nurses (AACN) was founded in 1969 as the American Association of Cardiovascular Nurses. The association was reincorporated in California in 1972 under its present name, which more accurately reflects the professional practice of its members. The present membership now totals 49,000, with over 200 chapters located throughout the United States and in other countries. AACN's major function is to provide CE for the critical-care nurse. Activities encompass clinical practice, nursing research, leadership, and administration.

The philosophy of AACN is that each critically ill person has the right to expect nursing care provided by a critical-care nurse. AACN provides regional programming and a four-day annual National Teaching Institute which cover all aspects of critical-care education, practice, research, administration, and leadership.

AACN has two official journals: *Heart & Lung: The Journal of Critical Care* and *Focus on Critical Care.* Both are included as benefits of membership. AACN encourages professional accountability and has established its *Standards for Nursing Care of the Critically Ill.* The *Standards,* together with AACN's Scope of Practice and Principles of Critical Care Nursing Practice, provide a definition and framework for nursing care of the critically ill.

Through its affiliate, the AACN Certification Corporation, CCRN certification is offered to critical-care nurses who meet eligibility criteria. Certification examinations and a recertification process occur every three years. Currently, over 15,000 critical-care nurses hold the CCRN credential.

Other membership benefits include reduced registration fees at AACN programs, professional liability and other group insurance programs, and professional discounts on AACN-authored textbooks. Membership and program information is available from AACN, One Civic Plaza, Newport Beach, California 92660. Certification information is available from the AACN Certification Corporation at the same address.

AACN maintains liaison relationships with other nursing specialty organizations through the National Federation for Specialty Nursing Organizations, with ANA, the Society of Critical-Care Medicine, the American College of Chest Physicians, and other health-related associations.

AMERICAN ASSOCIATION FOR THE HISTORY OF NURSING

The American Association for the History of Nursing (AAHN), formerly the International History of Nursing Society, was incorporated October 1982 in Kansas. Its purpose is to educate the public regarding the history and heritage of the nursing profession by stimulating interest and national/international collaboration in promoting the history of nursing; supporting research in the history of nursing; promoting the development of centers for the preservation and use of materials of historical importance to nursing; serving as a resource for information related to nursing history; and producing and distributing to the public educational materials regarding the history and heritage of the nursing profession. Membership is open to individuals interested in the purpose and work of the association. The AAHN's *Bulletin* is published quarterly. AAHN is located at: College of Nursing, University of Illinois, 845 South Damen Ave., Chicago, Illinois 60612.

AMERICAN ASSOCIATION OF NEUROSCIENCE NURSES

The American Association of Neuroscience Nurses (AANN) was founded in 1968 as the

American Association of Neurosurgical Nurses. Its purposes are to foster and promote interest, education, research, and high standards of practice in neurosurgical and neurological nursing, and to promote the growth of nursing as a profession.

Criteria for membership include:

1. Active involvement or primary interest in neurosurgical or neurological nursing
2. A license to practice as an RN in the United States or Canada
3. Letters of reference from nurses or physicians in neurosurgery or neurology

AANN currently has a membership of 1,700, and all members who are neurosurgical nurses are also members of the World Federation of Neurosurgical Nurses.

Major publications of AANN include the *Journal of Neurosurgical Nursing* (six issues a year); "Synapse," the membership newsletter, also published bimonthly; and two core curricula, one clinically oriented and the other related to the operating room. Other materials include a research directory, which lists nurses involved in neuroscience research; a speakers' bureau; *Standards of Neurological and Neurosurgical Practice* (published with ANA); and an audiovisual list and bibliography. CE programs are offered nationally and through a series of regional chapters (over forty) throughout the country. AANN is approved by ANA/NAB as a provider and an approval body in CE.

Certification is provided through the American Board of Neurosurgical Nursing, which offers examinations twice a year. Information may be obtained from ABNN, 7500 Old Oak Boulevard, Cleveland, Ohio 44130.

AANN holds its annual meeting each April in conjunction with that of the American Association of Neurological Surgeons, with which it is affiliated. AANN is headquartered at 22 South Washington Street, Suite 203, Park Ridge, Illinois 60068.

THE AMERICAN NEPHROLOGY NURSES ASSOCIATION

The American Nephrology Nurses Association (ANNA) was founded in 1969 (under the name, the American Association of Nephrology Nurses and Technicians) as an organization of nurses, technicians, social workers, and dietitians interested in the care of patients with renal disease. It was reorganized and retitled in 1984 and a second organization for the technicians was formed. The purpose is primarily educational with numerous national, regional, and local programs, seminars, and conferences given. Other major activities include a registry for continuing education credit, and provision of standards of nursing practice in the hemodialysis and transplantation areas. The objectives of ANNA are to develop and update standards for the practice of nephrology nursing, provide the mechanisms to promote individual growth, and promote research, development, and demonstration of advances in nephrology nursing.

There are approximately 3300 members of the national organization, a large majority of whom are registered nurses. AANNT began as a nationally based association and established five regional groups the following year. Several chapters have been established within each region. Any RN interested in the care of patients with renal disease is eligible for full membership. Dietitians, social workers, LPNs and technicians may participate as associate members. Major publications are *ANNA Update, Standards of Clinical Practice,* a journal entitled *ANNA Journal,* and a number of monographs. ANNA headquarters is located at North Woodbury Road/Box 56, Pitman, N.J. 08071.

AMERICAN ASSOCIATION OF NURSE ANESTHETISTS

Organized in 1931, the American Association of Nurse Anesthetists (AANA) is for professional nurses who are qualified by training and experience to give anesthesia. Nurse anesthetists become members of AANA by graduating from an accredited school of nurse anesthesia and passing a national certifying examination given by the Council on Certification of Nurse Anesthetists. Members of AANA automatically become members of their state associations.

The objectives of AANA are to advance the science and art of anesthesiology; to develop standards and techniques in the administration of anesthetics; to promote cooperation between nurse anesthetists and members of allied professions; to publish materials to aid in the association's activities and keep members informed; and to conduct an educational program stressing the importance of proper administration of anesthetics.*

With the assistance and encouragement of the American Hospital Association, AANA developed an accreditation program for schools for nurse anesthetists that went into effect in 1952. It is now administered by the Council on Accreditation. Only graduates of AANA-approved schools are now eligible to take the certifying examination for association membership. Nurse anesthetists are required to be recertified by the Council on Recertification every two years, which is accomplished by earning CE credits and fulfilling other requirements.

The association holds an annual convention. The sessions are open to AANA members, as well as others in the health care field.

The *Journal of the American Association of Nurse Anesthetists* is published bimonthly. *The AANA Newsbulletin* is published monthly for members only. The headquarters office is at 216 West Higgins, Park Ridge, Illinois 60068.

---

*Originally, the objectives of AANA included program accreditation and certification of practitioners. These activities are now carried out by autonomous councils.

AMERICAN ASSOCIATION OF NURSE ATTORNEYS

The idea of organizing nurses who were attorneys was proposed in 1977, when it became apparent that no national association addressed the needs and interests of this growing group of professionals. Meetings were held in areas where nurse attorneys were clustered. The American Association of Nurse Attorneys (AANA), was incorporated in 1982.

The aims and purposes of the association are to better nurse attorneys and to educate the public on matters of nursing, health care, and law. Specific goals are to educate the membership on relevant issues; to facilitate information sharing among nurse attorneys and with related professional groups; to establish an employment network; to provide mutual support among nurse attorneys; to develop the nurse attorney profession; to become well-known experts, consultants, and authors in nursing and law; to educate nurses about legal aspects of the profession; and to offer educational seminars and workshops for nurse attorneys.

An annual meeting whose educational component addresses issues of national concern to nurse attorneys occurs every fall in different areas of the country. Educational and social gatherings are held at regular intervals in approximately fifteen metropolitan areas. Entitled *in brief,* the official newsletter of AANA, is published no less than semiannually.

Current membership is over 170. Membership is open to any nurse attorney, nurse in law school, or attorney in nursing school. Information regarding AANA or its activities may be obtained from the national office at P.O. Box 5564, Washington, D.C. 20016.

AMERICAN ASSOCIATION OF OCCUPATIONAL HEALTH NURSES

The American Association of Occupational Health Nurses (AAOHN), organized in 1942, is an association of professional RNs employed in occupational health. Its purposes are to constitute a professional association of nurses engaged in the practice of occupational health nursing; to maintain the honor and character of the nursing profession; to improve community health by bettering nursing service to workers; to develop and promote standards for nurses and occupational health nursing services; to stimulate interest in and provide a forum for the discussion of problems in the field of industrial nursing; and to stimulate occupational health nurse participation in all nursing activities at local, state, and national levels. AAOHN's major activities are to formulate and develop principles and standards of occupational health nursing practice so that the nurse in occupational health may utilize more fully his or her professional knowledge and training in the service to workers and management and to the community; to promote, by means of publications, conferences, workshops, and symposia, both formal and informal programs of education designed specifically for the nurse in occupational health; to identify the rightful place of nursing in the occupational health program and to encourage cooperation among all groups engaged in protecting the health and welfare of the worker; and to impress upon management, physicians, and allied groups the importance of integrating into the activities of industry the services to be rendered by the occupational health nurse.

AAOHN is built upon its 115 local, state, and regional constituent associations, which have more than 9,000 members. A nonprofit organization, AAOHN derives its operating income from membership dues.

AAOHN may represent occupational health nurses in public policy discussions that affect their day-to-day practice. It also studies and attempts to influence legislative actions. However, the organization believes that increased professional competency, not collective bargaining, is the method for the occupational health nurse to achieve economic opportunity and security. Its goal is to pro-

mote the occupational health nurse as an impartial professional worker.

AAOHN's annual meeting is held in conjunction with that of the Occupational Medical Association, the combined meeting being called the American Occupational Health Conference. Symposia and workshops are also held on other occasions.

In addition to its official monthly magazine, *Occupational Health Nursing,* AAOHN issues special manuals, brochures, and guides for promoting nursing excellence in occupational health, including practice standards and occupational nursing service objectives. The organization's headquarters is located at 3500 Piedmont Road, N.E., Atlanta, Georgia 30305-1513.

AMERICAN ASSOCIATION OF PEDIATRIC ONCOLOGY NURSES

The American Association of Pediatric Oncology Nurses (APON) is an organization of RNs who are either interested in or engaged in pediatrics, oncology, and/or pediatric oncology nursing. The group was formally begun with election of officers in 1974, as a result of increasing demands for education and support for nurses who care for and about children with cancer and their families.

The overall objective of APON is to improve the care given to children who have cancer and to their families. This is achieved through an annual national educational meeting, the quarterly *Journal of the Association of Pediatric Oncology Nurses,* and publication of a literature review and a bibliography. In addition, APON promotes implementation of standards of pediatric oncology nursing practice and encourages research in nursing care of children with cancer.

Membership is open to all RNs in the United States, Canada, and foreign countries, and is currently over 500. New members receive a copy of APON's *Standards of Care for the Child with Cancer* and a chemotherapy booklet, both developed by APON.

The most frequently expressed benefit of APON membership is the opportunity to network with nurses with common goals, interests, values, as there is a continuing improvement in the quality of life and life expectations for children with cancer. The current address of APON changes with the election of officers and can best be found in the *AJN Directory*.

AMERICAN COLLEGE OF NURSE-MIDWIVES

The philosophy of the American College of Nurse-Midwives (ACNM) is based on the beliefs that every childbearing family has a right to a safe, satisfying experience with respect for human dignity and worth; for variety in cultural forms; and for the parents' right to self-determination. ACNM defines a certified nurse-midwife (CNM) as an individual educated in the two disciplines of nursing and midwifery, who possesses evidence of certification according to the requirements of the organization. Accreditation and certification activities are now carried out by autonomous entities. In pursuit of its goals, and working frequently in cooperation with other groups, ACNM identifies areas of appropriate nurse-midwifery practice; studies the activities of the nurse-midwife; establishes qualifications for those activities; administers a national program for certification of nurse-midwives; approves educational programs in nurse-midwifery; sponsors research and develops literature in this field; and serves as a channel for communication and interpretation about nurse-midwifery on regional, national, and international levels.

The American College of Nurse-Midwifery was established in 1955; it merged in 1969 with the American Association of Nurse-Midwives, founded in 1929, to become the American College of Nurse-Midwives. Membership is limited to ACNM-certified nurse-midwives, although they do not have to live in the United States.

ACNM is governed by an elected board. The president, vice president, secretary, treasurer, and the six regional representatives serve two-year terms. A national convention is held annually.

ACNM and its members conduct or take part in conferences, institutes, and workshops concerned with the practice of nurse-midwifery and with the improvement of services in the maternal and child health field. The official bimonthly newsletter of the college is *Quickening*; the official publication is *The Journal of Nurse-Midwifery*. ACNM is located at 1522 K Street, N.W., Suite 1120, Washington, D.C. 20005.

AMERICAN HOLISTIC NURSES' ASSOCIATION

The American Holistic Nurses' Association (AHNA) was organized in 1980 by a group of nurses and others dedicated to the principles and practice of holistic nursing. Its purposes are to promote the education of nurses in the concepts and practice of the health of the whole person and to serve as an advocate of wellness. AHNA strives to support the education of nurses, allied health practitioners, and the general public on health related issues; to examine, anticipate, and influence new directions and dimensions of the practice and delivery of health care; and to improve the quality of patient care through research on holistic concepts and practice in nursing.

Local, area, regional, and national educational programs, workshops, seminars, and conferences are presented. *Beginnings,* the official newsletter of AHNA, is published ten times each year. *The Journal of Holistic Nursing* is published annually.

Membership is open to nurses and others interested in holistically oriented health care practices. AHNA can be contacted at Box 116, Telluride, Colorado 81435.

AMERICAN INDIAN/ALASKAN NATIVE NURSES' ASSOCIATION

Established in 1972 as the American Indian Nurses' Association, the American Indian/Alaskan Native Nurses' Association (AIANNA) is a professional association of American Indian and Alaskan Native RNs. The purposes of the association are to promote optimum health among these people; to promote a more equitable number within the nursing profession; to educate all populations about the specific health needs of Indian and Alaskan Native people; and to recommend proper solutions to their health needs.[6]

To achieve these purposes, AIANNA wishes to develop awareness of the true history and cultural differences of the Indian/Native people, promoting and evaluating research of these groups, encouraging and assisting Indian/Alaskan Native consumers to become more involved in the delivery of health care services, and recommending various governmental and private agencies in developing programs designed to improve the total health of these people.

In order to promote a more equitable number of American Indians within the nursing profession, AIANNA works with schools of nursing, Indian and Alaskan Native communities, and federal and private agencies. The AIANNA/Allstate Scholarship is administered by the AIANNA staff. This scholarship was originally for associate degree programs but is now used equally for baccalaureate funding. The Margaret Prunty Scholarship funds are for American Indian students enrolled in baccalaureate programs who will return to work in Indian communities. In addition, American Indian nursing students are eligible to apply for loans from the Dr. Ethel E. Wortis Emergency Fund on a loan-at-no-interest basis. In 1975, the association initiated a directory of Indian nurses. In 1978, the organization's name was changed to include the Alaskan Native nurses. The national office address is P.O. Box 3908, Lawrence, Kansas 66004.

AMERICAN SOCIETY OF OPHTHALMIC REGISTERED NURSES

Organized in 1976, the American Association of Ophthalmic Registered Nurses, Inc. (ASORN) is open to all professional RNs engaged in ophthalmic nursing. ASORN's purpose is to unite professional ophthalmic RNs in order to promote excellence in ophthalmic nursing for the better and safer care of the patient with an eye disorder or injury. Specific objectives are to study, discuss, and exchange knowledge, experience, and ideas related to ophthalmic nursing in order to provide CE to its members; to hold regular meetings to advance the purpose of the society; and to cooperate with other professional associations, hospitals, universities, industries, technical societies, research organizations, and governmental agencies in matters affecting the purposes of the society.

A national meeting is held annually in conjunction with the American Academy of Ophthalmology meeting. *Insight,* the official newsletter of ASORN, is published bimonthly. Local chapters, which are independent of the national organization, meet at regular intervals in ten regional areas.

Current membership is 650. The address of ASORN, Inc., is P.O. Box 3030, San Francisco, California 94119.

AMERICAN SOCIETY OF PLASTIC AND RECONSTRUCTIVE SURGICAL NURSES

The American Society of Plastic and Reconstructive Surgical Nurses (ASPRSN) is an organization of nurses actively engaged in the field of plastic and reconstructive surgery. Its purposes are to promote the highest professional standards for the better and safer care of the patient and to provide CE programs in order to study, discuss, and share information, experiences, and ideas.

An annual convention is held each fall. Local and regional chapters provide supplementary seminars throughout the year. *The Journal of Plastic and Reconstructive Surgical Nursing* is published by ASPRSN. ASPRSN *Definitions and Scope of Practice* are available from the national office, which is located at 23341 North Milwaukee Avenue, Half Day, Illinois 60069.

AMERICAN SOCIETY OF POST ANESTHESIA NURSES

The American Society of Post Anesthesia Nurses (ASPAN) is a national association of nurses whose primary duties are in the postanesthesia care unit. The purposes for which ASPAN was organized are exclusively educational, scientific, and charitable, and include the following: to join in one organization all nurses who are engaged or interested in the care of patients in the immediate postanesthesia period; to provide education through conferences, courses, symposia, and the publication of articles, bulletins, and periodicals which will maintain and upgrade standards of patient care and promote professional growth; to study, discuss, and exchange knowledge, expertise, and ideas about patient care; to facilitate cooperation between nurses, physicians, and others concerned with caring for the postanesthesia patient; to encourage specialization and research in the field; and to promote public awareness.

Founded in 1980, ASPAN currently has 3,100 members representing thirty-two components in forty-four states. *Breathline,* the society's newsletter, is published and distributed quarterly to the membership. ASPAN has also issued *Guidelines for Standards in the Post Anesthesia Care Unit.* An annual meeting, held in April, draws an average attendance of 600. National headquarters is located at P.O. Box 11083, 2315 Westwood Avenue, Richmond, Virginia 23230.

AMERICAN UROLOGICAL ASSOCIATION, ALLıED

Organized in 1972, the American Urological Association, Allied (AUAA) is an organization dedicated to advancing the cause of professionalism and better patient care in the field of urology. The care of the urologic patient requires a high degree of education, skill, and dedication. Education is the key to achieving these objectives; thus, AUAA was organized to supplement and extend the urology curriculum provided by nursing schools.

It is the purpose of AUAA to serve as a vehicle for the distribution of all available information in the field of urology; to point the way to advanced nursing technique and new equipment; and to help those who wish to become urology specialists.

The AUAA council plans educational meetings on national, regional, and local levels. An annual national meeting is held in conjunction with that of the American Urological Association.

Active membership is open to persons in the health care professions who are engaged in care of the urologic patient.

AUAA provides certification and recertification for members. The certification board is separate from the American Urological Association. Certification is based on assessment of knowledge, demonstration of current clinical practice, and endorsement by colleagues. A newsletter, *Urogram,* is published four times a year, as is the *AUAA Journal.*

Current membership is over 1,000. AUAA is divided into eight geographic sections with a total of thirty-three chapters.

The administrative offices are located at 6845 Lake Shore Drive, P.O. Box 9397, Raytown, Missouri 64133.

ASSOCIATION OF OPERATING ROOM NURSES

The Association of Operating Room Nurses (AORN) is an organization of professional operating room (OR) nurses with both national and international members and a universal interest in encouraging cooperative action by RNs to improve the quality of perioperative nursing care by nurses in the operating room.

AORN was founded in 1954 in New York City. It currently has over 30,000 members and more than 300 chapters throughout the United States. The association moved its headquarters from New York City to Denver in 1969.

AORN believes that the OR nurse must be responsible and accountable in assuring high-quality nursing care for patients undergoing surgery. The association's stated philosophy recognizes its responsibility to health care and the OR nurse by setting standards of practice, contributing to essential nursing education, and providing an opportunity for continuous learning through a broad program of educational activities.

AORN recognizes that education is a continuous process and that the OR nurse must be committed to lifelong learning for continued competency. AORN's activities are structured to meet the needs and demands of society, as well as the constantly changing practice of perioperative nursing. Objectives of the association include:

1. To advance the concept of perioperative nursing as the role of the nurse practicing in the operating room
2. To enhance the knowledge, skills, and performance of perioperative nurses
3. To increase awareness of socioeconomic and governmental influences in nursing
4. To maintain cooperative relationships with other professional organizations
5. To evaluate existing practices and new developments in the field of OR nursing and education

AORN sponsors activities to meet the educational needs of its members and the objectives of the association. CE offerings are sponsored throughout the United States and in foreign countries. These include national congress, world conferences, other educational offerings, and self-directed study materials. Educational courses are held at AORN headquarters in Denver. AORN offers an approval process for CE activities of its chapters. The Education Department staff offers educational and hospital consultation. AORN continues to work with ANA, NLN, the American College of Surgeons, and other professional organizations on various issues. The AORN National Certification Board offers a certification program for professional achievement in perioperative nursing.

A professional RN who is currently employed in the OR, either full- or part-time, in a supervisory, teaching, or general staff capacity, is eligible for active membership. Associate membership is available to professional RNs who are inactive in nursing but who were OR nurses immediately prior to becoming inactive, and to professional RNs engaged in an allied field of nursing who have special skills or knowledge relative to perioperative nursing.

The official AORN organ is the monthly *AORN Journal,* which publishes original articles on OR nursing and key nursing issues as well as local chapter news and reports of national activities. A list of other publications currently available may be obtained from AORN, whose headquarters is at 10170 E. Mississippi Avenue, Denver, Colorado 80231.

ASSOCIATION FOR PRACTITIONERS IN INFECTION CONTROL

The Association for Practitioners in Infection Control (APIC) grew out of a need for an organization to provide communication and education to those professionals involved in infection control activities. In 1972, a steering committee met and established APIC. In 1983, the first international elections were held to elect members of the board of directors and officers.

The purpose of APIC is to improve patient care by serving the needs and aims common to all disciplines united by infection control activities. Its goals are to develop and initiate effective communication; to support the development of effective and rational infection control programs in health care facilities; to encourage standardization and critical evaluation of infection control practices; and to promote quality research in practices and procedures related to infection control.

Membership, currently in excess of 6000 practitioners, is open to all individuals involved in infection control activities. There are more than ninety chapters and numerous local groups representing all fifty states and an increasing number of foreign countries. A certification process has been established, and a curriculum for infection control practice has been developed. The *American Journal of Infection Control* is the official publication of APIC. Members also receive the APIC newsletter. An annual international educational conference brings practitioners together to exchange ideas and problem solving techniques.

The APIC national office is located at 23341 N. Milwaukee Avenue, Half Day, Illinois 60069.

ASSOCIATION OF REHABILITATION NURSES

The Association of Rehabilitation Nurses (ARN) was founded in 1974 to advance the quality of rehabilitation nursing services by offering educational opportunities to promote an awareness and interest in rehabilitation nursing and to facilitate the exchange of ideas in rehabilitation programs. The association has established itself as the representative organization for professional rehabilitation nurses, and has become involved in legislative and professional issues affecting the specialty of rehabilitation nursing.

Regional seminars emphasizing nursing expertise in dealing with topics of broad interest to various levels of rehabilitation nursing are offered in several of the ARN's seven geographic regions. National educational conferences deal with concepts and trends of importance to rehabilitation nursing. Local chapters provide opportunities for geographically accessible meetings, workshops, and discussions of professional problems with peers.

Rehabilitation Nursing, written for nurses who work with physically or emotionally disabled patients, is the official journal of ARN. Published bimonthly, it provides scientific and professional data to its readers. *Rehabilitation Nursing: Concepts and Practice—A Core Curriculum* has been published by ARN. *Standards of Rehabilitation Nursing,* authored jointly by ARN and ANA, sets forth standards of rehabilitation nursing practice.

Voting membership is open to RNs concerned with or engaged in the active practice of rehabilitation nursing. Nonvoting membership is available to those in other health care disciplines and to any others interested in rehabilitation and in the activities of ARN. There are currently 2,900 members and thirty-six chapters. The organization's headquarters is located at 2506 Gross Point Road, Evanston, Illinois 60201.

CHI ETA PHI SORORITY

Chi Eta Phi Sorority, Inc. is an international sorority of registered and student nurses, primarily black. Founded in 1932, its purposes are to encourage the pursuit of CE among members of the nursing profession; to have a continual recruitment program for nursing and the health profession; to stimulate a close and friendly relationship among the members; and to constantly identify a corps of nursing leaders within the membership who will function as agents of social change on national, regional, and local levels.

Its national projects include those designed to stimulate interest in nursing; facilitate recruitment and educational preparation for nursing and the health professions; increase retention of students in nursing programs; and provide scholarship funding for educational advancement. Service programs involve health screening, health education, and tutorial programs.

There are seventy chapters throughout the United States and in Africa. The national headquarters is located at 3029 13th Street, N.W., Washington, D.C. 20029.

COMMISSION ON GRADUATES OF FOREIGN NURSING SCHOOLS

The Commission on Graduates of Foreign Nursing Schools (CGFNS) was established in January 1977 as a nonprofit, independent organization sponsored by ANA and NLN. CGFNS supports the United Nations Declaration of Human Rights, which affirms the individual's freedom to migrate; however, CGFNS neither encourages nor discourages immigration. The purpose of CGFNS is to prevent the exploitation of graduates of foreign nursing schools who come to the United States to practice nursing, but are prevented from doing so as a result of failure to pass state licensing examinations. (Less than 20 percent passed on the first try.) Another purpose is to help assure safe patient care for the American public. To attain these purposes, CGFNS screens and examines foreign nursing school graduates while they are still in their own countries. Passing the CGFNS examination is now a federal requirement in order for a foreign nurse graduate to obtain an occupational preference visa and a labor certificate for employment in the United States. An examination is given twice each year.

The commission received a grant from the W. K. Kellogg Foundation to provide eight worldwide screening examinations testing both English comprehension and nursing proficiency in 1979–1982. The commission's governing body is a board of trustees of seven nurses and four trustees at large who specifically represent the interest of the general public. An executive director assumes the administrative responsibilities of the organization. CGFNS is located at 3624 Market Street, Philadelphia, Pennsylvania 19104.

DERMATOLOGY NURSES' ASSOCIATION

The Dermatology Nurses' Association (DNA) was established in 1982. Its purposes are to develop and foster the highest standards of dermatologic nursing care; to enhance professional growth through education and research; to facilitate communication among members; and to promote interdisciplinary collaboration.

An annual convention, combining an educational program and a business meeting, is held each December. *Focus,* the official newsletter, is published bimonthly. Membership, currently numbering nearly 400, is open to nurses and technicians involved in dermatology. DNA's offices are at North Woodbury Road, Box 56, Pitman, New Jersey 08071.

EMERGENCY DEPARTMENT NURSES' ASSOCIATION

The Emergency Department Nurses' Association (EDNA) was incorporated in December 1970, and since that time has grown to an active membership in excess of 11,000. It was founded to represent nurses faced with all the problems of providing emergency care so that these nurses could pool their knowledge and seek solutions to these problems, set standards, and develop improved methods for practicing efficient emergency medicine. Eligible for membership are RNs engaged in emergency care who have special skills or knowledge related to emergency nursing. Any other health professional may join the association as an affiliate member.

The major objective of EDNA is to provide optimum emergency care to patients in emergency departments. Members are urged to promote a positive attitude toward education on all levels within the emergency department by continuing study through the EDNA organization, to support formal programs of instruction for emergency techniques and for postgraduate courses on the professional level, and to participate in community planning of total emergency care.

Since 1975, EDNA has published *The Journal of Emergency Nursing,* which provides articles on all aspects of emergency nursing. The association has published a *Continuing Education Curriculum,* with teaching guidelines for twenty-six areas of emergency nursing. During the Annual EDNA Scientific Assembly, both business and clinical programs are presented, as well as postgraduate courses. Instructor certification courses for participants who have the responsibility of training both medical personnel and the community are also offered. The EDNA national office is located at 666 N. Lake Shore Drive, Suite 1131, Chicago, Illinois 60611.

NATIONAL ASSOCIATION OF
HISPANIC NURSES

The National Association of Hispanic Nurses (NAHN) was formed in June 1976 in Atlantic City, New Jersey, under the name National Association of Spanish Speaking/ Spanish Surnamed Nurses (NASSSSN). Evolving from an ad hoc committee of the Spanish Speaking/Spanish Surnamed caucus formed at the 1974 ANA convention, it brought together for the first time Hispanic nurses from all Hispanic subgroups—Mexican-American, Puerto Rican, Cuban, and Latin American—to provide a forum for exchange of information and experiences about health care services to the Hispanic community. Its name was changed in 1979.

The objectives of NAHN are to provide a forum in which Hispanic nurses can analyze, research, and evaluate the health care needs of the Hispanic community; to disseminate research findings and policy perspectives dealing with Hispanic health care needs to local, state, and federal agencies so as to impact policymaking and the allocation of resources; to identify Hispanic nurses throughout the na-

tion to ascertain the size of this work force available to provide culturally sensitive nursing care to Hispanic consumers; to identify Hispanic nurses throughout the nation in order to monitor the size and growth of this group of health care professionals; to collaborate, assist, and provide technical assistance to other Hispanic health-oriented professionals; to identify barriers to the delivery of health services for Hispanic consumers and recommend appropriate solutions to local, state, and federal agencies; to identify barriers to quality education for Hispanic nursing students and recommend appropriate solutions to local, state, and federal agencies; to assess the safety and quality of health care delivery services for the Hispanic community; to work for the recruitment and retention of Hispanic students in nursing educational programs, so as to increase the number of bilingual and bicultural nurses who can provide culturally sensitive nursing care to Hispanic consumers; to develop, test, and promote culturally sensitive models of intervention and approaches that will provide effective nursing care for Hispanic consumers; to ensure that Hispanic nurses have equal access to educational, professional, and economic opportunities; and to provide an opportunity for Hispanic nurses from all over the United States and Puerto Rico to share information dealing with their professional concerns, experiences, and research.

Membership is open to any Hispanic nurse in the United States, the Commonwealth of Puerto Rico, or other jurisdiction of the United States. Non-Hispanic nurses interested and concerned about the health delivery needs of the Hispanic community as well as the professional needs of Hispanic nurses are welcome to apply for associate membership.

The NAHN publishes a newsletter (*El Faro*) and a *Directory of Hispanic Nurses in the United States.* The organization holds biennial national conferences (even years). NAHN's mailing address is 114 Magnolia Drive, San Antonio, Texas 78212.

NATIONAL ASSOCIATION OF NURSE RECRUITERS

The National Association of Nurse Recruiters (NANR), founded in 1975, seeks to promote and exchange principles of professional nurse recruitment. The association maintains appropriate but separate relationships with voluntary and government hospitals, leading community health care organizations, educational institutions, nursing societies, and all advertising media. NANR serves its members by strengthening the recruiting and managerial skills needed to be effective in the profession, and gives nurse recruiters an opportunity to meet with their peers to exchange ideas and discuss mutual concerns. An annual conference featuring speakers, exhibits, and workshops is held. Problem solving is the emphasis of free, informal discussions held frequently in each of NANR's nine regions.

NANR News, published bimonthly, reports on industry events and association happenings. An annual nurse recruitment survey provides up-to-date data of importance to nurse recruiters.

Membership, currently numbering over 1,300, is open to those working in a hospital or health care agency who are actively involved in nurse recruiting. Nonvoting associate membership is available to individuals interested in supporting NANR activities. Institutional membership is open to organizations interested in promoting and supporting the association's development. NANR is located at 111 East Wacker Drive, Suite 600, Chicago, Illinois 60601.

NATIONAL ASSOCIATION OF PHYSICIAN NURSES

The National Association of Physician Nurses, Inc. (NAPN) is an association of professional people who, by the nature of their chosen profession, are affiliated with the medical profession. Its purposes are to bring professional stature through CE to this profession and to create for its members the benefits that are normally limited to members of specialized professional and fraternal groups.

The Nightingale, an informative, educational newsletter, is the official journal. Published monthly, it is written to help members grow both personally and professionally. An annual conference is also designed to accelerate the professional growth of members. Membership, currently 3,000, is open to all persons employed by physicians, including nurses, medical assistants, and office personnel. NAPN, Inc., is located at 3837 Plaza Drive, Fairfax, Virginia 22030.

NATIONAL ASSOCIATION OF SCHOOL NURSES

The National Association of School Nurses, (NASN) is the only organization in the United States today that represents only school nurses. It was formed in 1969 as a department of the National Education Association (NEA). In 1977, the name was changed from the Department of School Nurses, NEA, to its current name. It is still an affiliate of NEA. The primary goal of NASN is to strengthen the education of children by providing leadership in the promotion and delivery of adequate health services by qualified school nurses to the nation's children and youth.

NASN is governed by a board of directors made up of four elected officers (elected yearly) and representatives of thirty-six state affiliate associations. Each affiliate state elects or appoints a director to represent it on the board of directors. Active membership in the association is composed of school nurses employed by boards of education, institutions of higher learning, and state departments of education. Associate membership is open to school nurses employed by other agencies. There are presently over 2,000 members.

NASN has initiated a number of projects aimed at educating school nurses, and has published numerous policy statements, position papers, and resolutions. These papers address all aspects of school health services and school nursing. For instance, NASN supports baccalaureate education for entry into nursing, with additional courses in education and child development required for preparation for school nursing. The association has also co-authored a position paper entitled *School Nurse and the Handicapped Child,* as well as *School Nurse Standards* with the American Nurses Association, the American School Health Association, the National Association of School Nurse Consultants, the American Public Health Association, and the National Association of Pediatric Nurse Practitioners. NASN also works cooperatively with other health and nursing organizations. It monitors all health legislation that pertains to school health and school nursing, keeps membership informed, and stands ready to testify on important health issues.

The official publication is *The School Nurse,* published in the fall, winter, and spring. A quarterly newsletter is mailed to the membership. An annual four-day conference includes educational sessions and the annual membership meeting.

NASN headquarters is at 7395 S. Krameria Street, Englewood, Colorado 80112.

NATIONAL COUNCIL OF STATE BOARDS OF NURSING

The National Council of State Boards of Nursing, (NCSBN) was created in 1978 by the state boards of nursing throughout the United States so that they could "act and counsel together on matters of common interest and concern affecting the public health, safety and welfare including the development of licensing examinations in nursing." Previously, the organization, under a slightly different name, had been a part of ANA, but because of possible conflict of interest under Federal Trade Commission rulings (see Chapter 20) and the desire to be totally independent, the state board representatives voted to separate from ANA (with considerable objection from the ANA members and board).

The National Council, under the direction of its member boards, developed the National Council Licensure Examinations for Registered Nurses (NCLEX-RN) and Practical Nurses (NCLEX-PN), which are used by each member board in testing the entry-level nursing competence of candidates for nursing licensure.

Each examination is administered twice a year by the member boards. The National Council assists the member boards in administering the examinations and works continuously to ensure that they are relevant to current nursing practice.

NCSBN also assists its member boards in collecting and analyzing information pertaining to the licensure and discipline of nurses, providing communications and consultative services, conducting research, developing model nursing legislation and administrative regulations, and sponsoring educational programs.

The membership of the National Council consists of fifty-nine boards of nursing from every state, the District of Columbia, and two U.S. territories, Guam and the Virgin Islands.

Once a year, delegates from every member board convene in a Delegate Assembly to determine the direction and policies of the National Council and to elect individuals to the National Council's board of directors.

NCSBN services include the development and evaluation of the RN and PN licensure examinations (NCLEX-RN and NCLEX-PN), including aid in administering the exams; a disciplinary data book; various publications, including the newsletter *Issues*; and the collection, organization, and analysis of data and other pertinent research.

The national board is located at 303 E. Ohio, Suite 2010, Chicago, Illinois 60611.

NATIONAL INTRAVENOUS THERAPY ASSOCIATION

The National Intravenous Therapy Association, Inc. (NITA) is a national nonprofit professional nursing association which represents the clinical intravenous (IV) nurse. The objectives of NITA are to provide the benefits and protection of a qualified IV nurse to the patient, to provide research in IV nursing practice, and to assist in providing specialty care in every health care facility.

NITA has established national nursing standards of practice related to all aspects of IV therapy, such as total parenteral nutrition, blood component therapy, and oncology. NITA has established a credentialing board to certify IV nurses nationally.

Membership is offered on both an active and an associate basis. Active members are RNs engaged in the specialty practice of IV therapy. There are currently about 3,000 members. The association has an annual four-day meeting. There are fifty local chapters throughout the United States, which have bimonthly meetings and annual seminars.

NITA provides a bimonthly journal entitled the *NITA Journal,* which is the official publication of the association, and a bimonthly newsletter entitled *NITA Update.*

The national headquarters is located at 87 Blanchard Road, Cambridge, Massachusetts 02138.

NATIONAL BLACK NURSES' ASSOCIATION

The National Black Nurses' Association (NBNA) was formed at the end of 1971 as an outgrowth of the Black Nurses' Caucus held during the 1970 ANA convention. These nurses believed that black Americans and other minority groups "are by design or neglect excluded from the means to achieve access to the health mainstream of America" and that black nurses have the "understanding, knowledge, interest, concern, and experience to make a significant difference in the health care status of the Black Community." The group's leaders have also cited failure of the integration of NACGN into ANA as a reason for beginning a new organization and state that such lack of integration is evidenced by the absence of black nurses in leadership positions, limited opportunities in policymaking, failure to recognize the quality of performance of black nurses, loss of identity of black nurses, tokenism, and failure to increase significantly the percentage of black RNs.[7]

The purpose and objectives of NBNA, as stated in the membership brochure, are to

Define and determine nursing care for Black consumers for optimum quality of care by acting as their advocates.

Act as change agent in restructuring existing institutions and/or helping to establish institutions to suit our needs.

Serve as the national nursing body to influence legislation and policies that affect Black people and work cooperatively and collaboratively with other health workers to this end.

Conduct, analyze, and publish research to increase the body of knowledge about health needs of Blacks.

Compile and maintain a National Directory of Black Nurses to assist with the dissemination of information regarding Black nurses and nursing on national and local levels by the use of all media.

Set standards and guidelines for quality education of Black nurses on all levels by providing consultation to nursing faculties and by monitoring for proper utilization and placement of Black nurses.

Recruit, counsel, and assist Black persons interested in nursing to ensure a constant procession of Blacks into the field.

Be the vehicle for unification of Black nurses of varied age groups, educational levels, and geographic locations to ensure continuity and flow of our common heritage.

Collaborate with other Black groups to compile archives relevant to the historical, current, and future activities of Black nurses.

Provide the impetus and means for Black nurses to write and publish on an individual or collaborative basis.

Membership is open to all RNs, LPNs, and nursing students, regardless of race, creed, color, national origin, age, or sex. The first national conference was held in 1973, and annual conferences have continued to be held. Further information may be obtained from the National Black Nurses Association, Inc., P.O. Box 18358, Boston, Massachusetts 02118.

NATIONAL NURSES' SOCIETY ON ADDICTIONS

The National Nurses' Society on Addictions (NNSA), formerly a component of the National Council on Alcoholism, is an association of nurses interested in chemical dependency problems. The purposes are to extend knowledge, to disseminate information and to promote quality nursing care for the addicted patients and their families, and to become involved with public policy and social issues concerning addiction. This organization serves as a forum for nurses who wish to share their knowledge and experience and to continue their education.

Membership is available to all currently licensed nurses in any of the fifty states, the District of Columbia, Puerto Rico, territories of the United States, and other countries of North America. Candidate membership may be given to student nurses in their senior year.

NNSA meets annually, and the National Forum proceedings, other than the business meetings, are open to nonmembers. NNSA participates in conferences, panel discussions, and teaching sessions. The society is governed by an elected board.

NNSA publishes the *NNSA Newsletter* quarterly for distribution to its members. The

society can be reached at Box 7728, Shawnee Mission, Kansas 66207.

NURSES ASSOCIATION OF THE AMERICAN COLLEGE OF OBSTETRICIANS AND GYNECOLOGISTS

The Nurses Association of the American College of Obstetricians and Gynecologists (NAACOG) was organized in 1969. The purposes of NAACOG are to promote the highest standards of obstetric, gynecologic, and neonatal nursing practice, education, and research; to cooperate at all levels with members of the health team; and to stimulate interest in obstetric, gynecologic, and neonatal nursing. There are currently over 17,000 members.

The association is divided into eight districts or regions and one armed forces district; sections, composed of states and provinces in Canada; and special interest or geographic chapters. Members elect section, district, and national officers. Membership qualifications include graduation from a state- (or province-) accredited school of nursing; current licensure as an RN; and active participation or interest in obstetric, gynecologic, or neonatal nursing. Associate membership is available to allied health workers who demonstrate primary interest in obstetric-gynecologic nursing. Election to membership is by action of the executive board.

Major activities are related to CE through conferences, CE courses, national meetings, home study modules, and update subscription series. The association has developed standards for obstetric-gynecologic nursing and publishes three to four practice resources annually. Legislative networks have been established by state and special interest. Supplements to the journal, targeted to special populations, are published annually.

The official publication of NAACOG is the *Journal of Obstetric, Gynecologic and Neonatal Nursing,* which reflects current research, trends, and policies in the specialty. The *Newsletter* contains news of section, district, and national association activities. Similar publications exist in sections and districts.

The administrative office of NAACOG is located at 600 Maryland Avenue, S.W., Washington, D.C. 20024.

Certification for the obstetric, gynecologic, and neonatal nurse is available through a separate corporation, the NAACOG Certification Corporation (NCC). Certification examinations are available for the inpatient obstetric nurse, obstetric-gynecologic nurse practitioner, neonatal intensive care nurse, and neonatal nurse clinician/practitioner. Examinations are administered annually at approximately thirty sites throughout the United States. The NCC corporate office is located at 645 N. Michigan Avenue, Suite 1058, Chicago, Illinois 60611.

NURSES CHRISTIAN FELLOWSHIP

The Nurses Christian Fellowship (NCF) established in 1948, is affiliated with the Inter-Varsity Christian Fellowship, a nonprofit religious organization. NCF is also a member of Nurses Christian Fellowship International. NCF exists to help both students and nurses grow spiritually as they mature professionally. It focuses on ministering to the whole person —physically, psychosocially, and spiritually— in health and illness or in the face of death.

Books such as *Spiritual Care: The Nurse's Role, Spiritual Care of Children,* and *Spiritual Dimensions in Mental Health,* and workshops and conferences, as well as nursing-oriented Bible studies and fellowship groups, help prepare students and nurses to assess spiritual needs and intervene appropriately in giving care to the whole person.

The Journal of Christian Nursing, published quarterly (begun spring 1984), is the official publication of NCF. Subscription information for the *Journal,* as well as other materials and information, is available from

NCF, 233 Langdon St., Madison, Wisconsin 53703.

ONCOLOGY NURSING SOCIETY

The Oncology Nursing Society (ONS) was founded in 1975. The purposes of the organization are to develop new knowledge leading to the earlier detection and improvement of care of persons at risk for, or diagnosed with, cancer; to disseminate knowledge and information to nurses involved in the care of such patients; to encourage nurses to specialize in the care of cancer patients; and to establish guidelines of nursing care for patients with cancer. There are over 5,000 members in ONS. All RNs engaged in or interested in oncology are eligible to petition for membership.

The *Oncology Nursing Forum,* published six times a year, is the official publication of ONS. The first board of directors was elected in 1977 and consists of four officers. ONS has published standards for oncology nursing care. Additional information may be obtained by writing to 3111 Banksville Road, Pittsburgh, Pennsylvania 15216.

NURSES' ENVIRONMENTAL HEALTH WATCH

Nurses' Environmental Health Watch, Inc. (NEHW) is a national nonprofit membership organization of nurses interested in educating their peers and the public about actual and potential environmental health threats. Through its publication, *Health Watch,* and other printed materials, NEHW provides resource materials which include the nursing implications of environmental health hazards, explores actions that can be taken to identify and correct these hazards, and presents educational programs on occupational as well as community environmental health hazards. On the local level, NEHW chapters focus on grass-roots involvement of nurses working on specific environmental health threats. Further information may be obtained by writing to P.O. Box 811, Nassawadox, Virginia, 23413.

SIGMA THETA TAU

Sigma Theta Tau is the national honor society of nursing in the United States, comparable to the national honor societies in other professions. Organized in 1922,[8] Sigma Theta Tau (the initials of the Greek words meaning ''love,'' ''courage,'' and ''honor'') had grown in 1985 to 191 chapters in colleges and universities offering baccalaureate and higher degree programs in nursing. Its membership of some 75,000 makes it the second largest individual member nursing association in the United States and the largest consisting of all baccalaureate and higher degree nurses.

Members are chosen from among students enrolled in NLN-accredited nursing programs leading to a baccalaureate or higher degree. Criteria for selection are high scholastic achievement, leadership qualities, and capacity for personal and professional growth. Graduate nurses who hold a baccalaureate or higher degree may also be selected on the basis of having shown marked achievement in the field of nursing. The overall purposes of the society are to recognize superior achievement and the development of leadership qualities, to foster high professional standards, to encourage creative work, and to strengthen commitment to the ideals and purposes of the profession.

The National Council, which is composed of Sigma Theta Tau's seven elected national officers, meets three times a year. The House of Delegates, composed of two delegates from each local chapter, plus the National Council, is the governing body of the society. It meets biennially. Local chapters hold at least four meetings during the academic year, usually of

an educational nature, and regional conferences are held in each of the seven regions in the years alternate to the national convention. In 1983 Sigma Theta Tau began to co-sponsor international research conferences and is committed to a conference in relation to the International Council of Nursing Quadrennial Congress. Research programs are also presented at the Sigma Theta Tau, ANA, and NLN conventions.

Many local chapters grant scholarships and research funds. A research fund has been established on the national level, from which grants are made to nurses engaged in research. Awards are also presented in recognition of creativity and excellence in practice, research, education, leadership, professional goals, and chapter programming. Other awards recognize outstanding programs or publications by nurses or nonnurses in the communication media.

In 1981, the society announced the launching of a significant undertaking aimed at improving the health of the public: the implementation of a ten-year plan to increase the scientific base of nursing practice and to sensitize the public to the need for the nursing research required to achieve it.

Sigma Theta Tau's ten-year plan, entitled Focus on Scholarship, has three distinct components to be developed sequentially as well as concurrently. These are resource development, knowledge expansion, and knowledge utilization.

In announcing this ten-year plan-blueprint for excellence, the members of Sigma Theta Tau commit themselves to strengthening the education of nurses, to creating a better world for nursing research and practice, to promoting international dialogue among nurses, and to improving the care and health of all peoples throughout the world.

Image: The Journal of Nursing Scholarship, a peer-review journal, is published four times annually, and *Reflections,* the society's newsletter, is published five times annually.

Sigma Theta Tau national headquarters is

located at 1100 Waterway Boulevard, Indianapolis, Indiana 46202.

MID-ATLANTIC REGIONAL NURSING ASSOCIATION

The Mid-Atlantic Regional Nursing Association (MARNA), funded for the first three years by the U.S. Department of Health and Human Services, Public Health Service, Division of Nursing, as a special project grant, began full operation on July 1, 1981. A continuing extension grant was awarded by DHHS for years four and five, 1984–1986. At the time the initial grant was awarded, the mid-Atlantic region was the only area of the country that did not have a regional planning group for nursing.

The purpose of MARNA is to coordinate nursing, education, service, and research activities for improved quantity and quality of nursing personnel in five jurisdictions in the mid-Atlantic region: Delaware, New Jersey, New York, Pennsylvania, and Washington, D.C. MARNA serves as a voluntary consortium of nursing education institutions and nursing service agencies. Eligibility for full membership is extended to those education programs with a major in nursing (associate degree, diploma, baccalaureate, higher degree) or health care agencies providing RN services. Liaison agency membership is provided for those organizations and associations within the region that wish to establish formal communication with MARNA but are not eligible for full agency membership. There are over 250 full-member participating agencies.

The specific priorities of MARNA are to confront issues and resolve problems of mutual concern that can best be addressed on a regional basis; to provide a forum for the sharing of ideas and a channel of communication for decision making about the future of nursing education, service, and research; and to encourage a productive, collaborative, and cooperative relationship within nursing, as well as with other health disciplines, other regional organizations, and appropriate community groups.

Meetings have been held throughout the region, co-sponsored and in cooperation with member agencies, to discuss ideas, issues, and problems best addressed on a regional basis. Data have been identified to ascertain the available supply of and demand for nursing personnel throughout the region. A Task Force on Regional Planning for Nursing is modifying the Western Interstate Commission for Higher Education (WICHE) national and state projection model to predict regional needs and resources for the next decade. Advisory councils within each jurisdiction provide a broad base of information and guidance to this task force.

MARNA has also promoted interdisciplinary research and replication of nursing studies. Co-project investigators in each jurisdiction have sought to replicate research conducted in Oregon on the implications of federal budget cuts on access to maternity care and perinatal morbidity within the region. Descriptive analyses which will lead to further nursing research have been undertaken, with Delaware receiving block grant monies to replicate the Oregon proposal.

MARNA's governing board is composed of members who represent the various types of nursing education programs and service agencies within all five jurisdictions of the region. Standing committees, ad hoc committees, and task forces of the association allow for members agencies' participation in organizational matters. The staff of MARNA includes an executive director, associate director, assistant to the director, research assistants, and secretarial support.

A MARNAgram is published in the spring and fall of each year, with four mini-MARNAgrams disseminated four times a year. Individual subscriptions for publications are available at nominal fees. The address of MARNA is Teachers College, Columbia University, 525 West 120th Street, Box 146, New York, New York 10027.

MIDWEST ALLIANCE IN NURSING

The Midwest Alliance in Nursing (MAIN) is a thirteen-state nonprofit association of nursing service and nursing education agencies whose common purpose is to enhance the health of persons in the Midwest region. MAIN works with its member agencies and others to advance education in nursing, improve nursing practice, and promote nursing research.

MAIN was organized in 1979 as a unique mechanism to serve the public good, following a two-year regionwide feasibility study supported by a grant from the Division of Nursing, DHHS, and by subsequent five-year funding by the W. K. Kellogg Foundation. The thirteen states in the MAIN region are Illinois, Indiana, Iowa, Kansas, Michigan, Minnesota, Missouri, Nebraska, North Dakota, Ohio, Oklahoma, South Dakota, and Wisconsin.

The primary mission of MAIN is to facilitate regional investigation, planning, communication, and collaboration toward obtaining shared goals and resolving issues and problems arising from health care delivery. The ultimate goal is maximum utilization of nursing resources to achieve cost-effective health care in communities in the region.

To fulfill this mission, the organization attempts to foster productive relationships and better communication between personnel in nursing education, nursing service institutions, and liaison agencies and organizations. MAIN's special status as a regional association with four kinds of member agencies—hospitals, nursing education institutions, community health agencies, and long-term care and rehabilitation facilities—provides a broad base for sharing nursing talents and resources.

MAIN agency membership includes agencies giving direct nursing care or teaching persons to give such care. Identified as liaison agencies are those groups not eligible for membership but wishing to establish formal liaison with MAIN, such as nursing, hospital, or other health professional organizations.

The Midwest Nursing Research Society (MNRS), formally established in 1980, is an independent affiliate of MAIN. The purpose of MNRS is to promote and improve the quality of nursing research. MNRS offers individual membership for persons living or working in MAIN's thirteen-state region.

Publications include a newsletter, *Mainlines,* proceedings of conferences, and reports of studies. A list can be obtained from MAIN headquarters, located in Room 108-BR, Indiana University, 1226 W. Michigan Street, Indianapolis, Indiana 46223.

NEW ENGLAND ORGANIZATION FOR NURSING

The New England Organization for Nursing (NEON) held its first organizational meeting in April 1983 and established bylaws in April 1984. NEON incorporates the regional approach of its predecessor, the New England Council for Higher Education in Nursing (NECHEN), but seeks to meet the challenges to nursing by more fully representing both nursing education and nursing service in the six New England states (Connecticut, Maine, Massachusetts, New Hampshire, Rhode Island, and Vermont).

The primary purpose of NEON is to bring about cooperative planning and collaboration between and among nursing service and nursing education agencies toward the ultimate goal of improving the quality of health care services available to the people of the New England region.

Two forms of membership are possible. Agency membership with voting privileges by a designated official agency representative is available to educational institutions that have programs with a major in nursing leading to an associate, baccalaureate, and/or higher degree and schools of nursing leading to a diploma, and to health care agencies which provide nursing services and have identifiable nursing departments administered by a registered nurse. Liaison membership (nonvoting) is available to individuals employed by a voting member agency and to retired persons who formerly qualified under the agency membership category. In addition, other nursing or related health care groups may join as liaison members.

A fall meeting and a spring conference are held annually. A newsletter is published two times a year following each of these meetings.

Further information can be received by contacting The Education Development Center, Inc., 55 Chapel Street, Newton, Massachusetts, 02160.

SOUTHERN REGIONAL EDUCATION BOARD (SOUTHERN COUNCIL ON COLLEGIATE EDUCATION FOR NURSING)

The Southern Regional Education Board (SREB), operating agency of the nation's first interstate compact for higher education, is a coalition of educators, government officials, and civic leaders working to advance knowledge and improve the social and economic life of the South. Created in 1948 at the direction of the southern Governors' Conference, the board's member states are Alabama, Arkansas, Florida, Georgia, Kentucky, Louisiana, Maryland, Mississippi, North Carolina, South Carolina, Tennessee, Texas, Virginia, and West Virginia.

The board conducts studies and reports on needs, problems, and developments in higher education; directs cooperative programs to improve education at undergraduate, graduate, professional, and technical levels; serves as the fiscal agency for interstate arrangements for regional educational services and institutions; and offers consultation to the states, their planning and coordinating agencies for higher education, and their institutions.

Membership on the board consists of the governor of each state and four other persons, one of whom must be a state legislator and another of whom must be an educator. All appointments are made by the governor for four-year staggered terms. SREB's basic operating support comes from the fourteen participating states. Federal agencies and foundations provide the majority of funds for program activity.

In 1954 SREB sponsored the first regional project in nursing education, a five-year project in graduate education and research. The project demonstrated the effectiveness of a regional approach to nursing problems by helping to develop six master's degree programs in a region where none had existed. Three other projects in nursing education followed, funded first by the W. K. Kellogg Foundation and then by the DHEW Division of Nursing. These projects resulted in the improvement and expansion of nursing education programs and faculty and the gathering of vital data.

The Council on Collegiate Education for Nursing was formed by SREB in 1962 to facilitate relationships between the regional nursing programs in higher education and SREB in implementation of the second nursing project. During the next decade, SREB and the council examined and took action on issues such as statewide planning, curriculum theory and development, and new instructional strategies and techniques, with support from a variety of projects. SREB did not sponsor the council per se but, rather, the project under which the council existed.

In 1972, a three-year grant from the Division of Nursing DHHS, facilitated the development of plans for ongoing regional activities. In 1975, the council became a dues-paying, self-supporting organization in affiliation with SREB. (*Southern* was added to the council's name in 1980.) In the new relationship, the council generates and helps implement special projects which are administered by SREB.

Participation in the council is open to regionally accredited colleges and universities in SREB states that offer nursing programs leading to associate, baccalaureate, master's, or doctoral degrees. There are now approximately 225 participating institutions. The council functions as a forum where heads of programs can obtain information, discuss developments at national, state, and local levels, and conduct regional planning.

A number of seminars, workshops, and conferences are held in relation to funded projects, chiefly involving faculty of the member schools. Other activities provide contact with nursing service personnel in hospitals and other agencies and staff in state organizations and agencies. Publications are related to the projects, papers presented at council meetings, annual research conferences, special studies, and reports. SREB and SCCEN headquarters is 1340 Spring Street, N.W., Atlanta, Georgia 30309.

WESTERN INTERSTATE COMMISSION FOR HIGHER EDUCATION (WESTERN COUNCIL ON HIGHER EDUCATION FOR NURSING)

The Western Council on Higher Education for Nursing (WCHEN) is a part of the Western Interstate Commission for Higher Education (WICHE). WICHE is a nonprofit agency created in the 1950s by governors and legislatures of the thirteen western states. WICHE helps states work together to provide high-quality, cost-effective higher education programs to meet the human resource needs of the states and the education needs of the citizens.

An interstate compact created and shaped WICHE; the compact is a commitment by member states to work together to meet the needs of the region and the western students. WICHE's role is to encourage and nurture this interstate cooperation. The program areas

are Nursing, Student Exchange, Mental Health and Human Services, Minority Education, Economic Development, and the Information Clearinghouse. Alaska, Arizona, California, Colorado, Hawaii, Idaho, Montana, Nevada, New Mexico, Oregon, Utah, Washington, and Wyoming are the member states.

The Western Council on Higher Education for Nursing (WCHEN) is an organization of the western collegiate schools of nursing and affiliated clinical agencies. WCHEN serves as an advisory board to the WICHE commission. The mission of WCHEN is to help the schools and agencies work together to provide high-quality programs in nursing that meet the needs of the states and to strengthen nursing in the West.

As a result of a recent restructuring of WCHEN, membership is now open to the 200 schools of nursing in the West, clinical agencies affiliated with the education programs, and individual nurses.

The WCHEN council, as the decision-making body, includes official representatives from schools and agencies. There are two divisions, the Division of Affiliated Clinical Agencies and the Division of Educational Programs, which has sections for associate degree, baccalaureate, graduate, and CE programs. The executive board is an elected group with a chair, chair-elect, and elected representatives from the division/sections.

The council meets yearly. The two-day conference includes an educational program, division/section meetings, and a business session. It provides the opportunity for interaction among educators from collegiate schools of nursing and nursing service personnel from a variety of health care agencies. Issues of mutual concern are discussed, and recommendations for action are made by nurses in the West.

Through the Annual Communicating Nursing Research Conference, sponsored by the Western Society for Research in Nursing (WSRN), nursing research is presented and discussed. Papers are selected for the quality of research and the impact of the research on the discipline of nursing. Over thirty research studies covering education, clinical practice, and administration are presented and then published in the conference proceedings. Membership in the society is open to all who are interested in nursing research.

WCHEN has carried out a number of projects related to curriculum development, research utilization, minority recruitment and retention and planning. Reports on the projects and other publications are available from WCHEN.

WCHEN is conducting a W. K. Kellogg Foundation project entitled "Improving the Preparation and Utilization of Associate Degree Nurses." Although the major focus of the project is on competency of associate degree graduates, the project will also address the competency of graduates of baccalaureate programs. Nurses from service and education will be involved in building consensus and recommending changes in education and practice based on the agreed-upon competencies.

The headquarters of WICHE/WCHEN is P.O. Box Drawer P, Butler, Colorado 80302.

HEALTH-RELATED ORGANIZATIONS

Many health-related organizations, both governmental and nongovernmental, frequently provide opportunities for participation by nurses through some form of membership, consultation, or inclusion on committees or programs. A number provide services specifically for nurses, such as workshops, conferences, publications, and audiovisual materials. Nurses may also be invited to attend other program sessions, present papers, or serve on panels. Some examples include the American Cancer Society, the American Heart Association, the American Medical Association, and the Catholic Hospital Association.

There are also organizations in which there are large, active nursing components. Some of the most visible of these are described here, as well as the two practical nurse organizations and DHHS's Division of Nursing.

THE AMERICAN HOSPITAL ASSOCIATION

The American Hospital Association (AHA) includes a number of groups and activities involving nursing. The primary functions of the Division of Nursing at the AHA include consultation, education, and information services on such topics as nursing management, information systems, financial systems, and nurse executive development. The division provides the umbrella organization for AHA nursing constituencies: AONE, ANSN, and the Council on Nursing. The Division of Nursing is headed by a director and is supported by staff members including RNs with expertise in specific areas.

The American Organization of Nurse Executives (AONE), formerly the American Society for Nursing Service Administrators is a personal membership organization in the AHA. The objectives of AONE are to provide a medium for the interchange of ideas and the dissemination of information on nursing service administration, provide consultation and direction on all matters relating to nursing and health care issues, and promote educational programs and activities to strengthen nursing service administration and to support a recognition program for professional excellence in the field of nursing service administration.

AONE consists of a board of directors, committees, members, and associates. To qualify as a member of AONE, an RN must be a nurse administrator holding the highest management position in the organization of nursing service in a health care institution. Associate membership is available to nurses holding line management positions who are directly accountable to the top nurse administrator.

Members have full use of AHA library facilities. In addition, they receive publications such as *Hospitals,* a weekly newsletter of health care news, the *AHA Guide to the Health Care Field,* and position papers published by AHA. Members may attend the annual AHA business and program meeting, as well as national, regional, and local institutes and workshops.

The purpose of the Assembly of Hospital Schools of Nursing is to represent and express the views of the members of the assembly and to assist the House of Delegates and Board of Trustees in the development and implementation of policies and programs designed to promote recognition, support, and improvement of hospital schools of nursing as part of the general education system. Membership is open to hospital schools of nursing of AHA institutional members.

The American Society for Health Care Education and Training was founded in 1970. Hospital-based educators and trainers are eligible for individual membership. About 50 percent of the group are nurses. A national meeting and concurrent conferences are held annually. Other conferences are held regionally, according to the needs cited by those in a particular area. *The Hospital Manager* is published for members.

AHA is located at 840 North Lake Shore Drive, Chicago, Illinois 60611.

THE AMERICAN PUBLIC HEALTH ASSOCIATION

The American Public Health Association (APHA), established in 1872, is the largest organization of its kind in the world, with a membership of some 30,000, in addition to the approximately 25,000 members of its affiliates. As a professional organization, it represents workers of forty-four health-related fields in shaping national and local public health policies; as a communications network, it circulates new knowledge through the internationally respected *American Journal of Public Health* and a publishing house operation of major proportions. *Nation's Health* is

the official monthly newspaper of the association.

Of the twenty-four specialized sections that comprise APHA, the Public Health Nursing Section is the second largest, with almost 3,000 members, and one of the oldest, having been established in 1923. Highly active and influential, the Public Health Nursing Section provides a voice for nursing interests within the APHA structure, and nationally through that structure. Section members participate on APHA's program development board, action board, task forces and committees, and with other sections of the association. Through cooperative relationships with other nursing groups, such as ANA, the Federation of Specialty Nursing Organizations, and NLN, it strives for improvement of nursing and education services within the broad perspective of public health.

Over the six decades of its existence, the Public Health Nursing Section has studied numerous aspects and issues of public health nursing, including organization and administration, relationships between hospitals and public health agencies, population planning, services for unwed mothers, team nursing, salaries, educational and professional qualifications, quality assurance and staffing issues. Recently, a primary concern of the section, as voiced in policy resolutions presented to the APHA policy development committee, has been the further study qf the expanded role of the nurse in health care. In its investigation of these issues, the Public Health Nursing Section has continuously been in the organizational forefront of the APHA structure. Over the years, numerous nurses have been elected members of APHA's governing council, including the executive board. Nurses Marion Sheahan and Margaret Dolan served as president of the APHA in 1960 and 1973, respectively, and several nurses have held the office of vice president. In addition, Marion Sheahan, Margaret Arnstein and Doris Roberts have won the Sedgwick Memorial Medal, one of APHA's highest citations; the Albert Lasker and Martha May Eliot Awards have been won by nurses several times; and the prestigious Bronfman Prize was given to Ruth B. Freeman, in 1971.

The APHA annual meeting provides an excellent forum for the Public Health Nurses' scientific and business exchanges and social events, but meetings of the various section councils and committees are also held throughout the year. Two awards are given by the section at each annual meeting to recognize nurses who have made outstanding contributions to public health nursing. A fascinating and detailed *History of the Public Health Nursing Section, 1922–1972,* by Ella E. McNeil, is now out of print but on file in the APHA archives. In 1977, the Margaret B. Dolan Lectureship Fund was established by the Public Health Nursing Section, and at the 1978 APHA convention, the first lecture was presented as the convention keynote address.

APHA headquarters address is 1015 15th Street, N.W., Washington, D.C. 20005.

PUBLIC HEALTH SERVICE, DEPARTMENT OF HEALTH AND HUMAN SERVICES

As its name implies, the Public Health Service (PHS) is not an organization but a federal government agency, and an exceedingly important one as far as health and nursing are concerned. Established in 1798 as a hospital service for sick and disabled seamen, the PHS has steadily expanded its scope and activities over the years and is now the federal agency charged with overall responsibility for promotion and protection of the nation's health. Since the Department of Health, Education, and Welfare (DHEW)* was created in 1953, the PHS has been a component of that department.

Among the many subdivisions of the PHS is

---

*When a separate Department of Education was created in 1980, HEW became the Department of Health and Human Services (DHHS).

the Division of Nursing, which is the one unit in the federal government concerned exclusively with nursing. It is within the Division of Nursing that the PHS focuses on the nation's nursing situation.[9] Its roots go far back into the history of nursing in PHS, however. In 1933, the first public health nursing unit was created within the PHS, primarily to implement the health provisions of the Social Security Act and to conduct the first national census of nurses in public health work. In 1941, PHS established a unit on nursing education to administer federal programs, among them the United States Cadet Nurse Corps, which produced nurses during the emergency caused by World War II. In 1946, the Division of Nursing was established within the Office of the Surgeon General. Formally, the Division of Nursing was known as the Division of Nurse Education. During 1949, PHS was reorganized to better coordinate its activities. The Division of Nursing in the Surgeon General's Office was abolished and its functions were taken over by the Division of Nursing Resources of the Bureau of Medical Services. In 1960, a restructuring of PHS again occurred, uniting the Division of Nursing Resources and the Division of Public Health Nursing into the present-day Division of Nursing.

The division's overall purpose is to work toward the achievement of high-quality nursing care for the nation's growing population and to approach this goal through aid to nursing education, consultation, support of research in nursing, and analysis and evaluations of nursing personnel, and preparation of nurses for expanded roles in the primary care and teaching of patients. The division "seeks to find out what exists in nursing care, what is needed, and how improvements can be made.[10] The Division of Nursing is a "catalyst for the . . . process . . . that begins with producing nurses (and) further entails keeping them in nursing and heightening their contribution to patients through nursing practice of a high new order."[11]

The division consists of four branches, each

primarily responsible for one of the following areas of program activity: the Nursing Education Branch supports programs related to the development, financing, and use of educational resources for the improvement of nurse training; the Nursing Practice Branch designs, conducts, and supports a national program to improve the quality of nursing practice and health care; the Nursing Research and Analysis Branch conducts and supports a nurse fellowship program, research projects to expand the scientific base of nursing practice and a program of studies and evaluations of nursing personnel supply, requirements, utilization, and distribution; and the Advanced Nurse Training Resources Branch provides support to develop or maintain graduate nursing education programs and to prepare RNs for expanded roles in primary health care in various health care settings.

Through research, the division (and its predecessor units) has exerted significant influence and leadership within the nursing profession. Not only does the division conduct research, but it contracts out special research projects in which it is interested and has also encouraged, promoted, and supported many research projects in nursing carried on by others. It is responsible for grant programs that assist nurses to acquire additional education in order to prepare themselves for research to increase the nursing contribution to health care. Still another grant program has helped to prepare nurses for teaching, supervision, administration, and clinical specialization.

Through the research program, the Division of Nursing personnel have placed considerable emphasis on the development of methodology—study and research procedures—that could be used by others in studying nursing problems. Over the years, the division has developed many significant publications to that end. Other publications have been based on the various research projects done by external groups, as well as significant reports of special committees, such as that on the extended role of the nurse (discussed in Chapter 5) that

helped launch federal financing for NPs.* Consultation services in many nursing areas are available through the division. For example, groups that wish to experiment with new teaching methods in a school of nursing or study the way nursing services are provided in a public health agency may receive help from the division.

DHHS has ten regional offices throughout the United States, each headed by a Regional Health Administrator. PHS has always recognized the importance of nursing in the total scheme of providing health services, and there is scarcely a PHS program that does not have a nurse involved in some way. At one time, there was a regional nursing program director in each region, but in the cutback of the 1970s, that was discontinued and now the assigned nurse acts as a general consultant. A look through the PHS listings in a directory issue of the *American Journal of Nursing* gives added insight into the programs of PHS and demonstrates the extent to which nursing is an integral part of them.

Further information may be obtained by writing the Division of Nursing, Bureau of Health Professions, Public Health Service, Health Resources and Services Administration, U.S. Department of Health and Human Services, 5600 Fishers Lane, Rockville, Maryland 20857.

AMERICAN RED CROSS

Founded in 1881 by Clara Barton, who had ministered to the sick and wounded on the battlefields of the Civil War, the American Red Cross operates under a congressional charter granted in 1905. The President of the United States serves as honorary chairman and appoints the chairman and seven other members of the volunteer fifty-member board of governors. To administer its activities,

---

*A complete list of publications and reports is available from the Division of Nursing.

there are 3 operations headquarters, 200 key resource chapters, and more than 3,000 local chapters. Internationally, the American Red Cross is a member of the League of Red Cross Societies and supports the International Committee of the Red Cross, which is the guardian of the four Geneva Conventions.

The aims of the American Red Cross are to improve the quality of human life and enhance individual self-reliance and concern for others. It works toward these aims through national and chapter services governed and directed by volunteers. American Red Cross services help people avoid emergencies and cope with them when they occur.

To accomplish its aims, the Red Cross provides volunteer blood services to a large segment of the nation, conducts community services and, as mandated by its congressional charter, serves as an independent medium of voluntary relief and communication between the American people and their armed forces; maintains a system of local, national, and international disaster preparedness and relief; and assists the government of the United States to meet its humanitarian treaty commitments. The Red Cross has a number of publications describing its programs.

Ever since the Red Cross was founded, Nursing and Health Services has been one of the important units in many Red Cross societies. In the United States, a Division of Nursing Services was established in the American Red Cross in 1909, with Jane A. Delano as its first director. The maintenance of a reserve of qualified professional nurses who could be mobilized quickly in emergencies such as disaster or war was the initial purpose of the Red Cross Nursing and Health Services. During World Wars I and II, these services recruited and certified the majority of the nurses assigned to the military nurse corps. In 1947, legislation was passed by Congress establishing a permanent nurse corps for the armed forces, including the maintenance of a nurse reserve, thus relieving the Red Cross of the responsibility of maintaining this service. How-

ever, the need for nurses to volunteer in community services remains as great as ever, and nurses are urged to enroll in the Red Cross for this purpose.

Red Cross Nursing and Health Services today are designed to extend community resources in helping to meet the health needs of people at home and in the community. Policies and standards for all Red Cross services are determined at the national level. At the local level, the chapter Nursing and Health Services committees are responsible for planning and implementing the nursing services. Not all chapters have identical services because community needs, resources, and interests vary. However, standardized educational courses are available throughout the nation. Although the services may vary, Nursing and Health Services maintains a reserve of volunteer nurses who become enrolled as Red Cross nurses for the following activities:

Disaster Health Services. One of the charter-mandated services provided by the Red Cross is to meet the human needs of the victims of disaster. Nurses are prepared through a series of training courses to adapt their nursing skills to meet nursing needs brought about by disasters and to serve at the time of local and national disasters. The basic training includes skills in providing health services in disaster areas, as well as meeting other immediate needs of disaster victims. Through advanced training and experience on disaster operations, nurses can be prepared to serve at the Disaster Health Services supervisory and director levels on national disasters.

Educational Courses. In order to assist the population to assume responsibility for their own health maintenance, encourage preventive health care, and increase self-reliance, Red Cross Nursing and Health Services courses are available to the general public, elementary and secondary schools, colleges and schools of nursing, military dependents on United States military establishments at home and abroad, and other special groups. These courses include "Providing Health Services in Disaster"; "Providing Red Cross Disaster Health Services in Radiation Accidents"; "Home Nursing"; "Preparation for Parenthood"; "Parenting"; "Vital Signs"; "Cardiopulmonary Resuscitation"; "Multiple Sclerosis (ARC-MS) Home Care"; "Good Grooming"; and "Mother's Aide." New courses are developed to meet specific needs, such as "The Lowdown on High Blood Pressure" and "Better Eating for Better Health." Nursing and Health Services is presently working with other agencies to provide a course in respite care. This course will prepare individuals to give respite to family members responsible for the long-term care of someone handicapped or with a chronic illness. Nursing and Health Services also works with other agencies in the development of training material for the preparation of home health aides and other courses. Continuing Education Units have been approved in many states to prepare instructors for the courses mentioned.

Direct Services. In providing direct services for individuals and community groups, Nursing and Health Services volunteers are involved in activities such as assisting in blood services; immunization, vision, and hearing clinics; hypertension detection and follow-up programs; testing for sickle cell anemia, diabetes, and lead poisoning; emergency aid stations; and counseling and school health programs. These services are provided in cooperation with state and local public and private agencies.

The American Red Cross Nursing and Health Services and the Red Cross Blood Services Nursing work closely with all local, state, and federal nursing services and national organizations in the advancement of nursing education and nursing services in general, as well as for Red Cross nursing in particular.

Nurses participating in any of the Red Cross activities are provided recognition as part of a humanitarian organization through nurse enrollment. The basic requirements for

enrolling as a Red Cross nurse are the following:

1. Graduation from a state-approved school of professional nursing.
2. Registration following graduation and current registration where it is required by law for the type of work the nurse expects to do for the American Red Cross.
3. Satisfactory personal, educational, and professional qualifications, and a state of health consistent with the work the nurse plans to do.

In addition to these basic requirements, the nurse will be asked to give some Red Cross service as evidence of his or her willingness and desire to be a member of the Red Cross organization.

Red Cross Nursing and Health Services provides an excellent opportunity for students in schools of nursing to participate in community health activities. Directors of schools of professional nursing frequently include Red Cross experience as part of the curriculum or encourage their students to participate in Red Cross activities. The participating student can become an enrolled Red Cross nurse following registration as a professional nurse by presenting the credentials received as a student to the local chapter. The nurse will receive the Red Cross nurse's badge when the request has been processed.

NATIONAL ASSOCIATION FOR PRACTICAL NURSE EDUCATION AND SERVICE

The National Association for Practical Nurse Education and Service (NAPNES) is the oldest organization for practical nurses (PNs) in the United States. It was founded in 1941 by a group of nurse educators for the purpose of improving and extending the education of the PN to meet the critical need for more nursing personnel. Founded as the Association of Practical Nurse Schools, the name was changed to the National Association for

Practical Nurse Education in 1942; *and Service* was added to the title in 1959.

Within a few years, after professionally planned curricula had been set up and duties of the PN defined, NAPNES expanded its activities to include a broad program of service to schools of practical nursing and the licensed practical/vocational nurse (LP/VN). Important among these was the establishment in 1945 of the first accrediting service for programs of practical nursing education now recognized by the United States Office of Education (USOE) and the Council on Postsecondary Accreditation (COPA) as one of the accrediting bodies for practical nurse education.

NAPNES activities include working closely with its constituent state associations to provide guidance and assistance in initiating and carrying out a wide range of programs; conducting workshops and seminars to keep LP/VNs abreast of new nursing and medical techniques; providing guidelines for courses to upgrade and expand the capabilities of the LP/VN; sponsorship of CE programs; evaluation of such programs sponsored by other agencies for CE credit; a computerized record-keeping system for maintaining an accurate record of an individual's CE activities; awarding of scholarships to deserving students; dissemination of recruitment materials; conducting an annual survey of state boards of nursing to gather data on LP/VN licensure; and information on and interpretation of PN education and practice to the public. NAPNES serves as one of the spokesmen of the LPN on federal and state levels on such matters as licensing, laws governing LP/VN practice, educational opportunities for the LP/VN, and matters of general welfare. NAPNES publishes the *Journal of Practical Nursing* monthly, which is geared exclusively to meeting the needs of LP/VNs, students, and practical/vocational nurse educators.

Membership is open to all LPNs/VNs, professional RNs, nurse educators, physicians, hospital and nursing home administrators, and lay citizens interested in practical nursing's role in the health field. Agency membership is open to hospitals, nursing homes, schools of practical nursing, alumni groups, civic organizations, and others interested in the objectives of NAPNES. Students in schools of practical nursing are welcomed as student members. NAPNES headquarters office is at 254 West 31st Street, New York, New York 10001.

NATIONAL FEDERATION OF LICENSED PRACTICAL NURSES

The membership of the National Federation of Licensed Practical Nurses (NFLPN), a federation of state associations organized in 1949, is made up entirely of licensed practical (LPNs) or vocational nurses (LVNs) as they are called in some states. In states with a PN association affiliated with the federation, members enroll through the state association. In other states, individual LPN/VNs may join NFLPN as members at large. Each member participates in formulating policies and programs through election of a House of Delegates, which meets during the annual convention. In 1980 there were 16,000 members and more than 3,000 student affiliates. The latter may attend meetings with voice but no vote.

Some of the major purposes of the NFLPN are to preserve and foster the ideal of comprehensive care for the ill and the aged; to bring together all LPNs or persons with equivalent titles; to secure recognition and effective utilization of the skills of LPNs; to promote the welfare and interests of LPNs; to improve standards of practice in practical nursing; to speak for LPNs and interpret their aims and objectives to other groups and the public; to cooperate with other groups and the public; to cooperate with groups concerned with better patient care; to serve as a clearinghouse for information on practical nursing; and to continue improvement in the education of LPNs. A code of ethics for LPNs that stresses many of the same points as the ANA code has been developed by the NFLPN as a "motivation for establishing and elevating professional standards."

To help carry out its objectives, NFLPN maintains a government relations consultant in Washington, D.C., and other consultants on labor relations. In 1962 NFLPN established the National Licensed Practical Nurses' Educational Foundation "for scientific, educational, and charitable purposes."

Seminars, workshops, and conferences are financed by the federation, as well as leadership training conferences for persons engaged in PN association activities at the national, state, or local level. NFLPN encourages CE through sponsorship of the Continuing Education Unit (CEU) system for measuring and permanently recording the participation of individual LPNs in continuing education activities. Adopted by the NFLPN House of Delegates in 1974, the CEU system involves program assessment and approval processes, and provides yearly uniform data to support specifics of CE program types, provider agency types, and program lengths in regional and national configurations. An individual CEU Data Bank Account is an automatic benefit of membership in NFLPN, and nonmember LPNs may also arrange for an account and service. Official transcript service is also available.

Both ANA and NLN work with NFLPN in matters of mutual concern, principally through liaison committees. NFLPN supports NLN as the recognized agency for accreditation. NFLPN also supports NLN efforts in the development and improvement of PN programs. Members of NFLPN staff or appointed representatives serve on committees with other health personnel and organizations.

Publications on practical nursing, such as the *Statement on Standards of Practice,* are available from NFLPN headquarters at 214 South Driver, P.O. Box 11038, Durham, North Carolina, 27703.

REFERENCES

1. "Nursing Organizations Meet at ANA Headquarters to Plan Greater Coordination of Activities," *Am. J. Nurs.,* **73**:7 (Jan. 1973).
2. "Nursing Groups Reject Umbrella Congress, Agree on Need for Talks, Support on Issues," *Am. J. Nurs.,* **73**:420 (Mar. 1973).
3. "Nursing Organizations Adopt Group Name," *Am. J. Nurs.,* **73**:1306 (Aug. 1973).
4. "Groups Call for Better Use of RN," *Am. Nurse,* **5**:8 (July 1973).
5. "ANA, Collegiate Schools Form Alliance," *Am. J. Nurs.,* **74**:215 (Feb. 1974).
6. "Indian Nurses Hold National Conference," *Am. Nurse,* **7**:8 (June 1975).
7. Gloria Smith, "From Invisibility to Blackness: The Story of the National Black Nurses' Association," *Nurs. Outlook,* **23**:225–229 (Apr. 1975).
8. Carolyn Widmer, "Sigma Theta Tau: Golden Anniversary," *Nurs. Outlook,* **20**:786–788 (Dec. 1972).
9. Philip Kalisch and Beatrice Kalisch, "Nurturer of Nurses: A History of the Division of Nursing of the U.S. Public Health Service and Its Antecedents 1798–1977—Summary Review," unpublished report to the Division of Nursing, March 1977.
10. Gladys Uhl, "The Division of Nursing, USPHS," *Am. J. Nurs.,* **65**:82–85 (July 1965).
11. Jessie M. Scott, "Federal Support for Nursing Education 1964 to 1972," *Am. J. Nurs.,* **72**:1855–1861 (Oct. 1972).

28

International Organizations

The organizations discussed in the preceding chapters have all been national ones, although some have international affiliations. Included in this chapter are the major international organizations related to nursing and health.

INTERNATIONAL COUNCIL OF NURSES

Nursing claims the distinction of having the oldest international association of professional women, the International Council of Nurses (ICN).[1] Antedating by many years the international hospital and medical associations, ICN is the largest international organization primarily made up of professional women in the world. (There are, of course, men in ICN member organizations.)

The originator and prime mover of ICN was a distinguished and energetic English nurse, Ethel Gordon Fenwick (Mrs. Bedford Fenwick), who first proposed the idea of an international nursing organization in July 1899.[2] Among the American nurses present in London at that time, attending a meeting of the International Council of Women, was one whose name figures prominently in the nursing history of our own country, Lavinia Dock.

She was quick to support Mrs. Fenwick's idea and, shortly thereafter, a committee of nurses from nine different countries began laying the groundwork and drawing up a constitution for the proposed new organization. When ICN was officially established in 1900, Mrs. Fenwick became its first president. Miss Dock became its first secretary, a position she held for the next twenty-two years. Annie Goodrich became the first ICN president from the United States.

The essential idea for which the ICN stands is, in Miss Dock's words,

> . . . self government of nurses in their associations, with the aim of raising ever higher the standards of education and professional ethics, public usefulness, and civic spirit of their members. The International Council of Nurses does not stand for a narrow professionalism, but for that full development of the human being and citizen in every nurse, which shall best enable her to bring her professional knowledge and skill to the manysided service that modern society demands of her.[3]

Today ICN is sometimes referred to informally as the "United Nations of Nurses," an appropriate enough title. Although nonpolitical, and certainly less affluent than the UN,

ICN does bring together persons from many countries who have a common interest in nursing and a common purpose, the development of nursing throughout the world.

Membership

From the beginning, ICN was intended to be a federation of national nursing organizations. The association was a little ahead of its time, however, because in 1900 very few countries had organized nursing associations. Until 1904, therefore, ICN had individual members. (These included male nurses, although the first time men were specifically mentioned as attending an ICN Congress was in 1912 in Cologne, where greetings were given from the president of the association of male nurses in Berlin.) In 1904 three countries reported that their national nursing organizations were "ready and eager to affiliate with the International Council of Nurses," and thus Great Britain, the United States, and Germany became the three charter members of ICN.[4]

ICN today is a federation of national nurses' associations in ninety-seven countries. The requirements for membership have been, essentially, that the national association be an autonomous, self-directing, and self-govern-ing body, nonpolitical, nonsectarian, with no form of racial discrimination, whose voting membership is composed exclusively of nurses and is broadly representative of the nurses in that country. Its objectives must be in harmony with ICN's stated objective: to provide a medium through which national nurses' associations may share their common interests, working together to develop the contribution of nursing to the promotion of the health of people and the care of the sick.[5] A majority vote by the ICN's governing body determines the admission of national associations into membership.

At the 1973 meeting of ICN, a constitutional change was made to broaden the criteria for membership to include nurses who constitute a section or chapter of a national organization composed of other health workers as well as nurses. The ICN definition of *nurse* (the basis for national membership eligibility) was also broadened.[6]

A reiteration of the principle of nondiscrimination was also reinforced at this meeting through a resolution requiring the South African Nursing Association (SANA) to take action to enable nonwhite nurses to serve on SANA's board of directors or face the possi-

ICN Member Countries (1985)

Argentina	El Salvador	Israel	Nigeria	Switzerland
Australia	Ethiopia	Italy	Norway	Taiwan
Austria	Fiji	Jamaica	Pakistan	Tanzania
Bahamas	Finland	Japan	Panama	Thailand
Barbados	France	Jordan	Paraguay	Tonga
Belgium	Gambia	Kenya	Peru	Trinidad/Tobago
Bermuda	German Federal	Korea	Philippines	Turkey
Bolivia	Republic	Lebanon	Poland	Uganda
Botswana	Ghana	Lesotho	Portugal	United Kingdom
Brazil	Greece	Liberia	Puerto Rico	United States
Burma	Guatemala	Luxembourg	Senegal	Upper Volta
Canada	Guyana	Malawi	Seychelles	Uruguay
Chile	Haiti	Malaysia	Sierre Leone	Venezuela
Colombia	Honduras	Mauritius	Singapore	Western Samoa
Cuba	Hong Kong	Mexico	Spain	Yugoslavia
Cyprus	Hungary	Morocco	Sri Lanka	Zaire
Czechoslovakia	Iceland	Nepal	St. Lucia	Zambia
Denmark	India	Netherlands	Sudan	Zimbabwe
Ecuador	Iran	New Zealand	Swaziland	
Egypt (UAR)	Ireland	Nicaragua	Sweden	

bility of expulsion from ICN. (This discrimination apparently exists because of certain clauses in that country's nursing practice act, which must therefore be changed.) Later that year, SANA withdrew from ICN because of its inability to comply with the mandate.

Each country may be represented in ICN by only one national nursing organization. For the United States, the ICN member is ANA, which allocates a small percentage of membership dues to the support of ICN. Thus, even though individual nurses are not ICN members, those who are SNA members can consider themselves part of this great international fellowship.

Organization

The governing body of ICN, according to a new constitution adopted in 1965, is the Council of National Representatives (CNR), consisting of the presidents of the member associations. This group meets at least every two years to establish ICN policies. It also has the responsibility of electing the members and appointing the chairpersons of standing committees.

ICN's board of directors consists of its four officers (president and three vice presidents), plus eleven additional members, all elected by the Council of National Representatives. As of 1973, nearly half of the board is elected by geographic area.[7] The board, which meets at least once a year, carries on the general business of ICN, reporting to the council. The ICN president and vice presidents constitute its executive and finance committee, responsible for general administration of ICN affairs and advice in relation to investments.

Finally, the ICN constitution calls for one standing committee on professional services. This committee studies and makes recommendations in relation to the three broad areas with which ICN is concerned—nursing education, nursing practice, and the social and economic welfare of nurses. The membership committee of the board investigates the eligibility of national associations applying for membership and makes appropriate recommendations to the Council of National Representatives. Continued eligibility is now handled administratively.[8]

Assisting the ICN executive staff, standing committees, and board in their work is an Expert Advisory Panel, consisting of nurses expert in various fields of nursing as well as persons expert in other appropriate fields. Members of this panel, appointed by the board of directors for four-year periods of service, provide information, advice, and consultant services and, through their specialized knowledge and experience, serve to facilitate the work of ICN.

Carrying out ICN's day-to-day activities is its headquarters staff—a group of professional nurses, including ICN's executive director. These nurses represent ICN's executive staff, but in their relationships with and services to the member associations, they serve in an advisory and consultative capacity. Staff members are selected from various member countries.* Usually all of them speak more than one language and have special qualifications in one or more of ICN's areas of activity and service.

ICN headquarters is located at 5 rue Ancien-Port, 1201, Geneva, Switzerland (mailing address: P.O. Box 42, CH–1211 Geneva 20, Switzerland). For many years, its headquarters had been in London. The move to Geneva, however, locates ICN close to the many other international bodies in that city.

ICN Congresses

Once every four years, the ICN holds what is always referred to as its Quadrennial Congress: a meeting of the members of the national nurses' associations in membership with ICN. Nursing students are usually eligible to attend ICN congresses, too, if they are sponsored, and their applications are processed, by their national nurses' association. Students have been meeting as a Student Assembly during the congresses, where they dis-

---

*In 1981, an American nurse became the executive director.

cuss issues of concern across national borders, such as students' rights.

The seventeenth congress was held in the United States in 1981; the 1985 congress was in Israel. ICN met less regularly in its early years, and the two world wars also caused the canceling of meetings during these periods. The first meeting, which was to have been held in the United States in 1915, was disrupted by World War I. Instead, the business of ICN was carried on during the ANA convention in San Francisco that year, attended by American nurses and a few intrepid English nurses who braved the submarine-infested Atlantic Ocean.

During the last several congresses, discussions and resolutions ranged from those focusing specifically on nursing issues to general social concerns. Included, for instance, were career ladders, socioeconomic welfare, educational and practice standards, research, autonomy, nurse's role in safeguarding human rights, nurse's role in the care of detainees and prisoners, and nurse participation in national health policy planning and decision making. Related to general health care were such topics as primary care, excision and circumcision of females, increased violence against patients and health personnel, the uncontrolled proliferation of ancillary nursing personnel, environment quality, care for the elderly, and affirmation of the World Health Organization's "Health for all by the year 2000" theme (HFA/2000). On an even broader scale were the concerns about refugees and displaced persons, nuclear war, poverty, and the status of women.

Functions and Activities

In the foreword to its 1981 constitution, ICN points out that the primary purpose of nurses the world over is "to provide and develop a service for the public," and that ICN, as a federation of national nursing associations, provides for sharing of knowledge so that "nursing practice throughout the world is strengthened and improved." In pursuit of this objective, ICN promotes the organization of national nurses' associations and advises them in developing and improving health service for the public, the practice of nursing, and the social and economic welfare of nurses; provides a means of communication, understanding, and cooperation among nurses throughout the world; establishes and maintains liaison and cooperation with other international organizations; and serves as a representative and spokesman for nurses at an international level.

From the very beginning, ICN has been concerned with three main areas—nursing education, nursing service, and nurses' social and economic welfare. Two of its first objectives were to provide for the registration of trained nurses in order to protect the public from practice by unqualified practitioners and to promote a standardized and upgraded system of nursing education. Important statements on basic beliefs about and principles of nursing education, practice, and service and social and economic welfare were agreed upon in 1969. The nursing education statement indicates that nursing education should be conducted in institutions where education is the primary concern and that supervised experience related to theory should be gained in preventive and curative facilities. The nursing practice statement stresses health care and security as a basic human right, and the economic welfare statement calls for joint consultation in determining conditions of employment and the right of nurses to participate in their national organization.

Those who have attended any of the congresses will testify to the fact that they fully live up to the pomp and ceremony of their name. Held in various countries, upon invitation of the national nurses' association of that country, the congresses are inspiring demonstrations of international communication and fellowship in nursing. In conjunction with each congress, the Council of National Representatives (CNR) holds its meeting, with all those in attendance at the congress free to ob-

serve open sessions of the ICN council's deliberations. The official language of the congress
is English, but facilitating communication is a
system of simultaneous translation into the
official congress languages, English, French,
and Spanish. Each seat in the conference hall
is usually provided with earphones tuned into
this system, and the individual nurse has only
to select the language of her or his choice.
There is also a daily convention paper in all
three languages distributed during the congress.

One of the interesting traditions of the congress is that each outgoing president leaves a
watchword for the next four years. The first,
left by Mrs. Fenwick in 1901, was *work*. That
left by an American, Dorothy Cornelius, in
1977, was *accountability*.[9] Each watchword is
engraved on a link of the silver chain of office
of the ICN president and becomes a permanent part of ICN history.

At the congress, special program sessions
are held, usually linked to one unifying theme.
Among the most outstanding achievements of
the CNR meetings at the 1973 congress was
the acceptance of a new code of ethics (see
Chapter 10), which makes explicit the nurse's
responsibility and accountability for nursing
care. Eliminated, for instance, were statements that abrogated the nurse's judgment
and personal responsibility and stressed a
dependency on physicians, which nurses
throughout the world no longer saw as appropriate. There was also a major statement on
the developing role of the nurse, which read:

> In the light of scientific and social change
> and the goals of social and health policy to ex-
> tend health services to the total population,
> nursing and other health professions are faced
> with the need to adapt and expand their roles.
>
> In planning to meet health needs it is imper-
> ative that nurses and physicians collaborate to
> promote the development and optimum utili-
> zation of both professions. A variety of prac-
> tices may evolve in different settings, includ-
> ing the creation of new categories of health
> workers.

> Although this may require nurses to dele-
> gate some of their traditional activities and
> undertake new responsibilities, the core of
> their practice and their title should remain dis-
> tinctly nursing, and education programs
> should be available to prepare them for their
> expanding role in the various areas of nursing
> practice.[10]

Whenever possible, ICN has sought common denominators in education and practice
throughout the world. One such common denominator, for instance, is the international
Code of Ethics adopted by ICN and equally
applicable to nurses in every country. Another
example is the ICN publication *ICN Basic
Principles of Nursing Care,* now available
in fifteen languages and useful to nurses
throughout the world.[11] At the same time,
ICN has always recognized the autonomy of
its member associations and the principle that
each country will develop the systems of education and practice best suited to its individual
culture and needs. The definition of *nurse* is
an example (Exhibit 28-1).

Throughout the years, ICN has collected
and disseminated data on patterns of nursing
education and service throughout the world
and provided information and advisory and
consultative services in both areas to member
associations requesting such service. In recent
years, ICN has given special attention to primary care as a means of achieving HFA/2000,
and a number of workshops have been held in
Asia, Africa, and South America.[12]

Some of ICN's activities in the educational
field are financed, in whole or in part, by the
Florence Nightingale International Foundation (FNIF), which is associated with it. FNIF
was established in 1934 as an educational trust
in honor of Miss Nightingale. FNIF trust
funds have also been used by ICN to encourage and stimulate research activities in nursing. A new document developed by FNIF is
"The Nurse's Dilemma, Ethical Considerations in Nursing Practice," published in
1977.

EXHIBIT 28-1

Definition of Nurse

ADOPTED BY ICN IN 1973

A nurse is a person who has completed a programme of basic nursing education and is qualified and authorized in her/his country to practise nursing. Basic nursing education is a formally recognized programme of study which provides a broad and sound foundation for the practice of nursing and for post-basic education which develops specific competency.

At the first level, the educational programme prepares the nurse, through study of behavioural, life and nursing sciences and clinical experience, for effective practice and direction of nursing care, and for the leadership role. The first level nurse is responsible for planning, providing and evaluating nursing care in all settings for the promotion of health, prevention of illness, care of the sick and rehabilitation; and functions as a member of the health team.

In countries with more than one level of nursing personnel, the second level programme prepares the nurse, through study of nursing theory and clinical practice, to give nursing care in co-operation with and under the supervision of a first level nurse.

Source: International Council of Nursing, 1973.

ICN administers two annual scholarships of $7,500 each plus $200 (U.S.) to each national winner submitted by national nurses' associations.

In recent years, ICN has been particularly active in the area of nurses' social and economic welfare, and its staff has carried on field work to assist national associations in this area. Published in 1977 was "An Underestimated Problem in Nursing: The Effect of the Economic and Social Welfare of Nurses on Patient Care," by Ada Jacox, and the economic and general welfare of nurses is still considered a concern of top priority.

ICN is ready to supply general information relative to new developments in this area, as well as guidance to national associations wishing to develop or strengthen their social and economic welfare programs. ICN has already collected data on employment conditions of nurses in selected European countries and will undoubtedly extend this data gathering in the future.

At one time, facilitating arrangements whereby nurses from one country could observe, study, or work in another was an ICN activity. As of 1969, direct participation in such arrangements was discontinued, and arrangements are now made with the individual countries. Each member association provides guidance and assistance for nurses planning to come into or go out of its particular country.

Providing liaison for nurses with other international groups is one of ICN's most significant contributions to world nursing. Among the organizations, governmental and nongovernmental, with which ICN is associated in some way are the World Health Organization, the World Federation of Mental Health, the International Labor Organization, the World Medical Association, the International Hospital Federation, the League of Red Cross Societies, the International Committee of the Red Cross, United Nations Educational, Scientific and Cultural Organization (UNESCO), and the Union of International Associations.

Publications

Since 1929, ICN's official organ has been the *International Nursing Review,* published six times a year from ICN headquarters in Geneva. In addition to reports of ICN activities, the *Review* carries nursing articles of international interest, usually written by nurses from the ICN member countries. Occasionally it reprints articles from the official or other publications of member countries. Its primary language is English, but some articles are published in other languages; sometimes an article may appear in several languages. Subscription requests to the *Review* should be addressed to ICN headquarters. The journals of member associations—the *American Journal of Nursing,* for instance—also carry reports of ICN activities and actions.

Issued every four years is the book *Reports of ICN Member Associations.* It contains up-to-date and detailed data on the national nurses' associations affiliated with ICN. ICN also publishes documents from time to time on various aspects of nursing. These publications, as well as a list of those available, can be obtained from ICN headquarters. Some are free; for others there is a charge.

The Past and the Future

The preamble to ICN's original constitution stated, "We, nurses of all nations, sincerely believing that the best good of our Profession will be advanced by greater unity of thought, sympathy and purpose, do hereby band ourselves in a confederation of workers to further the efficient care of the sick, and to secure the honour and interests of the Nursing Profession."[13] From the beginning, ICN and its officers were farsighted and pioneering. Included were members of every race and creed. The courageous Mrs. Fenwick stood firmly for her beliefs in women's suffrage and often spoke of the organization as a federation of women's organizations (for all its male members), with women's suffrage as one of its objectives. In 1901 she also stated a need for nursing education to be in colleges and universities and for nurses to be licensed. (Lavinia Dock missed one major ICN meeting because she was too busy lobbying for women's suffrage.)

In conservative 1900, at the ICN program meeting in London, one subject discussed was venereal disease. Nurses demanded early sex education for children and accessible treat-

ment with no moral stigma attached. The members greeted this with a storm of applause. At other meetings they tackled such subjects as criminal assault on young girls, the role of nurses in prisons, and many other taboo topics. They reached out to effect change and for more than seventy years have been carrying on activities to meet their broadening objectives. It is impressive to see how an international group of nurses with such diverse membership can agree on common goals on education, practice, and economic security when often nurses within an individual country, including the United States, cannot agree.

In 1983, CNR adopted a blueprint for the long-term future. Among the areas of ICN involvement specified were the status and quality of life of women and better health care for mothers, children, and the aged. The Blueprint identified nine key priorities:

1. Developing the role and programmes of national nurses' associations influencing the development of health policy, standard-setting for nursing education and practice developing appropriate research activities and programme development for socio-economic welfare appropriate to that country;
2. influencing the development of policy affecting health and all health workers through work with WHO, ILO, UNICEF and other international bodies;
3. maintaining the impetus of the socio-economic welfare programme for nurses;
4. Implementing selected programmes of international organizations as they relate to national nurses' associations and ICN's priorities;
5. developing efforts to convey realistic and positive images of today's nurses to the media;
6. maintaining links with other nursing groups;
7. reviewing the Code for Nurses to ensure continued relevance;
8. monitoring of legislative issues of importance to nursing and nurses;

9. focusing ICN publications and programme efforts on these priority areas.[14]

Fulfilling these objectives will require the same innovative and challenging spirit shown by the founders of ICN. There are clear financial problems with which ICN must cope, reflecting perhaps the financial problems of each country's association, and there are disagreements about policy. However, the blueprint is a good example of cooperative thinking and goal setting.

At times, it may be questionable whether the nations of the world are coming closer together for human betterment, but it is possible that ICN can play a significant role in improving the health of mankind.

INTERNATIONAL ASSOCIATION FOR ENTEROSTOMAL THERAPY

The International Association for Enterostomal Therapy (IAET) is the professional association for enterostomal therapy (ET). Currently, one must be an enterostomal therapist to be a member of IAET. As of September 1978, only RNs are permitted to pursue ET education. In addition, candidates must have two recent years of full-time clinical experience prior to admission.

Membership in the IAET totals approximately 1,800. Current activities include involvement in advancing CE, studying the cost effectiveness of ET services, securing reimbursement for care of their clients, and certification.

The scientific publication, *Journal of Enterostomal Therapy,* is published quarterly. In an effort to advance education and research activities, the Enterostomal Therapy Foundation was established. Headquarters is located at One Newport Place, Suite 970, Newport Beach, California 92660.

WORLD FEDERATION OF NEUROSURGICAL NURSES

The World Federation of Neurosurgical Nurses (WFNN) was formed during the 1969

World Congress of Neurological Services in New York at the suggestion of the president of the International Congress of Neurological Surgery. It is affiliated with the World Federation of Neurosurgical Societies, and its first international meeting was in conjunction with that of the surgeons at the Fifth International Congress of Neurosurgical Surgery in Japan in 1973.

The organization is devoted to the improvement of neurosurgical patient care, the exchange and dissemination of knowledge and ideas among neurosurgical nurses around the world, and the fostering of research in clinical nursing. Membership in the federation is open to neurosurgical nurses through membership in national neurosurgical nursing societies; individual membership is accepted if such a national organization does not exist.

Because the address for communication with WFNN changes in relation to the officers elected, the best contact is probably made through the national constituent member or the AJN directory of organizations.

WORLD HEALTH ORGANIZATION

The World Health Organization (WHO) is one of the largest of the specialized agencies of the United Nations. Established in 1948, WHO's constitution states as one of its beliefs: "The enjoyment of the highest attainable standard of health is one of the fundamental rights of every human being without the distinction of race, religion, political, economic or social condition" and defines *health* as "a state of complete physical, mental, and social well-being and not merely the absence of disease."

Membership in WHO is open to all countries, including those that do not belong to the United Nations. WHO is organized on a regional basis; the regions are subdivided into zones, so that WHO and the nations within each region or zone can work together on matters of mutual concern. The six regions are Southeast Asia, the Eastern Mediterranean, Western Pacific, Africa, Europe, and the

Americas. The American region is served by the Pan American Health Organization, (PAHO), which also acts as the WHO regional organization.

An executive board directs the work of WHO, which is administered by a director general. Among its working force, known as the *secretariat,* are members of the health professions, including nurses. (However, at WHO headquarters, physicians outnumber nurses by about 100 to 1.) WHO's activities are largely financed by assessments on the member countries, on the basis of a scale authorized by the World Health Assembly.

World Health Assembly

WHO's governing body is the World Health Assembly. It is made up of delegates from all member countries and meets once a year. The United States was the only country to include a nurse (Lucile Petry Leone) in its delegation to the first World Health Assembly and has generally followed this practice ever since. Some other countries now include nurses in their delegations, too.

In her report on the first World Health Assembly, Mrs. Leone commented:

> Nursing was mentioned in many ways by a large number of the delegates. Everywhere there seemed recognition of the importance of nurses in the health activities which are recommended by the WHO. I was frequently consulted by delegates of many countries when they found that a nurse was present in the assembly. . . . The delegations of Ireland and the United States presented [a] resolution on nursing which formed the basis for the inclusion of nursing in WHO.[15]

The first World Health Assembly planned to include nurses only on specialized teams concerned with such health problems as malaria, tuberculosis, venereal diseases, and maternal and child health. Within a year, however, the importance of having nurses help with all phases of world nursing was recognized, and in 1949 a nurse consultant was appointed to WHO's headquarters staff, and an Expert Committee on Nursing was appointed to consider nursing education and nursing service on a worldwide basis. Since then, nursing has been an integral part of many WHO programs, with WHO's nursing staff including not only those nurses assigned to the headquarters and regional offices but also those providing direct assistance with health and nursing projects in many countries throughout the world. Nevertheless, there are still few nurses (or even women) on expert committees, and there is no woman regional director.

National and International Services

WHO's services are divided into three broad areas: (1) assisting governments, on request, with their health problems, (2) providing a number of worldwide health services, and (3) encouraging and coordinating international research on health problems. The trained staff of technical advisors, doctors, dentists, sanitary engineers, nurses, and others who are dispatched to help and advise any nation requesting aid works with the national ministry of health, the main emphasis being on making health care available to all persons.

Personnel are trained to initiate problem-solving programs and, when progress toward solution is assured, to teach people in the locality or country to carry on by themselves. WHO personnel recognize the influence of a people's social and economic status on health practices and attempt to effect improvement in those areas also.

Among WHO's major programs in individual countries are aid to strengthen local health services through better administration; eradication or control of such communicable diseases as malaria, typhoid fever, tuberculosis, syphilis, trachoma, and yaws; provision of better care for mothers and babies; development of better sanitation facilities; and improvement of mental health. WHO also provides fellowships, usually short-term, to enable health workers to observe or study in other countries, with the goal of improving practice or services in their own country. U.S.

nurses are among those eligible for these fellowships.

WHO, in cooperation with member nations, collects and disseminates epidemiological information, develops and administers international quarantine regulations, establishes a uniform system of health statistics, promotes standards of strength and purity for drugs and recommends names for pharmaceutical products, keeps countries advised of the possible dangers in the use of radioisotopes and helps train personnel in protection measures, and institutes international vaccination programs as, for example, those against poliomyelitis.

Within the last several years, WHO has emphasized primary care. At the WHO/UNICEF Alma-Ata (USSR) conference in 1978, primary health care was introduced as the key approach to achieving an acceptable level of health throughout the world. The HFA/2000 goal introduced at that meeting was adopted by the World Health Assembly in 1979, and member nations have been encouraged and assisted in various ways to work toward that goal. In 1983 a proposal was adopted to monitor and evaluate progress.

ICN, which has supported the primary care concept, was among the first to follow up on the Alma-Ata conference through a workshop that identified and recommended changes required in nursing education, practice, and legislation to prepare nurses for primary health care. In 1983, when the executive director reported to the WHO secretariat on these ICN activities and recommendations, many members from around the world noted the importance of nursing in primary health care.

In other actions WHO has also intensified its promotion of the medical systems used by the majority of people. In the Third World countries, most people depend on traditional healers, who have often been quite effective in caring for people. Their integration into the general health system is considered essential at this point of development and health care delivery.[16]

Nursing within WHO

As mentioned earlier, delegates at the first World Health Assembly realized that nursing was of worldwide interest and concern. More and better nurses were needed in every area of the world.[17] In some countries—in 1948—there was not a single fully qualified nurse. Health care was given entirely by aides, who often had little or no training. In other countries, as in the United States, there were adequate nursing services that could have been even better if more nurses were available. Between these two extremes were countries with widely varying numbers of nurses and vastly different educational patterns for preparing them. The largest part of WHO's nursing assistance has naturally been directed toward the relatively less developed, underprivileged countries with the most urgent health and nursing needs.

WHO nurses work primarily in an advisory capacity, helping the nurses in a country with their specific problems. Sometimes, however, WHO nurses must temporarily assume operational responsibilities until one of the country's own nurses has been prepared for the job. Thus, in establishing a postgraduate nursing program in a university, the WHO nurse may have to serve as director of the program in its early stages.

The areas in which WHO is called upon to provide assistance cover practically all of nursing—nursing education, organization and administration of hospital and public health nursing services, mental health, maternal and child health, clinical nursing specialties, and community health care planning. Improved midwifery services and education are vitally needed in many countries; so are programs to increase the number and upgrade the training of auxiliary nursing personnel. WHO helps in these areas by cooperating with manpower planning. Assistance from WHO is also available to governments and their nursing divisions (if any) to plan for the development of nursing in those countries and to promote nursing legislation in the interests of both nurses and the public.

Another WHO nursing activity is the sponsorship, sometimes in cooperation with other agencies, of regional conferences and seminars that focus on the changing role of the nurse in relation to current health policies. These enable nurses with similar backgrounds and problems to exchange information and work toward solutions, under the guidance of expert nurses from WHO or other international health agencies. Many of these nurses have never before had an opportunity to meet with members of their profession from other countries, and they derive not only knowledge but encouragement and moral support from such conferences.

It is obvious that WHO's nursing activities call for highly qualified nurses, expert in at least one of the fields in which WHO offers advisory services. Language requirements depend upon the country of assignment, but it is desirable for a nurse to be proficient in at least one language other than her own. The official languages of WHO are Spanish, English, French, Russian, Chinese, and Arabic. In addition to its more or less regularly employed nursing staff, WHO engages nurses for limited periods of time to carry out special projects in various countries. WHO nurses often work in collaboration with nurses from other agencies who are also helping with nursing development in a given country.

In addition to its advisory services, WHO has published a variety of documents in relation to nursing, most of them basic and intended to be widely applicable in many countries. WHO also publishes *World Health,* a monthly magazine on world health intended for the lay public, *International Digest of Health Legislation, World Health Statistics Annual,* directories of schools of the health professions, and a variety of technical papers, journals, and reports.

WHO has had a part in many of the major developments in the international health field such as increase in the average life span; decrease in infant mortality; total eradication of smallpox; major reduction in poliomyelitis and malaria; and increase in medical and other health profession schools.

The WHO address is Avenue Appia, 1211 Geneva 27, Switzerland. The Pan American Health Organization address is Pan American Sanitary Bureau, WHO Regional Office for the Americas, 525 23rd St. N.W., Washington, D.C. 20037.

AGENCY FOR INTERNATIONAL DEVELOPMENT

The Agency for International Development (AID), administered by the U.S. Department of State, is one of a succession of agencies through which the United States has assisted other countries in their social and economic development, with nursing one of the areas in which assistance has been provided. AID is a national rather than an international agency, but is included in this section because of the worldwide nature of its activities.

The distinguishing feature of the health and other technical assistance programs that have been carried out by AID and its predecessor agencies is that they have been bilateral—that is, undertaken cooperatively with the government of the country being assisted, upon the request of that country and with both nations sharing in the determination of the programs to be carried out and the goals to be achieved. These bilateral health programs had their beginnings in 1942 with the establishment of the Institute of Inter-American Affairs to work cooperatively with Latin American countries in improving their health and welfare services. Since that time, U.S. technical assistance in nursing has been provided under a variety of administrative auspices (Economic Security Administration, Foreign Operations Administration, International Cooperation Administration, and others), culminating in the establishment of AID in 1961.

The early nursing assistance projects were highly concerned with the development and improvement of public health nursing services; this was the most pressing health need in Central and South America in the 1940s. The U.S. nurses working in these programs, however, soon discovered that public health nursing services could not be permanently strengthened without a continuing supply of well-prepared nurses, which would, of course, require improved nursing school systems and facilities. In turn, if nursing students were to have their clinical experience in a true learning environment, hospital nursing services also needed improvement.

These three areas—public health nursing, nursing education, and hospital nursing services—have been the target of most nursing assistance projects carried out under AID's auspices. Like WHO, however, AID has also provided assistance in other nursing areas, such as midwifery services, the preparation of auxiliary personnel, and the establishment of postgraduate programs to prepare nurses for teaching and administrative responsibilities, among others. AID also operates a participant training program whereby qualified individuals—nurses among them—in the assisted countries are given an opportunity to get the basic or advanced education they need in educational institutions in this country or elsewhere.

AID employs nurses on a short- or long-term basis to carry out its nursing assistance projects. Some AID nurses have been with the agency or one of its predecessors for many years, assisting with projects in various countries. Others are recruited on a more limited basis or act as consultants.

SUMMARY

The purpose of this chapter was to provide an overview of international health and nursing activities. Therefore, only the largest and most significant organizations and agencies operating in this area were included. There are many other organized groups—religious and lay, private and governmental, societies and foundations—carrying on similar or related functions. For additional information, the heading *international* in any nursing, hospital, or medical literature index will provide additional information about the activities being carried on around the world in behalf of the health and nursing needs of its people.

REFERENCES

1. Daisy C. Bridges, "Events in the History of the International Council of Nurses." *Am. J. Nurs.,* **49**:594–595 (Sept. 1949).
2. Margaret Breay and Ethel Bedford Fenwick, *The History of the International Council of Nurses. 1899–1925* (Geneva: The International Council of Nurses, 1931). This is a detailed, fascinating, and informative account of ICN's founding and first twenty-five years, throwing considerable light on the nursing problems and personalities of this period.
3. According to ICN records, Miss Dock wrote these words as part of a foreword to the program of ICN's Second Quinquennial Meeting, held in London in 1909.
4. Mary M. Roberts, *American Nursing: History and Interpretation* (New York: Macmillan Publishing Company, Inc., 1954), pp. 80–81.
5. International Council of Nurses, *Basic Documents: Constitution and Regulations, Rules, Procedure at Meetings* (Geneva: The Council, 1966), p. 8.
6. "ICN," *Am. J. Nurs.,* **73**:1388, 1352 (Aug. 1973).
7. Ibid., 1352.
8. Ibid.
9. "ICN '77," *Am. J. Nurs.,* **77**:1303–1310 (Aug. 1977).
10. "ICN" op. cit. p. 1352.
11. Virginia Henderson, *ICN Basic Principles of Nursing Care* (London: International Council of Nurses, 1958).
12. Entire issue on primary health care, *Int. Nurs. Rev.,* **29** (Nov.–Dec. 1982).
13. Breay and Fenwick, op. cit., p. 12.
14. "Long Term Plans for ICN," *Int. Nurs. Rev.,* **31**:30 (Jan.–Feb. 1984).

15. Lucile Petry, "World Health Organization and Nursing," *Am. J. Nurs.,* **48**:611 (Oct. 1948).

16. "WHO Pushes Traditional Healing,"

The Nation's Health, **9**:3 (May 1979).

17. World Health Organization, *The First Ten Years of WHO* (Geneva: WHO, 1958), pp. 391ff.

29

The Professional Literature

Nursing is no exception to the publication explosion that is affecting all professions today. New nursing knowledge is accumulating rapidly, partly as a result of the extensive research now being carried on. Rapid advances in scientific knowledge and in medical therapies call for the development of corresponding nursing care techniques. New fields of nursing practice and new ways of delivering nursing services continue to emerge. More and more, as the nursing profession becomes increasingly mature and sophisticated, nurses recognize the need to share their concepts, research findings, and nursing care knowledge with their colleagues.

The result is a proliferation of nursing literature—books, periodicals, and monographs, as well as many specialized publications. Not too long ago, text or reference books in nursing were generally limited to the major clinical fields. Now there is scarcely any area relating to nursing that does not have books on the subject. New titles show the extremely diverse nature of the subjects that nurses must read and write about today. Many of these books (this one, for instance) must be frequently revised and published in new, updated editions to keep up with new knowledge and expanding concepts.

Reading the book advertisements in the nursing magazines is almost an education in itself; by doing this, the nurse is reminded of the pressing topics of the day—or of tomorrow. Even more important is reading the reviews of these books, also published in the nursing journals. That way, the reader will gain a better knowledge of their content and the reviewer's estimate (and he or she is usually an expert in the field) of their value. Then it is easier to decide whether to buy it, borrow it from the library, glance through it there, or forget about it. Certainly it is impossible to read all the books published in the nursing field today, so nurses will want to select those that promise to hold the most value for them and their individual interests.

It is the nursing journals, however, that will keep the nurse up-to-date and well informed. Usually at least six months passes between the writing of a book and its appearance in print, and a few more months may pass before it is reviewed. But the nursing journals, especially those that are published monthly, make available news, reviews, and information promptly. Within the past ten years alone, there has been a remarkable increase in the numbers and kinds of nursing magazines (over eighty in 1985). Some the nurse will undoubtedly want to subscribe to and keep for reference, others to look at each month in the library. It is helpful to have at least an idea of the content, purpose, and approach of all of them.[1]

In academia, there is some tendency to consider as more scholarly and prestigious those journals that are refereed, that is, have peer review. This means, in general, that the article (paper) written has been reviewed by other experts in the field before being published. These reviewers may be called an *editorial board, advisory board, editorial advisors, associate editors, co-editors,* or *assistant editors.* They are usually volunteers and generally are not involved in the production of the journal. There are mixed opinions as to whether these journals are really of better quality.[2-4] At times there is also a problem determining just how much involvement these expert volunteers have; some never see a manuscript, but their names are on the magazine's masthead.

It is not feasible to review the content of all these periodicals, so attention is directed primarily to the periodicals and services presented by the American Journal of Nursing Company, which was the first nursing journal company in the United States and is still owned by nurses—the American Nurses' Association (ANA).

AMERICAN JOURNAL OF NURSING

Oldest of the nursing periodicals now in existence and first started by and for nurses, the *American Journal of Nursing (AJN)* first appeared in October 1900, and has been published monthly ever since.* *AJN* is the professional journal of ANA and is published by the American Journal of Nursing Company, a nonprofit corporation owned by ANA, which also publishes *Nursing Research, Nursing Outlook, MCN, Geriatric Nursing,* and *International Nursing Index.*

AJN, intended for all nurses, cuts across all fields and levels of nursing practice, administration, and education, with special emphasis on the clinical practice of nursing. As fast as new nursing care principles or techniques evolve, they are reported in the *Journal* in clinical news reports gathered by nurse editors or in articles written by nurse experts in each area.

New ideas about nursing in general—its scope, its definition, and its problems—are found in the pages of *AJN.* And, not least important, *AJN,* as the official journal of nursing's professional organization, ANA, carries up-to-date information about ANA's programs and activities. *AJN* news ranges from local (legislative efforts of individual states, for instance) to international (reports of ICN congresses and interim activities). In recent years, there has been special emphasis on clinical problems and new technology, including articles for intensive care nurses on such topics as the intra-aortic balloon and the use of the electrocardiogram to detect myocardial infarction. The annual Drug Update (each July), equipment supplements, and columns on ethical dilemmas, legal decisions, pain interventions, computers, books, and films are other examples of the diversity of vital information available to readers. *AJN* also broke new ground by publishing programmed instruction on subjects before nursing books were available on the topic, beginning with a series on physical assessment in February 1974.

AJN also provides other professional services, such as a yearly listing of the addresses of nursing and health organizations; annual and five-year cumulative indexes; lists of major meetings and CE programs; and classified and other advertisements of job opportunities.

Through the years, *AJN* has done more

The Trained Nurse and Hospital Review (later *Nursing World*) antedated the *Journal* by twelve years but was not nursing owned and nursing run. It ceased publication in 1960.

than reflect changes and trends in nursing as a clinical practice and as a profession. It frequently has helped shape those changes. The most recent example of this is the publication in *AJN* of material through which nurses can earn CE contact hours by home study. As the trend toward CE gains momentum and certain states require documentation of CE for relicensure, a major problem facing the profession is availability of offerings through which nurses can obtain the credits as well as the knowledge they need. *AJN* was the first nursing publication to offer such material. CE units, approved for contact hours under the ANA Mechanism for Approval of Continuing Education in Nursing, have been published in four issues each year since March 1977. Nurses wishing to acquire CE contact hours through these home-study units, which are always on clinical topics, can do so by passing an examination on the material. *AJN*'s CE program includes the preparation, scoring, and handling of these exams. For this service to its readers, unique at the time, *AJN* won the 1979 National Magazine Award, in competition with consumer, business, and professional publications. The National Magazine Awards are regarded as the most prestigious in the magazine field.

Unlike many other nursing journals, the *AJN*'s editorial staff is largely, but not exclusively, made up of nurses chosen because of their expertise in a given nursing specialty plus journalistic ability. *AJN,* unlike most official magazines of a professional association, does not come automatically with membership in the association; it must be subscribed to and paid for independently. However, its lowest subscription rates are reserved for ANA members.

The history of *AJN*'s founding and subsequent development as a publication owned, managed, and edited by the profession is one of which nurses can be proud. This is related in *The American Journal of Nursing and its Company: A Chronicle, 1900–1975,* and various histories of nursing.

NURSING OUTLOOK

Nursing Outlook, also published by the American Journal of Nursing Company, was, until 1979, the official publication of the National League for Nursing (NLN). It is much younger than *AJN,* its first issue having appeared in January 1953, less than a year after NLN was organized. It is the successor to *Public Health Nursing,* which had been the official journal of the National Organization of Public Health Nursing, one of the associations that disbanded and became an integral part of NLN.

Outlook's content was originally directed toward the concerns of the NLN—nursing service and education, especially their administrative and community aspects. However, the journal is now broadly based, frequently focusing on controversial or new issues in nursing and health, such as institutional licensure, independent nursing practice, HMOs health economics, physician's assistants, and mandatory CE. For those interested in current trends in education, there are articles on curriculum development, theoretical models, approaches to teaching, and development of new nursing programs. There is also information on current community, hospital, nursing home, clinic, and independent nursing practice. Each issue contains articles on these topics, as well as special departments often focusing on current controversial issues.

As with *AJN,* book reviews, educational programs, and notices of major meetings are published, in addition to classified and other advertisements.

In 1982, *Nursing Outlook* became a bimonthly peer review journal with a panel of over 100 reviewers, as well as a distinguished editorial advisory board.

NURSING RESEARCH

Still another publication of the American Journal of Nursing Company is *Nursing Research,* a bimonthly journal established in

1952 for the purposes of stimulating and reporting research and scientific studies in nursing. *Nursing Research* has an editorial advisory committee and nurse editors who are qualified nurse researchers. *Nursing Research* carries reports of research projects, articles on research methods, and news about research activities.*

MCN, THE AMERICAN JOURNAL OF MATERNAL CHILD NURSING

MCN, The American Journal of Maternal/ Child Nursing, first appeared in January 1976 and quickly acquired interested subscribers. It is a bimonthly publication established to help the practicing nurse so that care given to individuals and families during the childbearing and childrearing phases of the life cycle can be of high quality. *MCN* is a refereed journal whose review panel is made up of practicing nurses and nurse researchers who are active in the field of maternal-child nursing. The editor is a clinical specialist in maternal-child nursing.

MCN primarily focuses on clinical practice, with particular emphasis on nursing intervention. The topics range from preconception through adolescence. Many issues have a special section that highlights such areas as human sexuality, mother–child relationships, or the school-age child. Occasionally, when merited, an entire issue of the journal is devoted to one subject, such as nutrition or the family. A recent addition is the development of a format to present pertinent research that focuses on those areas. In addition, every issue carries a column on research authored by a noted nurse researcher and one that focuses on a particular drug. Equally important, space is devoted to the discussion of other issues about

which practicing nurses must be knowledgeable. One section, "Professionally Speaking," includes such topics as how to write to a legislator, how to bring about change, and how to testify as an expert witness. Each issue also carries book reviews and notices of major meetings in the field of maternal/child care.

GERIATRIC NURSING

The newest of the AJN company refereed journals is *Geriatric Nursing,* which began publication with the May/June 1980 issue. Emphasis is on clinical articles on common diseases, disabilities and living problems of the aged, including ways to meet their visual, hearing, mental-emotional, and nutritional needs, as well as nurses' needs to capitalize on the strengths of older adults. News, current events, drug information, and a regular profile of an active, contributing elder over 70 are included.

OTHER AMERICAN JOURNAL OF NURSING COMPANY SERVICES

The *American Journal of Nursing, Nursing Outlook, MCN: The American Journal of Maternal Child Nursing, Geriatric Nursing,* and *Nursing Research* might be considered the official publications of the nursing profession. Their official status derives from the fact that they are all published by the American Journal of Nursing Company, a nonprofit corporation owned by ANA. The magazines are not published as commercial ventures, but as a service to the nursing profession. In addition to the magazines, the AJN Company publishes the quarterly *International Nursing Index* and the annual *AJN Guide: A Review of Nursing Career Opportunities*. It also provides a variety of other services related to the publications and communications fields.

For example, since 1973, the AJN Company has provided quarters and, until re-

---

*The idea for a magazine such as *Nursing Research* came initially from the Association of Collegiate Schools of Nursing, an organization that was merged into NLN in 1952.

cently, staff for the Nurses' Educational Funds (NEF), Inc. However, NEF remains a separate organization, its functioning enhanced by these services.

As a nonprofit entity, the AJN Company also supports, through grants, various nursing activities, including the American Nurses' Foundation, NEF scholarships, and the Nursing Archive Collection of Mugar Library at Boston University.

Microfilm or Microfiche Issues

To meet the demand for unavailable back issues of its publications, the AJN Company has given University Microfilms permission to reproduce on microfilm or microfiche out-of-print volumes of the magazines. Some organizations, individuals, and libraries also like microfilm/microfiche volumes because they require less storage space than original magazines.

University Microfilms also reproduces current out-of-stock issues of the magazines, on order, by photocopy, producing a very readable facsimile of the original publication, but with some limitations. Inquiries about prices and other details of this service should be sent directly to University Microfilms, 300 North Zeeb Road, Ann Arbor, Michigan 48106.

The AJN Company has a policy governing the reproduction of material on which it holds copyright. Generally, permission is granted except when the material is available from its Educational Services Division. Material may not be reproduced without written permission. Requests should be directed to the permissions department at the company address, 555 West 57th Street, New York, New York 10019. A charge may be made to commercial organizations.

The company has a special policy covering the reproduction of its material for library reserve collections. Interested organizations should write for copies of this policy.

Educational Services Division

The Educational Services Division was established in 1970, when the AJN Company absorbed the ANA-NLN Film Service and combined it with the existing service of providing reprints of articles from company periodicals. In 1973 Video Nursing, Inc., a nonprofit corporation which produced audiovisual educational tools, was acquired and merged with the division.

Since then, these activities have expanded through the company's production of multimedia and print materials and the acquisition of distribution rights to audiovisual materials produced by others.

Today, the Educational Services Division distributes a wide range of multimedia programs for generic and inservice nursing education. These programs are listed for purchase or rental in a catalog which is available on request.

In 1979, the division established the AJN Nursing Boards Review in answer to a growing demand from new graduates for an organized study program to assist them in preparing for the state board examination. This comprehensive, five-day program reviews the clinical nursing subjects covered in the state board exam. The program is offered each January and June in various cities throughout the United States.

To further assist students preparing for state boards, the company publishes a review book, *AJN Nursing Boards Review Book,* which is used in the course but can be purchased separately, and a companion question-and-answer book for students wishing to study on their own.

Writing Awards

In 1950, when *AJN* celebrated its fiftieth anniversary, the company established the Mary M. Roberts Fellowship (later, the Mary M. Roberts Writing Awards) in honor of Miss Roberts, who had retired the previous year after serving as editor of *AJN* for twenty-eight years (1921–1949). The purpose of these awards, as originally described, was to "afford specialized training in writing and other journalistic skills to a nurse [now, nurses] who has demonstrated talent for writing about subjects significant to nursing, addressed to nurses and other professional groups, and the general public.''

The nature of these awards has varied over the years since they were first established. For some ten years, six or more nurses attended annually, with all expenses paid, a writers' conference workshop or program that lasted for periods ranging from two weeks to one month. Today, the annual nurse writing awards, co-sponsored by participating state nurses' associations (SNAs), are intended primarily to encourage nurses to sharpen their skills in order to promote better communication within the profession and with the general public. Promotion and judging of the competition within each state is handled by the SNA; the AJN Company provides an award certificate and a monetary prize for each state competition.

State Publication Awards

To recognize excellence in the official publications of all professional SNAs, the AJN Company makes awards every two years to state publications for excellence in five categories: total editorial content, best feature article written by a member, best legislative coverage, best coverage of economic and general welfare issues, and best coverage of CE activities. To achieve fairness in making the awards, the association publications are grouped according to the size of association membership.

Outstanding editors and professional nurses serve as judges in the various categories, and awards are presented at a company awards banquet held in conjunction with each ANA biennial convention. They are not financial awards but, rather, certificates of merit.

Two other AJN Company services are provided during the ANA convention. The Educational Services Division conducts a Media Festival, awarding plaques to producers of films, videotapes, and slide tape programs judged to be outstanding. These are screened throughout the convention week, providing educators and other interested persons with

the opportunity to view them for possible later use.

The AJN Company also publishes *Convention News,* a newspaper which is distributed free to all participants and reports convention programs and business on a daily basis. For years, the company has provided editorial services to produce the daily publication distributed at the ICN congress and finances the daily bulletin at the National Student Nurses' Association (NSNA) convention as well.

Sophia F. Palmer Memorial Library

For many years, the AJN Company has maintained a library at its headquarters. Intended originally for the use of the magazines' editors and the staffs of ANA and NLN, the library's facilities have for some years been available to a limited number of nurses and graduate students. They must make an appointment to use the library, however; there is no mail or loan service, and no material may be taken out of the library.

In 1953 the library was named the Sophia F. Palmer Memorial Library in honor of *AJN*'s first editor. Under the administration of a professional librarian, the library contains a wealth of nursing literature, including textbooks, periodicals, numerous bulletins, reports, and official publications of all kinds, as well as rare and old material about nursing not available elsewhere. A Reader Service answers letters and other requests for information in all areas of nursing.

International Nursing Index

One of the AJN Company's most significant services to the profession is the *International Nursing Index (INI),* which it publishes in cooperation with the National Library of Medicine. This quarterly publication, whose first issue appeared in the spring of 1966, provides a categorized listing of the articles published in some 200 nursing journals throughout the world, many of them in languages other than English, plus articles relevant to nursing that appear in journals indexed in *Index Medicus.* The first three issues of *INI* each year are paperbound and noncumulated; the fourth issue is a cloth-bound cumulation of the three previous issues plus new material to the end of the year.

Representing a comprehensive and continuing index of the world literature pertaining to nursing, *INI* is important to nursing and nurses. In the words of the Journal Company's publishing director, in announcing the inauguration of *INI:*

> On the practical level, it means that the nurse looking for material on, say, the supervision of nursing services in a psychiatric hospital will no longer have to search through a whole battery of separate indexes; instead, she will find all the relevant references brought together in a single place: the *International Nursing Index.* And, on the professional level initiation of INI mans that nursing, like other professions, has a bibliographic instrument for the control of its scholarly record.[5]

INI has a circulation of about 1,900; copies are found in many nursing school and health profession (and probably hospital) libraries, and nurses will want to become familiar with it. It gives an idea of the scope, quantity, and variety of material about nursing being published today.

OTHER NURSING JOURNALS

There has been a dramatic increase in the number of nursing journals published in the last decade. Most welcome and often solicit manuscripts from nurses. A few have staff writers of their own but may, on occasion, solicit a particular kind of article. Exhibit 29-1 includes the major national nursing journals and serials in the United States (except the AJN Company journals previously discussed), some key journals from England and Canada, and several international journals. Not included are the national journals of other countries, the journals of the SNAs, and the journals of the organizations described in Chapters 24–27 if they are published by their

headquarters. It is worthwhile to review these journals, if possible (they are not subscribed to by many libraries), as well as the other health-related journals, because they also contain useful information. All nursing journals and serials are listed in *INI.* A listing of nursing and allied health periodicals, with addresses, is given in the *Cumulative Index to Nursing and Allied Health Literature.*

OTHER REFERENCE SOURCES

Most schools of nursing today do not have a collection adequate enough to meet the needs of a serious scholar or even of someone who wants to go beyond the major nursing journals and books. Because of limitations of space and money, a decision is usually made by faculty and library staff about what is most essential for that particular nursing program. Interprofessional health sciences libraries in medical centers and professional schools have collections that cover the various health professions, including international journals and other publications. Other disciplines also have their specialized libraries. What about access? A nurse enrolled in an educational program has access to all of that institution's learning resources, including libraries, audiovisual centers, faculty, and staff. Those same resources may be completely off limits for one who is not enrolled; at times, even those in university CE programs have only limited access. If the nurse is permitted to read and browse, chances are that nothing can be taken out.

Hospitals usually have some kind of medical library. Even if its acquisitions are useful to the nurse (and often they are), the librarian, too, has a primary responsibility to others—physicians, medical students (rarely other students), and perhaps administrative personnel and clinical specialists. Nevertheless, nurses who learn how to use the library, the interlibrary loan service, and the various computer information retrieval services will find a new world of reference sources.

EXHIBIT 29-1

Major Nursing Journals

Advances in Nursing Sciences (ANS)
Aspen Systems Corporation
16792 Oakmont Avenue
Gaithersburg, MD. 20760

Canadian Journal of Psychiatric Nursing
Psychiatric Nurses' Association of Canada
1854 Portage Ave.
Winnepeg, Manitoba
R3J 0G9, Canada

Canadian Nurse
Canadian Nurses' Association
50, The Driveway
Ottawa, Ont., K2P 1E2
Canada

Cancer Nursing
Masson Publishing, Inc.
14 East 60th Street, Suite 1101
New York, NY 10022

Cardiovascular Nursing
American Heart Association
7320 Greenville Avenue
Dallas, TX 75231

Computers in Nursing
2350 Virginia Avenue
Hagerstown, MD 21740

CONA Journal
Canadian Orthopaedic Nurses Association
43 Wellesley Street East
Toronto, Ontario M4Y 1H1
Canada

Critical Care Nurse
Simms Associates, Inc.
680 Route 206 North
Bridgewater, NJ 08807

Critical Care Quarterly
Aspen Systems Corporation
16792 Oakmont Avenue
Gaithersburg, MD 20760

Heart & Lung: Journal of Critical Care
Official Publication of the American
   Association of Critical-Care Nurses
C.V. Mosby Company
11830 Westline Industrial Drive
St. Louis, MO 63141

Home Healthcare Nurse
Home Healthcare Nurse, Inc.
680 Route 206 North
Bridgewater, NJ 08807

Issues in Mental Health Nursing
Hemisphere Publishing Corp.
Global Building
1025 Vermont Avenue, N.W.
Washington, DC 20005

International Journal of Nursing Studies
Pergamon Press
Maxwell House, Fairview Park
Elmsford, NY 10523

International Nursing Review
International Council of Nursing
Imprimeries Reunies SA
33 Avenue de la Gare
CH-1001 Lausanne, Switzerland

JEN: Journal of Emergency Nursing
C.V. Mosby Company
11830 Westline Industrial Drive
St. Louis, MO 63141

Journal of Continuing Education in Nursing
Charles B. Slack, Inc.
6900 Grove Road
Thorofare, NJ 08086

Journal of Gerontological Nursing
Charles B. Slack, Inc.
6900 Grove Road
Thorofare, NJ 08086

Journal of Neurosurgical Nursing
American Association of Neurosurgical
  Nurses
428 E. Preston Street
Baltimore, MD 21202

Journal of Nursing Administration
J.B. Lippincott Company
East Washington Square
Philadelphia, PA 19105

Journal of Nursing Education
Charles B. Slack, Inc.
6900 Grove Road
Thorofare, NJ 08086

Journal of Nurse-Midwifery
Elsevier North Holland, Inc.
52 Vanderbilt Avenue
New York, NY 10017

**Journal of Psychosocial Nursing and
  Mental Health Services**
Charles B. Slack, Inc.
6900 Grove Road
Thorofare, NJ 08086

Maternal–Child Nursing Journal
437 Victoria Bldg.
3500 Victoria Street
Pittsburgh, PA 15261

Neonatal Network
Journal of Neonatal Nursing
25 Valletta Court
San Francisco, CA 94131

Nephrology Nurse
Simms Associates, Inc.
680 Route 206 North
Bridgewater, NJ 08807

Nurse Educator
J.B. Lippincott Company
East Washington Square
Philadelphia, PA 19105

Nursing 85 (Year changes)
Intermed Communications, Inc.
111 Bethlehem Pike
Springhouse, PA 19477

Nursing Administration Quarterly
Aspen Systems Corp.
16792 Oakmont Avenue
Gaithersburg, MD 02760

**Nursing Careers: Continuing Education in
  Nursing**
P.O. Box 145
Pacific Palisades, CA 90272

Nursing Clinics of North America
W.B. Saunders Company
West Washington Square
Philadelphia, PA 19105

Nursing Economics
Anthony J. Jannetti, Inc.
North Woodbury Road, Box 56
Pitman, NJ 08071

**Nurse Practitioner—American Journal of
  Primary Care**
109 West Mercer Street
Seattle, WA 98119

Nursing Forum
Nursing Publications
P.O. Box 218
Hillsdale, NJ 07642

Nursing Leadership
Charles B. Slack, Inc.
6900 Grove Road
Thorofare, NJ 08076

Nursing Life
1111 Bethlehem Pike
Springhouse, PA 19477

Nursing Management
8 South Michigan Avenue
Chicago, IL 60603

Nursing Times
Macmillan Journals Limited
4 Little Essex St.
London, WC2R 3LF, England

Occupational Health Nursing
Charles B. Slack, Inc.
6900 Grove Road
Thorofare, NJ 08086

Oncology Nursing Forum
9913 Pomona Drive
Bethesda, MD 20817

Orthopedic Nursing
Anthony J. Jannetti, Inc.
North Woodbury Road, Box 56
Pitman, NJ 08071

Perspectives in Psychiatric Care
Nursing Publications, Inc.
Box 218
Hillsdale, NJ 07642

Public Health Nursing
Blackwell Scientific Publications
52 Beacon St.
Boston, MA 02108

Reagan Report On Nursing Law
Medica Press
1231 Industrial Bank Bldg.
Providence, RI 02903

Research in Nursing and Health
John Wiley & Sons, Inc.
605 3rd Avenue
New York, NY 10016

RN Magazine
Medical Economics Co.
550 Kinderkamack Road
Oradell, NJ 07649

Today's OR Nurse
Charles B. Slack, Inc.
6900 Grove Road
Thorofare, NJ 08086

Topics in Clinical Nursing
Aspen Systems Corp.
16792 Oakmont Avenue
Gaithersburg, MD 20760

There are a number of ways to become knowledgeable about these sources. One that is readily available is the "Selected List of Nursing Books and Journals"[6] published periodically in *Nursing Outlook,* which provides necessary or helpful sources that all libraries serving nurses should have, and informs nurses and others of what is potentially available. Included are listings of books considered essential in the clinical specialties, administration, communication, education, ethics, nursing law, science, nutrition, nursing trends, issues, and theories, transcultural nursing, and practical nursing. Also included are dictionaries and nursing reviews, as well as a basic list of nursing journals. References are made to other sources of information, including au-

diovisual materials. Both U.S. and Canadian listings are given.

A more extensive compilation, also published periodically in *Nursing Outlook,* is "Reference Sources for Nursing," which includes both nursing and biomedical reference works.[7]

These references are prepared by the Interagency Council on Library Resources organized in 1960. Seven national nursing organizations in the United States are represented on the Council, as well as the American Journal of Nursing Company, the Canadian Nurses' Association, the Nursing Archive Collection of the Mugar Memorial Library of Boston University (which houses the ANA's Archives), three national hospital associations, three national library associations, the Nursing Division of the United States Public Health Service, and the National Library of Medicine. This Interagency Council has no budget and no executive function, but its recommendations to the agencies represented on it carry weight.[8]

Interlibrary loans extend not only to other on-campus or intracity libraries, but include the vast resources of the National Library of Medicine and designated regional medical libraries.

Of course, all the reference sources in the world are of little value if an individual cannot utilize them properly. Taylor provides some good guidelines,[9] and Henderson delineates specific skills.[10]

1. Searching a card catalogue to find books and pamphlets.
2. Using indexes to find journal and serial publications.
3. Finding and using abstracting and excerpting journals, or serials that shortcut finding, scanning, or reading books, pamphlets, or journals on a given subject.
4. Finding and using lists and bibliographies that enable each worker to build on the searches of others. (Such lists or bibliographies may cite exclusively books and pamphlets, journal articles, or audio-visual materials, or any combination of these.)
5. Finding and using dictionaries, encyclopedias, directories, statistical and legal guides, fact books, and yearbooks.
6. Making correct citations for each item of information sought or found and preparing a file of these items organized in such a way that the maker of the file and any trained filing clerk can find (or retrieve) the item.
7. Finding nonprint learning media in catalogues, indexes, and lists.
8. Using viewers, projectors, and other mechanical devices for reading or looking at both print and nonprint media.
9. Making full (but considerate) use of the services of librarians and other members of the learning center staff in:

a. Seeking general information in the use of the resources.
b. Asking for bibliographical help.
c. Getting an interlibrary loan.
d. Using retrieval systems such as AV-LINE. CANCER LINE. MED-LINE or TOXLINE.[11]

Well-informed nurses will not want to confine themselves to the limits of their own profession's literature. The publications of medical and hospital groups, allied professions, education, administration, the social services, and other related fields frequently contain material of interest to the nurse as a member of the health team. Understanding of social, economic, educational, and other issues is as important to understanding current and future changes in nursing as knowledge of medical and scientific progress. Professional nurses never limit their interests and activities to their own field, but maintain active participation in broader areas as well.

WRITING FOR PUBLICATION

The nursing profession needs nurse writers to write articles about nursing for publication in professional journals and in magazines read by the general public; to write books on nursing and allied subjects; and to prepare pamphlets, releases, and other written communications for publication and distribution as indicated. Nurses who have any inclination at all toward writing should begin to develop this ability early in their career.

Why write? There are, of course, personal/professional reasons, and the most obvious is that a person has something to say, something to share with others. Sometimes it is to react to an issue, a concern, an event, or situation in nursing or elsewhere that affects nursing. It may be in response to an article read that could result in a letter to the editor, a reaction paper, or a follow-up article. A logical reason is that there has been little if anything in the literature on that particular topic, especially if this is in the area of clinical practice. Or a nurse may be involved in development of new techniques, use of new equipment, or an innovative approach to caring for a particular kind of patient. Sharing such information is satisfying in itself, but it is also a contribution to the profession. The most important reason for nurses to write (always assuming, of course, that what is written has substance) is the survival of the profession.

A profession must have an adequate body of literature documenting the theoretical and philosophical base of its practice and how its practitioners operate to provide the service that is the essence of professionalism. Informational voids encourage the multiple misconceptions and stereotypes of nursing that already exist and tempt others to fill the void on the basis of their own prejudices and interests.

It is true that both the quantity and quality of the nursing literature have grown in all its dimensions. In journals alone, the increase in clinical articles attests to nurses' interest in improving their clinical practice. More journals concentrating on a clinical specialty have sprung up. Functional specialties such as administration and education or the broad specialties of school and occupational nursing also have their journals and their interest groups. New authors are emerging. Many nurses, who were traditionally not seen as writers, through a broader formal educational base or writing workshops, have discovered that they have something to say and are learning to express it in writing. Usually they do not yet have a long wait from the time of submission of an article to publication, as is true of many other disciplines, although some journals are developing backlogs.

Nevertheless, there are still a number of informational gaps in the nursing literature in the clinical area, because research and practice follow-through are just beginning to hit their stride. But some other deficiencies may not be as easily detected. Consider the legislator who remarked coldly to a group of nurses, "Don't tell me about the need for baccalaureate education; there's nothing much in your own literature that gives *objective* evidence of the benefits to the public." Doubtless, other instances come to mind. Yet, in meetings, workplaces, and schools, some nurse is talking about a concept, an experiment, or a practice that excites a whole group.[12]

So why don't nurses write? Or at least as much as other professionals do? Perhaps the first reason is that too many nurses think that writing is for the academician, who must function in a "publish or perish" environment, or for the researcher who, in somewhat obscure language, adds to the theory of nursing. The average nurse has a string of excuses, "I don't have anything to say"; "I don't have a degree"; "I don't have time"; "I don't know how." All those *don'ts* can be overcome. A person has to start somewhere, and except for the handful who have an innate talent and inclination for writing, a little self-discipline and maybe some tutoring are needed. There are great satisfactions. As Styles says,

> the thrill of expressing oneself (and perhaps even gaining nursing immortality); of seeing one's ideas applied; of learning that one's published work is the basis of teaching, of seeing that it has stimulated or contributed to the work of others; of finding one's circle of professional friends and scope of influence extending, of being invited to speak, of being recognized by awards, not to mention possibly receiving promotions, better jobs and increased income.[13]

No doubt the writing novice will not find all these rewards immediately, but for the professional career nurse, writing is an essential step up the ladder of success.

It may not be easy, as shown by this litany of pains—the need for discipline, finding the time, searching out and documenting sources, having one's cherished ideas (or pet phrases) criticized, finding the right editors, even being rejected.[14] For those who want to write but feel that they don't know how, there are various practical steps. Anyone who has graduated from a nursing program should have the basic tools of writing: a firm grasp of grammar, punctuation, spelling, and word usage. If not, an embarrassment is created for the individual and the profession, and there is little excuse for not remedying the situation. To go a step further, for the purpose of writing, there are three indispensable tools: a good dictionary; *Roget's Thesaurus* (a dictionary of synonyms and anonyms to turn to when one knows the meaning but can't think of the word); and William Strunk Jr. and E. B. White's *The Elements of Style,* third edition (New York: Macmillan Publishing Co., Inc., 1979), which is easily read and includes basic rules of composition, grammar, punctuation, and word usage. In addition, there is a new surge of "how to" articles and books that can be extremely helpful, some of which, directed specifically to nurses, are cited in the references and bibliography of this chapter.

A word about style is appropriate: the best writers write so that they are understood; there is little that cannot be said without the use of long words, and there is absolutely no excuse for pretentious prose.[15] This does not mean that the technical words that may be essential to a clinical article should be omitted. It does mean that a simple collection of noun, verb, participle, clause, or whatever makes sense serves as well as, if not better than, a convoluted sentence that says nothing more.* The most common writing weaknesses cited by a group of editors were overly formal and pedagogic writing; poor organization; absence of an introduction and summary; poor sentence structure (too long and "doesn't flow"); poor or fabricated documentation; and use of jargon.[16] Today, the use of nonsexist gender is also desirable, whenever possible.

Most nurses start their writing ventures with letters to the editor or articles in state or national journals, although there are some who,

with or without a co-author, may publish a book first.

Another way to be published is to write a book review. Although someone who presents papers or has already written articles may be invited by an editor to review a book in his or her area of expertise, it is not necessary to wait to be asked. It is perfectly acceptable to write to the editors of one or more journals, in care of the book review editor, and describe one's qualifications and interests. It is *not* appropriate to send a self-selected book review. The book and the reviewer may already have been selected, or the book may not be slated for review. Most editors will follow up. There may or may not be reimbursement for the review, and the decision on whether you may keep the reviewed book (which is sent you) or must return it varies with the publisher. Although most reviewers develop their own style of reviewing, some journals have a general format and desired length. It is also useful to review the guidelines suggested by book review editors,[17] or at least read reviews already published in the selected journal.

For those who are ready to write an article, one editor suggests certain basic guidelines as a beginning:

1. Know as much as possible about your subject (review the literature). Research those areas you're not sure about (library, interviewing people involved or who have an opinion to offer). Make careful notes as you do this.
2. List all the ideas, arguments, facts, and illustrations you can think of.
3. Establish the what, where, when, why, how, and who for your beginning paragraphs.
4. Sort out your ideas, putting them in order so you provide continuity as you write.
5. Come to a logical conclusion—and make a note of that too.[18]

The article can be written first in draft form and then polished (a second look brings amazing insights). Sometimes a friend who writes or who is an editor can be helpful in making

---

*For some amusing examples, check the *Nursing Outlook* editorials and cartoons on the subject, some of which are collected in *Toward Getting Published: Guidelines for Nurses Who Want to Write* (New York: AJN Co., 1979).

suggestions. However, it is the writer's responsibility to see that the content is accurate and that the references and bibliography are properly cited.[19]

Selecting the appropriate journal for submission of an article is crucial. Some editors will return an article with a suggestion that another journal might be better for that type of paper,* but most do not. (Nor do most bother to critique it, in part because of the volume of mail they must deal with.) One way to determine which journal is right is to check several recent issues of the journals that might be suitable, or at least the major journals listed in respected indexes. The table of contents presents a quick overview, and several issues should give a fairly clear picture of that journal's areas of interest. In addition, some publish authors' guidelines that include their mission or purpose. Leah Curtin, a noted editor, also suggests checking the masthead for the credentials of the editors and of an editorial advisory board and peer review panel, if any. Colleagues can also give information, or at least an opinion, on the quality and reputation of the journal. It is always useful to read some of the articles; this not only gives some indication of the journal's quality, but also provides some information on its style (since most journals are edited by their editorial staff). A potential author who has a major disagreement with the style or philosophy of a journal should probably not send a manuscript there. Whether to choose a journal with a large circulation or a specialized journal that reaches the particular audience desired is another important decision. In the last few years, there have been some helpful publications that compare the various journals in which nurses may want to publish.[20,21]

However, one ethical point is overriding: a manuscript should be sent to *only one journal at a time*. If rejected, it can then go to another. Acceptance and publication by two journals (this does not refer to reprinting by

permission) is considered a serious embarrassment. For one thing, the author has then presumably given the copyright to two separate owners.

At times, authors, especially if they have no track record, may choose to approach an editor first to see whether there is any interest in a particular type of article. This procedure is called a *query*.[22] Opinion is mixed as to whether this is worthwhile, especially if the author has followed the previous steps, and is reasonably sure that the article is suitable for that journal and that a similar one has not been published within the last few years. However, should such an article be in the editor's file for future publication, it saves the author time and money to know it.

The usual procedure is as follows:

1. Write to the editor. If you know a particular editor of that journal, address it to him or her. However, check a recent journal for accuracy. Editors do not appreciate getting letters addressed to a long gone predecessor, and it does imply that you have not even looked at a current issue. Explain what you would like to write about; send an outline of major points; give brief autobiographical information to indicate that you are qualified to write on the subject; list previous writings, if any; and state whether or not you expect remuneration other than what the journal usually pays. (Only if you feel strongly about the last; nursing journals are not noted for extravagant fees, and may pay no cash fee.)

2. Wait for the editor's reply. If your idea is appealing, a letter or telephone call will follow with instructions regarding the length and sometimes the due date, and possibly with suggestions about content, development, and style.

3. In preparing the manuscript, follow the journal's guidelines. If no details are given, it is usually appropriate to type the manuscript, double-spaced, leaving 1-inch margins at the top, bottom and right-hand side and a 1½-inch margin at the left. Include

---

*Before publication, an article is properly called a *paper* or *manuscript*.

the references or bibliography and your (brief) autobiography as you would like to have it published with your article, but using that journal's style.

4. Send the article with as many copies as specified (often at least three) to the editor, via first class mail, together with pictures or other illustrations, protected with cardboards, and a covering letter. Keep a copy.

5. You should receive an acknowledgment of receipt of the manuscript and, later, a letter stating whether or not your article has been accepted for publication. How long that will be depends on how the article is reviewed—by one or more editors or a peer review panel, whether it appears to be a clear-cut winner, or whether it will require additional editorial conferences or reviews.[23] Probably three months should be allowed before inquiring about the manuscript's status. It is permissible to withdraw it if you wish. Some journals return declined manuscripts with the critiques of the reviewers and/or editors. If a revision and resubmission is requested, suggestions (or directions) for revision are made.

6. If the manuscript is accepted, the editor may or may not be able to give you a publication date, but you can ask. Much depends on the timeliness of the article, the production plans for future journal issues, and the number of articles on hand.

7. The magazine's editorial staff will edit and prepare the article for the printer. They may send the edited copy for you to check and approve, or they may send you the galley proofs after the article is set in type. Sometimes both the edited copy and proof are sent. Read the copy promptly, request only such changes as you feel are necessary for clarity and accuracy, and return it to the editor's office right away. Delay may mean that your article will not appear in the issue it was planned for and may disrupt the magazine's production schedule.

8. One or more complimentary copies of the issue in which your article is published will be mailed to you. If you wish extra copies, you will usually find the cost per copy noted on the magazine's table of contents page. If you want reprints, write at once to the magazine's business office for information regarding the policy for ordering and the price.

9. Much the same process occurs when an unsolicited manuscript is submitted. For those scholars who wish to publish their research, a similar approach is used, but depending on where and how the research is to be published (as a research paper or a narrative article), the style may vary. Again, it is wise to check with potential publishers; especially if the research is a thesis or dissertation, it is helpful to look at strategies that make the research publishable.[24]

A very brief article or lesser item, such as a letter to the editor, a news item, or a book review, also requires careful planning, organizing, and writing. It, too, must be acceptable to the editors of a publication, or it will never appear in print.

The procedure for writing a book is similar to that for a magazine article, but it is often more exacting and usually much more time-consuming.[25] There is more of everything, including satisfactions and remuneration. In addition to the manuscript for the main portion or body of the book, the author is usually responsible for writing the foreword or preface, preparing the index, and reading the galley proof. She or he must obtain written permission to use material quoted or adapted from other sources, being sure that credits are included in the book as indicated in order to avoid any embarrassment or difficulty for all concerned.

The editorial staff of a book publishing company is willing to help the author in every way possible. But only in unusual instances does the staff relieve the author of the responsibility of checking data and presenting them in proper form.

It is customary for a book publisher and an author to negotiate a contract covering the main considerations in the preparation of the manuscript, responsibilities for illustrative materials, revisions, and royalty rates. Because royalties, support or advances, and marketing vary among publishers, it is wise to "shop around" to find the one most suitable. Sometimes a lawyer or someone who has had considerable experience with publishers can be extremely helpful.[26]

Not all nurses have writing skills, but many do have ideas that are worth sharing. There are two solutions—developing those skills through practice, study, and workshops, or joining forces with someone who does write well, with one taking primary responsibility for the research or background and the other writing the article. Many research publications have multiple authors, only one of whom may do the actual writing; the others have contributed various aspects of the research. The important point is that the person who has something worthwhile to say finds a way to say it; this is a professional responsibility and a satisfying one.

REFERENCES

1. Joanne McClosky and Elizabeth Swanson, "Publishing Opportunities for Nurses: A Comparison of 100 Journals," *Image,* **14**:50–56 (June 1982).
2. Franz Ingelfinger, "Peer Review in Biomedical Publication," *Am. J. Med.,* **56**:686–692 (May 1974).
3. "A Peerless Publication," Editorial, *Nurs. Outlook,* **28**:225–226 (Apr. 1980).
4. Alfred Yankauer, "Editor's Report— Peer Review Again," *Am. J. Pub. Health,* **72**:239–240 (Mar. 1982).
5. Philip E. Day, "The International Nursing Index," *Am. J. Nurs.,* **66**:783–786 (Apr. 1966).
6. Alfred Brandon and Dorothy Hill, "Selected List of Nursing Books and Journals," *Nurs. Outlook,* **32**:92–101 (Mar.–Apr. 1984).
7. Interagency Council on Library Resources for Nursing, "Reference Sources for Nursing," *Nurs. Outlook,* **32**:273–277 (Sept.–Oct. 1984).
8. Virginia Henderson, "Awareness of Library Resources: A Characteristic of Professional Workers, an Essential in Research and Continuing Education," in *Reference Sources for Research and Continuing Education in Nursing* (Kansas City, Mo.: American Nurses' Association, 1977), p. 3.
9. Susan Taylor, "How to Search the Literature," *Am. J. Nurs.,* **74**:1457–1459 (Aug. 1974).
10. Henderson, op. cit., pp. 11–12.
11. Susan Sparks, "The National Library of Medicine's Bibliographic Databases: Tools for Nursing Research," *Image,* **16**:24–27 (Winter 1984).
12. Lucie Kelly, "Voices for Nurses," *Image,* **10**:4 (Feb. 1978).
13. Margretta Styles, "Why Publish?" *Image,* **10**:30–31 (June 1978).
14. Ibid., 31.
15. Ellen Goldensohn, "Acute, Fulminating Jargonitis," *Nurs. Outlook* **30**:541 (Nov.–Dec. 1982).
16. Jane Berger, "Writing for Publication: A Survey of Nursing Journal Editors," *J. Nurs. Admin.,* **9**:50–52 (Jan. 1979).
17. Melanie Dreher, "What Is a Book Review?" *Nurs. Outlook,* **31**:64 (Jan.–Feb. 1983).
18. Alice Robinson, "Want to Get Your Message Across? Write About It," *Imprint,* **23**:45 (Oct. 1976).
19. Arnold Relman, "Responsibilities of Authorship: Where Does the Buck Stop?" *New Eng. J. Med.,* **310**:1048–1049 (Apr. 1984).
20. McCloskey and Swanson, op. cit.
21. Steven Warner and Kathryn Schweer, *Author's Guide to Journals in Nursing and Related Fields* (New York: Haworth Press, 1982).
22. Marta Vivas, "Getting into Print," *Nurs. Outlook,* **30**:484 (Sept.–Oct. 1982).
23. Elizabeth Swanson and Joanne McCloskey, "The Manuscript Review Process of Nursing Journals," *Image,* **14**:72–75 (Oct. 1982).
24. Elizabeth Tornquist, "Strategies for Publishing Research," *Nurs. Outlook,* **31**:180–183 (May–June 1983).

25. Gail Stuart et al., "Getting a Book Published, *Nurs. Outlook,* **25**:316–318 (May 1977).

26. Suzanne Perry, "Dealing with Publishers: Suggestions from a Study of Academic Authors," *Chr. Higher Ed.,* **27**:19–22 (June 22, 1983).

TRANSITION
INTO
PRACTICE

Employment Guidelines

Graduation at last! And now what? For most nurses, "what" means it's now time to get a job. For some, the job is predetermined—commitment to the armed services, the Veterans Administration, or another agency that funded their education. Another group may have decided early on exactly the kind of nursing they prefer and the place they want to do it. If all goes well and there are no problems, such as an oversupply of nurses for that specialty or geographic area, at least one major decision is made. But for all graduates, choosing that crucial first job and preparing for it are big considerations.

There are many employment opportunities for nurses today, although the place of employment preferred may not offer the exact hours, specialty, opportunities, or assistance a new graduate might want. Pockets of unemployment most often result from budgeting factors and a tightening of the economy. Although nurses may be *needed,* sometimes seriously, some employers tend to retain those on lower salaries, although less qualified, and to eliminate patient care services. Another problem is maldistribution, with not enough nurses opting to work in ghettos or poor rural areas, although the need there is serious. Conversely,

small communities may be flooded by nursing graduates of a community college who wish to stay in that area.*

Even with these social and economic factors, new nursing opportunities are constantly emerging. And certainly there is no overabundance of nurses with graduate degrees (or baccalaureate degrees, for that matter). How, then, can you decide what is the best job for you? How do you maximize the chances of getting it?

SOME BASIC CONSIDERATIONS

Personal and Occupational Assessment

It's a good idea to start thinking about career choices while you are still in your educational program. Since most schools have rotations through the various clinical specialty areas, this gives you a chance to compare as you learn. Generally, there is also access to someone who can advise you about the pros and cons of certain types of nursing—or at

---

*See Chapter 15 for a discussion of career opportunities, along with issues and concerns about nurse employment.

least there's a more experienced nurse, often a faculty member, to talk to.

More important than anything else, though, is to take a considered look at yourself—your own qualities and what you want out of life. There are a variety of approaches to this sort of self-assessment that are interesting to explore in depth,[1,2] but there are generally certain commonalities. Some questions you might ask are:

What are my personality characteristics? Do I like to do things with people or by myself? Am I patient? Do I like to do things quickly? Am I good at details, or do I like to take the broad view? Do I like a structured and quiet environment or one that is constantly changing? Am I relatively confident in what I undertake or do I look for support? Am I easily bored? Do I like to tackle problem situations or avoid them? Do I have a sense of humor? Am I emotional? Am I a risk taker? Do I care about the way I look? Do I care what others think of me?

What are my values? Do I believe in the right to life or the right to die? Do I think everyone should have access to health care? Do I have some religious orientation? Do I think that too many people today are too rigid or too loose in their beliefs and behavior? Can I accept and work with those who have very different values? How do I feel about my responsibility to myself, my employer, my patient, the doctors, my profession, society? Do I believe strongly that my way is the right way? Am I intolerant of others' beliefs?

What are my interests? In the broad field of nursing? In certain specialties? In the health field? In my private and social life? In the community? Do I like to travel?

What are my needs? Am I ambitious? Do I like to boss? Is money important to me? Status? Do I need intellectual stimulation? Is academic success important? What about academic credentials? Am I willing to relocate? Does a city, suburb, or rural area fit

my desired life-style? Is success in my field important? Am I willing to sacrifice personal and family time for success? Do I think that my first responsibility is to my family at this point? Is part-time work an option? Do I want plenty of time for family, friends, and leisure activities? Do I see nursing as a career or a way to earn a living as long as that is necessary? Do I really like nursing? If not, why not, and what can I do about it?

What kinds of abilities do I have? In manual skills? In communication? In intellectual/cognitive skills? In analyzing? In coordinating? In organizing? In supervising? In dealing with people? Do I have a great deal of energy and stamina? Are there certain times, situations, or climate conditions in which I have less? Am I good at comforting people? Am I able to give some of myself to others?

It's good to prioritize some of these lists, since life and a job are usually a compromise. What's most important? What would make you miserable? It might also be very helpful to share this list with others. Is this the way you are seen by them? Have you missed something? If some of your friends and peers are involved in their own decision making, get together with them and/or a trusted teacher or mentor to brainstorm about the possibilities in the field now or later in order to match your own profile most accurately with nursing opportunities. When compromises are necessary, you can decide ahead of time which ones are tenable or even perfectly acceptable at that point.

Since there will probably be economic constraints in the health care system for a long time, one way to look at the job market is in terms of future growth. For instance, you may choose a hospital for a first job in order to hone your new skills, but have you considered an investor-owned hospital or, later, a long-term care facility, home care, or an ambulatory-care outreach center? All are part of a trend in health care. You should examine those job prospects as carefully as any other. They may have components that do not fit in with your own self-assessment. But don't close doors because of preconceived notions.

Licensure

Regardless of the results of your self-study, a basic and essential step in your professional nursing career is becoming licensed, since you cannot practice in any state without an RN. Information about how to apply to take the state board examination leading to licensure and other significant information is found in Chapter 20. The procedure for becoming licensed, either initially or later, may take from four to six months. State boards of nursing in most states permit nurses to practice temporarily while their application for licensure is being processed. You can usually be employed as a *graduate nurse* until you pass the licensure exam. In some places, you can continue in that status, if you fail, until you take the next scheduled examination. More frequently now, this is not done, and you are dismissed or must work as some type of nursing assistant.

What if you decide not to work right away? Stay home with your husband and children? Take a long vacation? It's probably wise to study for and take the exam anyway. Unused knowledge has a way of disappearing from the mind, and it might be much more difficult to pass the exams later, without intervening learning and practice. Should you take a nursing board review course? It depends on the confidence you have in your nursing knowledge and test-taking ability. The *good* courses can be very helpful, and may provide backup materials as well as lectures. However, be careful that you select a reputable company. Remember that these are profit-making operations, expensive to you, and always attract some borderline operators. Another way of preparing is to study with a group of peers, perhaps using board review workbooks or texts designed for that purpose.

PROFESSIONAL BIOGRAPHIES AND RÉSUMÉS

Now that you have done your self-assessment and thought about career alternatives, it's time to write your résumé. No matter how you obtain a position in nursing, you will probably be asked to submit a résumé or summary of your qualifications for the job. This might include a personal history, education and experience, character and performance references, professional credentials such as the license registration number, and a transcript of your education records.

Some universities and other educational programs still maintain a file with updated information about your career provided by you, and references that you have solicited. This has the advantage of eliminating the need to ask for repeated references from teachers who may scarcely remember you or to write again and again to a variety of places for records. However, this service is gradually fading away, and that may not be bad. As you and your career develop, a reference from your first teacher or your first staff position says little other than how you were perceived at that time. Newer references may be far more useful. Your academic record or simply evidence of your graduation may still be requested, and your school always provides that information, but today a well-prepared résumé is considered more appropriate.

A résumé is a relatively short professional or business biography. In academia, a curriculum vitae (CV), which is somewhat lengthier and contains different and more detailed information, is the appropriate form of professional biography.[3] Résumés are usually shorter than CVs.

The résumé should be businesslike, typed neatly on one side of good-quality plain white, off-white, or light gray paper measuring 8½ by 11 inches, with a good margin all around. No more than two pages are usually recommended. A word processor is useful in writing résumés because it allows you to tailor the résumé to a particular job opportunity without making a total revision. However, make sure that the word processor prepares a good-looking résumé.

There are various ways to write a résumé.[4-6] Remember that it is a marketing tool and should show you to advantage. Therefore, while you must never be dishonest,[7] the way you present your talents and credentials, especially after you have had additional work experience, may make the difference between whether you are even interviewed or ignored, especially in a competitive situation. While format is a matter of taste, a sample résumé is shown in Exhibit 30-1.

Some points can be made. The professional objective is not a must, especially if you are not sure exactly what you want to do. It should match the job for which you are applying, and thus may need to be changed accordingly. For instance, someone with a master's degree in perinatal nursing may be interested in either a teaching or a clinical specialist position. Both the objective and the emphasis in the résumé must focus on the position for which the person is applying. Needless to say, if you are applying for your first or second staff nurse position in a hospital, the decision on what to write is less complex.

All relevant work experiences should be included, with the most recent listed first. The usual format is to list the agency and date, followed by a brief description of duties performed, using "action" verbs—*developed, initiated, supervised*. Some experts suggest that if you have not had impressive positions, you should attempt to bury this fact in statements that focus on your personal qualities, such as: "Leadership—Demonstrated my ability to lead others—as night nurse on a pediatric unit at X hospital, such and such address." No one really knows whether this is more effective, but again, style is a matter of personal choice.

The education section should also begin with the most recent academic credential, and should include the major and such additions as research projects, special awards, academic honors, extracurricular activities, and offices held. Information on other honors, professional memberships and activities, and community activities might also be given in separate sections.

Under federal law, you cannot be required to include personal data such as your age, marital status, place of birth, religion, sex, race, color, national origin, or handicap. If you choose to do so, decide whether this makes you a more desirable candidate. For instance, a second language or extensive travel might be a plus in certain situations. When you are licensed as an RN, or if you later become certified in a specialty, that can be listed as well. It is usually best not to list specific references on your résumé, since this omission allows you to select the most appropriate reference for a particular position. If your school does maintain a file, you can state this, giving the correct address. When you do give the references, include the full names, titles, and business addresses of about three persons who are qualified to evaluate your professional ability, scholarship, character, and personality. Most suitable are teachers and former employers. Ask permission to use their names as references in advance. Choose carefully.[8]

LOOKING OVER THE JOB MARKET

The potentials for a particular job are assessed both before and after applying for and/or being offered a nursing position. Chapter 15 should be helpful as an overview of the opportunities available in terms of both specialties and professional development (career ladder, internships), but reading the literature, talking to practitioners in the field, and, if possible, getting exposure to the actual practice some time during your educational program will help answer some specific questions.

Today, even if an employer is actively recruiting for nurses, an application, a formal letter of interest, and often a résumé are nec-

EXHIBIT 30-1

RESUME

LESLIE B. SMITH

120 Pine Street   Home Phone (213) 456-7890
North Ridge, CA 91110   Message Phone (213) 482-6132

PROFESSIONAL
OBJECTIVE: Staff nursing in community hospital.

EXPERIENCE:
1979-1982   University Hospital Los Angeles

                Unit clerk on medical surgical units,
                evening shift. Assisted charge nurse
                in (list activities); trained new clerks;
                developed end of shift report between
                clerks.

1981   Williams General Hospital, Williams, Maine
(Summer)
                Nurses aide on medical surgical units.
                Responsible for care of thirty patients
                under direction of RNs including (list
                major activities.)

EDUCATION:
1983-1985   Blank University School of Nursing

                Bachelor of Science (to be awarded May, 1985)

1981-1983   Blank Community College

                Associate in Science (1983)

HONORS: 1984-1985

                Dean's List
                Member, Sigma Theta Tau, National Honor
                Society for Nursing

1983-1984   Honor Scholarship

1983   Outstanding Student Leader Award, Blank
                Community College

PROFESSIONAL
ACTIVITIES:
1983-1985   Member, National Student Nurses' Association

1985   Chair, Program Committee
March 1985   Presented paper "When Students Teach Patients."
1984   Chair, Program Committee at University
1984   Attended ANA convention
1982   Debate: "Be It Resolved: Everyone Has a Right
                       to Health Care." NSNA convention,
                       Los Angeles
COMMUNITY
ACTIVITIES:
1984-1985   Volunteer for public television telethon
1983-1985   Volunteer for March of Dimes
1981-1983   Candy-striper at Blank Hospital, Blank Town

                References will be provided upon request

essary before a position is actually offered. Although there are those who feel that going through the entire process is worthwhile for the experience alone, unless you have at least some interest, it is rather unfair to take an employer's time to review an application and go through an interview for nothing. Therefore, after self-assessment, it is useful to do at least a potential job assessment in advance. The first logical consideration is a place with which you have already had experience.

Hospitals or other agencies affiliated with schools of nursing may offer new graduates staff positions. That has several advantages for the employer and usually for the student as well. Nurses who are familiar with the personnel, procedures, and physical facilities may require a shorter orientation period, which saves time and money. There are also benefits for new graduates. During these first months after graduation, you can gain valuable experience in familiar surroundings. There are opportunities to develop leadership and teaching skills and to practice clinical skills under less pressure because the people, places, and routines will not be totally unknown. The potential trauma of relocating and readjusting your personal life is not combined with the tension of being both a new, untried graduate and a new employee. And it may be a wonderful place to work.

However, if the experiences offered do not help you to develop, if the milieu is one that eventually makes you resistant, resentful, indifferent, unhappy, or disinterested, the tone may be set for a lifetime of nursing jobs, not a professional career. Of course that can also happen in other places, but if you're alert, you can often get a pretty good notion of how it would be to work at the agencies in which you have had student or work experience. This evaluation can be a little more difficult if you don't know a place at all, but the opinion of someone you respect, word-of-mouth information, the institution's newsletter, brochures, and even the way someone replies to

your inquiry provides indirect as well as direct information.

On a more concrete level, you can give some thought to what you are willing to accept in terms of salary, shifts, benefits, and travel time. (Don't underestimate the value of the fringe benefits, which may not be taxable.) Balancing these with other advantages and disadvantages as determined by your self-assessment is important. And realistically, if the job market is tight, your choices may be fewer than they would be in times of nursing shortage.

All of these factors must be considered seriously. You'll never have another first job in nursing, a job that could set the tone of your professional future. At best, you'll have wasted time. It's much better to move carefully and make sure that your choice is the best possible one for moving you toward your goal whatever it may be.

SOURCES OF INFORMATION ABOUT POSITIONS

Three principal sources of information are available to nurses who are looking for a position: (1) personal contacts and inquiries; (2) advertisements and recruiters; and (3) commercial placement agencies.

Personal Contacts and Inquiries

The nursing service director or someone on the nursing staff of a student-affiliated agency, instructors, other nurses, friends, neighbors, and family may suggest available positions in health agencies or make other job suggestions. Hospitals not affiliated with schools of nursing sometimes ask the heads of nursing schools to refer graduates to them for possible placement on their staff. Often, letters or announcements of such positions are posted on the school bulletin board or are available in a file. Your own inquiries are likely to be equally productive in turning up the right position.

Never underestimate the value of personal contacts. People seldom suggest a position unless they know something about it. That gives you the opportunity to ask questions early on, and the information can help you decide as well as prepare you better for the interview. Moreover, if your contact knows the employer and is willing (better yet, pleased) to recommend you, your chances of getting the position are immediately improved. (This kind of networking, discussed more fully in Chapter 31, will be useful throughout your career.) One business executive has said, "Eighty percent of all jobs are filled through a grapevine . . . a system of referrals that never see the light of day." When equally qualified people compete for the same position, the network recommendation could make the crucial difference. Asking for job-seeking help is neither pushy nor presumptuous, but you should be prepared to discuss your interests intelligently. A résumé will help too. Most people like to be asked for advice and want to be helpful, but they have to be asked. On the other hand, you need to use some common sense in deciding how much and how often you ask for help from whom.

Advertisements

Local newspapers and official organs of district and state nurses' associations often carry advertisements of positions for professional nurses. National nursing magazines list positions in all categories of employment, usually classified into the various geographic areas of the country. National medical, public health, and hospital magazines also carry advertisements for nurses, but they usually are for head nurse positions or higher, or for special personnel such as nurse anesthetists or nurse consultants.

All publications carry classified advertisements for information only, and, of course, as a source of revenue. Rarely, if ever, does the publisher assume responsibility for the information in the advertisement beyond its conformity to such legal requirements as may apply. If you accept an advertised position that does not turn out to be what was expected, you cannot hold the publication responsible. Read the advertisement very carefully. Is the hospital or health agency well known and of good reputation? Is the information clear and inclusive? Does it sound effusive and overstress the advantages and delights of joining the staff? What can be read between the lines? How much more information is needed before deciding whether the job is suitable? Some of these questions can be resolved through correspondence or telephone contact or your network.

At some time, you may want to place an advertisement in the "Positions Wanted" column of a professional publication. In that event, obtain a copy of the magazine and read the directions for submitting a classified advertisement. They will be very explicit, and should be followed to the letter; otherwise publication of the advertisement may be delayed. The editor will arrange the information to conform to the publication's style, but will not change the material sent unless asked to. Therefore, all the information needed to attract a prospective employer within the limits of professional ethics should be included clearly and concisely.

Career directories published periodically by some nursing journals or other commercial sources are free to job seekers. They have relatively extensive advertisements with much more detailed information than appears in the usual ad. The other advantage is instant comparison and geographic separation, with pre-printed, prepaid postcards that can be sent to the health agency of interest. (Most are geared to hospital recruitment.) Directories are frequently available in the exhibit section of student and other nursing conventions. Some carry reprints of articles on careers, licensure, job seeking, and other pertinent information. Some journals also do periodic surveys on job salaries and fringe benefits that can be useful when considering various geographic areas.

Recruiters for hospitals and other agencies

are usually present at representative booths in the exhibit areas of conventions; some also have suites where they have an open house. Recruiters, who may or may not be nurses, also visit nursing schools or arrange for space in a hotel for preliminary interviews. Notices may be placed in newspapers or sent to schools. There are advantages to the personalized recruiter approach because your questions can be answered directly, and you can get "a feel" for the employer's attitude, especially if nurses accompany the recruiter. However, remember that recruiters are selected for their recruiting ability.

Commercial Placement Agencies

At one time, registries for private duty nurses were part of the services offered by state or local nurses' associations. These registries had a list of nurses available for private duty and sent them to hospitals or homes at the request of patients. This situation is almost nonexistent now, but there are still some commercial agencies for that purpose. Some also maintain a list of nurses who are looking for part-time work or who are job hunting. As might be expected, some are reliable and some are not. They can be checked out with the Better Business Bureau and your network. Almost always a fee must be paid to the registry, sometimes based on a percentage of the nurse's earnings. At another level of job seeking—executive positions—well-known agencies of good reputation (headhunters) are used by both employers and potential employees to match the best possible person to a suitable position.

Under ordinary circumstances, however, the so-called temporary nurse service is another option (see Chapter 15). These services function quite differently from agencies or registries, since they themselves employ the nurses and then, according to requests and a nurse's choices, send her or him to an institution or other agency for a specific period of time. Nurses are usually placed in short-term situations in hospitals, but some services advertise home care. The single most important factor that seems to attract nurses to temporary nurse services is control over working conditions, including the time, place, type of assignment, and so on. New graduates may find this type of employment attractive as a temporary measure, since the nonavailability of fringe benefits may not be important to them. There is also an opportunity to try out different types of nursing, but for the new nurse, the lack of individual support and supervision is a disadvantage.

PROFESSIONAL CORRESPONDENCE

New nursing graduates today have a wider variety of personal and educational backgrounds than they did a few years ago. Many have held responsible positions in other fields, and even more have worked part- or full-time before or during their educational programs.

Therefore, the suggested procedures for application and resignation presented are just that. They review generally accepted ways to handle certain inevitable professional matters in a sophisticated and businesslike way, and may serve as a refresher for those already familiar with these or other equally acceptable ways of relating and communicating in professional business relationships. For the younger, less experienced nurse, this material provides a convenient reference and guide.

The first contact with a prospective employer is usually made by letter, followed by a personal interview, telephone conversation, and, occasionally, telegrams or mailgrams. Every business letter makes an impression on its reader, an impression that may be favorable, unfavorable, or indifferent. To achieve the best effect, the stationery on which it is written should be in good taste; the message accurate and complete, yet concise; the tone appropriate; and the form, grammar, and spelling correct.

Stationery and Format

Business letters should be neatly and legibly typed or handwritten in black or blue ink on unlined white stationery. Single sheets no smaller than 7 by 9 inches or larger than 8½ by 11 inches are more suitable than folded sheets. Personal stationery is acceptable if it is of the right size; white, light gray, or off-white; and used with unlined envelopes. Notebook paper should never be used for business correspondence; neither should someone else's personal stationery or the stationery of a hospital, hotel, or place of business. Good-quality typing paper is always in good taste if a suitable envelope is used with it.

If you type the letter, which is often considered most desirable, use a fresh black typewriter ribbon and avoid erasures or carelessness in the general appearance of the letter. Use of a word processor is becoming more common. There is mixed feedback on its acceptance in formal correspondence, in part because of the variability in appearance. If it looks good, it's worth considering; it can certainly save a lot of time.

An attractive handwritten letter may have certain advantages over a typed one. For example, it can show your ability to prepare neat and legible records and reports, and can indicate precision and careful attention to details. A nicely handprinted letter may also make a good impression, perhaps because so few individuals have the patience and skill to do it. However, regardless of what you do, keep a copy for future reference.

Books on English composition and secretary's handbooks include correct forms for writing business letters. Two or more variations may be given; the choice is yours.

The block form is employed most widely in business correspondence, and therefore is selected for illustration here (Exhibit 30-2). The left-hand words or margins are aligned throughout the letter, with extra space between paragrphs. Commas are used sparingly in this form, and a colon is used following the salutation. No abbreviations are used. If personal stationery on which the name and address are engraved or printed is used, this information should be omitted from the heading of the letter and only the date given.

In doing business correspondence, it is always advisable to address a person exactly as the name appears on her or his own letters. The full title and position should be used, no matter how long they may be. It is better to place the lengthy name of a position on the line below the addressee's name, and break up a long address, in the interest of a neat appearance, remembering to indent continuation lines as follows:

Miss Selma T. Henderson, RN
Director, School of Nursing and Inservice
  Education Program for Nurses
The Reddington J. Mason Memorial Hospital
  School of Nursing
1763 Avenue of the Nineteenth Century
Chesapeake-on-Hudson, Ohio 00000

If the name of the person to whom you are writing to inquire about a position is not known, the letter may be addressed to the director or supervisor of the appropriate division, for example, "Director of the Department of Nursing." The salutation could then be "Dear Director." (Using "Dear Sir" or "Dear Madam" may be incorrect, since you don't know whether the recipient is male or female.) The inside address and the envelope address should be identical. People are sensitive about their names and titles; be accurate.

It is correct to give a title before the name in an address in the heading and on the envelope—not in the form of initials after the name—for example, "Dr. Constance E. Wright" rather than "Constance E. Wright, EdD." In a signature, however, it is preferable to reverse this order and place the degree initials after the name of the signer of the letter. Never use both the title and the initials in an address; "Dr. Constance E. Wright, EdD" is incorrect.

It is quite suitable, and even desirable, for a (licensed) nurse to use "RN" after his or her name, particularly in professional correspondence. Many nurses with doctorates sign their names with "RN, PhD," or "RN, EdD," added to clarify that they are nurses as well as

EXHIBIT 30-2

```
                              COVER LETTER


        Applicant's address
        Applicant's phone number
        Date of letter

        Employer's name and title        (Use complete title and address)
        Employer's address

        Salutation:                      (If you know name, use it rather
                                            than "Dear Sir/Madam")


        Opening paragraph:  State why you are writing.  Name the position or

        type of work for which you are applying.  Mention how you learned of

        the opening.  If appropriate, state your academic preparation and how

        it relates to the job description.

        Middle paragraph:  Explain your interest in working for this employer

        and specific reason for desiring this type of work.  Describe relevant

        work experience and be sure to point out any other job skills or

        abilities that relate to the position for which you are applying.  The

        reader will view the letter of application as an example of your writ-

        ing skills.  Strive for originality.  Be brief but specific.  Your

        resume contains details.  Do not reiterate the entire resume.

        Closing paragraph:  Have an appropriate closing to pave the way for an

        interview and indicate dates and times of availability.

        Sincerely,

        Signature

        Name typed

        Enc.                             (If a resume or other enclosure
                                            is used note in letter)
```

Source: Mary C. Parker, "How to Write Your Resumé," Am. J. Nurs. **79**:1741 (Oct. 1979).

holders of a doctorate. They should be addressed as "Dear Dr. Whatever":

A professional or business woman usually does not use her husband's name at all in connection with her work. However, she can use the title "Mrs." to identify herself as a person who is, or has been, married if she desires. "Mrs." goes in parentheses before her typed name.

Content and Tone

The information included in a business letter should be presented with great care, giving all pertinent data but avoiding unnecessary details and divulging nothing that would be better withheld, at least until a later date. It is often helpful to outline, draft, and edit a business letter, just as you would a term paper. This requires you to think it through from beginning to end in order to ensure completeness and accuracy. It is also helpful to tailor it to fit a well-spaced single page, if possible, or two at the most.

Your writing style is your own, and how you word your message may be part of what you are judged on. The tone of a business letter has considerable influence on the impression it makes and the attention it receives. It is probably better to lean toward formality rather than informality. Friendliness without undue familiarity, cordiality without overenthusiasm, sincerity, frankness, and obvious respect for the person to whom the letter is addressed set the most appropriate tone for correspondence about a position in nursing. Although there are those who suggest very unusual dramatic, or "different" formats, the reality is that they may backfire.

If you feel that you need more information before seriously considering a position (for instance, whether tuition reimbursement is a benefit or a particular specialty area has an opening), you can indicate your interest in a separate letter, simply asking for the information, or ask directly within the same application letter. The kind of response you get in terms of courtesy, promptness, and general

tone will tell you a lot about the prospective employer.

If you decide not to apply for the position after all, or not to follow through with an interview, it is courteous to inform the person with whom you have corresponded. Specific reasons need be given (briefly) only if such a decision is made after first accepting the position. This is not only courteous, but advisable, because you may wish to join that staff at another time or may have other contacts with the nurse administrator.

Applications

Applications are not just routine red tape. Whether or not a résumé is requested or submitted, the formal application, which is developed to give the employing agency the information it wants, can be critical in determining who is finally hired. Even if the information repeats information offered in the résumé, it should be entered. It is usually acceptable to attach the résumé or a separate sheet if there is not adequate space to give complete information. It's a good idea to read through the application first so that the information is put in the correct place. Neatness is essential. Erasures, misspellings, and wrinkled forms leave a poor impression. Abbreviations, except for state names and dates, should not be used as a rule.

If the form must be completed away from home, think ahead and bring anticipated data—Social Security and registration numbers, places, dates, and names. Although occupational counselors say that it is not necessary to give all the information requested (such as arrests, health, or race, some of which are illegal to request),* it is probably not wise to leave big gaps in your work history without explanation.

Personal Interview

An interview may be the deciding factor in getting a job. Anyone who has an appoint-

*See Chapter 19 regarding federal legislation on employment rights.

ment for a personal interview should be prepared for it physically, mentally, emotionally, and psychologically. The degree of preparation will depend on the purpose of the interview and what has preceded it. Assuming that you have written to a prospective employer about a position and an interview has been arranged, preparation might include the following:

Physical Preparation. Be rested, alert, and in good health. Dress suitably for the job, but wear something in which you feel at ease. It is important to be well groomed and as attractive as possible. First appearances are important, and given a choice, no one selects a sloppy or overdressed person in preference to someone who is neat and appropriately dressed. Have enough money with you to meet all anticipated expenses. If you are to be reimbursed by the employing agency, keep an itemized record of expenses for submission later. Arrive at your destination well ahead of time, but do not go to your prospective employer's office earlier than five minutes before the designated time.

Mental Preparation. Review all information and previous communications about the position. Showing that you know about the hospital or agency is desirable and impressive. Make certain that you know the exact name or names of persons whom you expect to meet and can pronounce them properly. Decide what additional information you want to obtain during the interview. Consider how you will phrase your leading questions. Carry a small notebook or card on which you have listed the names of references and other data that you may need during the interview. If you bring an application form with you, place it in a fresh envelope which you leave unsealed, and have it ready to hand to the interviewer when she or he asks for it, if it seems indicated; offer it at the appropriate time.

Emotional and Psychological Preparation. If you have any worries or fears in connection with the interview, try to overcome them by thinking calmly and objectively about what is likely to take place. (Role playing an interview with a colleague who may have been through the experience can be helpful.) Be ready to adjust to whatever situation may develop during the interview. For example, you may expect to have an extended conversation with the director of nurses and find when you arrive that a personnel officer who is not a nurse will interview you. She or he may interview you in a very few minutes and in what seems to be an impersonal way. Or you may have visualized the job setting as quite different.

Accept things as you find them, reserving the privilege of making a decision after thoughtful consideration of the total job situation. If a stimulating challenge is inherent in the position, you will sense it during the interview, or you may have reason to believe that it will develop after you assume your duties. However, you cannot demand a challenge, and if one is "created" for you spontaneously by the interviewer, take the promise with the proverbial grain of salt, knowing that an employment situation rarely adjusts to the new employee.

During the Interview

Usually, the interviewer will take the initiative in starting the conference and closing it. You should follow that lead courteously and attentively. Shake hands. Be prepared to give a brief overview of your experiences and interests, if asked. At some point, you will be asked if you have any questions, and you should be prepared to ask for additional information if you would like to have it. Should the interviewer appear to be about to close the conference without giving you this opportunity, say, "May I ask a question, please?" It is perfectly acceptable to ask, before the interview is over, about salary, fringe benefits, and other conditions of employment, if a contract or explanatory paper has not been given to you. In fact, it would be foolish to appear indifferent. A contract is desirable (see Chapter

22), but if that is not the accepted procedure, it is important to understand what is involved in the job. The job description should be accessible in writing, and it is best that you have a copy.

Most interviewers agree that an outgoing candidate who volunteers appropriate information is likeable. On the other hand, many use the technique of selective silence, which is anxiety provoking to most people, to see what the interviewee will say or do. A good interviewer will try to make you comfortable, in part to relax you into self-revelation; most do not favor aggressive methods. Good eye contact is fine, but don't stare. Be sensitive to the interviewer's being disinterested in a certain response; maybe it's too lengthy. Don't interrupt. Don't smoke.

When the interview is completed, thank the interviewer, shake hands, and leave promptly. You may or may not have been offered the position, or you may not have accepted it if it was offered. If it was offered to you, it is usually well to delay your decision for at least a day or two until you have had time to think the matter over carefully from every practical point of view. Perhaps you will want more information, in which case you may write a letter, send a telegram or mailgram, or make a phone call to your prospective employer. It is always courteous and sometimes acts as a reminder to send a thank-you letter.

Telephone Conversations, Mailgrams, and Telegrams

Sometimes during the procedure of acquiring a position, you may have occasion to discuss some aspect of it over the telephone with the prospective employer. If you make the call, be brief, courteous, and to the point, with notes handy, if needed. It may be helpful to make notations on the conversation. It is sensible to listen carefully and not interrupt. If you receive a call and are unprepared for it, be courteous but cautious and, perhaps, ask for time to think over the proposal—or whatever may have been the purpose of the call.

Agreements about a position made over the phone should be confirmed promptly in writing. If it is your place to do so, you might say, while speaking with the person, "I'll send you a confirming letter tomorrow." If it is the responsibility of the other party to confirm an agreement but she or he does not mention it, ask, "May I have a letter of confirmation, please?"

After any interview or conversation, it is useful to make notes about what happened for future use and reference. If any business arrangements are made by mailgram or telegram, file this information with other related correspondence.

For positions sought through a registry or employment agency, the same courteous, thorough, and businesslike procedures used when dealing directly with a prospective employer are appropriate. A brief thank-you note for help received shows consideration of the agency's efforts in your behalf.

Evaluation

What if you didn't get the job you wanted? There may simply have been someone better suited or better qualified. Still, it is helpful to review the experience in order to refine your interview skills. Were you prepared? Did you present yourself as someone sensitive to the employer's goals? Did you articulate your personal strengths and objectives? Did you look your best? Sometimes discussing what happened with another person also gives you a different perspective. And there's no reason why you cannot reapply another time.[9]

CHANGING POSITIONS

There seems to be an unwritten rule that nurses should remain in any permanent position they accept for at least a year. Certainly, this is not too long—except in the most unusual circumstances—for you to adjust to the employment situation and find a place on the staff in which to use your ability and talents to their fullest. Furthermore, persons who change jobs frequently in any profession or occupation soon gain a reputation for being "flitters," and some employers are reluctant to hire them. However, should it be desirable or necessary to change positions, a number of points might be observed. Consider your employer and co-workers as well as yourself, and leave under amicable and constructive circumstances. Try to finish any major projects you have started, such as the revision of written directives; arrange in good order the books, equipment, and materials your successor will inherit; and prepare memos and helpful guides to assist the nurse who will assume your duties. Tell your immediate superiors about aspects of your work that may be helpful to them. If requested by the administration, help select the person who will succeed you, being extremely careful to be objective. If this is impossible because of personal considerations, ask to be excused from this obligation.

Terminal interviews are considered good administrative practice, and are sometimes used for a final performance evaluation and/or a means to determine the reasons for resignation. There is some question of how open employees are about discussing their resignation (unless the reason is illness, necessary relocation, and so on), perhaps because of fear of reprisal in references or even a simple desire to avoid unpleasantness. This is a decision you must make in each situation.

If you plan to continue to work, be reasonably sure that you have a new position before resigning from the current one. Depending on the reasons for leaving and how eager you are to make a change, some writers suggest that before you definitely accept a new position, the present employer should be informed about your desire to leave and why. It may be that, depending on the employer's concept of your value to the institution, a new, more desirable position might be offered.

It is important to give reasonable notice of your intention to resign. If there is a contract, the length of the notice will probably be stipulated. Two weeks to a month is the usual period, depending principally upon the position held and the anticipated difficulty in hiring a replacement.

A letter of resignation is always indicated when leaving a position, unless you are asked to leave or dismissed. In that case, it is vital to know why. If a problem situation has existed and you are at fault, this should be known, with some understanding about avoiding similar situations. If you are not at fault, a full effort should be made to remedy the situation, particularly in light of probably unfair negative references. If the situation is serious and you are a member of an SNA, you may wish to seek the help of the state organization's economic security division. If the dismissal is a lay-off for economic reasons, it is wise to have a letter to this effect, both in terms of professional security and in order to obtain unemployment benefits, if necessary (see Chapter 19).

A letter of resignation should state simply and briefly, but in a professional manner, your intention of leaving, the date on which the resignation will become effective, and the reasons for making the change. A sincere comment or two about the satisfactions experienced in the position and regrets at leaving will close the letter graciously. There should be no hint of animosity or harbored resentment, because this will serve no constructive purpose and may boomerang.

One nurse author commented appropriately:

> When the nurse leaves a position, she does not burn her bridges or close a chapter. The reputation she made will go with her. Her old employer will be asked many times for comments on her performance, on her professional and social conduct, on her character and integrity. Her contribution in the nursing group and in the community will be scrutinized and evaluated and her readiness and ability to take over a new appointment will be judged largely in terms of what she did in the old one. Did she leave in a huff? Was she difficult to get along with? Or did she fill a difficult spot capably and is she missed? No

greater compliment can be paid a person than to say that the agency concerned not only regrets her leaving, but would be glad of an opportunity to reemploy her.[10]

REFERENCES

1. Mary Reres, "Assessing Growth Potential," *Am. J. Nurs.*, **74**:670–676 (Apr. 1974).
2. Joseph Price and Gretchen Randolph, "Career Trajectory in Nursing: The Randice Approach," *Nursing Success Today,* **1**:21–25 (Mar.–Apr. 1984).
3. Joan Newcomb and Patricia Murphy, "The Curriculum Vitae—What It Is and What It Is Not," *Nurs. Outlook,* **27**:580–583 (Sept. 1979).
4. Mary Parker, "How to Write Your Résumé," *Am. J. Nurs.*, **79**:1739–1741 (Oct. 1979).
5. Marilyn Edmunds, "Developing a Marketing Portfolio," *Nurse Practitioner*, **5**:41–46 (May–June 1980).
6. Rosemary Esler, "Getting a New Job," *Am. J. Nurs.*, **81**:758–760 (Apr. 1981).
7. Lucie Kelly, "The Pinocchio Principle," *Nurs. Outlook*, **32**:307 (Nov.–Dec. 1984).
8. Betty Cuthbert, "Please List Three Names," *Am. J. Nurs.*, **77**:1596–1599 (Oct. 1977).
9. Tanya Hanger, "How to Market Yourself," *Am. J. Nurs. Guide*, 18–23 (1984).
10. Frances M. McKenna, *Thresholds to Professional Nursing Practice*, 2nd ed. (Philadelphia: W. B. Saunders Company, 1960), p. 78.

The Challenge of Professionalism

SOCIALIZATION AND RESOCIALIZATION

The transition from student to RN is a psychological, sociological, and legal phenomenon. The student has spent two to four years being socialized into nursing in the education setting; now resocialization into the work world is necessary. Socialization into a new role is not usually a conscious process, although both the individual being socialized and those doing the socializing consciously make certain efforts. Hinshaw describes socialization as a sequential set of phases, a "chain of events." In an adaptation from Simpson,[1] she identifies the phases as:

1. Transition from anticipatory expectation of role to specific expectations of role as defined by the societal group.
2. Attachment to significant others in the social system milieu; labeling incongruencies in role expectations.
3. Internalization, adaptation, or integration of role values and standards.[2]

A further delineation of this process and the resocialization is described by Hinshaw,[3] us-

ing Davis' classical description of the doctrinal conversion process among student nurses.

Stage One. Initial innocence: students enter the profession with an image of what they expect to become and how they should behave, often based on public stereotypes. Most have had some degree of a "serving humanity" mentality, with emphasis on touching and doing. In the educational system, they are praised for presenting an analysis of the action more than the action itself.

Stage Two. Recognition of incongruity: students sharing their concern can begin to recognize what is different from their expectations.

Stages Three and Four. "Psyching out" and role simulation: those individuals who want to continue in nursing must identify appropriate behaviors and role model them. Soon those behaviors become part of those persons' own repertoire of how to act.

Stages Five and Six. Provisional and stable internalization. First, nurses vacillate between behaviors now attached to the new professional imagery and those reflecting previous lay imagery. But as they become more comfortable in practicing those behaviors and have increasing identification with nurse-teacher role models, they move to stage six, in which the imagery and behavior of the newly socialized nurse-student reflect the professionally, educationally approved model.

However, for all but a few new graduates, the first job is as an employee in some bureaucratic setting, the antithesis of professionalism. A comparison of characteristics of a profession and a bureaucracy clearly shows the differences.

Characteristics of a Bureaucracy

Specialized of roles and tasks.

Autonomous rational rules.

Overall orientation to rational, efficient implementation of specific goals.

Organization of positions into a hierarchical authority structure.

The impersonal orientation of contacts between officials and clients.

Characteristics of a Profession

Specialized competence having an intellectual component.

Extensive autonomy in exercising this special competence.

Strong commitment to a career based on a special competence.

Influence and responsibility in the use of special competence.

Development of training facilities that are controlled by the professional group.

Decision making governed by internalized standards.[4]

Kramer, in an extensive longitudinal study, has identified the problems of new graduates in resolving their role in a bureaucratic-professional conflict and has termed it *reality shock,* "the specific shocklike reactions of new workers when they find themselves in a work situation for which they have spent several years preparing and for which they thought they were going to be prepared, and then suddenly find that they are not."[5] The phenomenon is seen as different from, but related to, both culture shock and future shock.[6]

Thus, when the new nurse, who has been in the work setting, but not of it, embarks on what is thought to be the first professional work experience, there is not an easy adaptation of previously learned attitudes and behaviors, but the necessity for an entirely new socialization. Kramer has categorized and described these as follows:

1. Skills and routine mastery: The expectations are those of the employment setting. A major value is competent, efficient delivery of procedures and techniques to clients, not necessarily including psychological support. The new graduate immediately concentrates on skill and routine mastery.

2. Social integration: getting along with the group; being taught by them how to work and behave; the "backstage" reality behaviors. If the individual stays at stage one, she/he may not be perceived as a competent peer; if she/he tries to incorporate some of the professional concepts brought over from the educational setting and adheres to those values, the group may be alienated.

3. Moral outrage: With the incongruencies identified and labeled, new graduates feel angry and betrayed by both their teachers and their employers. They weren't told how it would be and they aren't allowed to practice as they were taught.

4. Conflict resolution: The graduates may and do change their behavior, but maintain their values; change both values and behaviors to match the work setting; change neither values nor behavior; or work out a relationship that allows them to keep their values, but begin to integrate them into the new setting.[7]

The individuals who make the first choice have selected what is called *behavioral capitulation.* They may be the group with potential for making change, but they simply slide into the bureaucratic mold, or more likely they withdraw from nursing practice altogether. Those who choose bureaucracy (*value capitulation*), may either become "rutters," with an "it's a job" attitude, or they may eventually reject the values of both. Others become organization men and women, who move rapidly into the administrative ranks and totally absorb the bureaucratic values. Those who will change neither values nor behavior, what might be called "going it alone," either seek to practice where professional values are accepted or try the "academic lateral arabesque" (also used by the first group), going on to advanced education with the hope of new horizons or escape. The most desirable choice, says Kramer, is *biculturalism*.

> In this approach the nurse has learned that she possesses a value orientation that is perhaps different from the dominant one in the work organization, but that she has the responsibility to listen to and seek out the ideas of others as resource material in effecting a viable integration of both value systems. She has learned that she is not just a target of influence and pressure from others, but that she is in a reciprocal relationship with others and has the right and responsibility to attempt to influence them and to direct their influence attempts on her. She has learned a basic posture of interdependence with respect to the conflicting value systems.[8]

THE REALITY OF REALITY SHOCK

Kramer, both in her book and in other articles, has documented that new graduates do indeed go through variations of the socialization process described.[9-12] One graduate linked the reality shock to physiological shock and drew up a list of "treatments," such as keeping communications open, arresting feelings of inadequacy, getting information and feedback, and watching for openings to inject your own ideas.[13] Others have cited the trauma of adjustment, the insecurities, the tensions with co-workers, the doctor–nurse games.[14-17]

That there has really been little change in the adjustment process for decades can be seen by reviewing journals in the interim and by the nomadic patterns of nursing that must reflect deep-seated job dissatisfaction. Until recently; some nurse turnover has been as high as 200 percent; it is said that 70 percent is not unusual, a higher rate than that of waitresses. Turnover and absenteeism are signs of boredom, lack of involvement, and apathy. New graduates are responsible for a larger part of these statistics, but it may be even more shocking to know that an unusually large percentage leave nursing altogether. Kramer reports that 29 percent of the baccalaureate graduates she studied left nursing within two years. This figure has improved, but even if new graduates stay in nursing, their disillusionment, if unchecked, does not bode well for the profession.

> "I think, in general, most of the nurses in the hospital are not really very happy as nurses; I think it's just more or less a job that they come to every day. They just don't seem to care. . . . "

> "A nurse I was talking with one night said 'Don't stay in hospitals. Get out as fast as you can because you're going to become bitter.' I can see her point; you do relax; you lower your standards a little bit when you get busy."

> "If I stay in the hospital much longer, I'll get into the same rut as the other nurses. You can't help yourself. I hope that I won't get like the rest of them, but I'm afraid I might."[18]

These statements, made by some of Kramer's subjects, were echoed by other new graduates more than ten years later.[19]

APPROACHES TO RESOLVING REALITY SHOCK

Kramer has suggested an anticipatory socialization program as one solution to reality shock. In brief, the intent is first to guide the student toward biculturalism while still in school through lectures, exposure to reality situations, discussion, and constant reinforcement and support in meeting and resolving reality shock issues.[20] A second aspect is to develop a postgraduate socialization process on the job as part of the orientation.[21] These approaches have been shown to work well.[22,23] The new graduates overwhelmingly agreed that they had been helped to adjust.

Others, recognizing that some of the problems are related to the new graduate's need to hone skills, have developed innovative orientation programs, internships or internship-type experiences planned cooperatively by the school and the service agency.*[24] One hospital created a nurses' ombudsman.[25]

There is some evidence that awareness of the stresses of transition may have improved the situation for new graduates. One study showed that new graduates working in two university-affiliated hospitals had a higher job satisfaction score than experienced nurses who had worked in at least one other hospital. The latter had a much higher resignation rate. Of the new graduates, more diploma nurses resigned than BSNs.[26] Clearly, even beyond those early years, nurses find problems of professionalism-bureaucracy that must be met.

BURNOUT AND OTHER OCCUPATIONAL HAZARDS

Burnout, considered by some as an occupational hazard for those in service occupations, has been described as a debilitating psychological condition resulting from work-related frustrations. Maslack and her colleagues who studied the dynamics of burnout list some of the symptoms and effects: lack of motivation, cynicism, negativism, an overwhelming sense of hurt, rejection, failure, and severe loss of self-esteem.[27] Among the early symptoms is emotional and physical exhaustion—not feeling good, not sleeping well, reluctance to go to

work, and being prone to all kinds of minor illnesses. Then the burned-out professional becomes negative and just wants to be left alone.[28] A final phase, terminal burnout, would be total disgust with everyone and everything.

Burnout is caused by various situations. Sometimes it happens because of the emotionally charged, stressful environment found in clinical units where death and pain are constant companions, added to understaffing and interpersonal staff tensions. It has also been found that when there are personal or home problems, the situation is aggravated. Maslack suggests that prevention or cure starts with simply "being good to yourself," taking time for yourself and a break when necessary, and taking care of physical problems. A "decompression routine" is also helpful—perhaps some physical activity such as swimming, walking, jogging (not competitive sports), or even doing "meditative kinds of things." Sharing feelings and problems with others is also important. Sometimes a change of job is necessary, but lateral job transfers or a period in another type of unit often provide the necessary change.[29]

Others suggest different approaches. Magill recommends adopting a concept from the electrical industry, where products are vigorously tested under simulated conditions that approximate reality to prevent later burnout. "Burnin can be defined as helping future nurses develop coping skills and assisting them to become effective change agents."[30] In a small study on those she called the "brightly burning," she found that they had a good self/professional image, were risk takers, had self-direction, had hopeful attitudes, had networks and support systems, were able to use stress for growth, and were able to decompress at home and at work.

This profile was almost the direct opposite of that of a burned-out nurse with thirty years' experience. The observer said that that nurse put burnout in words, with her sureness that nothing would change. Says Storlie, "Burnout is resignation to a lack of power,

---

*Chapters 12 and 15.

the perception that no matter what you do or how hard you try, you cannot make a difference in the situation."[31] To prevent this negative attitude, she also makes useful suggestions and includes the need for inner strength and determination.

An interesting approach recognizes the importance of that inner determination and suggests an analysis of your own feelings:

What can I do to help myself?
Who will support me?
Whom can I support?
What is the potential outcome?
How will I benefit or be affected?
How much of myself and my time am I willing to give?

The author notes, "The term, 'burnout' is a label for feelings. It is something all of us could use as an excuse for giving up control of our lives—or just plain copping out. It's the only life you'll ever have. Why not take charge, instead?"[32]

Stress

In the 1980s, stress appears to be the universal condition. The director of the American Institute of Stress noted that where stress might once have taken the form of an occasional calamity, it is now a "chronic, relentless, psychosocial condition."[33] A number of psychologists have listed stresses and developed scales[34] so that people can determine if they are likely to be stressed and can prepare. Dr. Hans Selye, the father of stress research, calls stress the nonspecific response of the body to demands made on it.[35] Some forty years ago, he mapped the hormonal pathways that occur in response to stress.[36] Stress can have both a positive and a negative side. In a positive sense, it can be, and often is, a great motivator. However, when the energy released by the stress response is turned inward, the result is negative. "The body turns on itself, so to speak, and in doing so, may cause serious physical or emotional disturbances."[37] Physiological indications of stress include anorexia, uncontrolled eating, urinary fre-

quency, insomnia, lethargy, muscular tension and aches, rashes, diarrhea, headaches, tachycardia, palpitations, tightness in the chest, increased blood pressure, blushing, twitching or trembling, nausea, increased perspiration, and hyperactivity. Psychologically the person may feel disoriented and disorganized, angry, frustrated, depressed, apathetic, helpless, indecisive, afraid, irritable, withdrawn, or unable to concentrate. If nothing is done about it, these symptoms or "cues" may develop into such physical disorders as colitis, ulcers, myocardial infarctions, or asthmatic attacks, or such emotional disorders as depression, addiction, or psychosis.[38]

An unusual amount of stress by any one individual or subgroup can cause pressure in the work situation. Scully points out that group indicators of stress are interpersonal and include such behaviors as snapping at and arguing with others; scapegoating staff members (for example, blaming another shift or the administration for unit tension); or responding to others with sullenness and silence, harried and "busy" behavior, defensiveness, and intolerance of others' ideas or behavior. Trends of tardiness, absenteeism, errors, inefficiency, and rapid staff turnover may also indicate the presence of stress in the group. If stress is not recognized and dealt with, poor morale and uncooperative behavior may progress to vindictive behavior, to apathy, and then to paranoia. The end result is a totally dysfunctional system.[39]

Some of the sources of stress can be related to the type of nursing done, such as intensive care or oncology, where part of nursing consists of dealing with the emotional concerns of very sick patients and their families. Other problems may be understaffing and the fear of not doing what is right or even safe. Dealing with physicians can cause stress as can a nonsupportive administration. Most experts feel that one factor is having unrealistic expectations of yourself.

Much advice has been given on dealing with stress. A noted cardiologist says, "Rule No. 1 is, don't sweat the small stuff. Rule No. 2, it's all small stuff. And if you can't fight and you can't flee, flow."[40] A yoga "scientist" says, "By understanding that *you* are the main source of your own stress, you can begin to alter and conquer it. The solutions to stress are amazingly simple. They aren't easy, but they're available. You need to experiment personally and try to see which ones work for you. The first is to gain self-knowledge."[41] He focuses on the individual's habits and gives suggestions for breaking or controlling poor eating habits, physiological habits, and tension habits. (Biofeedback and yoga are approaches suggested by a number of people.[42])

Some psychologists have demonstrated that the interpretation of an event, not the event itself, produces emotions. They suggest controlling stress by understanding how you label an event, and give advice on gaining control over irrational thoughts and combating distortions.[43]

Job dissatisfaction is one outcome of stress and burnout in the workplace,* or perhaps vice versa. The feelings of role deprivation or alienation (powerlessness, meaninglessness, normlessness, isolation, self-estrangement), often felt by nurse professionals in a bureaucracy, have often been described.[44,45] As with any of these conditions, there is no pat answer, but self-management efforts made by nurses are a key to overcoming them. Self-pity is foolish. It's quite possible to bring about change, to develop a peer support system, and to achieve autonomy.† It does take commitment, effort, and caring.

One nurse suggests that you can't accomplish any of your goals if you don't care for *yourself*. Her "tips that will help you take better care of yourself—and others"—are

- Check your immediate work setting and ask for it to be upgraded if necessary.
- Find a quiet place to retreat when you are overstressed.
- Examine the peer support you give and get.

- Let go of routine tasks.
- Take some time away from the patient-care area.
- Start a mentor system.
- Don't be satisfied with easy answers.
- Help your coworkers and your students to grow.
- Check the messages you are sending.
- Trust your instincts.[46]

STRATEGIES FOR SUCCESS

Dealing with Realities

Student who have survived what might have been a reality shock in nursing education can adopt the strategies learned and use them to meet the challenges of the work world.

Gortner makes some useful suggestions:

1. Become competent in what you do.
2. Know well the organization in which you work.
3. Be a master of the art of the possible.
4. Recognize and seize the opportunity for doing more.
5. Consider few problems to be original. Hence, the solution is somewhere and that is the challenge.
6. Recognize the value of support systems. Build and use some for yourself.
7. Know yourself well.[47]

Probably the first thing that you, as a new graduate, must realize is that you may not have chosen or been able to choose an institution that wants to or knows how to help an entering employee to adjust. An early problem could arise from your belief in a printed job description. Too often, having one does not preclude the possibility of being asked (or assigned) to responsibilities not included in these job descriptions. The first consideration should be the safety of the patient, and you must determine whether you are prepared and able to carry out such a function, and legally permitted to do so. If not what will you do about it? There are legal considerations* as

---

*See Chapters 5 and 15.

†See especially Chapter 16 for a discussion of how this can be accomplished.

---

*See Chapter 21.

well as ethical problems, and a good nurse administrator will recognize the importance of having you trained in that area. Should this not be so, you have a decision to make. The decision to refuse may cost you the job, but will also be only the first of many ethical decisions to be made. (Needless to say, this does not refer to the learning of new techniques of nursing care that evolve with advances in medical and nursing care.)

It is also not unusual for new graduates to be put temporarily in the position of charge nurse or team leader, for which they may not be prepared. This is especially likely to occur on the evening or night shift. In a good orientation or inservice program, this possibility is foreseen, and you will be given the appropriate learning experiences in such situations under supervision or guidance. When this kind of preparation is not included, you should at least be assigned with a more experienced nurse to share the responsibilities. (In anticipation of such assignments, you might have inquired of the prospective employer as to the availability of such training and supervision and indicate willingness to learn and practice such responsibilities before assignments using them are made. The response of the employer could well be one means of judging the working environment.)

It may be necessary to learn new techniques to cope with unexpected assignments, such as learning to manage time and people[48-51] and to activate beginning leadership skills. In some cases, assertiveness training, consciousness-raising groups, and internal support systems make the difference between disillusionment and challenge.[52-54]

Harmonious Relationships with Others

Nursing students are usually taught to respect the individuality of the patient/client and his or her family and to maintain therapeutically effective relationships with them. Not as much attention is given to human relationships with co-workers in the employment setting. However, lack of harmony in a work situation where the nurse must relate to every-

one is not easy to ignore. Anyone who has worked in an employment situation with tensions and pressures caused by personality conflicts and lack of respect for others knows the destructive nature of such an atmosphere. Whether it is caused by a sense of competition, disenchantment with the job, personal, mental, physical, or social problems; whether it emanates from authority groups or peer groups is irrelevant; the end result is not only an unhappy atmosphere, but often a poorer quality of nursing care.[55]

Harmonious interpersonal relationships are essential to one's growth, yet the stimulation of controversy is an added growth essential. Though the two may appear contradictory, ideally they should go hand in hand, provided, of course, that the controversies are not based on petty, personal disagreements, and stubborn behavior, but rather are the outgrowth of objective and constructive thought. Nurses can develop in their profession through healthy interpersonal relationships with their colleagues, or their paths can be obscured by personality limitations. Today's nurse is being educated to be a change agent; to be successful in this role requires the ability to relate well to others.[56]

Continuing Education*

Life without the stimulation of continued learning would be pretty dull. In a general way, you can continue to grow through reading, travel, community activities, and home study. Maintaining professional competency, however, takes a little more effort.

The term *continuing education (CE)* has been interpreted many ways. Most agree that it includes any learning activity after the basic educational program. However, most often those programs leading to an academic degree are separated out. There is still much confusion among nurses who are sure that the renewed social and legal pressures for CE mean

---

*See Chapter 13 for more detailed information about CE.

that they must enroll in a baccalaureate program. This is not so.

The basic and overriding purpose of CE in nursing is the maintenance of continued competence so that the care of the patient is safe and effective. The rapid changes in society, the emergence of new knowledge and technologies, make it impossible to function effectively with only the knowledge and skills gained in your basic program, no matter how outstanding the program.

In the course of your career, which might well cover a forty-year span, the knowledge needed to function effectively during the last years, or even earlier, will encompass only a fraction of that available at the beginning. The rest is all new.

Although the tremendous advance in the sciences has provided an added impetus to the need for CE, the concept goes back to Florence Nightingale, who said:

> Nursing is a progressive art, in which to stand still is to go back. A woman who thinks to herself, "Now I am a full nurse, a skilled nurse, I have learnt all there is to be learnt"—take my word for it, she does not know what a nurse is, and never will know; she is gone back already. Progress can never end but with a nurse's life.

Who should bear the cost of the nurse's CE is a controversial issue. Formalized programs in CE are offered as inservice education in places of employment, through conferences, workshops, institutes, and other program meetings of professional or other health organizations, or in CE programs offered by colleges and universities. Only inservice education is always free. The other programs frequently charge at least a token fee of some kind because the cost of providing quality programs is high.

As a professional nurse, you should expect to assume at least part of the cost. There are those who feel that because the employers ultimately benefit from the employee's improved performance, they should provide such support as partial or full tuition payment, sabbat-

icals, or short-term leaves. On the other hand, hospitals and like institutions often maintain that these additional costs must be passed on unfairly to the patient, and that they have a right to expect competent practitioners. With current tight money restrictions, that philosophy is bound to prevail, although some employers do offer opportunities for CE as a fringe benefit.

Another controversial issue is whether CE should remain on a voluntary basis or whether, in order to make sure that nurses (and others) do continue their education, it should be a requirement for relicensure. This issue is discussed in Chapter 20. What is not controversial is the responsibility of the nurse, as a professional practitioner, to maintain competence in whatever area of practice is being engaged in: clinical, administrative, or other. Some nurses maintain that working in a patient setting is CE. Of course it can be, depending on the setting, the opportunity for learning, and the nurse's inclination to use these opportunities. There are also nurses who merely repeat past experiences and do not recognize or choose to utilize available learning experiences.

There is some concern as to the content of CE for nurses. Arguments range from the stand that anything which adds to the development of the nurse in any way is CE to the equally firm stand that only clinical or directly related scientific studies should be acceptable. This argument may never be resolved, for it is primarily philosophic. What benefits any specific nurse in improving practice is probably as individual as that nurse, and the conscientious nurse will seek out the educational experience needed whether it "counts" toward required hours or not.

Possibly a significant message is relayed in a key governmental report, which states, "Continuing education in its present form—the bulk of which remains traditional—is destined for change; only those forms clearly related to continued competence should be maintained."[57] Eventually, it is clear, there must be some type of peer review of practice.

Little research has been done to determine the direct effects of CE on competency. Of the small studies done, the findings are sometimes contradictory, with improvement in practice either evidenced or absent. When nurses' participation is active and the program meets specific stated needs of the nurse, the result is likely to be more positive. The majority of programs offered in the last few years stress updating skills, gaining new skills (particularly in preparation for the NP role), and clinical knowledge.

With CE programs proliferating (and getting more expensive), better give some thought to what is worth spending time and money on. One suggested plan for diagnosing your continuing education needs is to develop a model of required competencies, assessing your practice in relation to the model, and identifying the gaps between your knowledge and skills and those required. Some of this preliminary testing can be done by taking some of the tests in journals, and by carefully evaluating your own practice and getting feedback from peers and supervisors as well.[58]

Other methods of CE learning, besides formal classes or conferences, are well worth investigating, although, of course, there is often the added value of interaction with other nurses in group activities.[59] One expert in CE suggests some useful ways of weighing the choices offered, including figuring the costs (registration, travel, time off); looking at objectives, intent, and learning methods in relation to your own specific needs; evaluating the quality of the program regarding speakers and sponsors; and finding programs that are suitable.[60]

Formal Higher Education

Besides participating in CE programs, the graduate of a diploma or associate degree program may want to give serious consideration to formal education leading to a baccalaureate degree, and the nurse with a baccalaureate degree may want to think about getting a master's. There is no question but that educational standards for all positions in nursing

are growing steadily higher. The nurse who really wants to advance professionally to positions of greater scope and challenge will, in the very near future, need at least a baccalaureate degree. The process of obtaining this and higher degrees not only will serve the nurse well professionally but will add considerably to the enrichment of his or her personal life and interests.

Although it would be difficult to denigrate the value to an individual of any good-quality educational program, give some thought to your future goals. The joy of exploring new fields and studying whatever you wish without the pressure of time or the need to fulfill requirements for a program may be especially tempting. If these interests are in any of the liberal arts or the social or physical sciences, which may be required, or can be used as electives in many programs, a dual purpose will be accomplished in that you are also started toward a degree.

Because baccalaureate programs with a nursing major are not always available (or affordable) to nurses in a particular geographic area, a number of programs have sprung up offering a degree in nursing or another field, giving credit for the lower-division nursing courses and offering no upper-division nursing courses. Evaluate them in relation to your career goals. This program is *not* usually acceptable for future graduate studies in nursing, and you may not be able to enroll in a graduate program without having taken upper-division nursing courses. Some nurses have found it necessary to complete a second baccalaureate program, this time with a nursing major, in order to continue into a master's program.[61]

If you are interested in a baccalaureate degree for personal development, any accredited baccalaureate program might, of course, meet these objectives. In some cases, individual courses would also enhance your understanding of nursing. The crucial question is whether you wish to enhance, deepen, and broaden the *nursing* knowledge you've already acquired and/or advance in newer nursing fields. If so, an accredited (or equivalent) nursing baccalaureate program is essential.

As noted in Chapter 12, RNs will find that they receive varying amounts of recognition or credit for their basic nursing courses, and may perhaps need to take challenge examinations. Nursing baccalaureate programs vary a great deal in this respect, but more and more nursing programs are offering some form of educational articulation, self-pacing, or other means of giving credit for previous knowledge, skill, and ability such as the external degree.[62] NLN publications listing baccalaureate, master's, and doctoral programs are helpful.

Many of the same points apply to graduate education. There are still some limitations in available nursing master's programs—limitations in their very existence or in the major within nursing which is available. Therefore, some nurses complete graduate programs in the various sciences or education, with or without any nursing input. Again, you must consider your specific career goals. Someone with a nursing major or at least a minor may be given preference in a position requiring a graduate degree, particularly in educational positions. Or if you are hired now, there is no guarantee that later, when there are more nurses with graduate nursing degrees, you may not be bypassed for promotion or may be required to take a second graduate degree in nursing in order to hold the current position.

These are practical considerations presented here for information. You must still make the educational decisions you wish, but with as complete a knowledge of the pros and cons as possible.

Suppose you simply don't want any degree? Or suppose you enroll in an accredited nursing program but then, in time, drop out? That's your decision. There is no reason why you can't function at an acceptable level of competence, maintaining and improving that competence through CE, thereby making a valuable contribution to the profession and society. If, however, you withdrew because of disappointment or lack of interest in that particular program, it may well be that the program is not congruent with your philosophy. Consider a second try, taking time to determine whether a program's philosophy, objectives, approaches to teaching, and attitudes are what you want. Some of this information can be obtained from the catalog, the faculty or advisor interviews, informal contact with students or *recent* graduates (programs do change). Sometimes, if some courses may be taken without need for full matriculation, a sampling of courses will prove especially informative.

Sources of Financial Aid

The problem of finances is undoubtedly the most common deterrent to advanced education for able professional nurses. Review your financial resources realistically before embarking on this new venture. If you are going to request financial aid, you will need to estimate as accurately as possible your expected income and expenses. Major educational expenses will include tuition, books, educational fees, and perhaps travel. Related personal expenses depend on where and how you live. Economizing may mean enrolling in a community college for the liberal arts and later transferring to a local or state college. Economy should not include enrolling in a poor program. Graduating from a nonaccredited nursing program may create difficulties in advancing to the next higher degree. Not all nonaccredited programs are poor, but this risk does exist.

The major sources of income for a self-supporting graduate nurse in an advanced educational program are savings or other personal resources, part-time work, scholarships, and loans. If you plan to do part-time work while attending college, make reasonably sure that a position is available at a satisfactory salary and that it seems to be professionally suitable, including enough flexibility to make it possible to take courses. Consider also your mental and physical health under this double load. Can you manage? One answer is cooperative education, part work and part school.[63]

There are a number of scholarships, fellowships, and loans earmarked for educational purposes for which professional nurses are often eligible if they seek them out and apply. Some sources of financial assistance are well known and used regularly; others are not used simply because people do not know about them. The financial aid officer at the institution where you plan to enroll is an excellent source of information.

In most instances educational scholarships, fellowships, and loans are defined as follows: (1) *scholarship*—a financial grant that does not involve repayment; (2) *fellowship*—a grant for graduate study not requiring reimbursement; (3) *loan*—a grant for educational purposes to be repaid by the recipient either with or without interest after completion of the course or education. Grants-in-aid are outright grants at both the undergraduate and graduate levels for accomplishment of a specific project. There may also be an outright grant to meet an immediate financial emergency or a grant to a student with a claim to a restricted scholarship fund. The term *traineeship* has also been used in recent years to denote federal grants with stipend and tuition costs, which need not be repaid, awarded to students in nursing programs, under the Nurse Training Act and its legislative successors.

Some funds are available to members of certain organizations or religious denominations or to students who meet other special requirements. Others are offered to any deserving person who has demonstrated such qualities as good character, leadership ability, and academic achievement. In general, scholarships, loans, and grants are available from both private and governmental sources and agencies.

The manner in which you apply for financial assistance may have considerable bearing on whether or not you obtain it. Correspondence, personal interviews, application forms, and references should all show the same meticulous attention that is given to an application for a new position.

Financial assistance may be found at the local, state, regional, national, or international level. Where you should apply will depend upon how you plan to use the money. For example, some funds are available for advanced study in mental health and psychiatry only, or for other clinical specialties; others are designed to prepare nurses for teaching, supervisory, or administrative positions; still others have different stipulations; and many are unrestricted as long as the applicant meets the designated personal qualifications.

The National League for Nursing, 10 Columbus Circle, New York, New York 10019, issues a pamphlet entitled *Scholarships, Fellowships, Educational Grants, and Loans for Registered Nurses.* This pamphlet contains a great deal of specific information that may help you decide where to apply first for financial assistance, thus saving valuable time in making applications.

The professional nursing journals frequently carry news items and articles[64,65] about such funds, which can be found through the annual and cumulative indexes. Most college catalogs also list sources of student financial support. Given here, in more general terms, are some of the possible sources of funds. Some give relatively small amounts of money, but these sums do add up.

Local Sources. Local sources of funds include both professional and civic groups in the nursing school, community, district, and state. The alumni association of a school of nursing often has appropriations for scholarships and loans that are available to graduates of the school. The president of the association or the director of the school will have information about such sources of financial assistance. Some district and state nurses' associations and NLN constituencies have funds for advanced study and other special purposes, either as direct gifts or on a reasonable interest and repayment basis. Some state legislatures have apportioned money to prepare selected professional nurses to work on state health problems and, more rarely, to provide loans and scholarships to nursing (and other) students. The state board of nursing and the operational institutions involved will have information about such appropriations.

Other local sources of funds include chapters of national sororities, fraternities, and clubs whose memberships are not restricted to nurses but offer financial aid to anyone who meets their qualifications. There are churches that have educational funds as do church-affiliated groups; the Elks, Masons, Altrusa Club, American Legion Auxiliary, and other similar organizations; unions; corporations; and private foundations and institutes.* Other good sources of information are local or state colleges or universities and the hospital associations. Your place of employment may also offer grants and loans, or pay part or all of the tuition fees.

In some instances, scholarships and loans are available to nurses in a region of the country comprising more than one state. Information about these funds is often carried in some of the previous sources mentioned.

National Sources. In recent years, professional nurses interested in applying for a national scholarship, fellowship, or loan would, with the assistance of the advanced nursing programs in which they were enrolled, have turned to the federal government. Both general scholarships and loans, as well as some designated especially for RNs, grants, fellowships, and full-time nurse traineeships, have been of increasing and invaluable aid to the RN. Although there are never enough to meet all needs, without them a large majority of RNs could not have completed advanced education. However, beginning in 1973, the administration became less interested in providing any financial aid to nurses and some loans and funds were cut back. Since 1975, funds for nurse traineeships have been progressively cut.† Loans and special scholarships for ser-

vice in underserved areas continue to be available, but there are predictions that federal money for all health professions will gradually dry up. Much depends on the amount of pressure put on Congress to legislate funds. Such congressional action appears to fluctuate from year to year but has been leaning in the direction of fewer and more restricted funds.

The Nurses' Educational Funds, Inc. (NEF), was established in 1954 to honor nursing pioneers. It was initiated largely through the efforts of NLN, which saw the need for centralized administration of the three separate educational allocations for nurses that existed at that time: the Isabel Hampton Robb Memorial Fund, the Isabel McIsaac Loan Fund, and the Nurses' Scholarship and Fellowship Fund. Since then, other funds have been initiated and turned over to NEF for administration. Many of the awards given are in the names of nurses who contributed greatly to the nursing profession. NEF is an independent organization that grants and administers scholarships and fellowships to RNs for post-RN study. It is governed by a board of trustees, mainly leaders in nursing education, and supported by contributions from business corporations, foundations, nurses, and persons interested in nursing.

In 1973 the American Journal of Nursing Company assumed the administrative, accounting, and secretarial responsibilities for NEF. Application forms and information about the necessary qualifications of applicants can be obtained from Nurses' Educational Funds, 555 W. 57th Street, New York, New York 10019.

Financial aid is also available from the National Student Nurses' Association (see Chapter 24), miscellaneous private foundations, and some health organizations that may give financial assistance to nurses for advanced work in that organization's major area of interest. In addition, the armed services and the Veterans Administration subsidize the advanced education of some nurses (see Chapter 15).

---

*Some of these are national and local sources.
†See Chapter 19.

International Sources. The national nursing organizations may be able to supply information about scholarships, fellowships, and loans accessible to RNs who wish to study abroad. It would be well to contact these organizations first, although the International Council of Nurses, the World Health Organization, and the U.S. Public Health Service are also possible sources of information. As more professional nurses become interested in international nursing, governmental, professional, educational, and philanthropic groups may originate new scholarships, fellowships, and loans to assist them. The competition for available funds for international study is likely to be increasingly keen, however, because many other professional and occupational groups also are becoming more eager for education and experience in other cuntries.

The UN's Educational, Scientific, and Cultural Organization (UNESCO) publishes an annual catalog entitled *Study Abroad,* which gives information on opportunities for financial assistance for international education. The fellowships and scholarships are awarded by governments, foundations, universities, and other institutions in almost every country in the world. The subjects of study cover nearly all fields of learning, including nursing. Complete data about the awards are given, such as the amount granted, qualifications, availability, length of study periods, and restrictions. Some funds are restricted; others are not. The common objective of the awards is to bring persons from different parts of the world into direct contact with each other and each other's cultures.

Although *Study Abroad* currently lists only a very limited number of sources of financial aid for U.S. nurses who wish to study abroad, it is hoped that such opportunities will increase in the future. A large general library in a city or university might have a copy of the catalog or it can be purchased for a nominal sum directly from UNESCO at UN headquarters in New York City.

Individuals and groups who contribute scholarships, fellowships, and loans want them to be used to the best possible advantage. If they are left unused for several years, the administering authority may decide to allocate the money elsewhere (if it is legally empowered to do so), or at least will be inclined to feel it unnecessary to try to increase the amounts or promote the establishment of new funds. Effective use of scholarships could increase the supply. Occasionally nursing and other journals list sources of educational funds, with guidelines for application and other useful information. These make good up-to-date references.

Professional and Community Activities

Active participation in community activities that allow you to share and utilize your professional background in full is very rewarding. Some activities are directly related to nursing, such as attending alumni and nurses' associations meetings and accepting appointments to committees and offices. Others include volunteer work on a regular or special basis, such as participating in student nurse recruitment programs or career days, soliciting donations for various health organizations, helping with the Red Cross blood program, assisting with inoculation sessions for children, acting as adviser to a Future Nurse Club, or volunteering time at a free clinic.

The importance of nursing input into the various community, state, and national joint provider-consumer groups which study means of improving the health care delivery system is obvious. Although participation at a state or national level may not be immediately feasible for a nurse who has not yet achieved professional recognition, just showing interest and volunteering your services will often open doors at a local level. Nurses involved in direct patient care activities are particularly welcome, because there is the feeling that they can more specifically delineate some of the problems and suggest logical, down-to-earth solutions. Participation of this kind is vital if nurses are to have a part in making policy decisions.*

Consumer activism has caused the formation of other groups concerned with health delivery, and nurses offering their expertise and understanding of health care services problems can make valuable contributions. Sometimes you need to convince these groups that you have a sincere interest in improved health care services and are willing to work cooperatively with the consumer to achieve that end. In some areas, ethnic and minority groups are especially suspicious of professional health workers outside of their own group, because unfortunate experiences have shown some of them to be more concerned with defending their own interests than the consumer's well-being, as the consumer sees it. In these groups, it is even more important to listen than to talk. Such participation can lead to development of free clinics, health fairs, health teaching classes, recruitment of minority students for nursing programs, tutoring sessions for students, liaison activities with health care institutions, programs for the aged, and legislative activities directed toward better health care. The opportunities, challenges, and satisfactions are unlimited.

Consumer health education is being stressed more and more today, and in what better area can professional nurses offer their expertise? Classes can be held under the auspices of health care institutions, public health organizations, and public and private community groups, and include teaching for wellness as well as teaching those with chronic or long-term illnesses. Nurses who like to teach and are skilled and enthusiastic can participate in programs already set up, and, and, equally important, can work to develop other programs and involve others on the health team.

Keeping the public informed about nursing and the changes that have occurred in recent years in both education and practice is a contribution to the community. Offers to present programs about modern nursing are often welcome in the many community, social, business, professional, and service groups that meet frequently and are interested in community service.

Activities such as these involve nurses in the community and are stimulating and satisfying. They also require time, effort, and often patience. But besides the satisfaction of being of service, the nurse gains in self-development and growth as a professional and as an individual, a dual reward that cannot be bought.

A FINAL WORD

There are many ways to conceptualize nursing. It is possible to think of nursing as a role, as an occupation, or as a career. Nursing, as a role, can be enacted within a family, a neighborhood, or in professional and civic associations. Some nurses who do not work or engage in professional activity see themselves as nurses and identify with the role of nursing. Many inactive nurses still hold licenses. For others, nursing is a job, defined by the scope of responsibilities to patients and the number of hours worked each day or week. Dedication to the job is limited by other interests, such as commitments to one's family, school, or personal interests. For others, nursing is a career—the work of one's life. Preparation, advancement, and concern with professional issues preoccupy nurse careerists.[66] Identifying with careerists in nursing opens up interesting professional and personal opportunities. It certainly places nurse careerists on the path with other men and women who plan to move up corporate hierarchies to positions of leadership and influence. People who are serious about their work and performance attract the attention of their executives. We may laugh at television advertisements about "impressing the boss." However, research in nursing shows that successful nurse executives had mentors who encouraged their development, sponsored their projects, and nurtured their ideas.[67]

*See Chapter 16.

Another characteristic of career-oriented nurses is the attention they give to educational and professional development. Advanced education is not a substitute for clinical skill, teaching ability, or administrative expertise. However, it is unlikely that anyone makes it to the top or to a good mid-level position without higher education. If you examine the educational and professional characteristics of the nurses you admire or review the qualifications of nurses who exercise authority in hospitals and in health and community organizations, you will have a better understanding of the education demanded by a career. The ambivalence within the profession about nursing education makes the decision to return to school more difficult than it need be. This is very interesting because physicians, social workers, physical therapists, hospital administrators—in fact, the whole health team—have master's-level preparation. Some feminist nurses suggest that discouraging intelligent young people from attaining the credentials they will need to get top jobs is a modern effort to subjugate women.[68]

There is renewed emphasis on political action and legislative awareness at each level of the nursing curriculum. This orientation is helpful because careerists give their time to professional, health, and civic organizations. In the 1970s, nurses were encouraged to make policy and to become engaged in public debates about social policy issues.[69] In the 1980s, several nurses held positions of influence in the Department of Health and Human Services. Another example of political activism is the growing number of nurses who are elected to legislatures.

These brief accounts of movement in professional, civic, and political spheres are presented to expand your awareness that being a career nurse means that you are committed to more than bedside nursing. It is not enough to say: "I am a good nurse; I take care of my patients." The changing political and economic environments, the development of multisystem corporations, and the new payment patterns that fix a price for care based on a diagnostic group require nurses to be professionally and politically sophisticated as well as clinically competent. Careerists are leaders in nursing.

Another dimension of the lives of successful career people is the attention they give to life-style. There is a new literature that markets strategies for success. It includes practical advice on dressing for success; balancing work and play; and integrating diet and exercise into your life-style. For years, nurses have balanced multiple and competing demands, often feeling that they never do anything as well as they could. Now that women are an active presence in the workplace, more attention and support are being given to families and working women.[70] No longer is the nurse the only woman in her neighborhood who works. New social support systems make careerism a real choice for the nurse who wants a family. Nursing is an exciting field that offers people a role and social status, a job, or a career. If your education or your present position does not challenge your potential, seek career counseling from your professional association, your school of nursing, or your nurse administrator.[71] One of the real benefits of living in a complex, changing world is that you are free to identify and select among multiple options. When you enter the world of practice, you will choose nursing as a role, a job, or a career. Some new graduates know where they will stand along nursing's continuum. Others are not so certain. Discussions with mature nurses indicate that they have occupied several positions along the continuum during their lives. Sometimes their orientation to nursing has not been a matter of choice. Rotational patterns and off-shift work in hospitals, coupled with the salaries of staff nurses, make scheduling and payment for child care difficult. These constraints often make the nurse with a young child change her place of work, change her specialty, or take a part-time position. These women's issues indicate that factors other than personal wish or ideology influence whether nursing is a role, a job, or a career.

As the new graduate enters practice, sociological and economic predictors become important. There is a consensus that the world of the 1990s will be radically different from life in the 1980s. The authors of *Megatrends*[72] and *The Third Wave*[73] identify the growth of an information society. Some writers stress the need for the development of third-wave nurses or knowledge workers who will be comfortable with high-tech, high-touch care.[74]

The changes in health care financing (prospective payment and diagnostic groups) mandated by PL 98-21, and the growth of multisystem and for-profit hospitals, have revolutionized the workplace. New graduates find that they can move within multihospital systems without losing benefits or status. Flat-rate reimbursement, which encourages the early discharge of patients, has the indirect effect of increasing the intensity of nursing care needed by inpatients. Changing health care financing has also stimulated new jobs in ambulatory centers, clinics, surgery, and/or emergency centers. New graduates find that new patterns of organization and financing of health care have changed their practices as much as the introduction of high-technology medicine revolutionized nursing care in the 1960s.

Today, more than ever before in modern history, your constructive talents and abilities are needed in full measure to help civilization advance on all fronts in every area of the globe, possibly of the universe. Nursing, with its unlimited frontiers and exciting future, also needs the full and unstinted output of its practitioners. The rewards promise to be many.

REFERENCES

1. Ida Simpson, "Patterns of Socialization into Professions: The Case of Student Nurses," *Soc. Inquiry,* **37**:47 (Winter 1967).
2. Ada Sue Hinshaw, "Socialization and Resocialization of Nurses for Professional Nursing Practice," in *Socialization and Resocialization of Nurses for Professional Nursing Practice* (New York: National League for Nursing, 1977), p. 2.
3. Ibid. pp. 5, 6.
4. Marlene Kramer. *Reality Shock* (St. Louis: C. V. Mosby Company, 1974), p. 15.
5. Ibid., pp. vii–viii, 3.
6. Ibid., pp. viii, 4–10.
7. Ibid., pp. 155–162.
8. Ibid., p. 162.
9. Margaret Treat and Marlene Kramer, "The Question Behind the Question," *J. Nurs. Admin.,* **2**:20–27 (Jan.–Feb. 1972).
10. Marlene Kramer and Constance Baker, "The Exodus: Can We Prevent It?" *J. Nurs. Admin.,* **1**:15–30 (May–June 1971).
11. Claudia Schmalenberg and Marlene Kramer, "Dreams and Reality: Where Do They Meet?" *J. Nurs. Admin.,* **6**:35–43 (June 1976).
12. Marlene Kramer and Claudia Schmalenberg, "Conflict: The Cutting Edge of Growth," *J. Nurs. Admin.,* **6**:19–25 (June 1976).
13. Linda Raker, "Treating Reality Shock," *Am. J. Nurs.,* **79**:688 (Apr. 1979).
14. Ginger Alhadeff, "Anxiety in a New Graduate," *Am. J. Nurs.,* **79**:687–688 (Apr. 1979).
15. Cynthia Schipani, "From the Ideal to the Real," *Am. J. Nurs.,* **78**:1034–1035 (June 1978).
16. Sandra Miller, "Letter from a New Graduate," *Am. J. Nurs.,* **78**:1688–1689 (Oct. 1978).
17. Sherril Santo, "A Beginning Nurse Reacts," *Am. J. Nurs.,* **78**:1032–34 (June 1978).
18. Marlene Kramer, "The New Graduate Speaks," *Am. J. Nurs.,* **66**:2420–2424 (Nov. 1966).
19. Claudia Schmalenberg and Marlene Kramer, *Coping with Reality Shock: The Voices of Experience,* (Wakefield, Mass: Nursing Resources, Inc., 1979).
20. *Reality Shock,* op. cit., pp. 67–77.
21. Ibid., pp. 137–190.
22. Ibid., pp. 315–329.
23. Suzanne Holleran et al., "Bicultural Training for New Graduates," *Nurse Educator,* **5**:8–14 (Jan.–Feb. 1984).

24. Joan Goldsberry, "From Student to Professional," *J. Nurs. Admin.,* **7**:46–49 (Mar. 1977).

25. Regina Block, "The Nurses' Ombudsman," *Am. J. Nurs.,* **76**:1631–1633 (Oct. 1976).

26. C. S. Weisman et al., "Employment Patterns Among Newly Hired Hospital Staff Nurses," *Nurs. Res.,* **30**:188 (May–June 1981).

27. Christina Maslack, "Burned Out," *Hum. Behavior,* **5**:16–22 (Sept. 1976).

28. Edwina McConnell, "How Close Are You to Burnout?" *RN,* **44**:29–33 (May 1981).

29. Seymour Shubin, "Burnout, the Professional Hazard You Face in Nursing," *Nurs. 78,* **8**:22–27 (July 1978).

30. Kathleen Magill, "Burnin, Burnout, and the Brightly Burning," *Nurs. Mgt.,* **13**:17–21 (July 1982).

31. Frances Storlie, "Burnout: Elaboration of a Concept," *Am. J. Nurs.,* **79**:2109 (Dec. 1979).

32. D. Lee Brown, "Burnout—or Cop-Out?" *Am. J. Nurs.,* **83**:1110 (July 1983).

33. "Stress: Can We Cope?" *Time,* **123**:48 (June 6, 1983).

34. Ibid., pp. 49–50.

35. Hans Selye, *Stress Without Distress* (Philadelphia: J.B. Lippincott Company, 1974).

36. *Time,* op. cit., p. 51.

37. Rosemarie Scully, "Stress in the Nurse," *Am J. Nurs.,* **80**:912 (May 1980).

38. Ibid.

39. Ibid.

40. *Time,* op. cit., p. 48.

41. Phil Nuernberger, "Freedom from Stress: A Holistic Approach," *Nurs. Life,* **1**:61–68 (Nov.-Dec. 1981).

42. *Time,* op. cit., pp. 52–54.

43. Matthew McKay et al., "Are You Listening to Yourself?" *Nurs. Life,* **3**:57–64 (Jan.-Feb. 1983).

44. Eileen Zungolo, "A Study in Alienation: The Nurse Practitioner," *Nurs. Forum,* **7**(1):38–48 (1968).

45. Mary Malone, "The Dilemma of a Professional in a Bureaucracy," *Nurs. Forum,* **3**(4):36–60 (1964).

46. Amy Haddad, "Caring for Yourself Comes First," *RN,* **47**:77–78 (June 1984).

47. Susan Gortner, "Strategies for Survival in the Practice World," *Am. J. Nurs.,* **77**:618–619 (Apr. 1977).

48. Marlene Kramer and Claudia Schmalenberg, "Constructive Feedback," *Nurs. 77,* **7**:102–106 (Nov. 1977).

49. Edwina McConnell, "What Kind of a Delegator Are You?" *Nurs. 78,* **8**:105–110 (Oct. 1978).

50. Robert Moskowitz, "Make the Most of Your Time," *Nurs. Life,* **2**:21–28 (Jan.-Feb. 1982).

51. Edwina McConnell, "Ten Tactics to Help Beat the Clock," *RN,* **46**:47–50 (Sept. 1983).

52. Rita Numeroff, "Assertiveness Training," *Am. J. Nurs.,* **80**:1796–1799 (Oct. 1980).

53. Marilyn Edmunds, "Assertive Skills," *Nurse Practitioner,* **6**:27–31, 39 (Nov.-Dec. 1981).

54. Bonnie Randolph and Clydere Ross-Valiere, "Consciousness Raising Groups," *Am. J. Nurs.,* **79**:922–924 (May 1979).

55. Frances Storlie, "Surviving on-the-Job Conflict," *RN,* **45**:51–53, 96 (Oct. 1982).

56. Robert Laser, "I Win—You Win Negotiating," *J. Nurs. Admin.,* **11**:24–29 (Nov.-Dec. 1981).

57. Harris Cohen and Lawrence Miike, *Developments in Health Manpower Licensure: A Follow-up Report to the 1971 Report on Licensure and Related Health Personnel Credentialing* (Washington, D.C.: Department of Health, Education and Welfare, June 1973), p. 42.

58. Andrea O'Connor, "Diagosing Your Needs for Continuing Education," *Am. J. Nurs.,* **78**:405–406 (Mar. 1978).

59. Gloria Hochman, "Continuing Education: How Can You Make the Most of It?" *Nurs. 78,* **8**:81–89 (Dec. 1978).

60. Dorothy del Bueno, "How to Get Your Money's Worth Out of Continuing Education," *RN,* **41**:37–42 (Apr. 1978).

61. Faye Carol Reed, "Education or Exploitation?" *Am. J. Nurs.,* **79**:1259–1261 (July 1979).

62. *Nursing Outlook,* September 1984, has a number of articles on education for RNs.

63. "Finding Funds for Education," Part 1, *Nurs. Life,* **1**:17–24 (Sept.-Oct. 1981).

64. "Finding Funds for Education," Part 2, *Nurs. Life,* **1**:21–28 (Nov.–Dec. 1981).

65. Katherine Detherage and Marshelle Thobaben, "Nursing Fellowship Opportunities for Advanced Studies," *Nurs. Outlook,* **30**:115–121 (Feb. 1982).

66. Marilyn Smith, "Career Development in Nursing: An Individual and Professional Responsibility," *Nurs. Outlook,* **30**:128–131 (Feb. 1982).

67. Connie Vance, "Women Leaders: Modern Day Heroines or Societal Deviants?" *Image,* **11**:37–41 (June 1979).

68. Jo Ann Ashley, *Hospitals, Paternalism and the Role of the Nurse* (New York: Teachers College Press, 1977).

69. Philip and Beatrice Kalisch, *The Advance of American Nursing* (Boston: Little, Brown and Company, 1978), pp. 615–649.

70. Ronnie Sandroff, "Nurse/Mother: How to Cope With a Double Career," *RN,* **43**:53–57 (July 1980).

71. Richard Nelson Balles, *What Color Is Your Parachute?* (Berkeley, Calif.: Ten Speed Press, 1981), p. 67.

72. John Naisbitt, *Megatrends* (New York: Warner Books, 1982).

73. Alvin Toffler, *The Third Wave* (New York: Bantam Books, 1980).

74. St. Rosemary Donley, "Nursing 2000: An Essay," *Image,* **16**:6 (Winter 1984).

Bibliography

This bibliography is organized in a way that should make it easy to find appropriate sources.

1. Under each part, title or section heading, general sources related to more than one chapter in that part of section are listed first. Then appropriate specific sources are listed under each chapter heading.
2. With rare exceptions, such as with books that cover the entire topic, citations already appearing in each chapter reference list are *not* reprinted in the bibliography. It is possible that some of these references are cited in more than one chapter, as appropriate.
3. As a rule, works published prior to 1978 are not included. Exceptions are publications of historical significance. Other useful works published prior to 1975 are cited in the third (1975) and fourth (1981) editions of *Dimensions of Professional Nursing.*
4. The selection of books and journals is broad in order to include other fields as well as nursing, so that readers who are interested may explore some other perspectives.
5. Many of the sources cited have extensive bibliographies.

PART I DEVELOPMENT OF MODERN NURSING

Austin, Anne L. *History of Nursing Source Book.* New York: G. P. Putnam's Sons, 1957.

Bingham, Stella. *Ministering Angels.* Oradell, N.J.: Medical Economics Company, 1979.

Bullough, Vern, and Bonnie Bullough. *The Care of the Sick: The Emergence of Modern Nursing.* New York: Prodist, 1978.

Carnegie, Elizabeth. "Black Nurses at the Front." *Am. J. Nurs.* **84** (Oct. 1984), 1250–1252.

Dolan, Josephine, Louise Fitzpatrick, and Eleanor Herrman. *Nursing in Society: A Historical Perspective*, 15th ed. Philadelphia: W. B. Saunders Company, 1983.

Ehrenreich, Barbara, and Deirdre English. *Witches, Midwives, and Nurses: A History of Women Healers.* Old Westbury, N.Y.: The Feminist Press, 1973.

Kalisch, Beatrice, and Philip Kalisch. *The Advance of American Nursing.* Boston: Little, Brown and Company, 1978.

The American Journal of Nursing Company has published a compilation of the articles on nursing history published in its journals: *Notes from Nursing History*, 1984.

SECTION 1 EARLY HISTORICAL INFLUENCES

Chapter 1 Care of the Sick: A Historical Overview

Ellis, Harold. "Royal Operations: A Contrast to Modern Surgery." *AORN J.,* **17** (May 1973), 101–108.

Mish, Ina. "Nursing Process—Medieval Style." *Nurs. Forum,* **18**(2) (1979), 196–203.

Chapter 2 The Influence of Florence Nightingale

Cope, Zachary. *Florence Nightingale and the Doc-*

tors. Philadelphia: J. B. Lippincott Company, 1958.

Herbert, Raymond. *Florence Nightingale: Saint, Reformer or Rebel?* Malabar, Fla.: Robert E. Krieger Publishing Company, 1981.

Kalisch, Beatrice, and Philip Kalisch. "Heroine Out of Focus: Media Images of Florence Nightingale, Part 1." *Nurs. and Health Care,* **4** (Apr. 1983), 181–187; Part 2, (May 1983), 270–278.

Levine, Myra E. "Florence Nightingale . . . the Legend That Lives." *Nurs. Forum,* **2,**4 (1963), 24–35.

Nuttal, Peggy. "The Passionate Statistician." *Int. Nurs. Rev.,* **31** (Jan.-Feb. 1984), 24–25.

Palmer, Irene. "Florence Nightingale: Reformer, Reactionary, Researcher." *Nurs. Res.,* **26** (Mar.-Apr. 1977), 84–89.

Palmer, Irene. "Florence Nightingale and International Origins of Modern Nursing." *Image,* **13** (June 1981), 28–31.

Palmer, Irene. "Nightingale Revisited." *Nurs. Outlook,* **31** (July–Aug. 1983), 229–233.

Seymer, Lucy. *Selected Writings of Florence Nightingale.* New York: Macmillan Publishing Company, Inc., 1954.

Thompson, John. "The Passionate Humanist: From Nightingale to the New Nurse." *Nurs. Outlook,* **28** (May 1980), 290–295.

Woodham-Smith, Cecil. *Florence Nightingale.* New York: McGraw-Hill Book Company, 1951.

See also the sections on Nightingale in the Bullough, Dolan, and Kalisch and Kalisch books. An outstanding collection of Nightingale's writings can be found in the Adelaide Nutting Historical Nursing collection at Teachers College, Columbia University, New York. Some of her most noted works are listed below in chronological order. Some of these are found in Seymer.

The Institution of Kaiserswerth on the Rhine for the Practical Training of Deaconesses under the Direction of the Rev. Pastor Fliedner, Embracing the Support and Care of a Hospital, Infant and Industrial Schools, and a Female Penitentiary, 1851.

Notes on Matters Affecting the Health, Efficiency, and Hospital Administration of the British Army. Founded chiefly on the Experience of the Late War. Presented by Request to the Secretary of State for War, 1858.

Subsidiary Notes as to the Introduction of Female Nursing into Military Hospitals in Peace and in

War. Presented by Request to the Secretary of State for War, 1858.

A Contribution to the Sanitary History of the British Army During the Late War with Russia, 1859.

Notes on Hospitals, 1859, 3rd ed., almost completely rewritten, 1863.

Notes on Nursing: What It Is, and What It Is Not, 1859.

Observations on the Evidence Contained in the Statistical Reports Submitted to the Royal Commission on the Sanitary State of the Army in India, 1863.

Suggestions on a System of Nursing for Hospitals in India, 1865.

Suggestions on the Subject of Providing, Training, and Organizing Nurses For the Sick Poor in Workhouse Infirmaries. Paper No. XVI in the 'Government Report of the Committee Appointed to Consider the Cubic Space of Metropolitan Workhouses, 1867.

Introductory Notes on Lying-In Institutions Together With a Proposal for Organizing an Institution for Training Midwives and Midwifery Nurses, 1871.

On Trained Nursing for the Sick Poor, 1876.

Nurses, Training of and Nursing the Sick, from *A Dictionary of Medicine,* edited by Sir Robert Qwain, Bart., M.D., 1882.

"Sick-Nursing and Health-Nursing" (paper read at the Chicago Exhibition 1893).

"Health Teaching in Towns and Villages—Rural Hygiene" (paper read at the Conference of Women Workers, Leeds, 1893), published 1894.

SECTION 2 NURSING IN THE UNITED STATES

Anderson, Nancy. "Ethel Fenwick's Legacy to Nursing and Women." *Image,* **13** (June 1981), 32–33.

Ashley, Jo Ann. *Hospitals, Paternalism, and the Role of the Nurse.* New York: Teachers College Press, 1976.

Brand, Karen, and Laurie Glass. "Perils and Parallels of Women and Nursing." *Nurs. Forum,* **14,**2 (1975), 160–174.

Christy, Teresa. "Portrait of a Leader: M. Adelaide Nutting." *Nurs. Outlook,* **17** (Jan. 1969), 20–24.

Christy, Teresa. "Portrait of a Leader: Isabel Hampton Robb." *Nurs. Outlook,* **17** (Mar. 1969), 26–29.

Christy, Teresa. "Portrait of a Leader: Lavinia

Lloyd Dock." *Nurs. Outlook*, **17** (June 1969), 72–75.

Christy, Teresa. "Portrait of a Leader: Isabel Maitland Stewart." *Nurs. Outlook,* **17** (Oct. 1969), 44–48.

Christy, Teresa. "Portrait of a Leader: Lillian D. Wald." *Nurs. Outlook,* **18** (Mar. 1970), 50–54.

Christy, Teresa. "Portrait of a Leader: Annie Warburton Goodrich." *Nurs. Outlook*, **18** (Aug. 1970), 46–50.

Christy, Teresa. "Equal Rights for Women: Voices From the Past." *Am. J. Nurs.*, **71** (Feb. 1971), 288–293.

Christy, Teresa. "Liberation Movement: Impact on Nursing." *AORN J.*, **15** (Apr. 1972), 67–72.

Christy, Teresa. "Entry into Practice: A Recurring Issue in Nursing History." *Am. J. Nurs.*, **80** (Mar. 1980), 485–488.

Christy, Teresa. "Clinical Practice as a Function of Nursing Education: An Historical Analysis." *Nurs. Outlook*, **28** (Aug. 1980), 493–497.

Christy, Teresa. "Portrait of a Leader: Sophia F. Palmer." *Nurs. Outlook,* **23** (Dec. 1975), 746–751.

Dock, Lavinia. "What We May Expect from the Law." *Am. J. Nurs.,* **50** (Oct. 1950), 599–600.

Heinrich, Janet. "Historical Perspectives on Public Health Nursing." *Nurs. Outlook*, **31** (Nov.–Dec. 1983), 317–320.

Kalisch, Beatrice, and Philip Kalisch. "An Analysis of the Sources of Physician–Nurse Conflict." *J. Nurs. Admin.*, **7** (Jan. 1977), 50–57.

"Lavinia L. Dock: Self-Portrait." *Nurs. Outlook,* **25** (Jan. 1977), 22–26.

"Lillian D. Wald," *Nurs. Outlook*, **19** (Oct. 1971), 659–660.

Lynaugh, Joan. "The Entry into Practice Conflict: How We Got Where We Are and What Will Happen Next." *Am. J. Nurs.*, **80** (Feb. 1980), 266–270.

Marshall, Helen. *Mary Adelaide Nutting: Pioneer of Modern Nursing.* Baltimore: Johns Hopkins Press, 1972.

Chapter 3 The Evolution of the Trained Nurse, 1873–1903

Alcott, L. M. *Hospital Sketches.* Boston: James Redpath, 1863.

Christy, Teresa. "Nurses in American History: The Fateful Decade, 1890–1900." *Am. J. Nurs.*, **75** (July 1975), 1163–1165.

Dolan, Josephine. "Nurses in American History:

Three Schools—1873." *Am. J. Nurs.*, **75** (June 1975), 989–992.

Parsons, Margaret, "Mothers and Matrons." *Nurs. Outlook*, **31** (Sept.–Oct. 1983), 274–278.

Shannon, Mary Lucille. "Nurses in American History: Our First Four Licensure Laws." *Am. J. Nurs.*, **75** (Aug. 1975), 1327–1329.

Chapter 4 The Emergence of the Modern Nurse, 1904–1965

Breckinridge, Mary. *Wide Neighborhoods: The Story of the Frontier Nursing Service.* New York: Harper & Row, Publishers, 1952.

Bullough, Bonnie. "Nurses in American History: The Lasting Impact of World War II on Nursing." *Am. J. Nurs.*, **76** (Jan. 1976), 118–120.

Donahue, M. Patricia. "Isabel Maitland Stewart's Philosophy of Education." *Nurs. Res.*, **32** (May–June 1983), 140–146.

Dreves, Katharine Densford. "Nurses in American History: Vassar Training Camp for Nurses." *Am J. Nurs.*, **75** (Nov. 1975), 2000–2002.

Fitzpatrick, M. Louise. "Nurses in American History: Nursing and the Great Depression." *Am. J. Nurs.*, **75** (Dec. 1975), 2188–2190.

Kalisch, Beatrice, and Philip Kalisch. "Nurses in American History: The Cadet Nurse Corps—in World War II." *Am. J. Nurs.*, **76** (Feb. 1976), 240–242.

Kalisch, Beatrice, and Philip Kalisch. "Nurses Under Fire: The World War II Experience of Nurses in Bataan and Corregidor." *Nurs. Res.*, **6** (Nov.–Dec. 1976), 409–429.

Kalisch, Philip. "How Army Nurses Became Officers: One Bar on a Shoulder Strap Is Worth Two Regulations in a Book." *Nurs. Res.*, **25** (May–June 1976), 164–177.

Kalisch, Philip, et al. "Louise Bourgeois and the Emergence of Modern Midwifery." *J. Nurse-Midwifery*, **26** (July–Aug. 1981), 3–17.

Lagemann, Ellen. *Nursing History: New Perspectives, New Possibilities.* New York: Teachers College Press, 1983.

Monteiro, Lois. "Lavinia L. Dock (1947) on Nurses and the Cold War." *Nurs. Forum*, **17**, 1 (1978), 46–54.

Watson, Joellen. "The Evolution of Nursing Education in the United States: 100 Years of a Profession for Women." *J. Nurs. Ed.* **16** (Sept. 1977), 31–38.

Chapter 5 Major Studies of the Nursing Profession

In the text of Chapter 5, the publisher and date of

publication are cited for older studies that were widely available. Many of these reports are now out of print. However, some libraries have photocopies, and microfilmed editions of most of them are also available. For information on the latter, address inquiries to University Microfilms, 300 N. Zeeb Rd., Ann Arbor, Michigan 48106.

Aiken, Linda. "Nursing's Future: Public Policies Private Actions." *Am. J. Nurs.*, **83** (Oct. 1983), 1440–1444.

Bowman, Marjorie, and William Walsh, Jr. "Perspectives on the GMENAC Report." *Health Affairs*, **1** (Fall 1982), 55–66.

Christy, Teresa, et al. "An Appraisal of 'An Abstract for Action,'" *Am. J. Nurs.*, **71** (Aug. 1971), 1574–1581.

Coelen, Craig, and Gary Gaumer. *Effects of Federal Support for Nursing Education in Admissions, Graduations, and Retention Rates at Schools of Nursing*. Cambridge, Mass.: Abt Associates, Inc., 1982.

"Commission Sums Up Findings in Eighteen Recommendations." *Am. J. Nurs.*, **83** (Sept. 1983), 1253.

"Credentialing in Nursing: A New Approach." *Am J. Nurs.*, **79** (Apr. 1979), 674–683. Also in *Nurs. Outlook*, **27** (Apr. 1979), 263–271.

"IOM Study Sees Need for Funds in Graduate Specialty Areas." *Am. J. Nurs.*, **83** (Mar. 1983), 343–344, 454.

Kelly, Lucie. "Endpaper: In Principle." *Nurs. Outlook*, **30** (June 1982), 370.

Kelly, Lucie. "No More Old News." *Nurs. Outlook*, **31** (July–Aug. 1983), 209.

Krekeler, Sister Kathleen. "The Detrimental Side of Tradition." *Sup. Nurs.*, **9** (Mar. 1978), 47–51.

Lysaught, Jerome P. *Action in Affirmation: Toward an Unambiguous Profession of Nursing*. New York: McGraw-Hill Book Company, 1981.

Mallison, Mary. "A New (Old) Prescription for Nursing." *Am. J. Nurs.*, **83** (Mar. 1983), 381.

Matejski, Myrtle. "Nursing Education, Professionalism, and Autonomy: Social Constraints and the Goldmark Report." *Adv. Nurs. Sci.*, **3** (Apr. 1981), 17–30.

Myths, Realities and Public Policy Dilemmas in Nursing. Interim Report. Washington, D.C. Institute of Medicine, July 1981.

Hospital Research and Educational Trust. *National Commission on Nursing Reports*. Chicago, Ill. The Trust, 1983.

Summary of the Public Hearings, July 1981 (Trust Catalog #9635).

Initial Report and Preliminary Recommendations, Sept. 1981 (Trust Catalog #654100).

Report of the Survey of Innovative Programs and Projects, Jan. 1982 (Trust Catalog #654640).

Nursing in Transition: Models for Successful Organizational Change Aug. 1982 (Trust Catalog #65450).

Summary Report and Recommendations, Apr. 1983 (Trust Catalog #654200)

"National Commission for the Study of Nursing and Nursing Education: Summary Report and Recommendations." *Am. J. Nurs.*, **70** (Feb. 1970), 279–294.

Nursing and Nursing Education: Public Policies and Private Actions. Washington, D.C.: National Academy Press, 1983.

Rawnsky, Marilyn. "The Goldmark Report: Midpoint in Nursing History." *Nurs. Outlook*, **21** (June 1973), 380–383.

"Report of the Task Force." *Nurs. Outlook*, **21** (Feb. 1973), 111–118.

The Study of Credentialing in Nursing: A New Approach, Vols. I and II. Kansas City, Mo: American Nurses' Association, 1979. Volume I presents a background of credentialing studies and recommendations. Volume II is a compilation of outstanding papers on credentialing and provides excellent references on the topic.

PART II CONTEMPORARY PROFESSIONAL NURSING

Aiken, Linda, ed. *Nursing in the 1980s: Crises, Opportunities, Challenges*. Philadelphia: J. B. Lippincott Company, 1982.

Aiken, Linda, ed. *Health Policy and Nursing Practice*. New York: McGraw-Hill Book Company, 1981.

Bullough, Bonnie, et al. *Nursing Issues and Nursing Strategies for the Eighties*. New York: Springer Publishing Company, 1983.

Chaska, Norma, ed. *The Nursing Profession: Views Through the Mist*. New York: McGraw-Hill Book Company, 1978.

Chaska, Norma, ed. *The Nursing Profession: A Time to Speak*. New York: McGraw-Hill Book Company, 1982.

Donnelly, Gloria, et al. *The Nursing System: Issues, Ethics, and Politics*. New York: John Wiley and Sons, Inc., 1980.

Duespohl, T. Audean. *Nursing in Transition*. Rockville, Md.: Aspen Systems Corporation, 1983.

McCloskey, Joanne, and Helen Grace, eds. *Current Issues in Nursing*. Boston: Blackwell Scientific Publications, 1981.

Nicholls, Marion, and Virginia Wessells, eds. *Nursing Standards and Nursing Process*. Wakefield, Mass: Contemporary Publishing Company, 1977.

SECTION 1 THE HEALTH CARE SETTING

Curtin, Leah. "Is There a Right to Health Care?" *Am. J. Nurs.*, **80**, (Mar. 1980), 462–465.

Donabedian, Avedis. "Quality, Cost and Cost Containment." *Nurs. Outlook*, **32** (May–June 1984), 142–145.

Fagerhaugh, Shizuka, et al. "The Impact of Technology on Patients, Providers, and Care Patterns." *Nurs. Outlook*, **28** (Nov. 1980), 666–672.

Friedan, Betty. *The Second Stage*. New York: Summit Books, 1981.

Gardner, Harold, and Marilyn Fiske. "Pluralism and Competition." *Am. J. Nurs.*, **81** (Dec. 1981), 2152–2157.

Ginzberg, Eli. "The Economics of Health Care and the Future of Nursing." *J. Nurs. Admin.*, **11** (Mar. 1981), 28–32.

Griffith, Hurdis. "Competition in Health Care." *Nurs. Outlook,* **31** (Sept.–Oct. 1983), 262–265.

Hadley, Jack. *More Medical Care, Better Health?* Washington, D.C.: Urban Institute Press, 1982.

Hawkins, Joellen, and Loretta Higgins. *Nursing and the American Health Care Delivery System*. New York: Tiresias Press, 1982.

"Health Care at the Crossroads: Competition or Regulation?" *Hospitals*, **56** (Feb. 1982), 28ff.

Jonas, Steven. *Health Care Delivery in the United States*. New York: Springer Publishing Company, 1981.

Krause, Elliott. *Power and Illness*. New York: Elsevier North-Holland, Inc., 1977.

Milio, Nancy. *Primary Care and the Public Health*. Lexington, Mass.: Lexington Books, 1983.

"Moving into the Second Stage: An Interview with Betty Friedan." *Nurs. Outlook*, **29** (Nov. 1981), 666–669.

Raffel, Marshall. *The United States Health System: Origins and Functions*. New York: John Wiley and Sons., Inc., 1980.

Roemer, Milton. *Comparative National Policies on Health Care*. New York: Marcel Dekker, Inc., 1977.

Sheridan, Donna. "The Health Care Industry in the Marketplace: Implications for Nursing." *J. Nurs. Admin.*, **13** (Sept. 1983), 36–40.

Smith, Judith. *The Idea of Health: Implications for the Nursing Professional*. New York: Teachers College Press, 1983.

Somers, Anne, and Herman Somers. *Health and Health Care: Policies in Perspective*. Germantown, Md.: Aspen Systems Corp., 1977.

Zwick, Daniel. "Establishing National Health Goals and Standards." *Pub. Health Rep.*, **98** (Sept.–Oct. 1983), 416–425.

Chapter 6 The Impact of Social and Scientific Changes

Armstrong, Myrna. "Paving the Way for More Effective Computer Usage." *Nurs. and Health Care*, **4** (Dec. 1983), 557–559.

Bayer, Ronald. "Women, Work, and Reproductive Hazards." *Hasting Center Rep.*, **12** (Oct. 1982), 14–19.

Boone, C. Keith. "Splicing Life, with Scalpel and Scythe." *Hastings Center Rep.*, **13** (Apr. 1983), 8–10.

Brownmiller, Susan. *Femininity*. New York: Simon & Schuster, Inc., 1983.

Cole, Thomas. "The 'Enlightened' View of Aging: Victorian Morality in a New Key." *Hasting Center Rep.*, **13** (June 1983), 34–40.

Computer Technology and Nursing. Conference Reports. Bethesda, Md. National Institute of Health, Department of Health and Human Services, 1983 and 1984.

Dagrosa, Terry. "Cancer in America: The Socialization and Promulgation of the Mystique." *Nurs. Forum.*, **19**, 4 (1980), 324.

Dean, Patricia. "Toward Androgeny." *Image*, **10** (Feb. 1978), 10–14.

Healthy People: The Surgeon General's Report on Health Promotion and Disease Prevention 1979. Washington, D.C.: Government Printing Office, 1983.

Kanter, Rosabeth. *The Change Masters: Innovations for Productivity in the American Corporation*. New York: Simon & Schuster, Inc., 1983.

Leavitt, Judith, ed. *Women and Health in America: Historical Readings*. Madison, Wisc.: University of Wisconsin Press, 1984.

Mattia, Michael. "Hazards in the Hospital Environment: Anesthesia Gases and Methylmethacrylate." *Am. J. Nurs.*, **83** (Jan. 1983), 73–77.

Mattia, Michael. "Hazards in the Hospital Environment: The Sterilants: Ethylene Oxide and

Formaldehyde." *Am. J. Nurs.*, **83** (Feb. 1983), 240–243.

McCormick, Kathleen. "Preparing Nurses for the Technologic Future." *Nurs. and Health Care*, **4** (Sept. 1983), 379–382.

Murray, Thomas. "Warning: Screening Workers for Genetic Risk." *Hasting's Center Rep.*, **13** (Feb. 1983), 5–8.

Schneir, Miriam, ed. *Feminism: The Essential Historical Writings.* New York: Vintage Books, 1972.

Sexton, Patricia. *The New Nightingales: Hospital Workers, Unions, New Women's Issues.* New York: Equity Press, 1982.

Sher, George, and Robert Lekachman. "Health Care and the Deserving Poor." *Hastings Center Rep.*, **13** (Feb. 1983), 9–14.

Skiba, Diane, and Mark Slichter. "Of Bits and Bytes." *Am. J. Nurs.*, **84** (Jan. 1984), 102–103.

Valentine, Jeanette, and Alonzo Plough. "Protecting the Reproductive Health of Workers: Problems in Science and Public Policy." *J. of Health Politics, Policy and Law*, **8** (Spring 1983), 144–163.

Much of the data on population and family planning were taken from reports of the Alan Guttmacher Institute, 360 Park Avenue South, New York, New York 10010. This institute also publishes *Family Planning Perspectives.* Also useful is *Population Reports* (Johns Hopkins University Population Information Program).

Several nursing journals have published issues with a major focus on computers. See *Nursing Outlook*, Jan. 1984; *Nursing Management*, July 1983.

There is also a computer column in the *American Journal of Nursing*, beginning in 1984, and an increasing number of such articles in many other nursing journals.

The Chronicle of Higher Education is a weekly newspaper that presents reports and discussions of the trends and issues in the field.

The publications of the World Health Organization are useful for their presentation of international health perspectives.

Both the *American Journal of Public Health* and *The Nation's Health*, publications of the American Public Health Association, publish numerous articles and reports on population, environmental hazards, and other aspects of public health.

Chapter 7 Health Care Delivery: Where

Bakken, Kenneth. "Integrated Health Care: The Whole Person in the Community." *Nurs. Economics*, **1** (Nov.–Dec. 1983), 178–180.

Carr, Charles, and Donna Carr. *Hospice Care: Principles and Practice.* New York: Springer Publishing Company, 1983.

Christman, Luther, and Michael Counte. *Hospital Organization and Health Care Delivery.* Boulder, Colo.: Westview Press, 1981.

Dayani, Elizabeth, et al. "Financing Health Promotion/Wellness." *Nurse Practitioner*, **6** (Aug. 1981), 37–42.

Dowling, Harry. *City Hospitals: The Undercare of the Underprivileged.* Cambridge, Mass.: Harvard University Press, 1982.

Feldman, Saul. "Out of the Hospitals, Into the Streets: The Overselling of Benevolence." *Hastings Center Rep.*, **13** (June 1983), 5–7.

Freshnock, L., and L. Jensen. "The Changing Structure of Medical Group Practice in the United States, 1969–1980." *J. Am. Med. Assn.*, **245** (June 1981), 2173.

Goodrich, Thelma, and G. Anthony Garry. "The Process of Ambulatory Care: A Comparison of the Hospital and the Community Health Center." *Am. J. Pub. Health*, **70** (Mar. 1980), 251–255.

Johnston, Maxene. "Ambulatory Health Care in the 80's." *Am. J. Nurs.*, **80** (Jan. 1980), 76–79.

Kerr, Frederick. "Considering a New Structure: The Health Services Holding Company." *Law, Med. and Health Care*, **11** (Oct. 1983), 214–219.

King, Carol. "The Self-Help/Self-Care Concept." *Nurse Practitioner*, **5** (May–June 1980), 34–35ff.

Mark, Barbara. "Investor-Owned and Nonprofit Hospitals: A Comparison." *Nurs. Economics*, **1** (July–Aug. 1984), 240–245.

Marszalek, Ellen. "Ambulatory Care Nursing: At the Crossroads." *Nurs. and Health Care*, **1** (Dec. 1980), 254–255.

Miller, C. Arden, et al. "A Survey of Local Public Health Departments and Their Directors." *Am. J. Pub. Health*, **67** (Oct. 1977), 931–939.

Mundinger, Mary. *Home Care Controversy: Too Little, Too Late, Too Costly.* Rockville, Md.: Aspens Systems Corporation, 1983.

Munley, Anne. *The Hospice Alternative: A New Context for Death and Dying.* New York: Basic Books, 1983.

Schwartz, R. "Multipurpose Day Centers: A Needed Alternative." *J. Gerontological Nursing*, **5** (1979), 48–53.

Shamansky, Sherry, and Cherie Clausen. "Levels

of Prevention: Examination of the Concept." *Nurs. Outlook*, **28** (Feb. 1980), 104–108.

Slavinsky, Ann, and Ann Cousins. "Homeless Women." *Nurs. Outlook*, **30** (June 1982), 358–362.

Smith, Shirley, and Nancy Bohnet. "Organization and Administration of Hospice Care." *J. Nurs. Admin.*, **13** (Nov. 1983), 10–16.

Thornton, Joyce. "Developing a Rural Nursing Clinic." *Nurse Educator*, **8** (Summer 1983), 24–29.

Vladeck, Bruce E. *Unloving Care*. New York: Basic Books, 1980.

Wald, Florence, et al. "The Hospice Movement as a Health Care Reform." *Nurs. Outlook*, **28** (Mar. 1980), 173–178.

Other good reference sources for current issues, problems, and trends in institutions are *Hospitals*, the AHA journal, *Hospital Progress*, the CHA journal, and other journals in the field, which always include nontechnical articles.

The best source of current, comprehensive data on health resources, although usually several years old, is the U.S. Department of Health and Human Services. The journal *Family and Community Health* puts great emphasis on innovative health care delivery. Almost every issue has several pertinent articles.

Chapter 8 Health Care Delivery: Who

Barney, Jane. "A New Perspective on Nurse's Aide Training." *Geriatric Nurs.*, **4** (Jan.–Feb. 1983), 44–48.

Copeland, Gary, and David Apgar. "The Pharmacist Practitioner Training Program." *Drug Intell. and Cl. Pharm*, **14** (Feb. 1980), 114–119.

Engel, Gloria. "A Longitudinal Investigation of Physician's Assistants' Perceptions as Members of a Health Care Team: A Preliminary Study." *Am. J. Pub. Health*, **70** (June 1980), 631–633.

Fraundorf, Kenneth. "Organized Dentistry and the Pursuit of Entry Control." *J. Health Politics, Policy, and Law*, **8** (Winter 1984), 759–781.

Friedman, Elliot. "Declaration of Interdependence." *Hosp.*, **57** (July 1983), 73–80.

Ginzberg, Eli. "The Future Supply of Physicians: From Pluralism to Policy." *Health Affairs*, **1** (Fall 1982), 6–19.

Grad, John. "Allied Health Professionals and Hospital Privileges: An Introduction to the Is-

sues." *Law, Med. and Health Care*, **10** (Sept. 1982), 165–167.

Grau, Lois, "Case Management and the Nurse." *Ger. Nurs.* **5** (Nov.–Dec. 1984), 372–375.

Hicks, Barbara, et al. "The Triage Experiment in Coordinated Care for the Elderly." *Am. J. Pub. Health*, **71** (Sept. 1981), 991–1003.

Jackson, Geraldine. *A Selected Bibliography on Nurse Practitioners and Physician Assistants*. Springfield, Va.: National Technical Information Service, 1981.

McGuire, Christine, et al. *Handbook of Health Professions Education*. San Francisco: Jossey-Bass Publishers, 1983.

"Medical Education in the United States 1982–1983," *J. Am. Med. Assn.*, **250** (Sept. 23 and 30, 1983), whole issue.

Oliver, Denis, et al. "Practice Characteristics of Male and Female Physician Assistants." *Am. J. Pub. Health*, **74** (Dec. 1984), 1398–1400.

Pesznecker, Betty, et al. "Collaborative Practice Models in Community Health Nursing." *Nurs. Outlook*, **30** (May 1982), 298–302.

Pigg, R. Morgan. "A National Study on Professional Preparation in Patient Education." *Am. J. Pub. Health*, **72** (Feb. 1982), 180–182.

Rauch, Terry. "Job Satisfaction in the Practice of Clinical Pharmacy." *Am. J. Pub. Health*, **71** (May 1981), 527–529.

Ritchey, Ferris, et al. "Physicians' Opinions of Expanded Clinical Pharmacy Services." *Am. J. Pub. Health*, **73** (Jan. 1983), 96–101.

Rosenstein, David, et al. "Professional Encroachment: A Comparison of the Emergence of Denturists in Canada and Oregon." *Am. J. Pub. Health*, **70** (June 1980), 614–623.

Silver, George. "Chiropractic: Professional Controversy and Public Policy." *Am. J. Pub. Health*, **70** (Apr. 1980), 348–351.

Smith, Marybelle. "A Team Approach to Health Care." *Nurs. Outlook*, **31** (Sept.–Oct. 1983), 271, 273.

Somers, Anne. "And Who Shall Be the Gatekeeper? The Role of the Primary Physician in the Health Care Delivery System." *Inquiry*, **20** (Winter 1983), 301–313.

Starr, Paul. *The Social Transformation of American Medicine*. New York: Basic Books, 1981.

Weston, Jerry. "Distribution of Nurse Practitioners and Physicians' Assistants: Implications of Legal Constraints and Reimbursement." *Pub. Health Rep*, **95** (May–June 1980), 253–258.

SECTION 2 NURSING IN THE HEALTH CARE SCENE

Chapter 9 Nursing as a Profession

Brodish, Mary. "Nursing Practice Conceptualized: An Interaction Model." *Image*, **14** (Feb.–Mar. 1982), 5–7.

Brown, Marie Scott, and Cathie Burns. "The Thinker-Doer Dual Nursing Role." *Nurse Practitioner*, **9** (Mar. 1984), 60–63.

Carlson, Judith, and Anne McGuire. *Nursing Diagnosis*. Philadelphia: W. B. Saunders Company, 1982.

Christman, Luther. "The Practitioner-Teacher." *Nurs. Educator*, **4** (Mar.–Apr. 1979), 8–11.

De Santis, Grace. "Power, Tactics, and the Professionalization Process." *Nurs. and Health Care*, **4** (Jan. 1982), 14–24.

Diers, Donna. "Between Science and Humanity: Nursing Reclaims Its Role." *Nurs. Outlook*, **39** (Sept.–Oct. 1982), 459–463.

Diers, Donna, and David Evans. "Excellence in Nursing." *Image*, **12** (June 1980), 27–30.

Donley, Sister Rosemary. "Why Has Nursing Been Slow in Developing a Theoretical Base?" *Image*, **12** (Feb. 1980), 2.

Engel, Nancy. "Confirmation and Violation: The Caring That Is Nursing." *Image*, (Oct. 1980), 53–56.

Engstrom, Janet. "Problems in the Development, Use and Testing of Nursing Theory." *J. Nurs. Ed.*, **23** (June 1984), 245–251.

Erickson, Helen, et al. *Modeling and Role Modeling: A Theory and Paradigm for Nursing.* Englewood Cliffs, N.J.: Prentice-Hall, Inc., 1983.

Fagin, Claire, and Donna Diers. "Nursing as Metaphor." *Am. J. Nurs.*, **83**: (Sept. 1983), 1362.

Fawcett, Jacqueline. "On Development of a Scientific Community." *Image*, **12** (Oct. 1980), 51–52.

Fawcett, Jacqueline. *Analysis and Evaluation of Conceptual Models of Nursing.* Philadelphia: F. A. Davis Company, 1984.

Flaskerud, Jacquelyn. "Avoidance and Distancing: A Descriptive View of Nursing." *Nurs. Forum*, **18** (1979), 158–173.

Hodgman, Eileen. "Excellence in Nursing." *Image*, **11** (Feb. 1979), 22–27.

Kim, Hesook Suzie. *The Nature of Theoretical Thinking*. Norwalk, Conn.: Appelton-Century-Crofts, 1983.

Kritek, Phyllis. "The Generation and Classification of Nursing Diagnoses." *Image*, **10** (1978), 33–40.

Masson, VeNeta. "Nursing: Healing in a Feminine Mode." *J. Nurs. Admin.* **11** (Oct. 1981), 20–25.

McMurrey, Phoebe. "Toward a Unique Knowledge Base in Nursing." *Image*, **14** (Feb.–Mar. 1982), 12–15.

Newman, Margaret. "Nursing Diagnosis: Looking at the Whole." *Am. J. Nurs.* **84** (Dec. 1984), 1496–1499.

Shamansky, Sherry, and Celeste Yanni. "In Opposition to Nursing Diagnosis: A Minority Opinion." *Image*, **15** (Spring 1983), 47–50.

Stevens, Barbara. *Nursing Theory: Analysis, Application, Evaluation.* Boston: Little, Brown and Company, 1979.

White, Caroline. "A Critique of the ANA Social Policy Statement." *Nurs. Outlook*, **32** (Nov.–Dec. 1984), 328–331.

Winstead-Fry, Pat. "The Need to Differentiate a Nursing Self." *Am. J. Nurs.*, **77** (Sept. 1977), 1452–1454.

Yura, Helen, and Mary Walsh. *The Nursing Process: Assessing, Planning, Implementing, Evaluating.* Norwalk, Conn.: Appleton-Century-Crofts, 1983.

Chapter 10 Professional Ethics and Accountability

American Nurses' Association. *Ethics in Nursing: References and Resources.* Kansas City, Mo.: The Association, 1979.

Aroskar, Mila. "Anatomy of an Ethical Dilemma—the Theory." *Am. J. Nurs.*, **80** (Apr. 1980), 658–660. "The Practice." 661–663.

Bandman, Elsie, and Bertram Bandman. *Bioethical and Human Rights.* Boston: Little, Brown and Company, 1978.

Bayles, M. D. "The Value of Life—By What Standard?" *Am. J. Nurs.*, **80** (Dec. 1980), 2226–2230.

Boyar, Dawn, and Joyce Avery. "Peer Review: Change and Growth." *Nurs. Admin. Q.*, **5** (Winter 1981), 59–66.

Chance, Kathryn. "Nursing Models: A Requisite for Professional Accountability." *Adv. in Nurs. Sci.*, **4** (Jan. 1982), 57–65.

Childress, James. *Who Should Decide? Paternalism in Health Care.* New York: Oxford University Press, 1982.

Christman, Luther. "Accountability and Autonomy Are More Than Rhetoric." *Nurse Educator*, **3** (July–Aug. 1979), 3–9.

Curtin, Leah. "A Proposed Model for Critical Ethical Analysis." *Nurs. Forum*, **17**(1) (1978), 12–17.

Daniel, Irvine. "Impaired Professionals: Responsibilities and Roles." *Nurs. Economics*, **2** (May-June 1984), 190-193.

Donahue, M. Patricia. "The Nurse—a Patient Advocate?" *Nurs. Forum*, **17**(2) (1978), 143-151.

Fry, Sara. "Dilemma in Community Health Ethics." *Nurs. Outlook*, **31** (May-June 1983), 176-179.

Fry, Sara. "Rationing Health Care: The Ethics of Cost Containment." *Nurs. Economics*, **1** (Nov.-Dec. 1983), 165-169.

Hawks, Jane. "Should Nurses Give Moral Advice?" *Image*, **16** (Winter 1984), 14-16.

Hull, Robert. "Responsibility and Accountability Analyzed." *Nurs. Outlook*, **29** (Dec. 1981), 707-712.

Kohnke, Mary. *Advocacy: Risk and Reality*. St. Louis: C. V. Mosby Company, 1982.

Levine, Myra. "The Ethics of Computer Technology in Health Care." *Nurs. Forum*, **19**(2) (1980), 193-198.

Marchewka, Ann. "When Is Paternalism Justifiable?" *Am. J. Nurs.*, **83** (July 1983), 1072-1073.

McClure, M. "The Long Road to Accountability." *Nurs. Outlook*, **26** (Jan. 1978), 47-50.

Mooney, Mary Margaret. "The Ethical Component of Nursing Theory." *Image*, **12** (Feb. 1980), 7-9.

Murphy, Catherine. "The Changing Role of Nurses in Making Ethical Decisions," *Law, Med. and Health Care*, **12** (Sept. 1984), 173-175, 184.

Prato, Sue Ann. "Ethical Decisions in Daily Practice." *Sup. Nurse*, **12** (July 1981), 18-20.

Smith, Christine. "Outrageous or Outraged: A Nurse Advocate Story." *Nurs. Outlook*, **28** (Oct. 1980), 624-625.

Steele, Shirley, And Vera Harmon. *Values Clarification in Nursing*, 2nd ed. Norwarlk, Conn.: Appleton-Century Crofts, 1983.

Thompson, Joyce, and Henry Thompson. *Ethics in Nursing*. New York: Macmillan Publishing Company, 1981.

Veatch, Robert. "Nursing Ethics, Physician Ethics, and Medical Ethics." *Law, Med. and Health Care*, **9** (Oct. 1981), 17-19.

Warren, J. J. "Accountability and Nursing Diagnosis." *J. Nurs. Admin.*, **13** (Oct. 1983), 34-37.

Weber, Leonard. "Ethics Commission Access Report Urges Adequate Care for Ill." *Hosp. Progress*, **65** (July-Aug. 1984), 62-65.

The entire March 1979 issue of *Nursing Clinics of North America* is devoted to bioethical issues. The *Hastings Center Report* consists totally of articles on ethics.

Chapter 11 Profile of the Modern Nurse

Dunkelberger, John, and Sophia Aadland. "Expectation and Attainment of Nursing Careers." *Nurs. Res.*, **33** (July-Aug. 1984), 235-240.

Greenleaf, Nancy. "Labor Force Participation Among Registered Nurses and Women in Comparable Occupations." *Nurs. Res.*, **32** (Sept.-Oct. 1983), 306-311.

Hardin, Sally, and Denise Benton. "Fish or Fowl: Nursing's Ambivalence Toward Its Symbols." *J. Nurs. Ed.*, **23** (Apr. 1984), 164-167.

Kalisch, Beatrice, and Philip Kalisch. "How the Public Sees Nurse-Midwives: 1978 News Coverage of Nurse-Midwifery in the Nation's Press." *J. Nurse-Midwifery*, **25** (July-Aug. 1980), 31-39.

Kalisch, Beatrice, and Philip Kalisch. "Perspectives on Improving Nursing's Public Image." *Nurs. and Health Care*, **1** (July-Aug. 1980), 10-15.

Kalisch, Beatrice, and Philip Kalisch. "An Analysis of News Flow on the Nation's Nurse Shortage." *Med. Care*, **19** (Sept. 1981), 938-950.

Kalisch, Beatrice, and Philip Kalisch. "Nurses on Prime-Time Television." *Am. J. Nurs.*, **82** (Feb. 1982), 264-270.

Kalisch, Beatrice, and Philip Kalisch. "Improving the Image of Nursing." *Am. J. Nurs.*, **83** (Jan. 1983), 48-52.

Kalisch, Beatrice, and Philip Kalisch. "An Analysis of the Impact of Authorship on the Image of the Nurse Presented in Novels." *Res. Nurs. and Health*, **6** (Mar. 1983), 17-24.

Kalisch, Beatrice, et al. "Reflections on a Television Image: The Nurses, 1962-1965." *Nurs. and Health Care*, **2** (May 1981), 248-255.

Kalisch, Beatrice, et al. "The Nurse as a Sex Object in Motion Pictures, 1930 to 1980." *Res. Nurs. and Health*, **5** (Sept. 1982), 147-154.

Kalisch, Beatrice, et al. "When Nurses Are Accused of Murder." *Nurs. Life*, **2** (Sept.-Oct. 1982), 44-47.

Kalisch, Philip, and Beatrice Kalisch. "The Image of Psychiatric Nurses in Motion Pictures." *Perspect. in Psych. Care*, **19**(3,4) (1981), 116-129.

Kalisch, Philip, and Beatrice Kalisch. "When Nurses Were National Heroines: Images of Nursing in American Film, 1942-1945." *Nurs. Forum*, **20**(1) (1981), 15-61.

Kalisch, Philip, and Beatrice Kalisch. "The Nurse-

Detective in American Movies." *Nurs. and Health Care*, **3** (Mar. 1982), 146–153.

Kalisch, Philip, and Beatrice Kalisch. "The Image of the Nurse in Motion Pictures." *Am J. Nurs.*, **82** (Apr. 1982), 605–611.

Kalisch, Philip, and Beatrice Kalisch. "The Image of Nurses in Novels." *Am. J. Nurs.*, **82** (Aug. 1982), 1220–1224.

Kalisch, Philip, et al. "World of Nursing on Primetime Television, 1950–1980." *Nurs. Res.*, **31** (Nov.–Dec. 1982), 358–363.

Murphy, Jeanne. "Seventeen Large Hospitals Surveyed: Trends Revealed." *Nurs. and Health Care*, **1** (July–Aug. 1980), 34–39.

Williams, Carolyn, ed. *Image-Making in Nursing.* Kansas City, Mo.: American Academy of Nursing, 1983.

Woolley, Alma. "Nursing's Image on Campus." *Nurs. Outlook*, **29** (Aug. 1981), 460–466.

The entire Feb.–Mar. issue of *Imprint* is focused on the nursing image. For follow-up letters, see the Sept.–Oct. issue, pp. 8–9.

SECTION 3 NURSING EDUCATION AND RESEARCH

Henderson, Margaret, ed. *Nursing Education.* New York: Churchill-Livingston Company, 1982.

Houle, Cyril. *Patterns of Learning.* San Francisco: Jossey-Bass Publishers, 1984.

Popiel, Elda. *Nursing and the Process of Continuing Education*, 2nd ed. St. Louis: C. V. Mosby Company, 1977.

Various nursing journals carry a large number of articles on nursing education and research: *Journal of Nursing Education, Nurse Educator, Journal of Continuing Education, Nursing Outlook*, and *Nursing and Health Care. The Chronicle of Higher Education* is an excellent weekly publication that carries both articles and news items related to education. ANA, NLN, and AACN have extensive publication lists that include books, proceedings, statistics, and position papers on nursing education. *Nursing Administration Quarterly*, **2** (Winter 1978): the entire issue is devoted to continuing education; **3** Spring, Summer (1979): the entire issue is devoted to nursing education from a nursing administration standpoint; the news section of *AJN* carries monthly news items on the progress and problems of the entry into practice issue. *American Nurse* also carries such news items, as well as editorials and articles on the subject.

Chapter 12 Major Issues and Trends in Nursing Education

Beckes, Isaac. "Toward an Understanding of Accreditation Practice." *Nurs. and Health Care*, **2** (Feb. 1981), 68–72.

Bower, Dolores. "Part-Time Faculty: Responsibilities, Opportunities, Employment Terms." *Nurs. Outlook*, **28** (Jan. 1980), 43–45.

Buckley, John. "Faculty Commitment to Recruitment and Retention of Black Students." *Nurs. Outlook*, **28** (Jan. 1980), 46–50.

Chamings, Patricia, and James Teevan. "Comparison of Expected Competencies of Baccalaureate and Associate Degree Graduates in Nursing." *Image*, **11** (Feb. 1979), 16–21.

Christy, Teresa. "Clinical Practice as a Function of Nursing Education: An Historical Analysis." *Nurs. Outlook*, **28** (Aug. 1980), 493–497.

Claerbaut, D. "New Directions in the Education of Minority Nursing Students." *J. Nurs. Ed.*, **19** (Mar. 1980), 11–15.

Dell, M., and G. Halpin. "Predictors of Success in Nursing School and on State Board Examinations in a Predominately Black Baccalaureate Nursing Program." *J. Nurs. Ed.*, **23** (Apr. 1984), 147–150.

De Marco, Nicholas, and Mildred Hilliard. "Comparisons of Associate, Diploma, and Baccalaureate Nurses' State Boards, Quality of Patient Care, Competency Rating, Subordinates' Satisfaction with Supervision and Self-Report Job Satisfaction Scores." *Int. J. Nurs. Stud.*, **15** (1978), 163–170.

de Tornyay, Rheba. "Changing Student Relationships, Roles, and Responsibilities." *Nurs. Outlook*, **25** (Mar. 1977), 188–193.

Ehrat, Karen. "Educational/Career Mobility: Antecedent of Change." *Nurs. and Health Care*, **2** (Nov. 1981), 487–499ff.

Galarowicz, Lea Rae. "Closing a Diploma School: A Time for Flexibility and Creativity." *Nurs. and Health Care*, **4** (Apr. 1983), 188–191.

Group, Thetis, and Joan Roberts. "Exorcising the Ghosts of the Crimea." *Nurs. Outlook*, **22** (June 1974), 368–372.

Heller, Barbara. "Associate Degree Nursing: Faculty Preparation and Commitment." *Nurs. Outlook*, **30** (May 1982), 310–311.

Lenburg, Carrie. "The External Degree in Nursing: The Promise Fullfilled." *Nurs. Outlook*, **24** (July 1976), 422–429.

Mauksch, Ingeborg. "Faculty Practice: A Professional Imperative.'' *Nurse Educator*, **5** (May–June 1980), 21–24.

Mooneyhan, Esther. ''The Demise of a Baccalaureate Program for Registered Nurses: Lessons Learned.'' *Nurs. and Health Care*, **4** (Apr. 1983), 192–197.

Muzio, Lois, and Julianne Ohaski. ''The RN Student—Unique Characteristics, Unique Needs.'' *Nurs. Outlook*, **27** (Aug. 1979), 528–532.

Nayer, Dorothy. ''Unification: Bringing Nursing Service and Nursing Education Together.'' *Am. J. Nurs.*, **80** (June 1980), 1110–1114.

''NLN Accreditation Study Report Approved—Major Improvements Forthcoming.'' *Nurs. and Health Care*, **2** (Dec. 1981), 565–568.

Petrie, John. ''Medicare Reimbursement for Nursing Education: Discriminatory?'' *Hosp. Prog.*, **62** (Dec. 1981), 50–52.

Soules, H. Maxine. ''Professional Advancement and Salary Differentials Among Baccalaureate, Diploma, and Associate Degree Nurses.'' *Nurs. Forum*, **17** (Feb. 1978), 184–201.

Starck, Patricia. ''Realism in Nursing Curricula.'' *Nurs. Outlook*, **32** (July–Aug. 1984), 220–224.

Styles, Margretta, and Holly Wilson. ''The Third Resolution.'' *Nurs. Outlook*, **27** (Jan. 1979), 44–47.

Trandel-Korenchuk, Darlene, and Keith Trandel-Korenchuk. ''Entry into Nursing Practice: Does Nursing History Repeat Itself? *Nurse Practitioner*, **9** (Mar. 1984), 15–25.

Wakefield-Fisher, Mary. ''The Issue: Faculty Practice.'' *J. Nurs. Ed.*, **22** (May 1983), 207–210.

Chapter 13 Programs in Nursing Education

''A Decade of Progress in Continuing Education in Nursing.'' *J. Cont. Ed. in Nurs.*, **11** (May–June 1980), 60–65.

Anderson, N. E. ''The Historical Development of American Nursing Education.'' *J. Nurs. Ed.*, **20** (Jan. 1981), 18–35.

Balint, Jane, et al. ''Job Opportunities for Master's Prepared Nurses.'' *Nurs. Outlook*, **31** (Mar.–Apr. 1983), 109–114.

Beare, Patricia, et al. ''Doctoral Curricula in Nursing.'' *Nurs. Outlook*, **29** (May 1981), 311–316.

Brimmer, Pauline, et al. ''Nurse Doctorates: Personal and Employment Characteristics.'' *Res. in Nurs. and Health*, **6** (Dec. 1983), 157–165.

Chatham, M. A. ''Discrepancies in Learning Needs Assessment: Whose Needs Are Being Assessed?'' *J. Cont. Ed. in Nurs.*, **10** (Sept.–Oct. 1979), 18–22.

Cooper, Signe, and Mary Neal. *Perspectives in Continuing Education in Nursing*. Pacific Palisades, Calif.: Nurseco, Inc. 1980.

Cox, Cheryl, and Baker, Marion. ''Evaluation: The Key to Accountability in Continuing Education.'' *J. Cont. Ed. in Nurs.*, **12** (Jan.–Feb. 1981), 11–19.

Curran, Connie, et al. ''Selecting a Doctoral Program for a Career in Nursing.'' *Nurse Educator*, **6** (Feb. 1981), 11–15.

Friedman, Freda. ''As the 'RN Gap' Becomes a Chasm, LPNs Move In.'' *RN*, **4** (Dec. 1981), 50–53.

Goldstein, Joan. ''Comparison of Graduating AD and Baccalaureate Nursing Students' Characteristics.'' *Nurs. Res.*, **29** (Jan.–Feb. 1980), 46–49.

Gorney-Fadiman, Mary Jo. ''A Student's Perspectives on the Doctoral Dilemma.'' *Nurs. Outlook*, **29** (Nov. 1981), 650–654.

Heller, Barbara. ''Associate Degree Nursing: Preparation and Practice.'' *Nurs. Outlook*, **30** (May 1982), 310–311.

Kramer, Marlene. ''Philosophical Foundations of Baccalaureate Nursing Education.'' *Nurs. Outlook*, **29** (Apr. 1981), 224–228.

Larocco, S., et al. ''A Study of Nurses' Attitudes Toward Mandatory Continuing Education for Relicensure.'' *J. Cont. Ed. in Nurs.*, **9** (Jan.–Feb. 1978), 25–35.

McElmurry, Beverly, et al. ''Resources for Graduate Education: A Report of a Survey of Forty States in the Midwest, West, and Southern Regions.'' *Nurs. Res.*, **31** (Jan.–Feb. 1982), 5–10.

Mathews, A. E., and S. Schumacher. ''A Survey of Registered Nurses' Conceptions of and Participation Factors in Professional Continuing Education.'' *J. Cont. Ed. in Nurs.*, **10** (Jan.–Feb. 1979), 21–27.

Montag, Mildred. ''Looking Back: Associate Degree Education in Perspective.'' *Nurs. Outlook*, **28** (Apr. 1980), 248–250.

Murphy, Nell, et al. ''A Data-Based Approach to Continuing Education.'' *J. Cont. Ed. in Nurs.*, **13** (Mar.–Apr. 1982), 4–9.

Norris, C. Gail. ''Characteristics of the Adult Learner and Extended Higher Education for Registered Nurses.'' *Nurs. and Health Care*, **1** (Sept. 1980), 87–93, 112.

Price, Sylvia. ''Master's Programs Preparing Nurse Administrators.'' *J. Nurs. Admin.*, **14** (Jan. 1984), 11–17.

Sweeney, Mary Ann, et al. ''Essential Skills for Baccalaureate Graduates' Perspectives of Education and Service." *J. Nurs. Admin.*, **10** (Oct. 1980), 37–44.

Welch, Deborah. "The Real Issues Behind Providing Continuing Education in Nursing." *J. Cont. Ed. in Nurs.*, **11** (Mar. 1980), 17–21.

Chapter 14 Nursing Research: Status, Problems, Issues

Cleland, Virginia. "Nursing Research and Graduate Education." *Nurs. Outlook*, **23** (Oct. 1975), 642–645.

Downs, Florence. "Caveat Emptor." *Nurs. Res.*, **33** (Mar.–Apr. 1984), 59.

Evans, David. "Everynurse as Researcher: An Argumentative Critique of *Principles and Practice of Nursing.*" *Nurs. Forum*, **11**(4) (1980), 335–349.

Fawcett, Jacqueline. "On Research and the Professionalization of Nursing." *Nurs. Forum*, **19**(3) (1980), 310–317.

Fawcett, Jacqueline. "Utilization of Nursing Research Findings." *Image*, **14** (June 1982), 57–58.

Fine, Ruth. "Marketing Nursing Research." *J. Nurs. Admin.*, **10** (Nov. 1980), 21–23.

Gortner, Susan R. "Scientific Accountability in Nursing." *Nurs. Outlook*, **22** (Dec. 1974), 764–768.

Hoskins, Carol. "Nursing Research: Its Direction and Future." *Nurs. Forum*, **13**(2) (1979), 175–186.

King, Daniel, et al. "Disseminating the Results of Nursing Research." *Nurs. Outlook*, **29** (Mar. 1980), 164–169.

Kramer, Marlene, et al. "The Teaching of Nursing Research—Part II: A Literature Review of Teaching Strategies." *Nurse Educator*, **6** (Mar.–Apr. 1981), 30–37.

Larson, Elaine, "Health Policy and NIH: Implications for Nursing Research. "*Nurs. Res.* **33** (Nov.–Dec. 1984), 352–356.

Lindeman, Carol, and Janelle Krueger. "Increasing the Quality, Quantity and Use of Nursing Research." *Nurs. Outlook*, **25** (July 1977), 450–454.

MacPherson, Kathleen. "Feminist Methods: A New Paradigm for Nursing Research." *Adv. Nurs. Sci.*, **5** (Jan. 1983), 17–25.

Murdaugh, Carolyn, et al. "The Teaching of Nursing Research: A Survey Report." *Nurse Educator*, **6** (Jan.–Feb. 1981), 29.

Nieswiadomy, Rose. "Nurse Educators' Involvement in Research." *J. Nurs. Ed.*, **23** (Feb. 1984), 52–56.

Oakley, Deborah. "The Case of Federal Funding for Nursing Research." *Nurs. Res.*, **39** (Nov.–Dec. 1981), 360–365.

Paletta, Jeanne Lynch. "Nursing Research: An Integral Part of Professional Nursing." *Image*, **12** (Feb. 1980), 3–6.

Parker, Meredith, and Georgie Labadie. "Demystifying Research Mystique." *Nurs. and Health Care*, **4** (Sept, 1983), 383–386.

Thomas, B., and M. Price. "Research Preparation in Baccalaureate Nursing Education." *Nurs. Res.*, **29** (July–Aug. 1980), 259–261.

The first two issues of *Advances in Nursing Science* focus entirely on practice-oriented nursing theory (Oct. 1978 and Jan. 1979). It is also useful to become acquainted with the books on nursing reseach and all the nursing research journals. The latter frequently have abstracts of research as well as detailed articles. The summer 1978 issue of *Nursing Administration Quarterly* is devoted to the impact of research on patient care, as is most of *Image* of Oct. 1979.

SECTION 4 THE PRACTICE OF NURSING

Mauksch, Ingeborg. *Primary Care: A Contemporary Perspective.* New York: Grune & Stratton, 1981.

Riccardi, Betty, and Elizabeth Dayani. *The Nurse Entrepreneur.* Reston, Va.: Reston Publishing Company, 1982.

Chapter 15 Areas of Nursing Practice

Adair, Melanie, and N. Korter Nygard. "Theory Z Management: Can It Work for Nursing?" *Nurs. and Health Care*, **3** (Nov. 1982), 489–491.

Aiken, Linda. "The Nurse Labor Market." *Health Affairs*, **1** (Fall 1982), 30–40.

Barnett, Sandra, and Pati Sellers. "Neonatal Critical Care Nurse Practitioner: A New Role in Neonatology." *MCN*, **4** (Sept.–Oct. 1979), 279–280ff.

Battista, Louise. "Careers in Nephrology Nursing." *Imprint*, **30** (Sept.–Oct. 1983), 29–32.

Betz, Michael, et al. "Cost and Quality: Primary and Team Nursing Compared." *Nurs. and Health Care*, **1** (Oct. 1980), 150–157.

Castiglia, Patricia, et al. "The Development and Operation of a Professional Nursing Corporation." *MCN*, **4** (July–Aug. 1979), 205–208.

Coleman, John, et al. "Nursing Careers in the Emerging Systems." *Nurs. Mgt.*, **15** (Jan. 1984), 19–27.

Duxbury, Mitzi. "You Can Be a Nurse Researcher." *MCN*, **3** (Jan.–Feb. 1978), 13–14.

Engelke, Martha. "Nursing in Ambulatory Services: A Head Nurse's Perspective." *Am. J. Nurs.*, **80** (Oct. 1980), 1813–1815.

Fleming, Juanita. "Tenure Today." *Am. J. Nurs.*, **83** (Feb. 1983), 279–280.

Fine, Ruth. "The Supply and Demand of Nursing Administrators." *Nurs. and Health Care*, **4** (Jan. 1983), 10–15.

Ford, Loretta. "A Nurse for All Settings." *Nurs. Outlook*, **27** (Aug. 1979), 516–521.

Hanks, Nancy. "The Future of Critical Care Nursing." *Crit. Care Focus*, **9** (Dec. 1982–Jan. 1983), 20–23.

"How Can I Get a Job on Capitol Hill?" *Am. J. Nurs.*, **81** (Jan. 1981), 112–116.

Igoe, Judith. "What Is School Nursing? A Plea for More Standardized Roles." *MCN*, **5** (Sept.–Oct. 1980), 307–311.

Lenz, Elizabeth, and Carolyn Waltz. "Patterns of Job Search and Mobility." *J. Nurs. Ed.*, **22** (Sept. 1983), 267–273.

Lewis, Mary Ann. "Managing Nurse Practitioners in Ambulatory Care: What Are the Issues?" *J. Nurs. Admin.*, **10** (July 1980), 11–16.

Marchione, Joanne, and T. Neal Garland. "An Emerging Profession? The Case of the Nurse Practitioner." *Image*, **12** (June 1980), 37–40.

Masson, Ve Neta. "International Nursing: What Is It and Who Does It?" *Am. J. Nurs.*, **79** (July 1979), 1242–1243.

Meleis, Afaf. "Oil Rich, Nurse Poor: The Nursing Crisis in the Persian Gulf." *Nurs. Outlook*, **28** (Apr. 1980), 238–243.

Morris, Ena. "Home Care Today." *Am. J. Nurs.*, **84** (Mar. 1984), 340–345.

Neal, Margo, ed. *Nurses in Business.* Pacific Palisades, Calif.: Nurseco, Inc., 1982.

Otto, Jeanne. "Be Prepared for Camp Nursing." *Am. J. Nurs.*, **80** (May 1980), 907–908.

Parsons, Margaret, and Ruth De Loor. ". . . to Care for Him Who Shall Have Borne the Battle. . . ." *Nurs. and Health Care*, **3** (Mar. 1982), 126–131.

Partridge, Rebecca. "The Decanal Role: A Dilemma of Academic Leadership." *J. Nurs. Ed.*, **22** (Feb. 1983), 59–61.

Pender, Nola, and Albert Pender. "Illinois Prevention and Health Promotion Services Provided by Nurse Practitioners: Protecting Potential Consumers." *Am. J. Pub. Health*, **70** (Aug. 1980), 798–803.

Price, Joseph. "So You Want to Try Consulting." *J. Cont. Ed. in Nurs.*, **15** (May–June 1984), 130–106.

Smith, Gayla. "Is Critical Care Nursing Right for You?" *Nurs. 80*, **10** (Sept. 1980), 97–104.

Spitzer, Walter. "The Nurse Practitioner Revisited: Slow Death of a Good Idea." *N. Eng. J. Med.*, **310** (Apr. 1984), 1049–1051.

Steel, Jean. "Putting Joint Practice into Practice." *Am. J. Nurs.*, **81** (May 1981), 964–967.

Stevens, Barbara. "The Role of the Nurse Executive." *J. Nurs. Admin.*, **11** (Feb. 1981), 19–23.

Stuart-Burchardt, Sandra, "Rural Nursing." *Am. J. Nurs.*, **82** (Apr. 1982), 616–618.

Taylor, Carl. "Changing Patterns in International Health: Motivation and Relationships." *Am. J. Pub. Health*, **69** (Aug. 1979), 803–808.

Tom, Sally. "Nurse-Midwifery: A Developing Profession." *Law, Med. and Health Care*, **10** (Dec. 1982), 262–266.

Wallace, Mary, and Linda Carey. "The Clinical Specialist as Manager: Myth Versus Realities." *J. Nurs. Ed.*, **13** (June 1983), 13–15.

Zachary, Fay. "Enjoy Professional Independence as an Insurance Physical Examiner." *Nurs. 79*, **9** (Feb. 1979), 96–99.

Several complete issues of *Nursing Administration Quarterly* have pertinent articles: "Maximizing Nursing Practice" (Fall 1979); "Primary Nursing Revisited: Part 1" (Spring 1981); "Part 2" (Summer, 1981), "Clinical Ladders and Professional Recognition" (Fall 1984). *The American Journal of Nursing*, Apr. 1981, includes a series of articles on correctional health nursing. Hundreds of articles on NPs have probably appeared since 1967 in nursing, medical, hospital, and public health journals, including information on education and practice, with evaluation research. Finally, for those who are interested in the variety of careers available to nursing, almost all the nursing journals publish articles on new careers periodically. See also the bibliography for Chapter 8 for references on NPs.

Chapter 16 Issues of Autonomy and Influence

Ahmed, Mary. "Taking Charge of Change in Hospital Nursing Practice." *Am. J. Nurs.*, **81** (Mar. 1981), 540–543.

American Nurses' Association. *Contemporary Minority Leaders in Nursing: Afro-American, Hispanic, Native American Perspectives.* Kansas City, Mo.: The Association, 1983.

Bigbee, Jeri. "Territoriality and Prescriptive Authority for Nurse Practitioners." *Nurs. and Health Care*, **5** (Feb. 1984), 106–110.

Brown, Billye. "Follow the Leader." *Nurs. Outlook*, **28** (June 1980), 357–359.

Carson, Frances, and Adrienne Ames. "Nursing Staff Bylaws." *Am. J. Nurs.*, **80** (June 1980), 1130–1134.

Challela, Mary. "The Interdisciplinary Team: A Role Definition." *Image*, **11** (Feb. 1979), 9–15.

Collins, Eliza, and Patricia Scott. "Everyone Who Makes It Has a Mentor." *Harvard Bus. Rev.*, **56** (July–Aug. 1978), 89–101.

Davis, Carolyne, and Pamela Maraldo. "Who Determines Health Policy?" *Nurs. and Health Care*, **1** (Aug. 1980), 27–33.

DeYoung, Carol et al. *Out of Uniform and Into Trouble—Again*. Thorofare, N.J.: Slack, Inc. 1984.

Diers, Donna. "Lessons on Leadership." *Image*, **11** (Oct. 1979), 67–71.

Diers, Donna. "Nursing as an Alternative to High-Cost Care." *Am. J. Nurs.*, **82** (Jan. 1982), 56–60.

Epstein, Charlotte. *The Nurse Leader: Philosophy and Practice*. Reston, Va.: Reston Publishing Company, 1982.

Griffith, Hurdis. "Strategies for Direct Third-Party Reimbursement for Nurses." *Am. J. Nurs.*, **82** (Mar. 1982), 408–414.

Griffith, Hurdis. "Nursing Practice: Substitute or Complement According to Economic Theory." *Nurs. Economics*, **2** (Mar.–Apr. 1984), 105–111.

Hughes, Elizabeth, and Joseph Pronex. "You Are What You Wear." *Hosp.*, **53** (Aug. 1979), 113–118.

Huntington, Judith, and Louise Shores. "From Conflict to Collaboration." *Am. J. Nurs.*, **83** (Aug. 1983), 1184–1186.

Isaacs, Marion. "Nurse Political Action: Interview with Marge Colloff." *Adv. Nurs. Sci.*, **2** (Apr. 1980), 89–94.

Kelly, Lucie. "How to Start a Counterculture." *Nurs. Outlook*, **27** (Feb. 1979), 149.

Kelly, Lucie. "Goodbye Appliance Nurse." *Nurs. Outlook*, **27** (June 1979), 432.

Kelly, Lucie. "The Missing Ingredient." *Nurs. Outlook*, **30** (Mar. 1982), 210.

Kelly, Lucie. "You Go First." *Nurs. Outlook*, **31** (Mar. 1983), 93.

Kennedy, Marilyn. *Powerbase: How to Build It/ How to Keep It*. New York: Macmillan Publishing Company, 1984.

Kleinman, Carol. *Women's Networks*. New York: Ballantine Books, 1980.

Kohnke, Mary. *The Case for Consultation in Nursing: Designs for Professional Practice*. New York: John Wiley and Sons, Inc., 1978.

Krueger, Janelle. "Women in Management: An Assessment." *Nurs. Outlook*, **28** (June 1980), 374–378.

Kudzma, Elizabeth. "Patterns for Effective Nursing Action within Health Bureaucracies." *Nurs. and Health Care.*, **3** (Feb. 1982), 68–72.

Kupchak, Sister Barbara. "Do Nurses Enjoy Appropriate Levels of Power?" *Nurs. Sci.*, **1** (Jan.–Feb. 1984), 4–8.

Little, Dolores. "The Strip Tease of Nurse Symbols or Nurse Dress Code: No Code." *Imprint*, **31** (Mar.–Apr. 1980), 49–52.

Little, Marilyn. "Nurse Practitioner/Physician Relationships." *Am. J. Nurs.*, **80** (Sept. 1980), 1642–1643.

McDonnell, Edwina. "Choosing a Leadership Style." *Nurs. 80*, **10** (Mar. 1980), 105–112.

Mechanic, David, and Linda Aiken. "A Cooperative Agenda for Medicine and Nursing." *N. Eng. J. Med.*, **307** (Sept. 1982), 747–750.

Missirian, Agnes. *The Corporate Connection: Why Executive Women Need Mentors to Reach the Top*. Englewood Cliffs, N.J.: Spectrum Books Prentice-Hall, Inc., 1983.

Moloney, Margaret. *Leadership in Nursing, Theory, Strategies, Action*. St. Louis: C. V. Mosby Company, 1979.

Mundinger, Mary. *Autonomy in Nursing*. Germantown, Md.: Aspen Systems Corporation, 1980.

Munn, Yvonne. "Power: How to Get It and Use It in Nursing Today." *Nurs. Admin. Q.*, **1** (Fall 1976), 95–102.

O'Connor, Andrea. "Ingredients for Successful Networking." *Nurse Educator*, **7** (Winter 1982), 40–43.

Rees, Barbara. "Television Talk Shows: An Untapped Resource for Nursing." *Nurs. Outlook*, **23** (Sept. 1980), 562–565.

Smith, Elizabeth Dorsey. "Nurses in Policymaking and Volunteerism." *Nurs. and Health Care*, **45** (Mar. 1983), 136–137.

Sovie, Margaret. "The Economics of Magnetism." *Nurs. Economics*, **2** (Mar–Apr. 1984), 85–92.

Stevens, Kathleen, ed. *Power and Influence: A Source Book for Nurses*. New York: John Wiley and Sons, 1983.

Tappen, Ruth. *Nursing Leadership: Concepts and*

Practice. Philadelphia: F. A. Davis Company, 1983.

Vance, Connie. "The Mentor Connection." *J. Nurse Admin.*, **12** (Apr. 1982), 7–13.

Welch, Mary Scott. *Networking*. New York: Harcourt Brace Jovanovich, 1980.

See also the entire issue of *Nursing Administration Quarterly*, "Leadership in Nursing Administration" (Fall 1976); "Politics and Power" (Spring 1978); "Influence and Action" (Summer 1982); "Nurse, Physician–Admistrator Relationship" (Summer 1983).

SECTION 5 LEGAL RIGHTS AND RESPONSIBILITIES

Listed here are a number of books on health and/or nursing law that are valuable for the following chapters. The styles and formats vary, but the basic information on law is the same. Later editions and the tremendous number of new books on nursing law are more current and therefore more accurate, but some earlier works are included because of their clarity of information on basic principles of law. To keep up-to-date on legal decisions and legislation concerning women's and children's rights, or any changes in basic principles of law, read major newspapers, news and business magazines, women's magazines, some health professional journals, and law journals. Especially useful is *Law, Medicine and Health Care*. See also columns on legal aspects of nursing in various journals, such as the *American Journal of Nursing, Nursing Life, RN,* and *Nursing Management*. Also useful are the public affairs pamphlets of the nonprofit Public Affairs Committee, which can be obtained from the committee at 381 Park Avenue South, New York, New York 10016.

Annas, George, et al. *The Rights of Doctors, Nurses and Allied Helath Professionals*. Cambridge, Mass.: Ballinger Publishing Company, 1981.

Cazalas, Mary. *Nursing and the Law*, 3rd ed. Germantown, Md.: Aspen Systems Corporation, 1978.

Creighton, Helen. *Law Every Nurse Should Know*, 4th ed. Philadelphia: W. B. Saunders Company, 1981.

Curran, Williams, and E. Donald Shapiro. *Law, Medicine and Forensic Science*, 3rd ed. Boston: Little, Brown and Company, 1982.

Hemelt, Mary, and Mary Ellen Mackert. *Dynamics of Law in Nursing And Health Care*, 2nd ed. Reston, Va.: Reston Publishing Company, 1984.

Hogue, L. Lynn, ed. *Public Health and the Law*. Rockville, Md.: Aspen Systems Corporation, 1980.

Lahen, Joyce, and Colleen McLean. *Legal Issues and Guidelines for Nurses Who Care for the Mentally Ill*. Thorofare, N.J.: Slack, Inc., 1984.

Mannino, Mary. *The Nurse Anesthetist and the Law*. New York: Grune & Stratton, 1982.

Miller, Robert. *Problems in Hospital Law*, 4th ed. Rockville, Md.: Aspen Systems Corporation, 1983.

Murchison, Irene, and Thomas Nichols. *Legal Foundations of Nursing Practice*. New York: Macmillan Publishing Company, 1970.

Murchison, Irene, Thomas Nichols, and Rachel Hanson. *Legal Accountability in the Nursing Process*, 2nd ed. St. Louis: C. V. Mosby Company, 1982.

Pozgar, George. *Legal Aspects of Health Care Administration*, 2nd ed. Rockville, Md.: Aspen Systems Corporation, 1983.

Rocereto, LaVerne, and Cynthia Maleski. *The Legal Dimensions of Nursing Practice*. New York: Springer Publishing Company, 1982.

Rothman, Daniel, and Nancy Rothman. *The Professional Nurse and the Law*. Boston: Little, Brown and Company, 1977.

Southwick, Arthur. *The Law of Hospital and Health Care Administration*. Ann Arbor: University of Mich. Press, 1978.

Wing, Kenneth. *The Law and the Public Health*. St. Louis: C. V. Mosby Company, 1976.

Chapter 17 An Introduction to Law

Annas, George. "How to Find the Law." *Nurs. Law and Ethics*, **1** (Dec. 1980), 5.

Rowe, Mary. "Dealing with Sexual Harassment." *Harvard Bus. Rev.*, **59** (May–June 1981), 42–46.

"How to Read Legal Citations: What Do All the Numbers Mean? Part 1." *NHLP Newsletter*, **125** (Oct. 1981), 5–6. "Part 2: Judicial Decisions." NHLP Newsletter, **126** (Dec. 1981), 4–5.

Chapter 18 The Legislative Process

Buckalew, Judy. "Federal Policy and the Lawmaking Process." *Nurse Practitioner*, **5** (Nov.–Dec. 1980), 7–8.

Buckalew, Judy, et al. "Policy Internships for Nurses." *Nurs. Outlook*, **32** (Mar.–Apr. 1984), 128, 123.

Congress and Health: An Introduction to the Legislative Process and Its Key Participants. New

York: National Health Council, revised periodically, sometimes with each Congress.

Donley, Sister Rosemary. "An Inside View of the Washington Health Scene." *Am. J. Nurs.*, **79** (Nov. 1979), 1946–1949.

Kalisch, Beatrice, and Philip Kalisch. "A Discourse on the Politics of Nursing." *J. Nurs. Admin.*, **6** (Mar.–Apr. 1975), 29–34.

Kalisch, Beatrice, and Philip Kalisch. *Politics of Nursing.* Philadelphia: J. B. Lippincott Company, 1982.

Lake, Rebecca. "Legislators' Opinions About Nursing: Results of a Pilot Study." *Nurs. and Health Care*, **5** (Apr. 1984), 204–207.

Lake, Rebecca, and Celia Lamper-Linder. "A Subject Bibliography in Legislative and Political Action." *Nurs. and Health Care*, **4** (June 1983), 334–337.

Maraldo, Pamela. "Politics: A Very Human Matter." *Am. J. Nurs.*, **82** (July 1982), 1104–1105.

Many publications of ANA, N-CAP, and NLN relate to legislation and politics, as do those of most other large health associations and the National Health Council. Useful government publications include *Congressional Record* (verbatim transcript of the proceedings of the Senate and House, (*Congressional Record* Office, H-112, Capitol, Washington, D.C. 20515) and annual subscription from the Superintendent of Documents, Government Printing Office, Washington, D.C. 20401; *Digest of Public General Bills*, also from the Superintendent of Documents; *Committee Prints and Hearing Records*, available about two months after the close of hearings, is free but requires a self-addressed label sent to the publications clerk of the committee from which the document is issued; and a *Catalogue of Washington Health Newsletters*, developed by some congressional staffs, available from the Health Policy Center, The Graduate School, Georgetown University, Washington, D.C. 20057. Major newspapers and news magazines always carry political-legislative news, with or without editorials. The entire issue of the Summer, 1984 *Nursing Administration Quarterly* is devoted to the "Legislative Impact on Nursing."

Chapter 19 Federal Legislation Affecting Nursing

Brett, Judy. "How Much Is a Nurse's Job Really Worth?" *Am. J. Nurs.*, **83** (June 1983), 877–881.

Brown, Lawrence. *Politics and Health Care Organization: HMOs as Federal Policy.* Washington, D.C.: Brookings Institute, 1983.

Caterinecchio, Russell. *DRGs: What They Are and How to Survive Them.* Thorofare, N.J.: Slack, Inc. 1984.

Creighton, Helen. "Recovery for on-the-Job Injuries or Illness." *Nurs. Mgt.*, **15** (Mar. 1984), 70–71.

Curtin, Leah. "Determining Costs for Nursing Services Per DRG." *Nurs. Mgt.*, **14** (Apr. 1983), 16–20.

Curtin, Leah, and Carolina Zurlage, eds. *DRGs: The Reorganization of Health.* Chicago: S-N Publications Inc., 1984.

Dolan, Andrew. "Antitrust Law and Physician Dominance." *J. Health Politics, Policy and Law*, **4** (Winter 1980), 675–690.

Duldt, Bonnie. "Sexual Harassment in Nursing." *Nurs. Outlook*, **30** (June 1982), 336–343.

Flagg, Joan. "Public Policy and Mental Health; Past, Present, and Future." *Nurs. and Health Care*, **4** (May 1983), 246–251.

Grimaldi, Pamela. "DRGs and Nursing Administration." *Nurs. Mgt.*, **13** (Jan. 1982), 30–34.

Huber, Douglas. "Restricting or Prohibiting Abortion by Constitutional Amendment: Some Health Implictions." *J. Reproductive Med.*, **27** (Dec. 1982), 729–736.

Johnson, Jean. "Comparable Worth: A Sleeping Giant." *Nurse Practitioner*, **9** (Sept. 1984), 11.

Livengood, Winifred. "The Impact of DRGs on Home Health Care." *Home Healthcare Nurse*, **1** (Sept.–Oct. 1983), 29–34.

Luft, H. S., and G. Frisvold. "Decisionmaking in Regional Health Planning Agencies." *J. Health Politics, Policy and Law*, **4**(2) (1979), 250–271.

Mancini, Marguerite. "Medicare: Health Rights of the Elderly." *Am. J. Nurs.*, **79** (Oct. 1979), 1810–1812.

Milio, Nancy. *Promoting Health Through Public Policy.* Philadelphia: F. A. Davis Company, 1981.

Pollard, Michael, and Patricia Schultheiss. "FTC and the Professions: Continuing Controversy." *Nurs. Economics*, **1** (Nov.–Dec. 1983), 158–163.

Regan, William. "So You Think You're Covered for Injuries at Work." *RN*, **46** (Jan. 1983), 91–92.

Robertson, Leon, and J. Philip Keeve. "Worker Injuries: The Effects of Workers' Compensation and OSHA Inspections." *J. Health Politics, Policy and Law*, **8** (Fall 1983), 581–597.

Rosenthal, Trudy. "Understanding Workers' Compensation: When You Get Hurt, Who Will Help?" *Nurs. Life*, **2** (May–June 1982), 39–42.

Rothman, Nancy, and Daniel Rothman. "Equal Pay for Comparable Work." *Nurs. Outlook*, **28** (Sept. 1980), 728–729.

Spitzer, Roxane. "Legislation and New Regulations." *Nurs. Mgt.*, **14** (Feb. 1983), 13–21.

"The FDA: What It Can and Cannot Do." *Ger. Nurs.*, **2** (Nov.–Dec. 1981), 418.

Trandel-Korenchuk, Darlene, and Keith Trandel-Korenchuk. "Medicare, DRGs and Nursing Practice." *Nursing Admin. Q.*, **8** (Summer 1984), 85–87.

Weingard, Margaret. "Establishing Comparable Worth Through Job Evaluation." *Nurs. Outlook*, **32** (Mar.–Apr. 1984), 110–113.

U.S. Department of Health and Human Services. *Your Medicare Handbook*. Washington, D.C.: Social Security Administration, 1982.

A great deal was written about DRGs and prospective payment in 1982–1984. See especially *Nursing and Health Care*, Sept.–Dec. 1983 and Jan.–Feb. 1984.

Chapter 20 Licensure and Health Manpower Credentialing

Baron, Charles. "Licensure of Health Professionals: The Consumer's Case for Abolition." *Am. J. Law and Med.*, **9** (Fall 1983), 335–356.

Bullough, Bonnie. *The Law and the Expanding Nursing Role*, 2nd ed. New York: Appleton-Century-Crofts, 1980.

Bullough, Bonnie. "State Certification of the Nursing Specialties: A New Trend in Nursing Practice Law." *Ped. Nurs.*, **8** (Dec. 1982), 1241–1247.

Chambers, Charles. "Confidentiality and Disclosure in Accreditation: A Précis of the Legal Issues and Risks." *Nurs. and Health Care*, **4** (Oct. 1983), 444–447.

Cohen, Harris. "On Professional Power and Conflict of Interest: State Licensing Boards on Trial." *J. Health Politics, Policy and Law*, **5** (Summer 1980), 291–308.

Creighton, Helen. "Physician's Assistant Medication Order." *Sup. Nurse*, **12** (Jan. 1981), 46–47.

Eichhorn, Elizabeth. "Continuing Education: Can It Be Legislated?" *Nurs. Forum*, **20**(1) (1981), 102–109.

Falk, Dennis. "The Challenge of Change." *Hospitals*, **57** (Apr. 1983), 92–98.

Grobe, Susan. "Sunset Legislation: Suggestions and Strategies." *Nurs. Admin. Q.*, **5** (Fall 1980), 64–71.

Isler, Charlotte. "The Alcoholic Nurse." *RN*, **41** (July 1978), 48–55.

Johnson, Mary Lou. "'I Don't Want to Be a Test Case.'" *Nurse Practitioner*, **5** (May–June 1980), 7–8.

Kay, Loraine. "If You Blow the Whistle on a Doctor." *RN*, **47** (Aug. 1984), 11–12.

Kelly, Lucie. "In Principle." *Nurs. Outlook*, **30** (June 1982), 370.

Kelly, Lucie. "Licensure Laws in Transition." *Nurs. Outlook*, **30** (July–Aug. 1982), 375.

Korolishen, Michael, and Terry Korolishen. "Two Willful Acts?" *Nurs. Life*, **4** (Oct. 1984), 80.

Markowitz, Lucille. "How Your State Board Works for You." *Nurs. Life*, **2** (May–June 1982), 25–32.

Regan, William. "License Suspended! A Nursing Board Bares Its Teeth." *RN*, **42** (Oct. 1979), 65–66.

Riesdorph, Linda. "Institutional Licensure: An Issue in Credentialing," in *Nursing in Transition*, ed. by T. Audean Duespohl. Rockville, Md.: Aspen Systems Corporation, 1983, pp. 41–50.

Rizzuto, Carmela. "Mandatory Continuing Education: Cost Versus Benefit." *J. Cont. Ed. in Nurs.*, **13**(3) (1982), 37–43.

Rose, Michael. "Laying Siege to Hospital Privileges." *Am. J. Nurs.*, **84** (May 1984), 613–615.

Trandel-Korenchuk, Darlene, and Keith Trandel-Korenchuk. "Current Legal Issues Facing Nursing Practice." *Nurs. Admin. Q.*, **4** (Fall 1980), 37–55.

White, William. "Why Is Regulation Introduced in the Health Sector? A Look at Occupational Licensure." *J. Health Politics, Policy and Law*, **4** (Fall 1979), 536–552.

See also the references and bibliography of Chapters 6, 13, and 16. News items on changes in licensure and appropriate articles appear in almost all nursing journals. ANA, NLN, and the National Council of State Boards of Nursing all have materials about licensure in their publications lists.

Chapter 21 Nursing Practice and the Law

Bernzweig, Eli. "When in Doubt—Speak Out." *Am. J. Nurs.*, **80** (June 1980), 1175–1176.

Bruce, Joan, and Marie Snyder. "The Right and Responsibility to Diagnose." *Am. J. Nurs.*, **82** (Apr. 1982), 645–646.

Cohn, Sarah. "Legal Issues in School Nursing Practice." *Law, Med., and Health Care*, **12** (Oct. 1984), 219–221.

Creighton, Helen. "Are Side Rails Necessary?"

Nurs. Mgt., **13** (June 1982), 45–48.

Cushing, Maureen. "A Judgment on Standards." *Am. J. Nurs.*, **81** (Apr. 1981), 797–798.

Cushing, Maureen. "When Medical Standards Apply to Nurse Practitioners." *Am. J. Nurs.*, **82** (Aug. 1982), 1274–1276.

Cushing, Maureen. "Cause of Death: Drug or Disease?" *Am. J. Nurs.*, **83** (June 1983), 943–944.

Cushing, Maureen. "Expanding the Meaning of Accountability." *Am. J. Nurs.*, **83** (Aug. 1983), 1202–1203.

Greenlaw, Jane. "Understaffing: Living with the Reality." *Law, Med. and Health Care*, **9** (Sept. 1981), 23–24, 33.

Greenlaw, Jane. "Communication Failure: Some Case Examples." *Law, Med. and Health Care*, **10** (Apr. 1982), 77–79.

Horsley, Jack. "MD Rape: Why *You* Can Be Indicted." *RN*, **43** (Jan. 1980), 71–72.

Horsley, Jack. "Beware: Your Hospital Could Turn on You!" *RN*, **43** (Aug. 1980), 65–66, 73.

Horsley, Jack. "Think Twice Before You Give Advice." *RN*, **43** (Sept. 1980), 95–96, 98.

Horsley, Jack. "Short-Staffing Means Increased Liability for You." *RN*, **44** (Feb. 1981), 73–74, 81–82.

Horsley, Jack. "Charting Nasty Truths with an Absence of Malice." *RN*, **46** (July 1983), 16.

Horsley, Jack. "How a Loose Tongue Can Land You in Trouble." *RN*, **46** (Sept. 1983), 23–24.

Kalisch, Beatrice, et al. "The 'Angel of Death' Case: The Anatomy of 1980's Major News Story." *Nurs. Forum*, **19**(3) (1980), 212–241.

Langdon, Carolyn. "The Legal Burden of Questionable Drug Orders." *Nurs. Life*, **4** (Oct. 1984), 23–25.

Lynn, Frances. "Incidents—Need They Be Accidents?" *Am. J. Nurs.*, **80** (June 1980), 1098–1101.

Rabinsow, Jean. "Delegating Safety within the Law." *Nurs. Life*, **2** (Sept.–Oct. 1982), 48–49.

Regan, William. "When Your Silence Is Tantamount to Fraud." *RN*, **43** (Oct. 1980), 87–88, 90.

Regan, William. "How to Cover Yourself When the MD's Wrong." *RN*, **44** (June 1981), 79–80.

Regan, William. "The Nurse as Expert Witness: Are You Ready?" *RN*, **45** (Apr. 1982), 75–76.

Rozovsky, Fay, and Lorne Rozovsky. "When Neighbors Ask Your Advice." *Nurs. Life*, **1** (July–Aug. 1981), 26–27, 29.

Trandel-Korenchuk, Darlene, and Keith Trandel-Korenchuk. "Borrowed Servant and Captain-of-the-Ship Doctrine." *Nurs. Practitioner*, **7** (Feb. 1982), 33–34.

Trandel-Korenchuk, Darlene, and Keith Trandel-Korenchuk. "Malpractice and Preventive Risk Management." *Nursing Admin. Q.*, **7** (Apr. 1983), 75–79.

Warling, Marilyn. "Legal Aspects of the Client's Record: A Guide for Community Health Nurses." *Caring*, **1** (Oct. 1982), 14–17.

Zaremski, Miles. "Hospital Corporate Liability: The Walls Continue to Tumble." *Law, Med. and Health Care*, **9** (Apr. 1981), 13–15, 20.

Books on hospital and medical law also have pertinent information. Parts of the Hemelt and Mackert book are reprinted in *Nurs. 79*, 9 (Oct. 1979), 57–64; (Nov. 1979), 57–64; and (Dec. 1979), 49–56. *Nursing Life*, Feb. 1981, also has a special section on law (pp. 61–68). The fall 1980 issue of *Nursing Administration Quarterly* focuses on legal aspects and legislation. In addition to these selected references, there are frequent articles on legal aspects of nursing and/or health care in *AJN, Nursing Outlook, JONA, RN, Nursing Management, Hospital Progress, Hospitals*, and other health journals. Some of these have been cited in the references to show the style and content. Some of Creighton's articles are reprinted in her book. Law journals almost always have articles about health law. Examples of those devoted exclusively to health law are *Journal of Law and Medicine* and *Law, Medicine and Health Care*.

Chapter 22 Health Care and the Rights of People

Annas, George. "Male Nurses in the Delivery Room." *Hastings Center Rep.*, **11** (Dec. 1981), 20–21.

Annas, George. "Prisoner in the ICU: The Tragedy of William Bartling." *Hastings Center Rep.*, **14** (Dec. 1984), 28–29.

Aroskar, Mila. "Institutional Ethics Committees and Nursing Administration." *Nurs. Economics*, **2** (Mar.–Apr. 1984), 130–136.

Besch, Linda. "Informed Consent: A Patient's Right." *Nurs. Outlook*, **27** (Jan. 1979), 32–42.

Caldwell, Janice, and Marshall Kapp. "The Rights of Nursing Home Patients: Possibilities and Limitations of Federal Regulation." *J. Health Politics, Policy and Law*, **6** (Apr. 1981), 40–48.

Childress, James. *Who Should Decide?* New York: Oxford University Press, 1982.

Connery, John. "The Clarence Herbert Case: Was

Withdrawal of Treatment Justified?'' *Hosp. Prog.*, **65** (Feb. 1984), 32–35, 70.

Creighton, Helen. ''Legal Concerns of Nursing Research.'' *Nurs. Res.*, **26** (Sept.–Oct. 1977), 337–341, 392.

Creighton, Helen. ''Recent Development in Consent to Treatment—Part II.'' *Sup. Nurse*, **12** (July 1981), 70, 74.

Creighton, Helen. ''Is Termination Proper?'' *Nurs. Mgt.*, **15** (Jan. 1984), 50–51.

Creighton, Helen. ''Decisions on Food and Fluid in Life-Sustaining Measures: Part II.'' *Nurs. Mgt.*, **15** (July 1984), 54–56.

Cushing, Maureen. '''No Code' Orders: Current Developments and the Nursing Director's Role.'' *J. Nurs. Admin.*, **11** (Apr. 1981), 22–29.

Cushing, Maureen. ''Treatment Beyond Death?'' *Am. J. Nurs.*, **81** (Aug. 1981), 1527–1528.

Dickman, Robert. ''The Ethics of Informed Consent.'' *Nurse Practitioner*, **5** (May–June 1980), 25–26, 32.

''Employee Rights vs. Hospital Prerogatives.'' *Nurs. Life*, **3** (Jan.–Feb. 1983), 80.

Feliu, Alfred. ''The Risks of Blowing the Whistle.'' *Am. J. Nurs.*, **83** (Oct. 1983), 1387–1388, and (Nov. 1983), 1541–1542.

Gaylin, Willard. ''The Competence of Children: No Longer All or None.'' *Hastings Center Rep.*, **12** (Apr. 1982), 33–38.

Greenlaw, Jane. ''Answers to 11 Pressing Questions About Terminal Care.'' *RN*, **46** (Dec. 1983), 21–23.

Greenlaw, Jane. *''Mississippi University for Women* v. *Hogan*: The Supreme Court Rules on Female-Only Nursing School.'' *Law, Med. and Health Care*, **10** (Dec. 1982), 267–269.

Hull, Kent. ''Limiting Davis: Educating Handicapped People for Health Care Professions.'' *Medicolegal News*, **8** (Feb. 1980), 12–13, 28.

Kapp, Marshall. ''Legal Guardianship.'' *Ger. Nurs.* **2** (Sept.–Oct. 1981), 366–369.

McCormick, Richard. ''Ethics Committees: Promise or Peril?'' *Law, Med. and Health Care.* **12** (Sept. 1984), 150–155.

Podratz, Rosalyn, ''A Student Sues.'' *Am. J. Nurs.*, **80** (Sept. 1980), 1604–1605.

Poteet, Gaye, and Clementine Pollak. ''When a Student Fails Clinical.'' *Am. J. Nurs.*, **81** (Oct. 1981), 1889–1890.

Regan, William. ''You *Don't* Have to Tolerate Substandard Hospital Practices.'' *RN*, **44** (Jan. 1981), 99–100.

Robertson, John. *The Rights of the Critically Ill.*

Cambridge, Mass.: Ballinger Publishing Company, 1983.

Storch, Janet. ''Consumer Rights and Health Care.'' *Nurs. Admin. Q.*, **4** (Winter 1980), 107–115.

Strong, Carson. ''Defective Infants and their Impact on Families: Ethical and Legal Considerations.'' *Law Med. and Health Care*, **11** (Sept. 1983), 168–172.

Trandel-Korenchuk, Darlene, and Keith Trandel-Korenchuk. ''Minor Consent in Birth Control and Abortion.'' *Nurse Practitioner*, **5** (Mar.–Apr. 1980), 47–50ff., and (May–June 1980), 48, 50ff.

Watson, Annita. ''Informed Consent of Special Subjects.'' *Nurs. Res.*, **31** (Jan.–Feb. 1982), 43–47.

Ziengenfuss, James. *Patients' Rights and Professional Practice.* New York: Van Nostrand Reinhold Company, 1983.

Zimmerman, Don. ''Trends in National Labor Relations Board Decisions for the Health Care Industry.'' *Law, Med. and Health Care*, **9** (Oct. 1981), 12–16.

See also the references and bibliography of Chapters 6, 10, 11, 16, 17, 19, 24, and 25. *Children's Rights Report*, issued by the Juvenile Rights Project of the ACLU Foundation in New York, usually includes health-related items. The summer 1979 issue of *Medicolegal News* has a series of articles on the legal rights of children. The May 1978 issue of AJN section on ethics includes articles that consider legal rights, as well. The nursing and hospital law books cited in this and preceding chapters vary in the depth of coverage of various topics; Creighton has a large section on contracts; Hemelt and Mackert, on child abuse. The Concern for Dying has a newsletter with continued update on right-to-die cases and issues, as well as a number of pertinent pamphlets. The *Hastings Center Report* and *Law, Medicine and Health* always have articles on rights. *AJN* has an ongoing series titled ''Dilemmas in Practice'' that frequently refers to rights issues. *Nursing Life* (Jan.–Feb. 1984), 18–27, focuses on right-to-die issues, including a poll of nurses' opinions. The winter 1982 issue of *Nursing Administration Quarterly* is devoted to collective bargaining.

Publications by the President's Commission for the Study of Ethical Problems in Medicine and Biomedical and Behavioral Research can be obtained from the Superintendent of Documents,

U.S. Government Printing Office, Washington, D.C. 20402. These are: *Defining Death; Implementing Human Research Regulations; Deciding to Forego Life-Sustaining Treatment* (may also be obtianed from Concern for Dying, 250 W. 57th Street, New York, New York 10019); *Protecting Human Subjects; Making Health Care Decisions; Screening and Counseling for Genetic Conditions; Spicing Life; Securing Access to Health Care; Whistleblowing in Biomedical Research;* and *Summing Up.*

PART III PROFESSIONAL COMPONENTS AND CAREER DEVELOPMENT

SECTION 1 ORGANIZATION AND PUBLICATIONS

Chapter 23 Organizational Procedures and Issues

Bliss, Edwin. "The Meeting Will Now Come to Order . . . or Will It?" *Assn. Mgt.*, **34** (Apr. 1982), 71–74.

Dunlop, James. "Responsibility and Authority: Out of Sync?" *Leadership*, 3 (June 1980), 34–39.

Falconer, Merry. "Life in the Fast Lane: Professional Societies Respond to the Demands of a Changing World." *Assn. Mgt.*, **33** (May 1981), 88–93.

Fox, Elliot. "How to Develop and Use an Agenda." *Leadership*, 3 (Sept. 1980), 43–45.

Grumme, Marguerite. *Basic Principles of Parliamentary Law and Protocol.* St. Louis: The author, 1973.

Jay, Antony. "The Meeting Chairperson: Master or Servant?" *J. Nurs. Admin.*, **11** (May 1981), 30–32.

Merton, Robert K. "The Functions of the Professional Association." *Am. J. Nurs.*, **58** (Jan. 1958), 50–54.

Merton, Robert K. "Dilemmas of Democracy in the Voluntary Associations." *Am. J. Nurs.*, **66** (May 1966), 1055–1061.

Peplau, Hildegard. "Dilemmas of Organizing Nurses." *Image*, 4(3) (1970–1971), 4–8.

Smith, David, and Richard Reddy. "Improving Participation in Voluntary Action." *J. Nurs. Admin.*, 3 (May–June 1973), 36–42.

See also the bibliography and references of the following chapters on the various organizations, as well as those related to Chapter 16. *Leadership*, "a publication for the effective association volunteer," is published intermittently by the American

Society of Association Executives; its articles are invaluable for both volunteers and staff. Included are short, pertinent how-to-do-it articles, as well as more thoughtful analyses of issues. *Association Management*, the monthly magazine of the society, also contains excellent articles of this kind, as well as articles geared to association staff. The society has also published a series of booklets to help volunteers function more effectively in associations (for example, "Getting Involved: The Challenge of Committee Participation" and "Moving Forward: Providing Leadership as the Chief Elected Officer").

Merton and other sociologists frequently write about associations and provide an in-depth understanding of their sociological implications.

Chapter 24 National Student Nurses' Association

The American Journal of Nursing and *Nursing Outlook* usually report on the annual NSNA conventions, in addition to providing news items and pertinent articles. Various publications of NSNA may be requested from its headquarters. *Imprint* is the best reference.

Chapter 25 American Nurses' Association

Information about the activities of ANA is found most extensively in the ANA publications described in Chapter 25 and the ANA publications list. In addition, ANA conventions are always reported in some detail in the *American Journal of Nursing, Nursing Outlook*, and *American Nurse*. Until 1985, when the first annual House of Delegates meeting was held, convention reports appeared in *AJN* in the even years, usually in the July or (for *Nursing Outlook*) later issues. Other journals may also give brief reports.

Chapter 26 National League for Nursing

The best source of current information about NLN can be found in the NLN publications noted in Chapter 26 and the NLN publications list. This includes data from many research projects and surveys, position papers, and conference proceedings. NLN conventions and meetings are usually reported in some depth in *Nursing and Health Care. Nursing Outlook* also reports on the conventions (odd years—June or later), and other journals may have brief news reports.

Chapter 27 Other Nursing and Related Organizations in the United States

"Federation Becomes Stronger Voice for Nursing

Groups." Editorial, *AORN J.*, **27** (Apr. 1978), 809.

Kalisch, Beatrice, and Philip Kalisch. *Nurturer of Nurses: A History of the Division of Nursing of the U.S. Public Health Service and Its Antecedents, 1798-1977.* Summary report of a study for the Division of Nursing, Mar. 1977.

Lindemann, Carol. "Implications of Social, Political and Economic Changes for Nursing and Nursing Organizations." *Washington State J. Nurs.*, **52** (1980), 40–46.

Scott, Jessie. "Federal Support for Nursing Education to Improve Quality of Practice." *Pub. Health Rep.*, **94** (Jan.–Feb. 1979), 31–35.

"Special Interest Groups or the ANA: An Analysis," in *Current Perspectives in Nursing: Social Issues and Trends.*, ed. by Michael Miller and Beverly Flynn. St. Louis: C. V. Mosby Company, 1977, pp. 111–119.

See also the journals, newsletters, and other published material of the various organizations for further information or updating on each. *AJN* usually reports meetings and/or statements of the Federation and often of other groups.

Chapter 28 International Organizations

Reports of ICN congresses are usually found in the *American Journal of Nursing, Nursing Outlook*, and other nursing journals that carry news items about ICN activities. Other news is carried in the *International Nursing Review.* The World Health Organization has a number of publications that report on its activities.

Chapter 29 The Professional Literature

Bernstein, Theodore. *The Careful Writer—A Modern Guide to English Usage.* New York: Atheneum Books, 1981.

Bestor, Dorothy. "Writing an Article for Publication: Part I." *Nurse Practitioner*, **1** (Mar.–Apr. 1976), 13–17; "Part II," (May–June 1976), 21–23.

Binger, Jane. "The Nursing Journal—Learning Resource, Professional Symbol, and Commodity." *Image*, **13** (Oct. 1981), 67–70.

Binger, Jane. "Nursing Journal Editors." *Nurs. Outlook*, **30** (Apr. 1982), 260–264.

Binger, Jane, and Lydia Jensen. *Lippincott's Guide to Nursing Literature.* Philadelphia: J. B. Lippincott Company, 1980.

Clayton, Bonnie, and Kathleen Boyle. "The Refereed Journal: Prestige in Professional Publication." *Nurs. Outlook*, **29** (Sept. 1981), 531–534.

Cormack, Desmond. *Writing for Nursing and Allied Professions.* Boston: Blackwell Scientific Publications, 1984.

Day, Robert. *How to Write and Publish a Scientific Paper*, 2nd ed. Philadelphia: ISI Press, 1983.

Dickerson, Janet. "Guidelines for Peer Reviewers." *Nurs. Outlook*, **32** (July–Aug. 1984), 232.

Diers, Donna. "Why Write? Why Publish?" *Image*, **13** (Feb. 1981), 3–8.

Evans, Nancy. "Author and Publishers: The Mutual Selection Process." *Am. J. Nurs.*, **81** (Feb. 1981), 350–352.

Fox, Richard, and Marlene Ventura. "Efficiency of Automated LIterature Search Mechanisms." *Nurs. Res.*, **33** (May–June 1984), 174–177.

Gandalfo, Anita, and Judy Romano. *The Nurses' Writing Handbook.* Norwalk, Conn.: Appleton-Century-Crofts, 1984.

Huth, Edward. *How to Write and Publish Papers in the Medical Sciences.* Philadelphia: ISI Press, 1982.

Johnson, Suzanne. "Organizing a Manuscript for Publication." *Nurs. Economics*, **1** (July–Aug. 1984), 283–286, 297.

King, Lester. *Why Not Say It Clearly—A Guide to Scientific Writing.* Boston: Little, Brown and Company, 1978.

Kolin, Philip, and Joneen Kolin. *Professional Writing for Nurses in Education, Practice, and Research.* St. Louis: C. V. Mosby Company, 1980.

Lewis, Edith. "For the Nurse Writer's Bookshelf." *Am. J. Nurs.*, **82** (July 1982), 1116–1118.

Long, Lois, and Debra Brady. "Writing a Book Proposal." *Nurs. Outlook*, **32** (Sept.–Oct. 1984), 288.

Maxwell, Mary. "The Agony and the Ecstasy: How to Write and Publish Your Paper." *Oncology Nurs. Forum*, **7** (Summer 1980), 41–47.

Mullins, C. *A Guide to Writing and Publishing in the Social and Behaviorial Sciences.* New York: John Wiley and Sons, Inc., 1977.

Strunck, William, Jr., and E. B. White. *The Elements of Style*, 3rd ed. New York: Macmillan Publishing Company, 1979.

Tornquist, Elizabeth. "Editors for Nurses." *Image*, **13** (Feb. 1984), 24.

Zinsser, William. *On Writing Well, An Informal Guide to Writing Nonfiction.* New York: Harper & Row, 1976.

Zinsser, William. *Writing with a Word Processor.* New York: Harper & Row, 1983.

See also the references and bibliography of Chapter 14 for research resources, as well as the various nonnursing manuals, articles, and books on writing.

SECTION 2   TRANSITION INTO PRACTICE

Nursing journals and the yearly *Career Guide*, published by some, periodically carry articles on career guidance and employment guidelines. (Some are in the reference lists and bibliography.) Business journals, and especially career women's magazines, have also been emphasizing these topics. Any bookstore has a section devoted to career development; some of the books are best-sellers and may be found in paperback.

Chapter 30   Employment Guidelines

Campbell, Laure. "Fired! What to Do If It Happens to You." *RN*, **47** (June 1984), 58–60.

Edmunds, Marilyn. "Developing a Marketing Portfolio." *Nurse Practitioner*, **5** (May–June 1980), 41–43, 46.

Ester, Rosemary. "Getting a New Job." *Am. J. Nurs.*, **81** (Apr. 1981), 758–760.

Godfrey, Marjorie. "Is Part-Time Nursing the Answer for You?" *Nurs. 80*, **10** (Oct. 1980), 65–72.

Gulack, Robert. "Are Your Fringes a Waste?" *RN*, **45** (July 1982), 33–39.

Gulack, Robert. "The Main Chance." *RN*, **45** (Mar. 1983), 35–41.

Kiely, Mary. "The Resume Writer's Task." *Focus on Crit. Care*, **10** (June 1983), 10–11.

Kroner, Kristine. "Changing Jobs—Take the Gamble Out of It." *Nurs. Life*, **2** (Mar.–Apr. 1982), 50–53.

Kurman, Annette. "Moving Up the Career Ladder." *Nurs. Life*, **2** (Jan.–Feb. 1982), 40–43.

Lewis, Howard. "Part-Time Nursing: How Much of a Career?" *RN*, **47** (Jan. 1984), 34–36.

Manley, Mary Jo et al. "The Bilateral Job Interview." *Am. J. Nurs.* **84** (Oct. 1984), 1237–1241.

See also the references and bibliography of Chapters 11, 15, 16, 21, 22, and 31.

Chapter 31   The Challenge of Professionalism

Anastas, Lila. *Your Career in Nursing.* New York: National League for Nursing, 1984.

Angel, Gerry, and Diane Petronko. *Developing the New Assertive Nurse: Essentials for Advancement.* New York: Springer Publishing Company, 1983.

Balassone, Patricia. "I Like Miss Piggy Too, But . . ." *MCN*, **7** (Jan.–Feb. 1982), 9–10.

Barritt, Evelyn. "Inbreeding, Infighting, and Impotence." *Am. J. Nurs.*, **84** (June 1984), 803–804.

Benner, Patricia. *From Novice to Expert.* Menlo Park, Calif.: Addison-Wesley Publishing Company, 1984.

Byrnes, Mary Ann. "Non-Nursing Functions: The Nurses State Their Case." *Am. J. Nurs.*, **82** (July 1982), 1089–1094.

Donnelly, Gloria, "Stop Driving Yourself Crazy." *RN*, **44** (Feb. 1981), 54–55, 100ff.

Duffy, Mary. "When a Woman Heads the Household." *Nurs. Outlook*, **30** (Sept.–Oct. 1982), 468–473.

Edelwick, Jerry, and Archie Brodsky. *Burn-Out.* New York: Human Sciences Press, Inc. 1980.

Fishel, Anne. "Graduation/Termination." *Am. J. Nurs.*, **81** (June 1981), 1156–1158.

Hamilton, Jane. "Effective Ways to Relieve Stress." *Nurs. Life*, **4** (July–Aug. 1984), 24–27.

Hoffman, Vicki. *New Directions for the Professional Nurse.* New York: Arco Publishing Company, 1984.

Kaye, Beverly. "Six Paths for Development." *Nurs. Mgt.*, **13** (May 1982), 18–22.

Kjervik, Diane, and Ida Martinson. *Women in Stress.* New York: Appleton-Century-Crofts, 1979.

Kövecses, Judith. "Burn-Out Doesn't Have to Happen." *Nurs. 80*, **10** (Oct. 1980), 105–111.

Laser, Robert. "I Win—You Win Negotiating." *J. Nurs. Admin.*, **11**, (Dec. 1981), 24–29.

Matthews, Ann, and Sally Schumacher. "A Survey of Registerd Nurses' Conceptions of and Participation Factors in Professional Continuing Education." *J. Cont. Ed. in Nurs.*, **10** (Jan. 1979), 2–27.

McDonald, Terry. "Facing Conflicts." *Nurs. Life.*, **4** (May–June 1984), 25–27.

Minehan, Paula. "Training Bicultural Leaders," *J. Nurs. Admin.*, **11** (Mar. 1981), 37–41.

Nowak, Janie, and Cecelia Grindel. *Career Planning in Nursing.* Philadelphia: J. B. Lippincott Company, 1984.

Putney, Janet. "Specializing without Going Back

to School.'' *Nurs. Life*, **1** (July–Aug. 1981), 30–35.

Rosenow, Ann. ''Professional Nursing Practice in the Bureaucratic Hospital—Revisited.'' *Nurs. Outlook*, **31** (Jan.–Feb. 1983), 34–39.

Shaffer, Mary, and Yvonne Moody. ''A Model for Career Development.'' *J. Nurs. Ed.*, **19** (Oct. 1980), 42–47.

Simpson, Ira et al. *From Student to Nurse: A Longitudinal Study of Socialization*, New York: Cambridge Univ. Press. 1979.

Smith, Elizabeth. ''Nurses in Policy Making and Volunteerism.'' *Nurs. and Health Care*, **4** (Mar. 1983), 135–137.

Smythe, Emily. *Surviving Nursing*. Menlo Park, Calif.: Addison-Wesley Publishing Company, 1984.

Swanburg, Russell, and Philip Swanburg. *Strategic Career Planning and Development for Nurses.*

Rockville, Md.: Aspen Systems Corporation, 1984.

Tavris, Carol. ''Feeling Angry? Letting Off Steam May Not Help.'' *Nurs. Life*, **4** (Sept.–Oct. 1984), 58–61.

Trotter, Carol. ''What Can We Do About Nursing Staff Burnout?'' *MCN*, **7** (May–June 1982), 153–155ff.

Turner, Saundra. ''Building a Nursing Support Group.'' *Nurs. and Health Care*, **4** (Sept. 1983), 387.

Valiga, Theresa. ''It's Time for Nurses to Begin Nursing Nurses.'' *Nurs. and Health Care*, **5** (June 1984), 330–335.

See also the references and bibliography of Chapters 5, 6, 10, 11, 12, 13, 15, 16, 19, 20, 22, and 30. The Fall 1982 issue of *Nursing Administration Quarterly* focuses on ''The Staff Nurse.''

Index

DATE DUE

APR 2 1986		
APR 1 9 1986		
APR 1 4 1987		
MAY 7 1987		
4/24/87		
JAN 2 0 1988		
MAR 1 7 1988		
APR 1 1988		
MAY 1 4 1988		
MAY 1 5 1988		
MAR 1 7 1989		
APR 0 6 1989		
APR 1 1 1994		
FEB 0 9 2001		
NOV 2 8 2010		
GAYLORD		PRINTED IN U.S.A.